Head and Face Medicine: Principles and Practice

Head and Face Medicine: Principles and Practice

Edited by Conner Bale

hayle
medical

New York

Hayle Medical,
750 Third Avenue, 9th Floor,
New York, NY 10017, USA

Visit us on the World Wide Web at:
www.haylemedical.com

ISBN: 978-1-63241-727-5

Cataloging-in-Publication Data

Head and face medicine : principles and practice / edited by Conner Bale.
     p. cm.
Includes bibliographical references and index.
ISBN 978-1-63241-727-5
1. Head--Diseases. 2. Face--Diseases. 3. Head--Diseases--Treatment. 4. Face--Diseases--Treatment.
5. Head--Diseases--Diagnosis. 6. Face--Diseases--Diagnosis. 7. Otolaryngology. I. Bale, Conner.
RC936 .H43 2019
617.51--dc23

Table of Contents

Permissions

List of Contributors

Index

Preface

The branch of medicine concerned with the conditions of the ear, nose and throat is known as otolaryngology. Some of its main sub-specialties include facial plastic and reconstructive surgery, head and neck oncologic surgery, neurotology, pediatric otolaryngology, otology, and rhinology and sinus surgery. Facial plastic and reconstructive surgery is a speciality of otolaryngology. This domain of medicine is concerned with the aesthetic and reconstructive surgery of the face, head and neck. This book attempts to understand the multiple branches that fall under the discipline of head and face medicine and how such concepts have practical applications. It studies, analyzes and upholds the pillars of otolaryngology and its utmost significance in modern times. Researchers, doctors and students actively engaged in this field will find this book full of crucial and unexplored concepts.

All of the data presented henceforth, was collaborated in the wake of recent advancements in the field. The aim of this book is to present the diversified developments from across the globe in a comprehensible manner. The opinions expressed in each chapter belong solely to the contributing authors. Their interpretations of the topics are the integral part of this book, which I have carefully compiled for a better understanding of the readers.

At the end, I would like to thank all those who dedicated their time and efforts for the successful completion of this book. I also wish to convey my gratitude towards my friends and family who supported me at every step.

Editor

Biocompatibility of three bioabsorbable membranes assessed in FGH fibroblasts and human osteoblast like cells culture

Michelle Pereira Costa Mundim Soares[1], Paulo Vinícius Soares[2], Analice Giovani Pereira[3], Camilla Christian Gomes Moura[4], Priscila Barbosa Ferreira Soares[3], Lucas Zago Naves[5] and Denildo de Magalhães[6*]

Abstract

Objectives: Specific physical and chemical features of the membranes may influence the healing of periodontal tissues after guided tissue regeneration (GTR). The aim of the present investigation was to analyze the biological effects of three bioabsorbable membranes. The hypothesis is that all tested membranes present similar biological effects.

Methods: Human osteoblast like-cells (SaOs-2) and gingival fibroblasts FGH (BCRJ -RJ) were cultured in DMEM medium. The viability of the cells cultured on the membranes was assesses using 3-(4,5-Dimethylthiazol-2-yl)-2,5-diphenyltetrazolium bromide (MTT). Quantitative determination of activated human Transforming Growth Factor beta 1 (TGF-β1) on the supernatants of the cell culture was observed. Samples were examined using scanning electron microscope (SEM).

Results: SaOs2, in 24 hours, PLA group showed higher values when compared to other groups (P < 0.05). All groups presented statistical significance values when compared two times. In 4 h and 24 h, for the fibroblasts group, significantly difference was found to PLA membrane, when compared with the other groups (p < 0.05). For TGFβ1 analyzes, comparing 4 and 24 h, for the osteoblast supernatant, COL1 and PLA groups showed statistically significant difference (p <0,008). On the analysis of culture supernatants of fibroblasts, in 24 hours, only PLA group presented significant difference (p = 0,008).

Conclusions: The biomaterials analyzed did not show cytotoxicity, since no membrane presented lower results than the control group. PLA membrane presented the best performance due to its higher cell viability and absorbance levels of proliferation. Both collagen membranes showed similar results either when compared to each other or to the control group.

Keywords: Membranes, Biosorbable, Regeneration, Fibroblast, Osteoblast

Background

Periodontal disease is very common in general population and is the major cause for loss of the tooth-supporting apparatus [1]. The goals of periodontal therapy have been described in many ways over the years. The key concept is to improve periodontal health and thereby to satisfy a patient's aesthetic and functional needs or demands [2,3]. Regeneration of the damaged structures using regenerative procedures present variable success rates,

depending on multiple factors such as defect size and type, patients' age, genetics [1].

Regeneration is defined as the reproduction or reconstitution of a lost or injured part [4]. Periodontal regeneration requires restitution of the periodontal attachment apparatus including new bone formation, new cementum deposition upon the denuded root surface, and reinsertion of functionally oriented new collagen fibers of the periodontal ligament, into the new bone and new cementum [1,5]. Cementoblasts, fibroblasts, and osteoblasts and their precursors are the principal cells found in periodontal ligament [2,6,7]. Physical barriers can be applied during regeneration procedures to exclude unwanted cells from the wound space to promote periodontal regeneration.

* Correspondence: denildo@foufu.ufu.br
[6]Associate Professor of Histology of Periodontics and Implant Dentistry Department at the Dentistry School of Federal University of Uberlandia, Av. Para 1720, Campus Umuarama, Zip Code 38400-000 Uberlandia, Minas Gerais, Brazil
Full list of author information is available at the end of the article

The desirable characteristics of barrier membranes include biocompatibility, cell occlusion properties, integration by the host tissues, ability to induce cellular proliferation and differentiation, clinical manageability and space making ability [3].

The use of barrier membranes has become a standard step on guided tissue regeneration (GTR) introduced in 1988, by Dahlin, as a therapeutic modality aiming, excluding epithelial and connective tissues, to enable bone progenitor cell proliferation and differentiation into the isolated area [8,9]. The aim of GTR is fully reestablish functional periodontium, including new cementum and periodontal ligament, as well as new bone regeneration. Since fibroblasts from the wound margins are able to attach to the membrane the proliferation of the epithelial cells is stopped in the presence of collagen [10,11].

Various biomaterials from natural and synthetic origin have been extensively investigated about biocompatibility, biodegradability, cell interaction, and mechanical properties. The prepared scaffolds with various shapes and structures have to suitable carry the cell, provide initial support similar to extracellular matrix and facilitate the nutrient and metabolite diffusion during *in vitro* culture. For *in vivo* cultures the membrane is expected to allow angiogenesis after transplantation, ensuring continuous viability and functionality of the regenerative cells [1,11]. Several materials have been tested for their effectiveness as barriers such as millipore filters, expanded polytetrafluoroethylene (ePTFE) membranes, collagen membranes, polygalactin, calcium sulfate and polylactid acid membranes [4,5,12].

A disadvantage of non-absorbable membranes is the need of a second-step surgery to remove the membrane. This procedure may injure the newly formed granulation tissue. Furthermore, early spontaneous exposure to the oral environment and subsequent bacterial colonization has been reported to be common problems of non-absorbable membranes [5,13,14]. Barrier materials derived from porcine or bovine collagen type I and III demonstrated their usefulness in GTR procedures. However, several complications such as early membrane degradation, epithelial down growth and premature loss of the material were reported following the use of collagen materials [5]. Besides the surgical aspects, specific physical and chemical features of the membranes may influence the healing of periodontal tissues after GTR therapy [15].

The purpose of the present investigation was to analyze the biological effects of commercially available bioabsorbable collagen and polylactic acid membranes in cultures of gingival fibroblasts, and human osteoblast-like cells. In particular, to analyze the proliferations rate/cell viability, TGFβ1 level and the adhesion/morphology of the cells in contact to the membranes by scanning electron microscopy (SEM).

Methods

The present study was performed as mastering dissertation at School of Dentistry of Federal University of Uberlandia under the approval of Post Graduate degree Program.

Membranes examined

Three commercially available bioabsorbable membranes with different composition and structures were examined: Gore Tex (polylactic acid - Resolut W L Gore and Associates Inc Flagstaff A Z), Gen Derm (type I bovine collagen – Genius biomaterials – Baumer SA Brazil), Surgidry Dental F (type I bovine collagen – TechoDry Liofilizados Médicos Ltda Brazil) (Table 1).

Cell cultures

A SaOs-2 cell line and gingival fibroblasts FGH, immortalized cell line obtained from the Banco de Células do Rio de Janeiro (BCRJ-RJ)were cultured in a humidified atmosphere (95% air, 5% CO_2) at 37°C, maintained in DMEM high glicose medium (DMEM, Cultilab, SP, Brazil) containing gentamicine sulfate and anfotericina B, supplemented with 10% fetal bovine serum. Tissue culture medium was changed every 2 days until confluence was reached. Upon reaching confluence, the cells were detached using trypsin-EDTA solution. Cells between the passages 2-3 were counted for viability using Trypan Blue.

The membranes (diameter 3,65 mm) were placed in 96-well plates and immersed in serum-free medium for 15 min. Then the medium was discarded and 1×10^5 SaOs-2 were seeded in the well plates. Cells plated on the well without barriers served as positive control. The same was carried for the fibroblasts FGH cells.

Viability test

The viability of the cells cultured on the membranes was assessed using 3-(4,5-Dimethylthiazol-2-yl)-2,5-diphenyltetrazolium bromide, a yellow tetrazole (MTT).

Table 1 Groups and membranes used in the study

Group description	Composition	Bioabsorbable membrane	Manufacturer
PLA	POLYLACTIC ACID	GORE TEX	W L Gore and Associates Inc Flagstaff A Z
CL1	TYPE I BOVINE COLLAGEN	GEN DERM	Baumer SA Brazil
CL2	TYPE I BOVINE COLLAGEN	SURGIDRY DENTAL F	TechoDry Liofilizados Médicos Ltda Brazil

The adhesion test was carried out in according to Mosmann [16]. The membranes were removed from the wells after 4 and 24 h, 100 μl of 1% MTT was added and then incubated at 37°C for 3 h. After incubation, the MTT containing medium was removed from the plate and 100 μl of solubilizing solution, consisting of 20% of Sodium lauryl sulfate in 50% dimethylformamide, was added to each well. This addition was performed to dissolve the formazan crystals formed from the tetrazolium salts. The optical density (OD) of the colored complex formed was read by spectrophotometer with 570 nm wavelength. The amount of viable cells adhered to the membranes (directly proportional to OD) was calculated by Digiread software based on the resultsobtained from the spectrophotometer. The experiments were performed five times for each sample. The Analysis of Variance Two-way test and Tukey's test (p < 0.05) were applied.

TGFβ1 Level

For quantitative determination of activated human Transforming Growth Factor beta 1 (TGF-β1) concentrations in cell culture supernatants ELISA test (Human/Mouse TGFβ 1 ELISA Ready-SET-Go! -eBioscience, San Diego,USA) was performed.

The cytokine TGFβ1 was assessed to indicate the presence of growth factor. ELISA plates were used for high-affinity. The plates were sensitized with anti-TGFβ1, kept overnight in refrigerator and then washed with PBS-Tween 5 times. The sites were blocked for 1 hour rinsed with PBS-T 3 times. The second detection antibody was added for 1 h washed with PBS-T 5 times, added AVIDIN HRP for 30 minutes, washed with PBS-T 5 times. Then Tetramethylbenzidine solution (TMB) was added. The optical density was determined using a microplate reader set to 450 nm. The results were compared with a wavelength control curve. The Kruskal Wallis One Way Analysis and Mann Whitney test (p < 0.05) were employed.

Scanning electron microscopy examination

Three membranes of each group was fixed and processed for electron microscopy 24 h after culture. Fixation was carried out with 2,5% glutaraldehyde at pH7,2 for 4 h. The fixed samples were washed twice with phosphate buffered saline (PBS) for 5 minutes each followed by immersion in 1% osmium tetra oxide, for 1 h. Then the samples were washed twice with PBS followed by serial dehydration in series of graded ethanol solutions ranging from 50 to 100%; dried over 15 minutes with 50% vol/vol mixture of hexamethyldisilazane (HMDS) and ethanol, and finally with 100% HMDS twice for 15 minutes. Finally the samples were air dried by leaving them partly covered for 4 h, mounted onto 12.5-mmdiameter carbon tabs and aluminum stubs and gold sputtered with 20 nm. Samples were examined using a scanning electron microscope (SEM).

Results

Viability test

Statistically significant differences were found between the periods 4 and 24 h evaluated for all osteoblasts groups. There was no statistical difference between the osteoblasts groups when compared in 4 h. For 24 h the PLA group showed significantly higher values when compared to the other groups (P <0.05) (Figure 1). From 4 to 24 h of culture, the MTT test did not show increasing metabolic activity of the fibroblasts in all groups of membranes. In 4 h, for the fibroblasts group, significantly difference was found for PLA membrane compared with control (p < 0,001), and PLA with COL2 (p = 0,006). In 24 h analysis, PLA presented significant difference when compared to COL2 (p < 0,001) and control (p = 0,010) (Figure 2).

TGFβ1 level

Comparing two times, 4 and 24 h, with the osteoblast supernatant, COL1 and PLA groups showed statistically significant difference (p <0.008). For 4 h COL1 and PLA groups showed significantly higher values when compared with control and COL2 (p <0.05). For 24 h the group COL2 showed significantly lower values when compared with other groups (Table 2). On the analysis of culture supernatants of fibroblasts, 4 and 24 h, only PLA group presented significant difference (p = 0.008). For 4 h all the groups showed similar results and for 24 h PLA group showed higher significant values when compared to other groups (Table 3).

Scanning electron microscopy

SEM examination showed attachment and physiologic morphology grown of the cells on the membranes. After 24 h culture SEM showed that both cells had attached to all groups of membranes. However, some cells had flattened

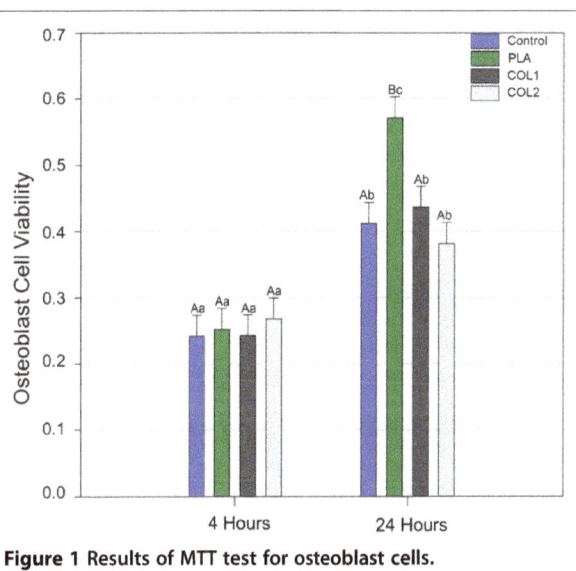

Figure 1 Results of MTT test for osteoblast cells.

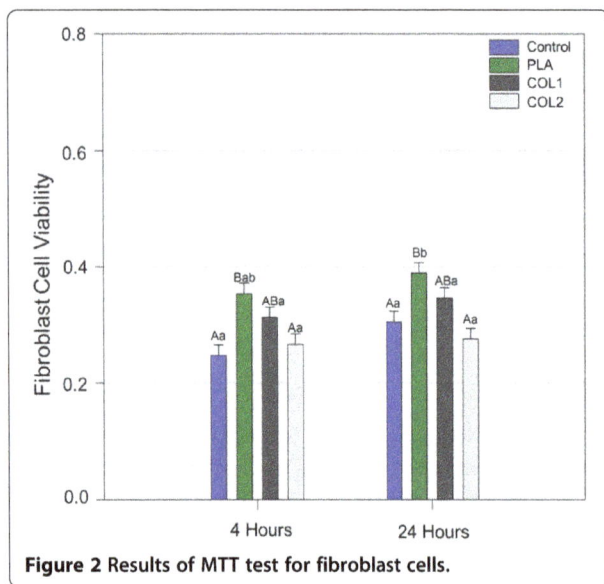

Figure 2 Results of MTT test for fibroblast cells.

onto the collagen membrane while those on PLA remained rounded. SEM examination of cells cultures revealed healthy cells populations (Figure 3).

Discussion

The use of GTR has proved to be a suitable technique when simulating regeneration, new connective tissue attachment and bone formation [17]. When a membrane is placed between the denuded root surface and the repositioned mucogingival flap, it provides a secluded space into which fibroblasts and osteogenic cells from the healthy apical portion of the periodontium may migrate [15].

The purpose of this study was to determine the biocompatibility of several barrier materials in human cell cultures, which are comparable to the periodontal regenerative cells. The cells selected for this study in vitro, were gingival fibroblasts and osteoblasts, since both are present in periodontal tissue regeneration.

The viability cell test showed that the absorbance level for osteoblasts increased for all groups between 4 and 24 h, indicating that the membranes did not exhibit cytotoxicity to cells. The PLA group showed better results when compared to other groups at 24 h. The cells probably reached the log phase showing higher viability and metabolic activity.

In the analysis of fibroblasts proliferation of using the MTT method, the membrane PLA, also presented better results than the other groups. However, in 24 h analysis

it was observed that COL1 and COL2 were similar to PLA. Fibroblasts and osteoblasts have different growth kinetics. Since fibroblasts have reached the log phase at 24 h assessment the absence of statistical difference between the groups between 4 and 24 h can be confirmed by the same behavior observed in the control group. Probably the characteristics of the PLA membrane favor cell proliferation.

The TGFβ1 test confirmed the ability of proliferation of both cells fibroblasts and osteoblasts. When in contact to PLA membrane a statistical significant difference was observed for two types of cells. For COL1 group the osteoblasts dosage of the supernatant were significant. Probably, the contact with the membranes further favors cell proliferation, since it was observed in greater proportion than in control group. The TGFβ1 is a proliferation factor that acts in the repair process. Besides assessing cell viability, the aim of the study also includes analysis of the cells ability to regenerate when in contact with the membranes. Another important factor is that TGFβ1 is present in the two types of cells evaluated.

SEM analysis showed that the cells had a rounded and flattened appearance on collagen membrane, associated with cellular health. The cells migrated horizontally on the collagen membrane. However, this pattern was not seen in PLA membrane, because of the high distance among the fibers that permitted cells to be in direct contact with only an individual fiber. SEM examination of the fibroblasts cells on the collagen revealed cytoplasmatic membranes and lamellipodia extension presence. Also the surface topography of the membranes plays an important role in cell's adhesion, rough or porous textured surfaces have been considered to promote attachment cell. Morphology can be regarded as an indicator of the affinity of the cells to a substratum [18].

The adhesion of mesenchymal cells to barrier membranes is dependent of the type and nature of the barrier and is thought to influence regenerative results positively [10]. These barrier membranes must, ideally, present the ability to allow cell's adhesion and induce cellular proliferation and differentiation [10].

The results of this study indicate that biomaterials do not affect the cellular proliferation, once all results were similar or better than control group. In the present study the results showed that collagen membrane presented lower values than PLA membrane which are similar to Chandrahasa, et al. 2011 [19], Parrish et al. 2009 [4] and [14]. Polylactic acid and collagen membranes'

Table 2 Results of ELISA test for osteoblast cells

Time	Control	PLA	COL1	COL2
4 hours	147,8 (0,3) Ba	4347,5 (723,5) Aa	5715,0 (1391,7) Aa	147,7 (0,8) Ba
24 hours	147,6 (0,50) Aa	147,9 (0,12) Ab	147,7 (0,10) Ab	147,7 (0,09) Ba

Uppercase letters indicate differences in the lines, lowercase letters indicate differences in columns.

Table 3 Results of ELISA test for fibroblast cells

Time	Control	PLA	COL1	COL2
4 hours	148,0 (1,10) Aa	148,0 (0,36) Aa	147,8 (0,12) Aa	147,7 (0,34) Aa
24 hours	148,0 (0.63) Aa	2972,9 (777,61) Ba	148,9 (0,29) Aa	148,0 (0.74) Aa

Uppercase letters indicate differences in the lines, lowercase letters indicate differences in columns.

biocompatibility was evaluated in vitro using osteoblast-like cells. The results showed proliferation capacity in both types of materials, but better results were found polylactic acid membrane PLA group [14]. In a systematic review, it was observed that the use of polylactic acid membrane even shows better results than open flap debridement with grafts [4].

The results of all experiments indicated that PLA membrane exhibited excellent biocompatibility in contradiction with other in vitro studies using polylactic acid membranes

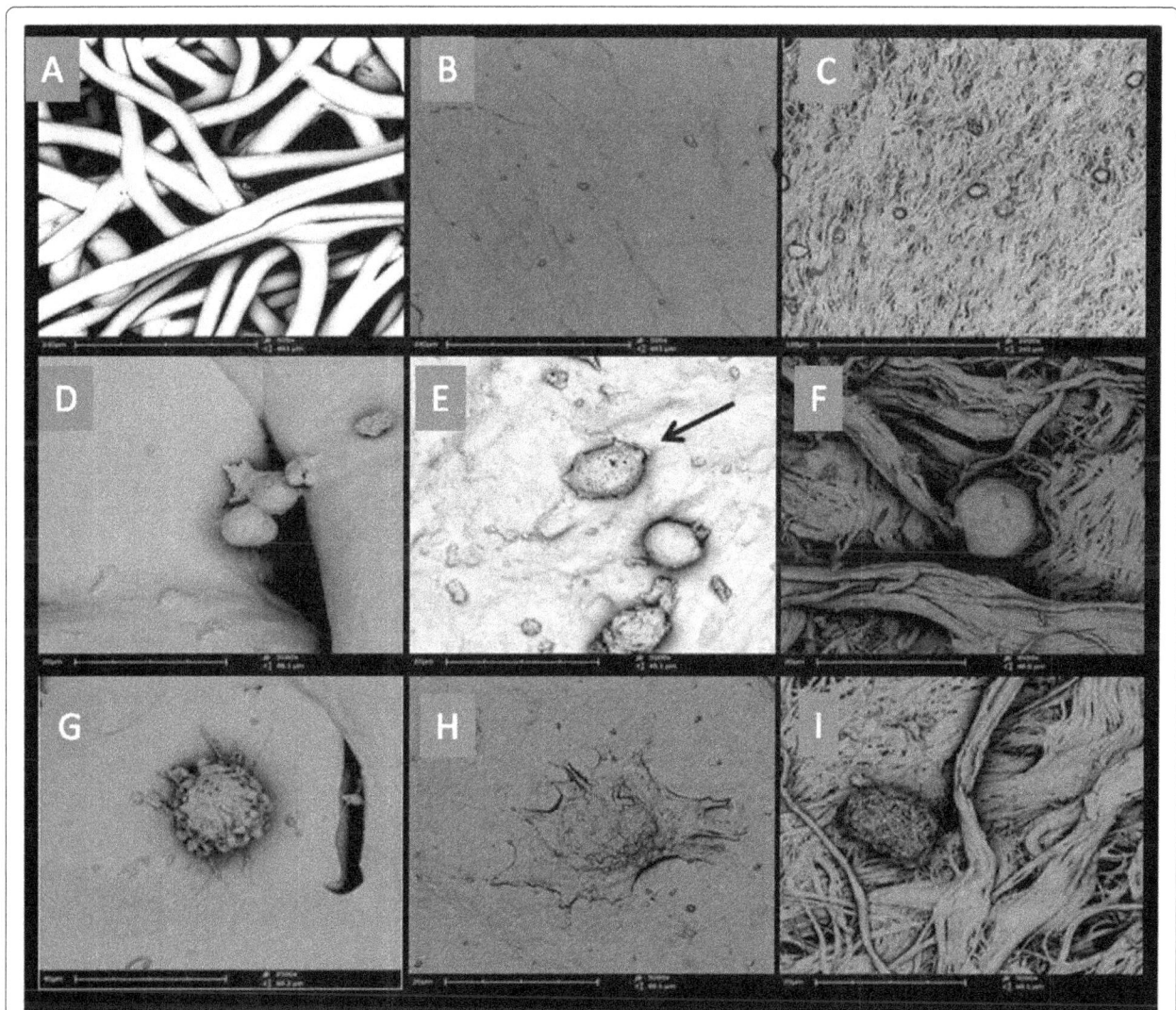

Figure 3 SEM analysis. (A) PLA membrane showing separation between the fibers. **(B)** COL1 surface showing more regular structure with some pores. **(C)** COL2 showing woof of small fibers and more layers. **(D)** Attachment time 24h osteoblast cell beginning to emit small cytoplasmic expansion in PLA. **(E)** Attachment time 24h COL1 and some rounded SaOs-2 cell with initial lamellopodia represented with arrow in the image. **(F)** Attachment time 24h COL2 revealing rounded osteoblast. **(G)** Attachment time 24h PLA showing fibroblast adhesion with cytoplasm expansion **(H)** Attachment time 24h COL1 fibroblasts were also observed flatted, beginning to look like a star format. **(I)** Attachment time 24h COL2 round shaped fibroblasts were observed.

[3,5,20]. Collagen membranes have shown regenerative favorable results, due to their excellent biocompatibility and cell affinity. Nevertheless, collagen based membranes show relatively poor mechanical and dimensional stability, due to its rapid degradation [10]. Among the papers of a systematic literature review performed to evaluate collagen membranes on the potential of different cells to attach to, proliferate on, and migrate over barrier membranes, an in vitro study showed that different cell types have different comportments on identical membranes [11].

Another factor that must be considered is that, despite having the same composition, biomaterials and treatments may have different morphologic structures (Figure 3). So, caution is essential while interpreting results obtained by using in vitro experimental model, since cell type, material characteristics and patient response may play an important role.

Further studies using controlled experimental models in vivo are needed in order to verify the present results. Guided tissue regeneration has different degrees of success, depending on the type of barrier selected, presence or absence of underlying graft material, type of graft, feasibility of the technique applied, and clinician's preference among other factors [13].

Conclusion

Within the limits of this study, it was concluded that biomaterials did not show cytotoxicity, since no membrane showed lower results than the control group. PLA membrane presented it's the highest biocompatibility and absorbance levels of proliferation and COL1 membrane showed similar results for the test with fibroblasts.

Competing interests
The authors declare that they have no competing interests.

Authors' contributions
DM and PBFS made substantial contributions to conception of the present study. MPCMS and CCGM performed analysis and interpretation of data besides drafting the manuscript. LZN had led acquisition of data. PVS and AGP involved in revising the manuscript critically and giving final approval of the version to be published. All authors read and approved the final manuscript.

Author details
[1]Master degree of Dentistry School of Federal University of Uberlandia, Uberlandia, Minas Gerais, Brazil. [2]Associate Professor of Operative Dentistry and Dental Materials Department at the Dentistry School of Federal University of Uberlandia, Uberlandia, Minas Gerais, Brazil. [3]Doctoral student of Dentistry School of Federal University of Uberlandia, Uberlandia, Minas Gerais, Brazil. [4]Adjunct Professor of Federal University of Triangulo Mineiro, Uberaba, Minas Gerais, Brazil. [5]Post Doctoral student of Dentistry School of Estadual University of Campinas, Piracicaba, São Paulo, Brazil. [6]Associate Professor of Histology of Periodontics and Implant Dentistry Department at the Dentistry School of Federal University of Uberlandia, Av. Para 1720, Campus Umuarama, Zip Code 38400-000 Uberlandia, Minas Gerais, Brazil.

References

1. Inanc B, Arslan YE, Seker S, Elcin AE, Elcin YM: Periodontal ligament cellular structures engineered with electrospun poly(DL-lactide-co-glycolide) nanofibrous membrane scaffolds. *J Biomed Mater Res A* 2009, **90**(1):186–195.
2. Needleman I, Tucker R, Giedrys-Leeper E, Worthington H: A systematic review of guided tissue regeneration for periodontal infrabony defects. *J Periodontal Res* 2002, **37**(5):380–388.
3. Thangakumaran S, Sudarsan S, Arun KV, Talwar A, James JR: Osteoblast response (initial adhesion and alkaline phosphatase activity) following exposure to a barrier membrane/enamel matrix derivative combination. *Indian J Dent Res* 2009, **20**(1):7–12.
4. Parrish LC, Miyamoto T, Fong N, Mattson JS, Cerutis DR: Non-bioabsorbable vs. bioabsorbable membrane: assessment of their clinical efficacy in guided tissue regeneration technique. A systematic review. *J Oral Sci* 2009, **51**(3):383–400.
5. Kasaj A, Reichert C, Gotz H, Rohrig B, Smeets R, Willershausen B: In vitro evaluation of various bioabsorbable and nonresorbable barrier membranes for guided tissue regeneration. *Head Face Med* 2008, **4**:22.
6. Isaka J, Ohazama A, Kobayashi M, Nagashima C, Takiguchi T, Kawasaki H, Tachikawa T, Hasegawa K: Participation of periodontal ligament cells with regeneration of alveolar bone. *J Periodontol* 2001, **72**(3):314–323.
7. Lekovic V, Camargo PM, Weinlaender M, Kenney EB, Vasilic N: Combination use of bovine porous bone mineral, enamel matrix proteins, and a bioabsorbable membrane in intrabony periodontal defects in humans. *J Periodontol* 2001, **72**(5):583–589.
8. Dahlin C, Linde A, Gottlow J, Nyman S: Healing of bone defects by guided tissue regeneration. *Plast Reconstr Surg* 1988, **81**(5):672–676.
9. Moses O, Vitrial D, Aboodi G, Sculean A, Tal H, Kozlovsky A, Artzi Z, Weinreb M, Nemcovsky CE: Biodegradation of three different collagen membranes in the rat calvarium: a comparative study. *J Periodontol* 2008, **79**(5):905–911.
10. Bornstein MM, Heynen G, Bosshardt DD, Buser D: Effect of two bioabsorbable barrier membranes on bone regeneration of standardized defects in calvarial bone: a comparative histomorphometric study in pigs. *J Periodontol* 2009, **80**(8):1289–1299.
11. Behring J, Junker R, Walboomers XF, Chessnut B, Jansen JA: Toward guided tissue and bone regeneration: morphology, attachment, proliferation, and migration of cells cultured on collagen barrier membranes. A *Syst Rev Odontol* 2008, **96**(1):1–11.
12. Retzepi M, Donos N: Guided Bone Regeneration: biological principle and therapeutic applications. *Clin Oral Implants Res* 2010, **21**(6):567–576.
13. Carpio L, Loza J, Lynch S, Genco R: Guided bone regeneration around endosseous implants with anorganic bovine bone mineral. A randomized controlled trial comparing bioabsorbable versus non-resorbable barriers. *J Periodontol* 2000, **71**(11):1743–1749.
14. Bilir A, Aybar B, Tanrikulu SH, Issever H, Tuna S: Biocompatibility of different barrier membranes in cultures of human CRL 11372 osteoblast-like cells: an immunohistochemical study. *Clin Oral Implants Res* 2007, **18**(1):46–52.
15. Alpar B, Leyhausen G, Gunay H, Geurtsen W: Compatibility of resorbable and nonresorbable guided tissue regeneration membranes in cultures of primary human periodontal ligament fibroblasts and human osteoblast-like cells. *Clin Oral Investig* 2000, **4**(4):219–225.
16. Mosmann T: Rapid colorimetric assay for cellular growth and survival: application to proliferation and cytotoxicity assays. *J Immunol Methods* 1983, **65**(1–2):55–63.
17. Simain-Sato F, Lahmouzi J, Kalykakis GK, Heinen E, Defresne MP, De Pauw MC, Grisar T, Legros JJ, Legrand R: Culture of gingival fibroblasts on bioabsorbable regenerative materials in vitro. *J Periodontol* 1999, **70**(10):1234–1239.
18. Rothamel D, Schwarz F, Sculean A, Herten M, Scherbaum W, Becker J: Biocompatibility of various collagen membranes in cultures of human PDL fibroblasts and human osteoblast-like cells. *Clin Oral Implants Res* 2004, **15**(4):443–449.
19. Chandrahasa S, Murray PE, Namerow KN: Proliferation of mature ex vivo human dental pulp using tissue engineering scaffolds. *J Endod* 2011, **37**:1236–1239.
20. Gebhardt M, Murray PE, Namerow KN, Kuttler S, Garcia-Godoy F: Cell survival within pulp and periodontal constructs. *J Endod* 2009, **35**(1):63–66.

2

Frontal facial proportions of 12-year-old southern Chinese: a photogrammetric study

Charles Yat Cheong Yeung[1], Colman Patrick McGrath[2], Ricky Wing Kit Wong[3], Erik Urban Oskar Hägg[4], John Lo[5] and Yanqi Yang[6*]

Abstract

This study aimed to establish norm values for facial proportion indices among 12-year-old southern Chinese children, to determine lower facial proportion, and to identify gender differences in facial proportions.

A random population sample of 514 children was recruited. Fifteen facial landmarks were plotted with ImageJ (V1.45) on standardized photos and 22 Facial proportion index values were obtained. Gender differences were analyzed by 2-sample t-test with 95 % confidence interval. Repeated measurements were conducted on approximately 10 % of the cases. The rate of adopted subjects was 52.5 % (270/514). Intraclass correlation coefficient values (ICC) for intra- examiner reliability were >0.87. Population facial proportion index values were derived. Gender differences in 11 of the facial proportion indices were evident ($P < 0.05$).

Upper face-face height (N- Sto/ N- Gn), vermilion height (Ls-Sto/Sto-Li), upper face height-biocular width (N-Sto/ExR-ExL) and nose -face height (N-Sn/N-Gn) indices were found to be larger among girls ($P < 0.01$). Males had larger lower face-face height (Sn -Gn/ N-Gn), mandibulo-face height (Sto-Gn/N-Gn), mandibulo-upper face height (Sto-Gn/N-Sto), nasal (AIR-AIL/N-Sn), upper lip height-mouth width (Sn-Sto/ChR-ChL), upper lip-upper face height (Sn-Sto/N-Sto) and upper lip-nose height (Sn-Sto/N-Sn) indices ($P < 0.05$).

Population norm of facial proportion indices for 12-year-old Southern Chinese were derived and mean lower facial proportion were obtained. Sexual dimorphism is apparent.

Keywords: Facial proportions, Southern Chinese, Photogrammetry, Population norm, Facial attractiveness, Diagnosis, Treatment outcome evaluation, Orthodontics, Orthognathic surgery, Plastic surgery, Cosmetic surgery

Introduction

Facial attractiveness has been a subject of interest since the beginning of recorded history. Bashour reviewed the historical and current literatures and concluded with four important cues that emerge as being the most important determinants of facial attractiveness [1]. They are: (i) averageness, (ii) sexual dimorphism, (iii) youthfulness, and (iv) symmetry. Averageness is regarded as one of the most important factors and supported by various studies [2–6].

Facial attractiveness has long been of central concern to orthodontic and surgical care given that treatments are capable of changing facial appearance and thereby improve

facial attractiveness [7]. It is therefore important to establish population norms to address the averageness cue, and provide insight on sexual dimorphism and youthfulness. Symmetry can be assessed clinically without the need of a norm.

Farkas suggested the use of facial proportion indices to assess aesthetics relating to facial proportions in different facial types [8]. Edler quantified facial attractiveness after orthognathic surgery and found, the greater the improvement in facial proportion indices, the better the aesthetic result as judged by orthodontists and maxillofacial surgeons [6]. These post surgical indices correlated closely to Farkas' findings. Facial proportion is, therefore, important in both clinical diagnosis and treatment outcome evaluation.

Photogrammetry is increasingly being employed to assess facial characteristics [6, 9–14]. It is reported to be

* Correspondence: yangyanq@hku.hk
[6]Department of Paediatric Dentistry and Orthodontics, Faculty of Dentistry, The University of Hong Kong, Hong Kong SAR, China
Full list of author information is available at the end of the article

valid for many measurements [15, 16], reliable [6, 10–13, 16, 17] and is a practical approach to clinical analyses and comparison [6, 14, 17].

While facial proportion norms are well-established for Caucasian populations [9], it remains paucity for southern Chinese.

The aims of this study were:

I. To provide a database of norm of facial proportion indices for 12-year-old southern Chinese for surgical and orthodontic diagnosis.
II. To determine sexual dimorphism in facial proportions.
III. To determine the lower facial proportion

Materials and method
Sample

This epidemiological study was conducted in Hong Kong SAR, China among 12-year-old children. Ethical approval was obtained by the local IRB committee (UW 09–453). Ten percent of all secondary schools in Hong Kong SAR were randomly selected and children within each selected school were invited to participate. Written informed consent was obtained from parents and children provided their ascent. A sample of 514 (259 males, 255 females) 12-year-old children was recruited. That was approximately 10 % of the Chinese birth cohort since all 12-year-old children in Hong Kong, spread over all secondary schools, are included in the cohort.

Photographic set up

A scale backdrop of 1 cm increments with a plumbline was set up for a camera-subject distance of around 170 cm. The camera used was Canon EOS 400D (Canon, Shimomaruko, Ohta-ku, Tokyo, Japan) with Canon EF-S 60 mm f/2.8 Macro USM Lens and Canon MR-14EX TTL Macro Ring Lite Flash. Subjects were first instructed to a stand with their eyes looking forward to a vertically standing mirror on the side for a natural head posture and then turn their whole body 90° to face the camera with the lip relax. Glasses or other accessories which may obstruct the face were taken away beforehand. The photo was then taken in natural head posture [18].

Selection of landmarks and proportion indices: (Fig. 1)

Fifteen landmarks (Fig. 1) as employed by Farkas and Munro [8] were considered; based on key variables considered by Bishara [10–12] (1) visibility in most frontal photographs (2) reliable identification (3) minimally affected by the subject's grooming, and (4) involved in the measurement of proportional indices of interest. Twenty-two proportion indices (Table 1) employed by Farkas and Munro [8] were selected to be investigated basing on key variables considered by Bishara [10–12],

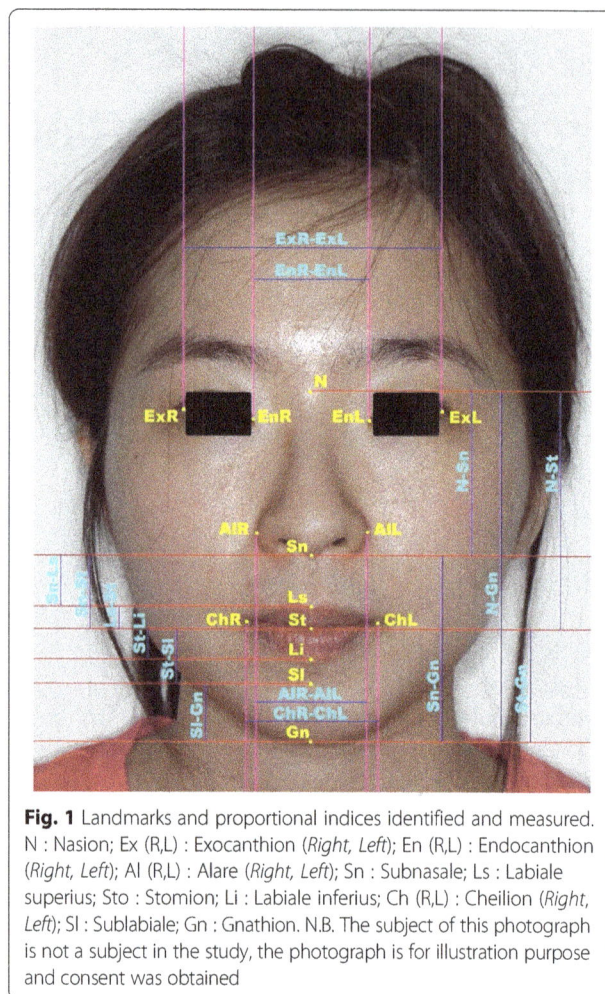

Fig. 1 Landmarks and proportional indices identified and measured. N : Nasion; Ex (R,L) : Exocanthion (*Right, Left*); En (R,L) : Endocanthion (*Right, Left*); Al (R,L) : Alare (*Right, Left*); Sn : Subnasale; Ls : Labiale superius; Sto : Stomion; Li : Labiale inferius; Ch (R,L) : Cheilion (*Right, Left*); Sl : Sublabiale; Gn : Gnathion. N.B. The subject of this photograph is not a subject in the study, the photograph is for illustration purpose and consent was obtained

and Edler [6] (1) Measurable on a frontal photographs; (2) reliability; and (3) be potentially changed by the effects of orthodontics and/or orthognathic surgery.

Selection of photos

Photos were inspected for their quality and usability in identification of landmarks and validity in measurement of the proportion indices. Photos were excluded if: (1) landmarks were obscured; (2) head tilted up or down significantly; (3) head turned left or right by assessing symmetrical structures; (4) out focused photo; (5) subject wearing glasses; (6) subject showing lip strain or obviously opened mouth; (7) subject smiled; (8) patient partly or completely closed their eyes; and (9) subject previously or currently having orthodontic treatment.

Digitalization of photos

The selected photos were cropped to show the head only. A tangent at superior palpebral sulci was used to determine the vertical level of Nasion [8, 19]. Landmarks were located with ImageJ (V.1.45) (USA National Institutes of Health) and position of each landmark was recorded as

Table 1 Descriptions of Facial Proportion Indices abd their respective intraclass correlation coefficients of intra examiner reliability

Index	Description	Intra-examiner reliability (ICC)
Upper face-face height index	N- Sto/ N- Gn ×100	1
Lower face-face height index	Sn -Gn/ N-Gn ×100	0.99
Mandibulo-face height index	Sto-Gn/N-Gn ×100	1
Mandibulo-upper face height index	Sto-Gn/N-Sto ×100	1
Mandibulo-lower face height index	Sto-Gn/Sn-Gn ×100	0.99
Nasal index	AIR-AIL/N-Sn ×100	0.88
Upper lip height-mouth width index	Sn-Sto/ChR-ChL ×100	0.98
Cutaneous-total upper lip height index	Sn-Ls/Sn-Sto ×100	0.95
Vermilion-total upper lip height index	Ls-Sto/Sn-Sto ×100	0.95
Vermilion-cutaneous upper lip height index	Ls-Sto/Sn-Ls ×100	0.95
Vermilion height index	Ls-Sto/Sto-Li ×100	0.96
Chin-mandible height index	Sl-Gn/Sto-Gn ×100	0.9
Upper face height-biocular width index	N-Sto/ExR-ExL ×100	0.99
Intercanthal-nasal width index	EnR-EnL/AIR-AIL ×100	0.99
Nose-face height index	N-Sn/N-Gn ×100	0.99
Nose-mouth width index	AIR-AIL/ChR-ChL ×100	0.98
Upper lip-upper face height index	Sn-Sto/N-Sto ×100	0.98
Upper lip-mandible height index	Sn-Sto/Sto-Gn ×100	0.99
Upper lip-nose height index	Sn-Sto/N-Sn ×100	0.97
Lower lip-face height index	Sto-Sl/Sn-Gn ×100	0.89
Lower lip-mandible height index	Sto-Sl/Sto-Gn ×100	0.9
Lower lip-chin height index	Sto-Sl/Sl-Gn ×100	0.91

a set of X-Y pixel coordinates by the same trained operator. The proportion indices were generated by Microsoft Excel® with the formulas in Table 1.

Statistical analysis

For each facial proportion index, descriptive statistics of mean, standard deviation and range (maximum, minimum) were generated by Statistical Product and Service Solutions (V20) (IBM Corporation, New York, USA). Two sample T- test (with 95 % confidence interval provided) were used to identify any gender difference. The intraclass correlation coefficients [20] were calculated by SPSS (V.19) to assess for intra-examiner reliability, among approximately 10 % of randomly selected subjects that were re-analyzed and compared to original assessments.

Results

Out of 514 subjects, 53 % (270) were included in the analysis, among that, 51 % (137) were female. 47 % (244) were excluded according to the exclusion criteria (as described above). Intra-examiner reliability is presented in Table 1. The intraclass correlation coefficients were all above 0.87 for intra examiner reliability, indicating very good/excellent reliability [20].

Facial proportion index norm values are presented in Table 2. Greatest variance were observed in vermilion cutaneous-upper lip height (Males: 29.58–145.59, Females: 28.81–124.32), vermilion height (Males: 55.26–120.75, Females: 44.59–175.00) and lower lip-chin height (Males: 36.25–135.63, Females: 25.44–131.40) indices. Lowest variances were observed in upper face-face height (Males: 56.73–70.79, Females: 58.35–70.19), lower face-face height (Males: 50.34–62.69, Females: 48.06–60.95) and mandibulo-lower face height (Males: 57.98–72.07, Females: 58.64–70.64) indices. From lower face-face height index, the proportion of lower face was 56 % of total face height. The proportion of upper lip height (Sn-Sto), lower lip height (Sto-Sl) and chin height (Sl-Gn) were found to be 35.12, 27.33 and 37.55 % respectively.

Gender differences in 11 of the 22 facial proportion indices assessments were apparent. For females, upper face-face height ($P < 0.05$), vermilion height ($P < 0.001$), upper face height-biocular width ($P < 0.01$) and nose -face height ($P < 0.001$) indices were larger. In contrast, lower face-face height ($P < 0.001$) mandibulo-face height ($P < 0.05$), mandibulo-upper face height ($P < 0.05$), nasal ($P < 0.001$), upper lip height-mouth width ($P = 0.001$), upper lip-upper face height ($P < 0.001$) and upper lip-nose height ($P < 0.001$) indices were larger in males. The index with the largest mean percentage difference (7.56 %) between genders was upper lip-nose height index.

Discussion

This study was conducted on a random population sample of 12-year-old children, as opposed to small, non-random, convenient samples as described in the majority of photogrammetric studies published to date [21–23]. With the rate of adopted subjects of 53 %, there are a number of factors to account for the loss of samples including less than ideal cooperation from 12 years old children, time constraint and past or current orthodontic treatment. This reflects the difficulties in performing population-wide photogrammetric studies under non-clinical/outreach settings in the community. Nevertheless, the sample size was sufficient to provide populations norms and to discover gender differences and it is one of the largest samples for photogrammetric study with random population

Table 2 Mean, standard deviation, maximum, minimum and p-values of statistical tests (2 sample t-test) of facial proportion indices

	Male (n = 133)				Female (n = 137)				
	Mean	SD	Min.	Max.	Mean	SD	Min.	Max.	P-value
Upper face-face height index	63.27	2.58	56.73	70.79	63.92	2.36	58.35	70.19	0.031*
Lower face-face height index	56.75	2.44	50.34	62.69	55.25	2.59	48.06	60.95	0.000***
Mandibulo-face height index	36.73	2.58	29.21	43.27	36.08	2.36	29.81	41.65	0.031*
Mandibulo-upper face height index	58.33	6.54	41.25	76.26	56.66	5.80	42.47	71.37	0.028*
Mandibulo-lower face height index	64.69	2.83	57.98	72.07	65.29	2.63	58.64	70.64	0.075
Nasal index	77.12	5.69	64.32	93.83	73.99	6.54	60.70	93.94	0.000***
Upper lip height-mouth width index	52.02	6.47	37.09	71.21	49.36	6.21	36.46	67.05	0.001**
Cutaneous-total upper lip height index	62.16	6.84	40.72	77.17	61.99	6.82	44.58	77.63	0.838
Vermilion-total upper lip height index	37.84	6.84	22.83	59.28	38.01	6.82	22.37	55.42	0.837
Vermilion-cutaneous upper lip height index	63.00	19.83	29.58	145.59	63.30	18.37	28.81	124.32	0.898
Vermilion height index	76.61	12.08	55.26	120.75	82.21	19.80	44.59	175.00	0.005**
Chin-mandible height index	58.12	5.57	42.44	73.39	58.78	6.03	43.22	79.72	0.352
Upper face height-biocular width index	85.33	5.01	73.41	98.37	86.92	4.54	74.69	98.24	0.007**
Intercanthal-nasal width index	95.22	6.70	79.48	112.82	95.37	7.75	77.32	113.96	0.871
Nose -face height index	43.25	2.44	37.31	49.66	44.75	2.59	39.05	51.94	0.000***
Nose-mouth width index	86.22	7.03	68.69	109.87	84.70	7.02	70.98	109.49	0.075
Upper lip-upper face height index	31.65	2.31	25.60	37.19	30.02	2.55	24.28	35.99	0.000***
Upper lip-mandible height index	54.87	6.76	38.75	72.48	53.42	6.22	41.57	70.55	0.067
Upper lip-nose height index	46.46	4.96	34.41	59.21	43.08	5.26	32.07	56.23	0.000***
Lower lip-face height index	27.05	3.43	17.07	35.81	26.87	3.80	12.91	36.22	0.693
Lower lip-mandible height index	41.88	5.57	26.61	57.56	41.22	6.03	20.28	56.79	0.352
Lower lip-chin height index	73.66	17.05	36.25	135.63	71.94	18.03	25.44	131.40	0.421

*P-value<0.05, **P-value<0.01, ***P-value<0.001

sample and largest range of assessment of proportion indices.

A smaller local study analyzed facial profiles with photogrammetry on only 82 12-year-old southern Chinese with just five proportion indices [21]. Findings were consistent with the present study, with mean differences less than 1 standard deviation for four indices: lower-face-face height index, mandibulo-lower face height, intercanthal-nasal width and lower lip-face height indices. The only inconsistency was reported for the lower lip-face height index, which they reported a statistically significant gender difference. In comparison with northern America Caucasian population [8], the only index that differed by more than 2 standard deviation is the nose-mouth width index for both males and females. This indicates that southern Chinese have a relatively wider nose (AlR-AlL) or narrower mouth (ChR-ChL) compared to Caucasians. The nasal index for males, upper face height-biocular width index and upper-lip-mandible height index for females were larger in southern Chinese by almost 2 standard deviations. The reverse was found for the female mandibulo-upper face height index.

Of a particular importance to orthodontics and orthognathic surgery is the lower face proportion. The lower face height in our study was found to be 56.7 %(male) and 55.3 %(female) of the total face height corresponding well to lateral cephalometric study [24] (M:56.5 %, F:55.7 %), photogrammetric study [25] in Nigerian adults (M:58.15 %, F:56.97 %) and anthropotmetric study [8] on 12-year-old Caucasian children (M:59.7 %, F:59.5 %). Regarding the proportions of the lower third of the face, Renaissance artist Francesca [8] suggested that the lower lip and chin should make up two thirds of the lower one third of face and lower lip and chin should have the same proportion, this is widely adopted in orthodontics and surgery text. Farkas had found proportionality from anthropometric study [8], which is 31.2, 26.2 and 42.6 % for Sn-Sto, Sto-Sl and Sl-Gn. In our study, the proportion was 35.1, 27.3 and 37.6 % respectively.

Farkas [8], Song [26] and Bao [27] reported that there gender difference in facial dimension and proportions but the average differences were small. The results from this study generally supports Farkas' conclusion. In this study,

11 (50 %) out of 22 facial proportion indices showed significant gender differences. All except 4 of the indices had a percentage difference of less than 5 %. They are upper lip-nose height (7.6 %), vermilion height (7.0 %), upper lip-upper face height (5.3 %) and upper lip height-mouth width (5.3 %) indices.

The norm facial proportion indices obtained can be used for clinical assessment and comparison with same analysis and photogrammetric technique. Frontal photogrammetry was widely used to assess treatment change [6, 9–12], attractiveness [13, 28, 29], comparisons between different ethnic groups [13, 14, 30] and growth [10–12, 31] in additional to daily use for clinical diagnosis and treatment planning.

To conclude, the following were the key findings of this study.

I. Population norm of facial proportion indices are obtained from the mean values of this study and can serve as a reference to evaluate facial proportions in treatment planning and treatment outcome assessment using the same frontal photogrammetric analysis.
II. Gender differences in facial proportion were found in 11 indices. Lower face-face height index, mandibulo-face height index, mandibulo-upper face height index, nasal index, upper lip height-mouth width index, upper lip-upper face height index and upper lip-nose height index were significantly larger in males. The findings were opposite for upper face-face height index, vermilion-height index, upper face height-biocular width index and nose -face height index.
III. The lower face height is found to be 56.7 %(male) and 55.3 %(female) of the total face height and proportions of lower facial height were 35.1, 27.3 and 37.6 % for Sn-Sto, Sto-Sl and Sl-Gn respectively.
IV. Ethnic differences were evaluated by comparing with a North American Caucasian population, southern Chinese was found to have a relatively wider nose (AlR-AlL) or narrower mouth (ChR-ChL) compared to the Whites.

Competing interests
The authors declare that they have no competing interests.

Authors' contributions
CY did all the measurements, calculations and drafted the manuscript. CM designed the study and amended the manuscript. RW helped with the arrangement of the survey and the manpower associated. UH set objectives for the study, calibrated the examiner and revised the manuscript. JL advised on the methodology and helped with data analysis. YY organized the survey, designed the study, helped with data analysis and revised the manuscript. All authors read and approved the final manuscript.

Acknowledgment
I would like to thank Mr Shadow Yeung for his technical and statistical support, Miss Angela for the permission of use of her frontal photo, Miss Karen Lau for editing and to all who have collaborated in any respects of this research project.

Author details
[1]Department of Paediatric Dentistry and Orthodontics, Faculty of Dentistry, The University of Hong Kong, Hong Kong SAR, China. [2]Department of Periodontology and Public Health, Faculty of Dentistry, The University of Hong Kong, Hong Kong SAR, China. [3]Department of Paediatric Dentistry and Orthodontics, Faculty of Dentistry, The University of Hong Kong, Hong Kong SAR, China. [4]Department of Paediatric Dentistry and Orthodontics, Faculty of Dentistry, The University of Hong Kong, Hong Kong SAR, China. [5]Department of Oral and Maxillofacial Surgery, Faculty of Dentistry, The University of Hong Kong, Hong Kong SAR, China. [6]Department of Paediatric Dentistry and Orthodontics, Faculty of Dentistry, The University of Hong Kong, Hong Kong SAR, China.

References
1. Bashour M. History and current concepts in the analysis of facial attractiveness. Plast Reconstr Surg. 2006;118(3):741–56.
2. Symons D. The evolution of human sexuality. 1st ed. New York: Oxford University Press; 1979.
3. Langlois JH, Roggman LA. Attractive faces are only average. Psychol Sci. 1990;1:115–21.
4. Strzalko J, Kaszycka KA. Physical attractiveness: interpersonal and intrapersonal variability of assessments. Soc Biol. 1991;39:170–6.
5. Grammer K, Thornhill R. Human facial attractiveness and sexual selection: the role of symmetry and averageness. J Comp Psychol. 1994;108:233–42.
6. Edler R, Agarwai P, Wertheim D, Greenhill D. The use of anthropometric proportion indices in the measurement of facial attractiveness. Eur J Orthod. 2006;28(3):274–81.
7. Mackley RJ. An evaluation of smiles before and after orthodontic treatment. Angle Orthod. 1993;63:183–9.
8. Farkas LG, Munro IR. Anthropometric facial proportions in medicine. 1st ed. Springfield: Thomas; 1987.
9. Gode S, Tiris FS, Akyildiz S, Apaydin F. Photogrammetric analysis of soft tissue facial profile in Turkish Rhinoplasty population. Aesthetic Plast Surg. 2011;35:1016–21.
10. Bishara SE, Jorgensen GJ, Jakobsen JR. Changes in facial dimensions assessed from lateral and frontal photographs. Part I-Methodology. Am J Orthod Dentofacial Orthop. 1995;108:389–93.
11. Bishara SE, Jorgensen GJ, Jakobsen JR. Changes in facial dimensions assessed from lateral and frontal photographs. Part II-Results and conclusions. Am J Orthod Dentofacial Orthop. 1995;108:489–99.
12. Bishara SE, Cummins DM, Jakobsen JR. "A computer assisted photogrammetric analysis tissue changes after orthodontic treatment. Part II: Results. Am J Orthod Dentofacial Orthop. 1995;108:38–47.
13. Rhee SC, Dhong ES, Yoon ES. Photogrammetric facial analysis of attractive Korean entertainers. Aesthetic Plast Surg. 2009;33:167–74.
14. Sim RS, Smith JD, Chan AS. Comparison of the aesthetic facial proportions of Southern Chinese and White women. Arch Facial Plast Surg. 2000;2:113–20.
15. Farkas LG, Bryson W, Klotz J. Is photogrammetry of face reliable? Plast Reconstr Surg. 1980;66:346–55.
16. Guyot L, Dubuc M, Richard O, Philip N, Dutour O. Comparison between direct clinical and digital photogrammetric measurements in patients with 22q11 microdeletion. Int J Oral Maxillofac Surg. 2003;32:246–52.
17. Muradin MSM, Rosenberg A, Bilt AV, Stoelinga JW, Koole R. The reliability of frontal facial photographs to assess changes in nasolabial soft tissues. Int J Oral Maxillofac Surg. 2007;36:728–34.
18. Cooke MS, Wei SH. The reproducibility of natural head posture: a methodological study. Am J Orthod Dentofacial Orthop. 1988;93:280–8.
19. Ashley-Montagu MF. The location of the nasion in the living. Am J Phys Anthropol. 1935;20:81–95.
20. Stanish WM, Taylor N. Estimation of the intraclass correlation coefficient for the analysis of covariance model. Am Stat. 1983;37:221–4.
21. Yuen SW, Hiranaka DK. A photographic study of the facial profiles of southern Chinese adolescents. Quintessence Int. 1989;20:665–76.
22. Porter JP. The average African American male face. Arch Facial Plast Surg. 2004;6:78–81.

23. Sepehr A, Mathew PJ, Pepper JP, Karimi K, Devcic Z, Karam AM. The Persian Woman's face: a photogrammetric analysis. Aesthetic Plast Surg. 2012;36:687–91.

24. Saksena SS, Walker GE, Bixler D. A Clinical atlas Roentgencephalometry in norma lateralis. New York: Liss; 1987.

25. Loveday OE. Photogrammetric analysis of soft tissue profile of the face of igbos in port harcourt. Asian J Med Sci. 2011;3(6):228–33.

26. Song WC, Kim JI, Kim SH, Shin DH, Hu KS, Kim HJ, et al. Female-to-male proportion of head and face in Koreans. J Craniofac Surg. 2009;20:356–61.

27. Bao B, Yu S, Cai Y. The analysis of frontal facial soft tissue of normal native adult of Han race of Guangdong Province by using the computer assisted photogrammetric system. Hua Xi Kou Qiang Yi Xue Za Zhi. 1997;15(3):266–75.

28. Kiekens RM, Kuijpers Jagtman AM, Van't Hof MA, Van't Hof BE, Straatman H, Maltha JC. Facial esthetics in adolescents and its relationship to "ideal" ratios and angles. Am J Orthod Dentofacial Orthop. 2008;133:188. 1-8.

29. Kiekens RM, Kuijpers-Jagtman AM, van't Hof MA, van't Hof BE, Maltha JC. Putative golden proportions as predictors of facial esthetics in adolescents. Am J Orthod Dentofacial Orthop. 2008;134:480–3.

30. Jeffries JM, DiBernardo B, Rauscher GE. Computer analysis of the African-American face. Ann Plast Surg. 1995;34:318–22.

31. Ferring V, Pancherz H. Divine proportions in the growing face. Am J Orthod Dentofacial Orthop. 2008;134:472–9.

3

A comparison of mandibular and maxillary alveolar osteogenesis over six weeks: a radiological examination

Marthinus J Kotze[1*], Kurt-W Bütow[1,2], Steve A Olorunju[3] and Harry F Kotze[4]

Abstract

Introduction: Insufficient information exists on comparing radiological differences in bone density of the regeneration rate in the alveolar bone of the maxilla and mandible following the creation of similar defects in both.

Methods: Alveolar bone defects were created from five healthy Chacma baboons. Standardized x-ray images were acquired over time and the densities of the selected defect areas were measured pre-operatively, directly post-operatively and at three- and six weeks post-operatively. Differences in densities were statistically tested using ANOVA.

Results: The maxilla was significantly more radiologically dense (p = 0.026) than the mandible pre- operatively. No differences were obtained between the maxilla and mandible directly postoperatively and three- and six weeks post-operatively respectively; i.e. densities were not significantly different at the different time points after the defects had been created (three weeks: t = 1.08, p = 0.30; six weeks: t = 1.35, p = 0.19; three to six weeks: t = 1.20, p =0.25). The increase in density in the mandible was 106% (8.9 ± 7.6%/time versus 4.3 ± 2.7%/time) over three weeks, 28% (15.0 ± 8.1%/time versus 11.7 ± 8.0%/time) over six weeks and 56% (12.5 ± 9.7%/time versus 8.0 ± 6.9%/time) over three-to-six weeks and was higher than in the maxilla over the same intervals.

Conclusions: Radiological examination with its standardized gray-scale analysis can be used to determine the difference in bone density of the maxilla and mandible. Although not statistically significant, the mandible healed at a faster rate than the maxilla, especially observed during the first three weeks after the defects were created.

Keywords: Regeneration, Alveolar bone, Radiological, Gray-scale

Introduction

Surgical procedures in the alveolar processes of the maxilla and mandible often lead to permanent loss of bone substance. This missing bone has to regenerate to restore normal function. Bone is distinctive in connective tissue healing because it heals entirely by cellular regeneration and production of a mineral matrix. The sequence of events that occurs after tooth extraction has been described previously in detail [1]. At an extraction site, the alveolar socket is filled with a blood clot, which is replaced by vascularized granulation tissue. During this regeneration process, intense osteoclastic bone resorption occurs to remove necrotic bone and bone debris. At the same time, osteoblast differentiation and proliferation start. New bony trabeculae are formed in the apical region at day five. Bone apposition in the extraction socket occurs along the lateral alveolar walls and at the fundus of the socket by means of new woven bone projecting until the socket is entirely filled between days 20 and 28. Bone remodeling occurs finally when the newly formed woven bone is replaced by mature lamellar bone [2]. No literature could be found on a comparison of the regeneration rate of the mandible and maxilla following trauma. In one study, the overall healing process following tooth extraction in the mandible and maxilla was evaluated but the rates of regeneration were not compared [2]. Different aspects of alveolar bone remodeling were investigated. Remodeling of alveolar bone subjected to orthodontic

* Correspondence: thinus.kotze@up.ac.za
[1]Department Maxillo-Facial and Oral Surgery, Faculty of Health Sciences, University of Pretoria, Pretoria, South Africa
Full list of author information is available at the end of the article

forces was evaluated and reported in the literature [3-6]. In one study significantly more orthodontic tooth movement was observed for maxillary than for mandibular teeth for the same time of force application. In the same study an overall decrease in bone volume for the first four weeks following the application of the orthodontic force and an increase in bone formation rate after 12 weeks were found [3]. Guided bone regeneration was also investigated in procedures such as bone augmentation [7,8], through the use of different membranes [9,10], and in implantology through observing osseointegration as well as bone quality [11-13]. Furthermore, investigations of alveolar regeneration in the mandible and maxilla were done using resorbable and non-resorbable plates and screws [14,15].

When alveolar cortical bone density of the maxilla was compared with that of the mandible [16], the mandibular measurements were statistically significantly higher than those of the maxilla, except at the incisor region measurements. For cancellous bone, the canine and retromolar areas of the mandible were statistically higher than those of the maxilla [16]. Huja *et al.* found that the average bone volume within the alveolar process of the mandible was 2.8 fold greater than in the maxilla [4].

The process of bone regeneration can be monitored radiologically as bone density becomes more detectable during the regeneration process [1,17,18]. A significant correlation between mineral bone density and bone structure exists when density is measured radiologically [19]. This correlation enables the rate of healing for the maxilla and mandible to be determined. A previous histomorphometric study indicated that the rate of healing of the mandible was approximately twice as fast as that of the maxilla [4]. However, there are no radiology studies that could substantiate these findings. Owing to the lack of information in comparing the healing rate after trauma between the maxilla and mandible, a radiological evaluation in determining alveolar bone density differences between the mandible and maxilla was decided on as an assessment tool.

Methods

Five healthy male Chacma baboons (*Papio ursinus*) were used. The average weight of the animals was 19.8 ± 4.3 Kg, which implied it is young animals, as the weight of an adult male Chacma baboon can reach up to 40 Kg in five years [20]. Approval for the study was granted by both the Animal Use and Care Committee (AUCC), and a subcommittee of the Committee for Research Ethics and Integrity at University of Pretoria and North West University. The animals were anaesthetized with intravenous ketamine hydrochloride (dose: 10 mg/kg). In order to control haemostases and pain, 1.8 mL (9 mg) Bupivacaine with 0.5% epinephrine 1:200,000 (as bitartrate) (Novocol,

Pharmaceuticals of Canada. Inc., Cambridge, Ontario, Canada) was injected intramuscularly.

Surgical intervention

Defects were created in the premolar areas of the mandible and maxilla by the same surgeon. The bone at the selected site being exposed by reflection of the overlying mucosa. Three alveolar bone defects, 3 mm deep, were created with a 3 mm diameter trephine bur, fitted onto a straight surgical hand piece connected to a surgical drilling unit. The defects were positioned 2 mm apart.

Radiology

Radiographs were taken pre-operatively, directly post-operatively and again after three and six weeks. Standardized reproducible radiographs for analysis was acquired for each of the four quadrants at each time point with an apparatus (Figure 1) constructed as follows: For each quadrant, maxillary and mandibular in each animal, a sectional tray was prepared by cutting in half a disposable mandibular impression tray (#21, Wright Cottrell Co., Kingsway West, West Dundee, Dundee). In each instance the tray was adjusted to fit properly over as many teeth as possible. A bite block (XPC-DS Digital Position System (Gendex, Lake Zurich, Illinois) was secured onto the tray with a self-tapping screw and cyanoacrylate cement. The block carried the cradle for the sensor (Gendex Visualix EHD Digital intra-Oral x-ray unit – Size 1 (universal size) with 25.6 line pairs/mm; KaVoDental, Gendex Imaging, Via Alessandro Manzoni, 44, 20095 Cusano Milanino, Milan, Italy) (Figure 1). A step wedge was made from a 3 mm x 6 mm strip of commercially

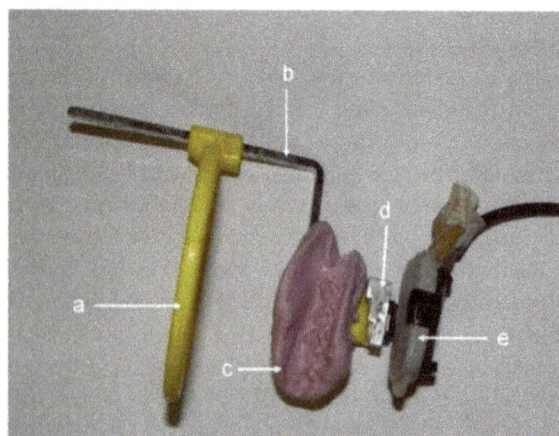

Figure 1 The apparatus after a lab putty impression was made. This impression was made to ensure that images were acquired in the same position every time an image of that quadrant was made. (a + b = Rinn apparatus; c = #21 mandible disposable impression tray with Lab Putty impression; d = aluminum step wedge; e = Gendex Visualix EHD Digital intra-Oral x-ray unit – Size 1 censor (universal size) attached to a XPC-DS Digital Position System.

available aluminium. Three steps were cut, 2 mm wide and 1 mm deep. The wedge was supported on the bite block so that it was parallel to and just touching the sensor. Removal and accurate replacement of the wedge in this position was achieved by an arrangement of location pins which fitted precisely into receptacle holes. A drill of the requisite diameter was used to make two small holes through the aluminium and into the bite block. Short straight sections of a paperclip were cut and glued into the holes in the bite block. These protruding pins fitted precisely into the holes in the aluminium wedge, enabling repeated removal of the wedge and its subsequent replacement in the same position. The procedure was repeated for every bite block, enabling ready transfer of the aluminium wedge for each radiograph. The bite block, sensor and tray were secured to a Dentsply-Rinn apparatus (Dentsply, Elgin, Illinois), consisting of a metal ring holder and plastic positioning ring.

The sectional tray was loaded with laboratory putty (Coltene/Whaledent, Switzerland), a silicone base and polysiloxane activator and positioned in the quadrant to include as much of the alveolar ridge as possible. While the laboratory putty was still in the soft stage of the setting process, an x-ray was taken to enable confirmation that the sensor was correctly positioned. Once the putty had set, the impression of the teeth and the alveolar ridge provided a secure key to accurate repositioning of the set up for subsequent radiographs. The position of the ring on the holder as well as the position in the bite block was identical for all the radiographs.

A Planmeca Intra Wallmount X-ray unit (Planmeca Oy, Asentajankatu 6, 00880, Helsinki, Finland.) was used to acquire the radiographs which were taken at 8 mA with 63 kV and an exposure time of 0.08 seconds. A Toshiba D-0711 SB x-ray tube was used and the focal spot was 0.7×0.7 mm. The focal distance for all the images was 110 mm.

The computer software program used for the radiology was Gendex VixWin Pro (Gendex Dental Systems 901 West Oakton Street Des Plaines, IL 60018).

Evaluation methods

Four digital images were acquired per quadrant on each occasion when records were taken i.e. 16 images per animal at each of the four time periods. The images were imported into Adobe Photoshop (V6.0; Adobe Systems Inc., San Jose, CA). An A4 transparent sheet was positioned on the computer screen and firmly secured. The first pre-operative image was imported on the screen and with the lasso tool of the program an area of interest (AOI) was selected on the image of the step wedge (Figure 2). The corners of the selected area were marked on the transparent sheet with a fine point permanent marker pen. Now each of the three postoperative images could sequentially be accurately positioned and oriented on the screen, using the drag and drop function, so that the marks on the transparent sheet precisely superimposed on the selected area on the image. The gray scale values for this defined area of the wedge were standardized across all four images recorded from each quadrant by using the

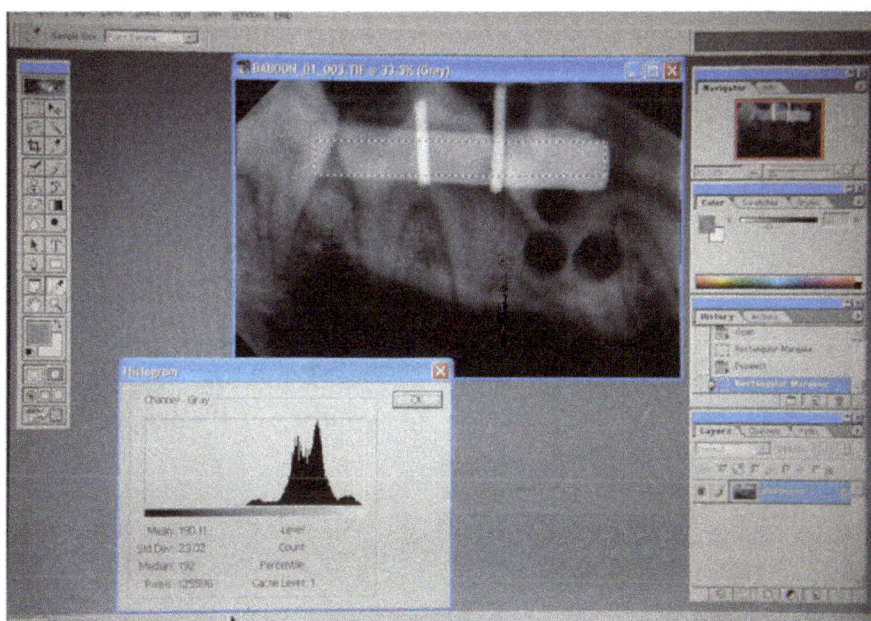

Figure 2 A histogram of a selected area on the aluminum step wedge.

histogram, contrast and brightness tools of the Photoshop software [21] to make the required point adjustments, ensuring that the density never differed by more than 12 data points Hence all images now reflected comparable degrees of gray scale. An AOI was selected on each of the biopsy sites on each of the images taken immediately post-operatively and marked on the transparent sheet (Figure 3). The average gray-scale values for these areas on each of the three defects on each image were determined and recorded.

This was done for all images of a quadrant acquired from each of the different time periods. The method used was described in a 2012 publication of Kotze *et al.* [17].

Statistical analyses

All the animals were within the same age, weight range and sex. Only one examiner took the measurement and recorded the results. The analysis of the data was standardized and repeatable which implies that there was no reason to measure inter-observer variation. ANOVA for repeated measures (analysis of variance considering more than one factor period) was used to test for possible differences in the data set. The variance ratio (F) can be defined as ratio of the effect of treatment to the unexplained variance is assumed to have F distribution. Periodic changes (actual and percentage) were analyzed using the two-sample t-test within each time point to compare mandible and maxilla. The t-statistic is a ratio of the departure of an estimated parameter (mean difference between Mandible and Maxilla in each time period) its standard error and is defined as the ratio of the difference between changes in

the measurements at two time intervals and the associated standard error.

Results

The results are summarized in Table 1. The calculations of the percentage change at three and at six weeks included the pre-operative values to exclude the effect of differences in bone density of the different animals. Through this approach, the pre-values were equal to zero and the percentage change expressed as the increase from pre-values.

With the use of ANOVA for repeated measures, there was a significant difference between the densities in the maxilla and mandible (F = 11.92, p = 0.0007) when the data were analyzed. No significant differences between animals were found (F = 2.18, p = 0.24). Periodic analysis indicated that the maxilla was significantly denser than the mandible before the defects were created (t = 2.4743, p = 0.0235). No significant difference was found between the post-operative densities of the maxilla and mandible (t = 1.3417, p = 0.20). Analysis showed that the percentage change in densities was not significantly different at any of the time points after the defects were created (three weeks: t = 1.08, p = 0.30; six weeks: t = 1.35, p = 0.19; three-to-six weeks: t = 1.20, p = 0.25). The rate of increase in density in the mandible was 106% (8.9% over three weeks versus 4.3% over three weeks), 28% (15.0% over six weeks versus 11.7% over six weeks) and 56% (12.5% over three to six weeks versus 8.0% over three-to-six weeks) more for the maxilla after three, six and three-to-six weeks respectively.

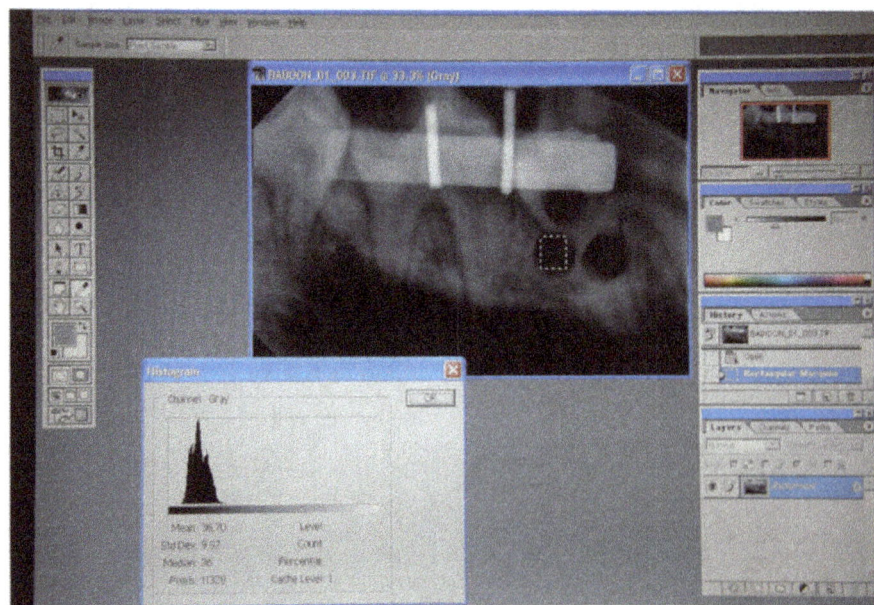

Figure 3 A histogram of a selected area on the created defect.

Table 1 The percentage changes in grey-scale values over six weeks

| | Grey-scale values | | Per Cent Change over Time | | |
	Pre-operative	Post-operative[a]	Three weeks[b]	Six weeks[c]	Three to Six weeks[d]
Maxilla	98 ± 26	54 ± 19	4.3 ± 2.7	11.7 ± 8.0	8.0 ± 6.9
Mandible	72 ± 22	53 ± 18	8.9 ± 7.6	15.0 ± 8.1	12.5 ± 9.7

[a]Post-operative change = (preoperative - postoperative) ÷ preoperative x 100.
[b]Three weeks = (3 weeks - postoperative) ÷ preoperative x 100.
[c]Six weeks = (6 weeks - postoperative) ÷ preoperative x 100.
[d]Three/six weeks = (3/6 weeks - postoperative) ÷ preoperative x 100.
Values are given as a mean ± 1SD.

Discussion

Bone regeneration in the premolar area of the maxilla and mandible using changes in average gray-scale value (AGV) derived from radiographs was investigated. The radiological changes in density of bone were compared with histological and histomorphometrical measurements and a correlation were found between the different approaches [22-24].

This principle of change in radiological density over time can be used as an indicator of bone turnover. The pre-operative AGV indicated that the maxilla was significantly denser than the mandible (Table 1; F = 11.92, p = 0.0007). This finding contrasts with previous findings that the density of the mandible is higher than that of the maxilla [25]. This can be due to the difference in position of the AOI, as the bone density measured on radiographs in the mouth is normally affected by surrounding structures in the length of the pathway of the x-ray and also the thickness of bone [22]. The AOI in our study was more apically located and included more of the dense palatal bone on the radiographic image. However, in the present study, the pre-operative difference in bone density of the maxilla and mandible is not of any significance, as the changes in density were measured over time with the post-operative value as the starting point. This pre-molar area included more bone volume and the denser soft tissue from the palate, as well as the thicker cortical bone of the palate. The pre-operative values were used for calculating the percentage change in bone density. The possible influence of differences in bone density between the maxilla and mandible and between animals before the defects were created was excluded by calculating the changes relative to the pre-operative densities. Through this approach, the post-operative values were normalized to zero. It was not surprising that the post-operative percentage density for the area of interest was similar for both the mandible and maxilla following the removal of the same volume of bone (Table 1). Any change to a number greater than the post-operative percentage AGV was regarded as a percentage increase in bone regeneration.

The increase in density of the mandible after the surgical intervention – was not significantly different from that in the maxilla at three-, six- and three-to-six weeks

(Table 1). This finding contrasts with that of a study using histomorphometric methods where the mandible healed twice as fast as the maxilla [26]. Similar results were found in our study comparing the rate of healing between the mandible and maxilla during the first three weeks period. The percentage increase in density in the mandible was 8.9% and 4.3% in the maxilla (Table 1) which represents a difference of approximately 106%. At six weeks the difference in percentage of the rate of healing between the mandible and maxilla decreased to an average of 20%. The time sequence of bone regeneration following an extraction is started with clot formation on the same day which is replaced by granulation tissue in the first week. The granulation tissue is replaced by connective tissue on day 20. Osteoid formation is evident from day seven and on day 38, two-thirds of the extraction socket is filled by connective tissue [27]. The sequence of the regeneration process indicates active cellular activity directly post-operative in the defect area which implies a quicker increase in density of the AOI on the radiological image. The tempo of the process of regeneration decreases from day 20 as connective tissue and osteoid is developing. As the mandibular alveolar bone is denser than the maxillary alveolar bone, it can be expected that more regeneration tissue will be present in the mandible bone, therefore the difference in the rate of healing between the maxilla and mandible in the first three weeks. The mandible is subjected to higher mechanical forces and consequently has a higher rate of healing than the maxilla [27]. The dynamism imposed by muscle force on the bone causes complex patterns of stress and strain in the mandible, such as sagittal and transverse bending and deformation from shear and torsion [28]. In contrast, the maxillary and pre-maxillary bones are primarily exposed to forces generated by occlusal contact with the mandibular teeth [29]. The bone quality for both anterior and posterior jaw regions are predominantly types 2 and 3 (Lekholm-Zarp classification) [30]. The anterior part of the mandible has the densest bone, followed by the posterior mandible, anterior maxilla, and posterior maxilla [31]. The area of interest was the pre-molar region of both the mandible and maxilla. Both regions were Lekholm-Zarp type II or III classification with the density of the cortical and trabecular bone in the mandible the highest [13,16].

One may speculate that the denser quality of bone in the mandible provided more bone cells for osteogenesis at the site of trauma. Bone cells respond to mechanical stimulation and induce new bone formation *in vivo* and also increase the metabolic activity and gene expression of osteoblasts [31]. However, the molecular events involved in the translation of mechanical stimulation into cell proliferation and bone formation are not yet well understood [32]. The more mechanical stimulation of the mandibular bone cells due to the denser bone and more forces influencing the mandible [28,29] may also contribute to the increase in the rate of bone healing, especially following the creation of defects at the postoperative three-week period.

Conclusions

There was no statistically significant difference in the density of the alveolar bone between the maxilla and mandible. Therefore, bone regeneration in the mandible and maxilla after similar defects were inflicted to both and a radiological evaluation carried out three weeks and six weeks post-operatively was not different. In contrast, the rate of regeneration of the mandible after three weeks was 106% higher than that of the maxilla. The literature review provided no studies that compared the rate of bone regeneration following the inflicting of defects without the need of osteointegration or stimulation by foreign biomaterials. With the aid of histology or histomorphmetry as a control, further investigation with a larger sample over longer periods of time is necessary before a definite conclusion can be reached on a comparison of alveolar bone regeneration of the mandible and maxilla.

Competing interests
The authors declare that they have no competing interests.

Authors' contributions
MJK, K-WB and HFK made substantial contributions to conception of the present study. SAO performed analysis and interpretation of data besides drafting the manuscript. MJK and HFK had led acquisition of data. K-WB involved in revising the manuscript critically and giving final approval of the version to be published. All authors read and approved the final manuscript.

Acknowledgements
The personnel of the Animal Facility of North West University who supplied the animals and the company Unique Dental, South Africa, for supplying the radiological equipment and computer software. The Dental Research Education & Development Trust of the South African Dental Association contributed financially. Barbara English of the research office of the University of Pretoria's faculty of health sciences is thanked for language editing. Permission was granted by the Managing Editor of The South African Dental Journal for the use of figures. (Kotze MJ, et al. SADJ 67:210–214)

Author details
[1]Department Maxillo-Facial and Oral Surgery, Faculty of Health Sciences, University of Pretoria, Pretoria, South Africa. [2]College of Health Sciences, University of KwaZulu-Natal, Durban, South Africa. [3]Medical Research Council of South Africa, Pretoria, South Africa. [4]Faculty of Health Sciences, University of The Free State, Bloemfontein, South Africa.

References
1. Rauch F, Schoenau E: Skeletal development in premature infants: a review of bone physiology beyond nutritional aspects. *Arch DisChild Fetal* 2002, **86:**F82–F85.
2. Cardaropoli G, Araujo M, Lindhe J: Dynamics of bone tissue formation in tooth extraction sites. an experimental study in dogs. *J Clin Periodontol* 2003, **30:**809–818.
3. Deguchi T, Takano-Yamamoto T, Yabuuchi T, Ando R, Garetto LP: Histomorphometric evaluation of alveolar bone turnover between the maxilla and the mandible during experimental tooth movement in dogs. *Am J Orthod Dentofacial Orthop* 2008, **133:**889–897.
4. Huja SS, Fernandez SA, Hill KJ, Li Y: Remodeling dynamics in the alveolar process in skeletally mature dogs. *Anat Rec A Discov Mol Cell Evol Biol* 2006, **288:**1243–1249.
5. Henneman S, Von den Hoff JW, Maltha JC: Mechanobiology of tooth movement. *Eur J Orthod* 2008, **30:**299–306.
6. Masella RS, Meister M: Current concepts in the biology of orthodontic tooth movement. *Am J Orthod Dentofacial Orthop* 2006, **129:**458–468.
7. McAllister BS, Haghighat K: Bone augmentation techniques. *J Periodontol* 2007, **78:**377–396.
8. Tanner KE: Bioactive ceramic-reinforced composites for bone augmentation. *J R Soc Interface* 2010, **7:**S541–S557.
9. Monteiro ASF, Macedo LGS, Macedo NL, Balducci I: Polyurethane and PTFE membranes for guided bone regeneration: Histopathological and ultrastructural evaluation. *Med Oral Patol Oral Cir Bucal* 2010, **15:**401–406.
10. Hämmerle CH, Jung RE: Bone augmentation by means of barrier membranes. *Periodontol 2000* 2003, **33:**36–53.
11. Schropp L, Isidor F: Timing of implant placement relative to tooth extraction. *J Oral Rehabil* 2008, **35:**33–38.
12. Peñarrocha-Diago MA, Maestre-Ferrín L, Demarchi CL, Peñarrocha-Oltra D: Immediate versus nonimmediate placement of implants for full-arch fixed restorations: A preliminary study. *J Oral Maxillofac Surg* 2011, **69:**154–159.
13. Fuh LJ, Huang HL, Chen CS, Fu KL, Shen YW, Tu MG, Shen WC, Hsu JT: Variations in bone density at dental implant sites in different regions of the jawbone. *J Oral Rehabil* 2010, **37:**346–351.
14. Quereshy FA, Dhaliwal HS, El SA, Horan MP, Dhaliwal SS: Resorbable screw fixation for cortical onlay bone grafting: A pilot study with preliminary results. *J Oral Maxillofac Surg* 2010, **68:**2497–2502.
15. Landes CA, Ballon A: Five-year experience comparing resorbable to titanium miniplate osteosynthesis in cleft lip and palate orthognathic surgery. *Cleft Palate-Craniofac J* 2006, **43:**67–74.
16. Park HS, Lee YJ, Jeong SH, Kwon TG: Density of the alveolar and basal bones of the maxilla and the mandible. *Am J Orthodont Dentofac Orthoped* 2008, **133:**30–37.
17. Kotze MJ, Bütow K-W, Kotze HF: A radiological method to evaluate alveolar bone regeneration in the Chacma baboon (Papio ursinus). *SADJ* 2012, **67:**210–214.
18. Kotze M, Bütow K-W, Olorunju SA, Kotze HF: Ozone treatment of alveolar bone in the Cape Chacma baboon does not enhance healing following trauma. *J Maxillofac Oral Surg* 2014, **13:**140–147.
19. Jonasson G, Jonasson L, Kiliaridis S: Changes in the radiographic characteristics of the mandibular alveolar process in dentate women with varying bone mineral density: A 5-year prospective study. *Bone* 2006, **38:**714–721.
20. Estes RD: *The Behavior Guide To African Mammals: Including Hoofed Mammals, Carnivores, Primates.* Berkely, California: University of California Press; 1992.
21. Bittar-Cortez JA, Passeri LA, Bóscolo FN, Haiter-Neto F: Comparison of hard tissue density changes around implants assessed in digitized conventional radiographs and subtraction images. *Clin Oral Impl Res* 2006, **17:**560–564.
22. Gulsahi A, Paksoy CS, Ozden S, Kucuk NO, Cebeci ARI, Genc Y: Assessment of bone mineral density in the jaws and its relationship to radiomorphometric indices. *Dentomaxillofac Radiol* 2010, **39:**284–289.
23. Cakıcı H, Hapa O, Gideroğlu K, Ozturan K, Güven M, Yüksel HY, Yılmaz F: The effects of leukotriene receptor antagonist montelukast on histological, radiological and densitometric parameters of fracture healing. *Eklem Hastalik Cerrahisi* 2011, **22:**43–47.

A comparison of mandibular and maxillary alveolar osteogenesis over six weeks: a radiological...

19

24. Campisi P, Hamdy RC, Lauzier D, Amak M, Schloss MD, Lessard ML: **Overview of radiology, histology, and bone morphogenetic protein expression during distraction osteogenesis of the mandible.** *J Otolaryngol* 2002, **31:**281–286.

25. Southard KA, Southard TE, Schlechte JA, Meis PA: **The relationship between the density of the alveolar processes and that of post-cranial bone.** *J Dent Res* 2000, **79:**964–969.

26. Huja SS, Beck FM: **Bone remodeling in maxilla, mandible, and femur of young dogs.** *Anat Rec A Discov Mol Cell Evol Biol* 2007, **291:**1–5.

27. Amler MH: **The time sequence of tissue regeneration in human extraction wounds.** *Oral Surg Oral Med Oral Pathol* 1969, **27:**309–318.

28. Jacobs FJ: *The effect of innovative screw angled mini implants on biomechanical stability of mono-cortical-fixation: An in vitro model in Maxillo-Facial and Oral Surgery.* Pretoria: PhD Thesis University of Pretoria; 2009.

29. Hylander WL: **Stress and strain in the mandibular symphysis of primates: A test of competing hypotheses.** *Am J Phys Anthropol* 1984, **64:**1–46.

30. Lekholm U, Zarb GA: **Patient selection and preparation.** In *Tissue Integrated Prostheses: Osseointegration in Clinical Dentistry.* Edited by Brånemark PI, Zarb GA, Alberktsson T. Chicago: Quintessence Publishing Company; 1985:199–209.

31. Truhlar RS, Orenstein IH, Morris HF, Ochi S: **Distribution of bone quality in patients receiving endosseous dental implants.** *J Oral Maxillofac Surg* 1997, **55**(12 SUPPL 5):38–45.

32. Lewinson D, Rachmiel A, Rihani-Bisharat S, Kraiem Z, Schenzer P, Korem S, Rabinovich Y: **Stimulation of Fos- and Jun-related genes during distraction osteogenesis.** *J Histochemist Cytochemist* 2003, **51:**1161–1168.

4

Comparative three-dimensional analysis of initial biofilm formation on three orthodontic bracket materials

Marc Philipp Dittmer[1†], Carolina Fuchslocher Hellemann[2†], Sebastian Grade[3], Wieland Heuer[3], Meike Stiesch[3], Rainer Schwestka-Polly[2] and Anton Phillip Demling[2*]

Abstract

Introduction: The purpose of the present study was to investigate and compare early biofilm formation on biomaterials, which are being used in contemporary fixed orthodontic treatment.

Methods: This study comprised 10 healthy volunteers (5 females and 5 males) with a mean age of 27.3 +−3.7 years. Three slabs of different orthodontic materials (stainless steel, gold and ceramic) were placed in randomized order on a splint in the mandibular molar region. Splints were inserted intraorally for 48 h. Then the slabs were removed from the splints and the biofilms were stained with a two color fluorescence assay for bacterial viability (LIVE/DEAD BacLight−Bacterial Viability Kit 7012, Invitrogen, Mount Waverley, Australia). The quantitative biofilm formation was analyzed by using confocal laser scanning microscopy (CLSM).

Results: The biofilm coverage was $32.7 \pm 37.7\%$ on stainless steel surfaces, $59.5 \pm 40.0\%$ on gold surfaces and $56.8 \pm 43.6\%$ on ceramic surfaces. Statistical analysis showed significant differences in biofilm coverage between the tested materials ($p=0.033$). The Wilcoxon test demonstrated significantly lower biofilm coverage on steel compared to gold ($p=0.011$).
Biofilm height on stainless steel surfaces was 4.0 ± 7.3 μm, on gold surfaces 6.0 ± 6.6 μm and on ceramic 6.5 ± 6.0 μm. The Friedman test revealed no significant differences between the tested materials ($p=0.150$). Pairwise comparison demonstrated significant differences between stainless steel and gold ($p=0.047$).

Conclusion: Our results indicate that initial biofilm formation seemed to be less on stainless steel surfaces compared with other traditional materials in a short-term observation. Future studies should examine whether there is a difference in long-term biofilm accumulation between stainless steel, gold and ceramic brackets.

Keywords: Biofilm, CLSM, Gold, Stainless steel, Ceramic, Orthodontics, Brackets

Introduction

Contemporary fixed orthodontic therapy comprises a variety of biomaterials, which have been introduced in orthodontics since the last century. In the early part of the 20th century, gold was routinely used for many orthodontic appliances like bands, wires and ligatures [1]. Since the 1930s stainless steel was available, but it was not until approximately 1960 that stainless steel was preferred to gold [2]. Thank the increasing esthetical demand of patients, in the 1980s ceramic brackets came into existence [3-5]. In the beginning of the new century, gold was reintroduced in fixed orthodontics due to its use in CAD-CAM design of customized lingual brackets [6-8].

Several clinical studies indicate that the nature of the used biomaterial has a significant impact on biofilm formation in the short-and long-term. Especially the physico-chemical properties of the surfaces are thought to be responsible for an influence on bacterial adherence and accumulation [9-13]. In multiple studies it was found that ceramic materials were covered less by microorganisms than gold, natural dental hard substances and composites

---

* Correspondence: demling.anton@mh-hannover.de
†Equal contributors
[2]Department of Orthodontics, Hannover Medical School, Carl-Neuberg-Strasse 1, Hannover 30625, Germany
Full list of author information is available at the end of the article

[14-18]. Furthermore, studies indicate that metals like gold and amalgam exert an influence against the adhering biofilm by damaging or killing bacteria to a certain extend [14,19].

Despite the antimicrobial potential of orthodontically used biomaterials, the side effects of fixed orthodontic therapy have been described comprehensively in the literature. Insertion of fixed appliances changes the oral microbiota by affecting its quantity, composition, metabolism and pathogenicity [20-23], which results in a higher incidence of gingival inflammation and caries lesions [23-27].

However, iatrogenic side effects of fixed orthodontic treatment might be reduced by the use of biomaterials with a lower biofilm formation. Changes in this variable might facilitate the prevention of caries and gingivitis in the long-term.

Therefore, the objective of the present study was to compare early biofilm formation on biomaterials which are used in contemporary fixed orthodontic treatment.

The null hypothesis of this study was that there would be no statistically significant difference between stainless steel, ceramic and gold in biofilm accumulation after a period of 48 hours.

Materials and methods

The present study was approved by the Ethics Committee of Hannover Medical School (ethical vote no. 4347) and comprised 5 females and 5 males with a mean age of 27.3 ± 3.7 years. The examination was preformed with the understanding and written consent of each volunteer.

Using nQuery Advisor 5.0 (Statistical Solutions, Saugus, MA, USA), power and sample sizes were calculated. The study was designed to detect a difference of 2.0 ɥm in height and 25% in biofilm coverage while assuming a standard deviation of 2.0 ɥm in height and 25% in biofilm coverage for the within subject differences. This corresponds to an effect size of 1.0. The sample size to achieve a power of 80% to detect an effect size of 1.0 in a pairwise comparison using the Wilcoxon-test at the level of alpha=0.05 was calculated as n=10.

All volunteers were clinically examined for the exclusion of periodontitis. Recorded parameters were Plaqueindex (PI), Pocket probing depth (PPD) and Bleeding on probing (BOP) [28,29]. Selection of first and third or second and fourth quadrants was performed in randomized order (block randomization with a block size of ten). Only volunteers with PI ≤ 25% and PPD ≤ 4 mm were included in the study. Further criteria for exclusion were systemic illness, pregnancy, removable partial dentures, smoking and antibiotic therapy during the last 6 weeks before the study. Volunteers were advised not to brush their teeth and not to use antimicrobial mouth rinses during the 48 hour period of the present study.

In the present study initial biofilm formation on three traditional biomaterials used in orthodontic treatment was investigated. These were stainless steel (Victory Series, 3 M Unitek, Monrovia, CA, USA), gold (Incognito 3 M Unitek, Monrovia, CA, USA), and ceramic (Clarity, 3 M Unitek, Monrovia, CA, USA). 10 samples per bracket material were obtained from commercially available stock and received a similar surface treatment: the slabs were grounded and polished with grinding paper (grit sizes P600, P1000, P1200, P2400, P4000, Buehler, Düsseldorf, Germany). After polishing all samples, the roughness depths of the different biomaterials were measured at a random area of 90 ɥm x 90 ɥm, using an Atomic Force Microscope (AFM) (MFP-3D, Asylum Research, Santa Barbara, CA, USA).

After clinical examination impressions of the lower and upper jaws were taken (Alginoplast, Heraeus Kulzer, Hanau, Germany). On the lower cast a splint was manufactured by use of a viscous hard transparent foil (Erkodur, Erkodent, Pfalzgrafenweiler, Germany; Palapress, Heraeus Kulzer, Hanau, Germany) using a thermoforming technique. The casts were mounted in an articulator (Protar 5, KaVo, Leutkirch, Germany) and the splint was grinded in uniform contact.

The three tested biomaterials (stainless steel, gold and ceramic) were mounted with Tetric Flow (Ivoclar Vivadent, Schaan, Liechtenstein) on the splint, placing these in the mandibular molar region on the buccal site. Afterwards, all specimens were degreased by alcohol. The selection of right and left quadrants was randomized by using a random list. Splints were inserted for 48 hours.

Afterwards splints were removed from the oral cavity and the samples were detached from the splints without destruction of the biofilm and stored in phosphate buffered saline (PBS).

For fluorescence staining of the bacteria an assay for bacterial viability (LIVE/DEAD BacLight–Bacterial Viability Kit 7012, Invitrogen, Mount Waverley, Australia) was used. After staining the samples according to the manufacturer protocol the biofilm formation was analyzed by using a confocal laser scanning microscope (CLSM) (Leica upright-MP Microscope, Leica Microsystems GmbH, Germany).

For analysis of biofilm coverage five randomized areas on each biomaterial were evaluated and from each area a surface picture was obtained in tenfold resolution. Ten pictures vertically to the surface were taken for the evaluation of biofilm thickness at the same area with a 40x resolution and a zoom level of 2.4 set by the software.

The quantitative biofilm surface coverage was calculated using surface-analysis software (Adobe Photoshop; Adobe Systems Inc., San Jose, CA, USA). The bright areas on these pictures represented biofilm coverage, non-covered surfaces appeared dark. Biofilm coverage was calculated concerning these different grey values. Biofilm thickness was measured at five defined coordinates per picture resulting in 250 measuring points for each biomaterial. The mean values and standard deviations of biofilm surface coverage and thickness were calculated for each area of all probes.

Documentation and statistical analysis was performed using the data processing program SPSS/PC-version 20.0 for windows (IBM, Armonk, NY, USA). The Kolmogorov-Smirnov test was applied to test for normal distribution. As data were not distributed normally, data were compared globally using the Friedman test. Pairwise comparison was performed with the Wilcoxon test. All tests were performed two-tailed with a significance level of p=0.05.

Results

No dropouts were recorded during the study. Periodontal parameters were as follows: PI (Plaque Index) was 23,2 ± 12,9%, PPD (Probing pocket depth) 1,6 ± 0,2 mm and BOP (Bleeding on probing) 3,9 ± 5,4%.

The roughness depths determined by AFM were Ra=0.2 µm on stainless steel, Ra=0.3 µm on ceramic and Ra=0.2 µm on gold.

Biofilm was detected by CLSM on all tested bracket materials after exposure to the oral cavity for 48 h. Figure 1 shows the results after analysis of biofilm height with respect to bracket material. On stainless steel surfaces average biofilm height was 4.0 ± 7.3 µm (Figure 2). Biofilm height on gold surfaces was 6.0 ± 6.6 µm (Figure 3), whereas ceramic showed biofilm heights of 6.5 ± 6.0 µm (Figure 4). The Friedman test revealed no significant differences between the tested materials (p=0.150). However, pairwise comparison demonstrated significant differences between stainless steel and gold (p=0.047).

Biofilm covered 32.7 ± 37.7% of stainless steel surfaces, 59.5 ± 40.0% of gold surfaces and 56.8 ± 43.6% of ceramic surface. Statistical analysis showed significant differences in biofilm coverage between the tested materials (p=0.033). The Wilcoxon test demonstrated a significantly lower biofilm coverage on steel compared to gold (p=0.011). Comparison of biofilm coverage between steel and ceramic (p=0.074) and ceramic and gold (p=0.285) showed no significant differences.

Discussion

Bracket debonding causes an enamel loss of about 50 µm [30] and the mechanical bracket debonding entails the risk of enamel fractures as well [31]. To avoid this enamel damage on permanent teeth and for a secure atraumatic removal, the samples were fixed on a splint. Different kinds of individual splints have been used to collect biofilm in the past [14,32-34]. For the present study, a simple individual removable model was used. Furthermore, accessibility of samples without destruction of fragile initial biofilm was ensured by using the splint model.

The amount of biofilm formation is influenced by the intraoral location [33], whereas posterior regions exhibit a higher plaque formation than anterior ones [35]. This effect is contributed to the self-cleaning mechanisms of the tongue, salivary flow and accessibility to oral hygiene. To avoid mechanical plaque removal by tongue activity in the present study samples were placed bucally

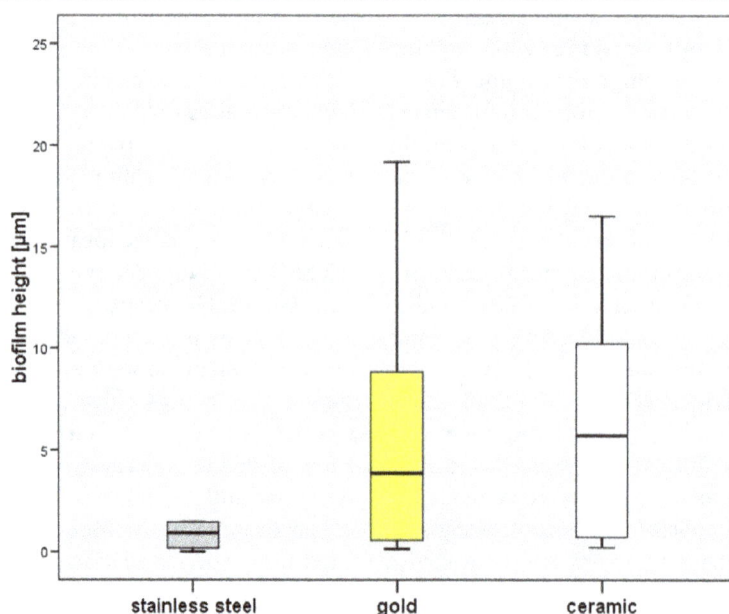

Figure 1 Boxplot presentation of biofilm height.

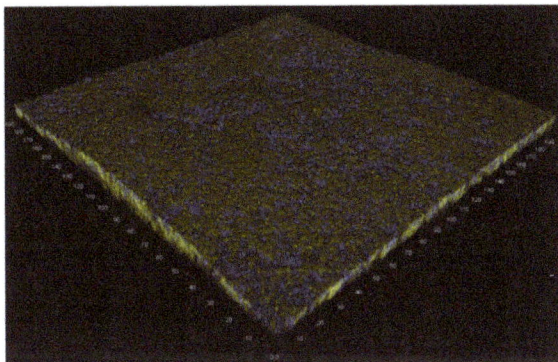

Figure 2 Three-dimensional reconstruction of biofilm accumulating on stainless steel.

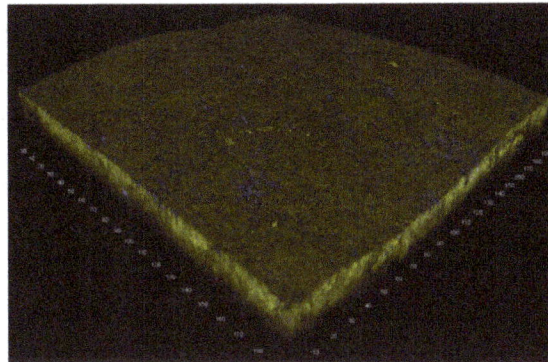

Figure 4 Three-dimensional reconstruction of biofilm accumulating on ceramic.

in the molar region on the splints. Furthermore, specimens were placed in a randomized order to eliminate the cofounder intraoral localization. In the present study no standardization of diet was applied, which could have influenced the interindividual differences in biofilm formation. Furthermore wearing time of the split was not monitored electronically. As data was only compared intraindividually, this aspect can be neglected in the interpretation of the results.

In vivo studies have shown no differences of the bacterial adhesion and colonization on surfaces with a roughness value ≤ Ra=0.2 μm [36,37]. As the surface roughness of the tested biomaterials was fairly 0.2 μm, the confounder "surface roughness" should not have influenced the results of biofilm thickness and coverage. The reported differences of the biofilm formation between the variety of bracket materials might to some extend be caused by different shapes of brackets. This confounder was avoided by using uniformly shaped test specimens in the present study.

The technique of confocal laser scanning microscopy has been proven to be particularly well suited for the

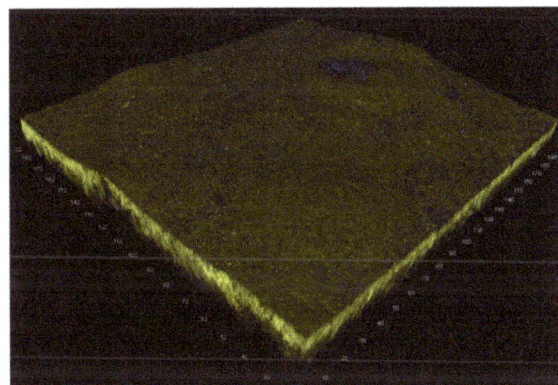

Figure 3 Three-dimensional reconstruction of biofilm accumulating on gold.

examination of fragile and thin initial microbial biofilms [38-40]. With the aid of CLSM, biofilm formation can be studied in their natural hydrated state, with no requirement of dehydration, chemical fixation or embedding techniques.

The height of biofilm on stainless steel was significant lower than with gold, and almost significant lower compared with ceramic. There is a controversial discussion in the literature which bracket material is more prone to biofilm adherence and plaque retention. To the best of our knowledge, there is a lack of information about in vivo short-term biofilm formation on orthodontic bracket materials. However, by means of mid-and long-term studies data base is inconsistent. A lower initial affinity to bacterial accumulation (Streptococcus mutans) was found in an in vitro study with metal brackets compared to ceramic or plastic brackets [41]. In contrast, no significant differences were found in the accumulation of caries-inducing bacterial species in vivo comparing the plaque-retaining capacity of metal vs. ceramic brackets by counting the levels of different bacterial species on the day of debonding [9]. Nevertheless, other studies indicate a higher plaque-retaining capacity of stainless steel brackets compared to ceramic or plastic brackets due to a higher critical surface tension and total work of adhesion [10]. Furthermore, Escherichia coli, Porphyromonas gingivalis and Streptococcus mutans exhibited a greater affinity to metal brackets compared to ceramics or plastic ones [42,43]. In an in vitro study brackets manufactured from gold were less prone to colonisation of streptococci species [44].

Conclusion

Comparing findings in literature with data of the present study, there is a significant difference in short-term and mid-or long-term biofilm formation. These differences might be explained by physico-chemical surface alterations that occur over time: Signs of wear caused by food, drink, oral hygiene and corrosion have an influence on surface roughness or surface free energy and would consequently have a significant impact on long-term biofilm formation [11,45,46].

Future studies should examine whether there is a difference in long-term biofilm accumulation between stainless steel, gold and ceramic brackets. Furthermore, the clinical impact on the development of decalcifications and periodontal parameters should be investigated.

Competing interests
The authors declare that they have no competing interests.

Authors' contributions
MPD performed the interpretation of data and wrote main parts of the manuscript. CFH carried out the clinical part of the study, performed the measurement of biofilms and wrote minor parts of the manuscript. SG implemented the method of biofim analysis. WH created minor parts of the study design and helped in the interpretation of data. MS and RSP provided the financial support and infrastructure, helped in the development of study design. APD was the head of the project team: definition of the topic, development of study design, coordination of co-workers, structure of the paper and finalisation. All authors read and approved the final manuscript.

Acknowledgments
We would like to thank Professor Dr. H. Hecker, Institute of Biostatistics, Hannover Medical School, for helping with the statistical analysis.

Author details
[1]Center of Dentistry, Oral and Maxillofacial Medicine, Hannover Medical School, Carl-Neuberg-Strasse 1, Hannover 30625, Germany. [2]Department of Orthodontics, Hannover Medical School, Carl-Neuberg-Strasse 1, Hannover 30625, Germany. [3]Department of Prosthetic Dentistry and Biomedical Materials Science, Hannover Medical School, Carl-Neuberg-Strasse 1, Hannover 30625, Germany.

References
1. Kusy RP. Orthodontic biomaterials: from the past to the present. Angle Orthod. 2002;72:501–12.
2. Thurow RC. Edgewise Orthodontics. 3rd ed. St. Louis: Mosby 1972, v-viii. p. 22–34,148,270.
3. Keith O, Kusy RP, Whitley JQ. Zirconia brackets: an evaluation morphology and coefficients of friction. Am J Orthod Dentofacial Orthop. 1994;106:605–14.
4. Kusy RP. Morphology of polycrystalline alumina brackets and its relationship to fracture toughness and strength. Angle Orthod. 1988;58:197–203.
5. Swartz ML. Ceramic brackets. J Clin Orthod. 1988;22:82–8.
6. Wiechmann D. A new bracket system for lingual orthodontic treatment. Part 1: Theoretical background and development. J Orofac Orthop. 2002;63:234–45.
7. Wiechmann D. A new bracket system for lingual orthodontic treatment. Part 2: First clinical experiences and further development. J Orofac Orthop. 2003;64:372–88.
8. Wiechmann D, Rummel V, Thalheim A, Simon JS, Wiechmann L. Customized brackets and archwires for lingual orthodontic treatment. J Orthod Dentofacial Orthop. 2003;124:593–9.
9. Anhoury P, Nathanson D, Hughes CV, Socransky S, Feres M, Chou LL. Microbial profile on metallic and ceramic bracket materials. Angle Orthod. 2002;72:338–43.
10. Eliades T, Eliades G, Brantley WA. Microbial attachment on orthodontic appliances: I. Wettability and early pellicle formation on bracket materials. Am J Orthod Dentofacial Orthop. 1995;108:351–60.
11. Quirynen M, Bollen CM. The influence of surface roughness and surface free-energy on supra-and subgingival plaque in man. A review of the literature. J Clin Periodontol. 1995;22:1–14.
12. Siegrist BE, Brecx MC, Gusberti FA, Joss A, Lang NP. In vivo early human dental plaque formation on different supporting substances. A scanning

13. Weerkamp AH, Quirynen M, Marechal M, van der Mei HC, van Steenberghe D, Busscher HJ. The role of surface free energy in the early in vivo formation of dental plaque on human enamel and polymeric substrata. Microb Ecol Health and Dis. 1989;2:11–8.
14. Auschill TM, Arweiler NB, Brecx M, Reich E, Sculean A, Netuschil L. The effect of dental restorative materials on dental biofilm. Eur JOral Sci. 2002;110:48–53.
15. Hahn R, Neutschil L, Loè STC. Initiale Plaquebesiedlung keramischer Restaurationsmaterialien. Dtsch Zahnarztl Z. 1992;47:330–4.
16. Savitt ED, Malament KA, Sokransky SS, Melcer AJ, Backman KJ. Effects on colonization of oral microbiota by a cast glass ceramic restoration. Int J Periodont Rest Dent. 1987;2:23–35.
17. Skjùrland KK. Bacterial accumulation on silicate and composite materials. J Biol Buccale. 1976;4:315–22.
18. Wise MG, Dykema RW. The plaque-retaining capacity of four dental materials. J Prosthet Dent. 1975;33:178–90.
19. Augthun M, Brauner A. Antimikrobielle Wirkung unterschiedlicher Dentallegierungen auf Keime oder oralen Mirkoflora in vitro. Dtsch Zahnarztl Z. 1988;43:869–73.
20. Diamanti-Kipioti A, Diamanti-Kipioti A, Gusberti FA, Lang NP. Clinical and microbiological effects of fixed orthodontic appliances. J Clin Periodontol. 1987;14:326–33.
21. Paolantonio M, Festa F, di Placido G, D'Attilio M, Catamo G, Piccolomini R. Site-specific subgingival colonization by Actinobacillus actinomycetemcomitans in orthodontic patients. Am J Orthod Dentofacial Orthop. 1999;115:423–8.
22. Chang HS, Walsh LJ, Freer TJ. The effect of orthodontic treatment on salivary flow, pH, buffer capacity, and levels of mutans streptococci and lactobacilli. Aust Orthod J. 1999;15:229–34.
23. Hägg U, Kaveewatcharanont P, Samaranayake YH, Samaranayake LP. The effect of fixed orthodontic appliances on the oral carriage of Candida species and Enterobacteriaceae. Europ J Orthod. 2004;26:623–9.
24. Atack NE, Sandy JR, Addy M. Periodontal and microbiological changes associated with the placement of orthodontic appliances. A review J Periodontol. 1996;67:78–85.
25. Naranjo AA, Trivino ML, Jaramillo A, Betancourth M, Botero JE. Changes in the subgingival microbiota and periodontal parameters before and 3 months after bracket placement. Am J Orthod Dentofacial Orthop. 2006;130:275e217–22.
26. Ahn SJ, Lim BS, Lee SJ. Prevalence of cariogenic streptococci on incisor brackets detected by polymerase chain reaction. Am J Orthod Dentofacial Orthop. 2007;131:736–41.
27. van Gastel J, Quirynen M, Teughels W, Coucke W, Carels C. Longitudinal changes in microbiology and clinical periodontal variables after placement of fixed orthodontic appliances. J Periodontol. 2008;79:2078–86.
28. Lang NP, Adler R, Joss A, Nyman S. Absence of bleeding on probing. An indicator of periodontal stability. J Clin Periodontol. 1990;17:714–21.
29. Silness J, Löe H. Periodontal disease in pregnancy. II. Correlation between oral hygiene and periodontal condition. Acta Odontol Scand. 1964;22:121–35.
30. Al Shamsi AH, Cunningham JL, Lamey PJ, Lynch E. Three-dimensional measurement of residual adhesive and enamel loss on teeth after debonding of orthodontic brackets: an in-vitro study. Am J Orthod Dentofacial Orthop. 2007;131:301e309–315.
31. Stratmann U, Schaarschmidt K, Wegener H, Ehmer U. The extent of enamel surface fractures. A quantitative comparison of thermally debonded ceramic and mechanically debonded metal brackets by energy dispersive micro-and image-analysis. Eur J Orthod. 1996;18:655–62.
32. Arweiler NB, Hellwig E, Sculean A, Hein N, Aushill TM. Individual Vitality Pattern of in situ Dental Biofilms at Different Locations in the Oral Cavity. Caries Res. 2004;38:442–7.
33. Auschill TM, Hellwig E, Sculean A, Hein N, Arweiler NB. Impact of the intraoral location on the rate of biofilm growth. Clin Oral Invest. 2004;8:97–101.
34. Hanning M. Transmission electron microscopy of early plaque formation on dental materials in vivo. Eur J Oral Sci. 1999;107:55–64.
35. Zachrisson S, Zachrisson BU. Gingival condition associated with orthodontic treatment. Angle Orthod. 1972;42:26–34.
36. Bollen CM, Papaioannou W, Van Eldere J, Schepers E, Quirynen M, van Steenberghe D. The influence of abutment surface roughness on plaque accumulation and peri-implant mucositis. Clin Oral Implant Res. 1996;7:201–11.

37. Quirynen M, Bollen CM, Papaioannou W, Van Eldere J, van Steenberghe D. The influence of titanium abutment surface roughness on plaque accumulation and gingivitis: Short-term observations. Int J Oral Maxillofac Implants. 1996;11:169–78.

38. Costerton JW, Lewandowski Z, Caldwell DE, Korber DR, Lappin-Scott HM. Microbial biofilms. Atm Rev Microbiol. 1995;49:711–45.

39. Shotton DM. Confocal scanning optical microscopy and its applications for biological specimens. £ Cell Sci. 1989;94:175–206.

40. Wood S, Kirkham J, Marsh PD, Shore RC, Naltress B, Robinson C. Architecture of Intact Natural Human Plaque Biofilms Studied by Confocal Laser Scanning Microscopy. J Dent Res. 2000;79:21–7.

41. Fournier A, Payant L, Bouclin R. Adherence of Streptococcus mutans to orthodontic brackets. Am J Orthod Dentofacial Orthop. 1998;114:414–7.

42. Knoernschild KL, Rogers HM, Lefebvre CA, Fortson WM, Schuster GS. Endotoxin affinity for orthodontic brackets. Am J Orthod Dentofacial Orthop. 1999;115:634–9.

43. Ahn SJ, Kho HS, Lee SW, Nahm DS. Roles of salivary proteins in the adherence of oral streptococci to various orthodontic brackets. J Dent Res. 2002;81:411–5.

44. Passariello C, Gigola P. Adhesion and biofilm formation by oral streptococci on different commercial brackets. Eur J Paediatr Dent. 2013;14:125–30.

45. Matasa CG. Pros and cons of the reuse of direct-bonded appliances. Am J Orthod Dentofacial Orthop. 1989;96:72–6.

46. Lin MC, Lin SC, Lee TH, Huang HH. Surface analysis and corrosion resistance of different stainless steel orthodontic brackets in artificial saliva. Angle Orthod. 2006;76:322–9.

5

In-vivo durability of a fluoride-releasing sealant (OpalSeal) for protection against white-spot lesion formation in orthodontic patients

Michael Knösel[1*], David Ellenberger[2], Yvonne Göldner[3], Paulo Sandoval[4] and Dirk Wiechmann[5,6]

Abstract

Background: Sealant application during fixed appliances orthodontic treatment for enamel protection is common, however, reliable data on its durability in vivo are rare.

Objective: This study aims at assessing the durability of a sealant (OpalSeal, Ultradent) for protection against white-spot lesion formation in orthodontic patients over 26 weeks in vivo, taking into account the provision or absence of an adequate oral hygiene. We tested the null hypothesis of (1) no significant abatement of the sealant after 26 weeks in fixed orthodontic treatment compared to baseline, and (2) no significant influence of the factor of brushing and oral hygiene (as screened by approximal plaque index, API) on the abatement of the sealant.

Methods: Integrity and abatement of OpalSeal applicated directly following bracketing was assessed in thirty-six consecutive patients (n_{teeth} = 796) undergoing orthodontic treatment with fixed appliances (male/female 12/24; mean age/SD 14.4/1.33 Y). Assessment of the fluorescing sealant preservation was by a black-light lamp, using a classification that was concepted in analogy to the ARI index: (3, sealant completely preserved; 2 = > 50% preserved; 1 = <50%; 0 = no sealant observable) immediately following application (Baseline, T0), after 2 (T1), 8 (T2), 14 (T3), 20 (T4) and 26 weeks (T5). API was assessed at T0 and T1. Statistical analysis was by non-parametric repeated measures ANOVA (α = 5%, power >80%).

Results: At baseline, 43.4% of teeth had a positive API. Oral hygiene deteriorated after bracketing (T1, 53%) significantly. Null hypothesis (1) was rejected, while (2) was accepted: Mean values of both the well brushed and non-brushed anterior teeth undercut the score "1" at T3 (week 14). Despite a slightly better preservation of the sealer before and after T3 in not-sufficiently brushed (API-positive) teeth, this finding was statistically not significant.

Conclusion: One single application of OpalSeal is unlikely to last throughout the entire fixed appliance treatment stage. On average, re-application of the sealant can be expected to be necessary after 3.5 months (week 14) in treatment.

Keywords: Orthodontic sealant, Durability, OpalSeal, White-spot lesions, In-vivo

Introduction

Prevention of white-spot lesions (WSL) during fixed appliances orthodontic treatment is still a challenge in today's orthodontic treatment: There is evidence that neglecting oral hygiene during orthodontic treatment with fixed appliances can cause WSL formation within weeks [1-4]. Other than mechanical plaque removal by tooth brushing,

local fluoridation by dentifrices and mouth rinses, or the use of fluoride-releasing bonding materials, major preventive strategies for a prevention of enamel demineralization during fixed orthodontic treatment focus on the application of fluoride-releasing sealants [5,6].

Sealant application for enamel protection is common in fixed appliances orthodontic treatment patients, however, reliable data on its durability in vivo are rare [7]. Tüfekçi et al. investigated the preservation of a sealant on extracted premolars 67 ± 28 days following bracket bonding and sealant application in vivo, and found that

* Correspondence: mknoesel@yahoo.de
[1]Department of Orthodontics, University Medical Center Göttingen (UMG), 37099 Göttingen, Germany
Full list of author information is available at the end of the article

layers of OpalSeal (Ultradent) remained on an average of 50% at the time of assessment, and found no correlation between sealant residues and the variation of time the teeth were in the mouth [7]. However, it is conceivable that the factors of oral hygiene and abrasion caused by mechanical tooth brushing, as well as acidic or mechanical assaults during consumption of food and beverages may have an impact on the sealant condition and durability in vivo: Varnish layers may be reduced in thickness and extension by daily mechanical wear. However, whilst there have been studies on reduction of WSL occurrence following fluoride-releasing sealant application, there is a lack of studies concerning an vivo-screening of the integrity or abatement of sealants, in interference with oral hygiene habits and observation time.

Study aims

This study aims at assessing the durability of a sealant (OpalSeal, Ultradent Products, South Jordan, Utah) for protection against white-spot lesion formation in orthodontic patients over more than six months (26 weeks) in vivo, taking into account the provision or absence of an adequate oral hygiene.

We tested the null hypotheses of (1) no significant abatement of the sealant (as screened by a score from 0–3) after 26 weeks in fixed orthodontic treatment compared to baseline, and (2) no significant influence of the factor of oral hygiene (as screened by approximal plaque index, API [8]) on the abatement of the sealant.

Subjects and Methods

Thirty-six consecutive patients undergoing orthodontic treatment with fixed appliances (male/female 12/24; age 12–17 years; mean age 14.44 Y; SD 1.33) were consecutively recruited at an orthodontic practice in Hannover, Germany, between Nov 1st, 2011 and April 30, 2012. Subjects were included upon meeting the following inclusion criteria:

- upcoming indirect Damon-3 (Ormco, Orange, CA, USA) bracket placement of least of sixteen teeth,
- application of a sealant (OpalSeal, Ultradent Products, South Jordan, Utah) on that same appointment, and
- having given consent for participation and accepting follow-up assessments during recall visits.

Subject were excluded upon refusal of sealant application, or less than sixteen teeth bracketed, or if they disagreed to participate. Other than exclusion of subjects, single teeth of included trial subjects were not assessed by this study in case they were not bracketed on the same appointment, or in case they were subject to upcoming

extraction. Of 864 potentially eligible teeth, a number of 796 trial teeth was included (drop-out: n = 68 teeth).

Standardized indirect bracket placement using a dry-field system for isolation was performed prior to sealant application, in order to allow for a removal of excessive adhesives without setting damages to sealant layers. Following cleaning of tooth surfaces with fluoride-free pumice, adhesive and sealant application routine was carried out following manufacturer's instructions and included a 15 s interval of etching with 37 % phosphoric acid of the complete labial enamel surface, followed by indirect bonding using chemically-cured Monolok2 composite adhesive system (Rocky Mountain Orthodontics, Denver, Colo, USA). Adhesive residues have been removed prior to sealant application. According to the manufacturer's instructions, OpalSeal was gently air-dried following application, prior to light-curing for 20s per tooth (Bluephase C8, 800 mW/cm2, IvoclarVivadent, Schaan, Liechtenstein).

Ethical approval

The study was performed in extension of an earlier positively voted study protocol (# 4/8/09). All procedures used in this prospective observational study had been presented to the ethics committee of the University of Göttingen, Germany, earlier. There were no objections against publication. The patients and their guardians gave informed consent for taking part in the study.

Parameter 1: Screening of oral hygiene

The approximal plaque index (API) has been introduced in dentistry for a quick assessment of oral hygiene status [8]. Although being based on more or less subjective decisions that are made chair-side, API assessments have been established as a basic clinical methodology used in research on the subject of cariology and periodontology [9]. Oral hygiene status was screened using the API for each bracketed tooth, as a yes/no decision (results given in % of teeth with plaque) prior to bracket placement and sealant application at T0, and after 14 days in treatment (T1). All patients received identical, standardized instructions on both tooth- and inter-bracket brushing during orthodontic treatment with fixed appliances, and were advised to do so three times daily, using typical commercially available 1,400-1,450 ppm fluoridated dentifrices. They were provided with the same type of tooth brushes with medium filaments, and interdental brushes (TePe, Malmö, Sweden).

Parameter 2: Scoring of sealant layer integrity

Integrity and condition of the OpalSeal-layer was assessed using a black-light UV lamp provided by the manufacturer for screening purposes of the fluorescing sealant. Similar to previous trials [4], assessments were done chair-side by a clinician who was blinded to the patient's trial time frame, while notes were made by a study nurse: Immediately after bonding and sealant application (Baseline, T0), after 14 days (T1), 8 weeks (T2), 14 weeks (T3), 20 weeks (T4) and 26 weeks (T5). Abatement of the varnish was parameterized using a classification from 0 to 3 that was concepted in analogy to the adhesive remnant index (ARI, [10]): (3 = sealant undamaged/completely preserved, 2 > =50% preserved, 1 < =50%, 0 = no sealant observable to the naked eye), assessed for every bracketed tooth (max. 24 per patient, Figure 1a, b and c).

Statistical analysis

The factor of 'oral hygiene' as assessed by API scores at Baseline (T0) and two weeks following bracketing (T1) was tested for potential changes (increases in API score = deterioration of oral hygiene) using a t-test for dependent samples. The status of the durability of the OpalSeal-layer as well as potential impacts and interactions of the initial API (T0), trial time elapse (T1-T5), tooth type (#1-#6; 1, central -; 2, lateral incisor; 3, canine; 4, first-; 5, second premolar; 6, first molar) and jaw (maxilla, mandible) were tested by non-parametric, repeated measures ANOVA, with the OpalSeal-Score as dependent variable. Correlated measurements within one patient as well as over time for each tooth were modeled by a random factor 'subject' along with a random factor 'tooth' yielding a nested compound symmetry structure. In the case of significant interactions between the experimental factors, the data were split and further analyzed in subgroups. The significance level was set to 5%. Sample size calculation according to O'Brien-Castelloe yielded a power in excess of 80% for an inclusion of 36 subjects/796 teeth. All analyses were performed using SAS 9.3 (SAS Institute, Cary, NC, USA) and Statistica 10 (StatSoft (Europe) GmbH, Hamburg, Germany).

Results

At baseline, 43.4% of teeth had a positive API (SD: 20.5%). Oral hygiene deteriorated after bracketing (T1, 53%, SD: 22.0%) significantly: The T-test for dependent samples API (complete, %) T0 vs T1 yielded p = 0.01.

Effect of oral hygiene (API) on sealant abatement

At T1, we found that teeth with positive API scores showed no significant differences in terms of sealant layer preservation, in contrast to teeth with negative API scores (Table 1). Generally spoken, there was an increase in the abatement of the sealant from front teeth 1–4 to posterior teeth #5 or #6, which is globally significant (Table 2) and was found to be more rapid in well brushed lower posterior teeth (teeth #5 and #6 with negative API). (Table 1, Figures 2a and b). Mean values of both the well brushed and non-brushed anterior teeth undercut the score "1" (<50% sealer left) at T3

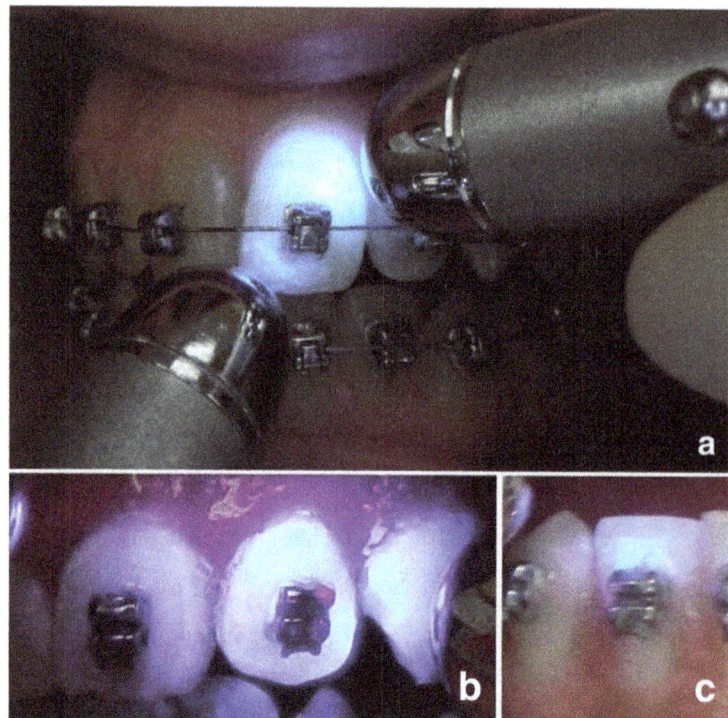

Figure 1 a Assessment of sealant integrity was done by black-light illumination, using the fluorescent properties of the OpalSeal. **b** and **c** give examples of sealant scores 3 (sealant undamaged/completely preserved), and 1 (<=50% of sealant left).

Table 1 As anterior teeth #1-#4 were found to be homogeneous in terms of abatement of the sealant score, pair-wise comparisons between this group of teeth with teeth #5 and #6 were implemented

Time	API (T0)	Tooth groups compared	Opalseal score difference	Standard error	p-value
1	positive	1-4	5	0.24	0.16	0.20
1	positive	1-4	6	0.26	0.12	0.07
1	positive	5	6	0.03	0.19	0.94
1	negative	1-4	5	0.21	0.08	0.02
1	negative	1-4	6	0.69	0.09	<.0001
1	negative	5	6	0.49	0.10	<.0001
2	positive	1-4	5	0.26	0.16	0.08
2	positive	1-4	6	0.41	0.12	0.001
2	positive	5	6	0.15	0.19	0.57
2	negative	1-4	5	0.39	0.08	<.0001
2	negative	1-4	6	0.69	0.08	<.0001
2	negative	5	6	0.31	0.10	0.005
3	positive	1-4	5	0.20	0.16	0.15
3	positive	1-4	6	0.45	0.12	0.0002
3	positive	5	6	0.25	0.19	0.25
3	negative	1-4	5	0.33	0.08	<.0001
3	negative	1-4	6	0.54	0.09	<.0001
3	negative	5	6	0.21	0.10	0.07
4	positive	1-4	5	0.22	0.16	0.17
4	positive	1-4	6	0.61	0.12	<.0001
4	positive	5	6	0.39	0.19	0.03
4	negative	1-4	5	0.21	0.08	0.003
4	negative	1-4	6	0.46	0.09	<.0001
4	negative	5	6	0.26	0.10	0.02
5	positive	1-4	5	0.30	0.16	0.04
5	positive	1-4	6	0.58	0.12	<.0001
5	positive	5	6	0.27	0.19	0.13
5	negative	1-4	5	0.00	0.08	0.79
5	negative	1-4	6	0.32	0.09	<.0001
5	negative	5	6	0.32	0.10	0.001

Especially during the first weeks in treatment, sealant preservation was better in API-negative teeth, although this finding was globally not significant when considering all time points (see also Table 3).

Table 2 Factors and interactions that have a potential impact on sealant durability scores

Effect	ANOVA p-Value
Jaw (Maxilla, Mandible)	<.0001
Tooth type (#1,#2,#3,#4,#5,#6)	<.0001
Jaw * Tooth type	0.01
Time (T 1,2,3,4,5)	<.0001
Jaw * Time	0.45
Tooth type * Time	0.69
Jaw * Tooth type * Time	0.83
Oral hygiene by initial API (0)	0.54
Jaw * Oral hygiene	0.24
Tooth type * Oral hygiene	0.73
Jaw * Tooth type * Oral hygiene	0.26
Time * Oral hygiene	0.10
Jaw * Time * Oral hygiene	0.08
Tooth type * Time * Oral hygiene	0.0002
Jaw * Tooth type * Time * Oral hygiene	0.83

The explained variance by within-subject measurements was found to be crucial with $R^2 = 0.34$ (p < .0001) for the random factor 'subject' and $R^2 = 0.27$ (p < .0001) for the random factor 'tooth'.

of the sealant. See (Figure 2a and b) for a visualisation of this effect.

Maxilla vs. Mandible

Pairwise comparisons indicate a more pronounced abatement of the sealant in the mandible than in the maxilla at T1, and it was significantly increased in mandibular teeth #1, #2, and #6 when compared to the maxillary equivalent (Figure 3).

Discussion

An inhibition of enamel demineralization during orthodontic fixed treatment can be achieved by the application of fluoride-releasing sealants [11,12], however, the efficacy of those sealants also depends on their integrity or durability [7]. It is a popular fallacy to assume that one sealant application at the start of fixed appliances orthodontic treatment will suffice for enamel protection throughout the entire fixed treatment stage, without a renewal [13,14]. In-vivo research yielded evidence that sealants offer some protection and are suitable for reducing frequencies of new WSL [12], but do not offer outright protection from WSL formation for the full duration of treatment [7]. Diligence during application and frequencies of re-application may be relevant in terms of sealant durability, as may be the presence of different levels of oral hygiene and intensities of tooth- and interbracket brushing as a factor that is potentially causing sealant abrasion. In-vivo data on the durability of those

(week 14) (Figure 2a and b). Percentages of teeth with a score higher than 0 are depicted by Table 3 and Figure 2c and d. Despite the overall slightly better preservation of the sealant before and after T3 in not-sufficiently brushed (API positive) teeth compared to API-negative teeth, this finding was statistically not significant (Table 2). That is, considering the total trial time, the factor oral hygiene itself has no global significant effect on the abatement

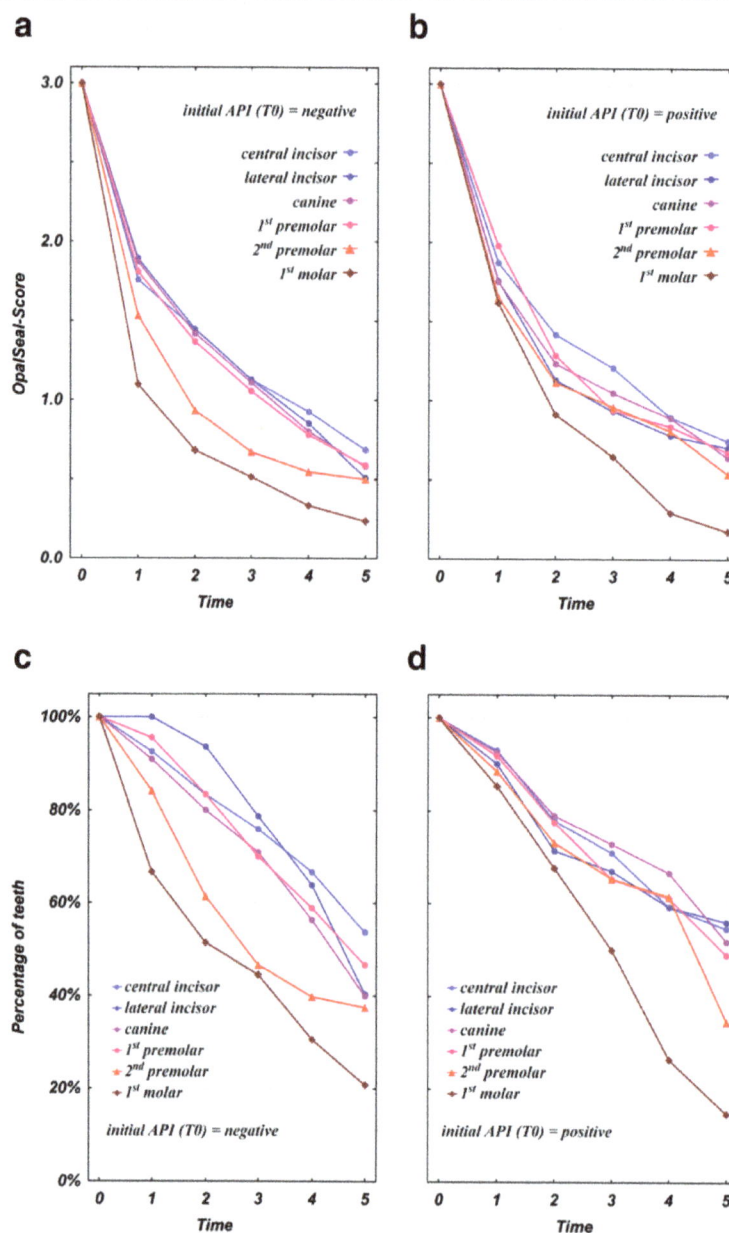

Figure 2 a, **b** Sealant layer abatement by mean OpalSeal-scores in sub-groups with positive or negative API scores indicate a significant increase in abatement from front teeth to posterior teeth (see also Table 1). On average, well brushed (left) and non-brushed (right) anterior teeth undercut the 50% sealant preservation (score "1) at T3 (week 14). The slightly better sealant preservation before and after T3 in API-positive teeth was globally not significant. On average, re-application of sealant can therefore be expected to be necessary after 3.5 months in active treatment. **c**, **d** Percentages of teeth with sealant scores higher than 0. At T5, approximately 50% of front teeth #1-#4 with positive API had at T5 a sealant score higher than 0, while in the case of well brushed teeth percentages were slightly lower. See also Table 3 for details.

sealants are scarce: A recent in vivo report on sealant preservation in premolars extracted following 67 ± 28 days found that an average of 50% of OpalSeal was left on the teeth [7]. Moreover, the authors reported the reduction of WSL frequencies in OpalSeal-treated teeth as being small, but not significant in comparison to a non-fluoride releasing bonding following 90 or more days; a beneficial effect in terms of a significant reduction of WSLs was only seen in teeth assessed within the first 3 months. They concluded that this result may have been due to an abatement of the sealant, indicating the necessity for multiple applications [7]. However, there is no clear guideline for the handling of sealant re-application based on the available evidence, particularly as it is not yet known how protective effects and durability of the fluoride-releasing sealants interact with additional etching intervals that may be

Table 3 Sealant abatement: Percentages of teeth with sealant scores higher than 0 in sub-groups with adequate or inadequate oral hygiene (negative or positive API scores)

Tooth type #	Time	Teeth with sealant score 1 or higher (%)	
		Negative API	Positive API
1	0	100	100
1	1	92.59	93.02
1	2	83.33	77.91
1	3	75.93	70.93
1	4	66.67	59.30
1	5	53.70	54.65
2	0	100	100
2	1	100	90.11
2	2	93.62	71.43
2	3	78.72	67.03
2	4	63.83	59.34
2	5	40.43	56.04
3	0	100	100
3	1	90.91	91.84
3	2	80.00	77.55
3	3	70.91	65.31
3	4	56.36	61.23
3	5	40.00	48.98
4	0	100	100
4	1	95.56	92.59
4	2	83.33	79.01
4	3	70.00	72.84
4	4	58.89	66.67
4	5	46.67	51.85
5	0	100	100
5	1	84.09	88.46
5	2	61.36	73.08
5	3	46.59	65.38
5	4	39.77	61.54
5	5	37.50	34.62
6	0	100	100
6	1	66.67	85.29
6	2	51.39	67.65
6	3	44.44	50.00
6	4	30.56	26.47
6	5	20.83	14.71

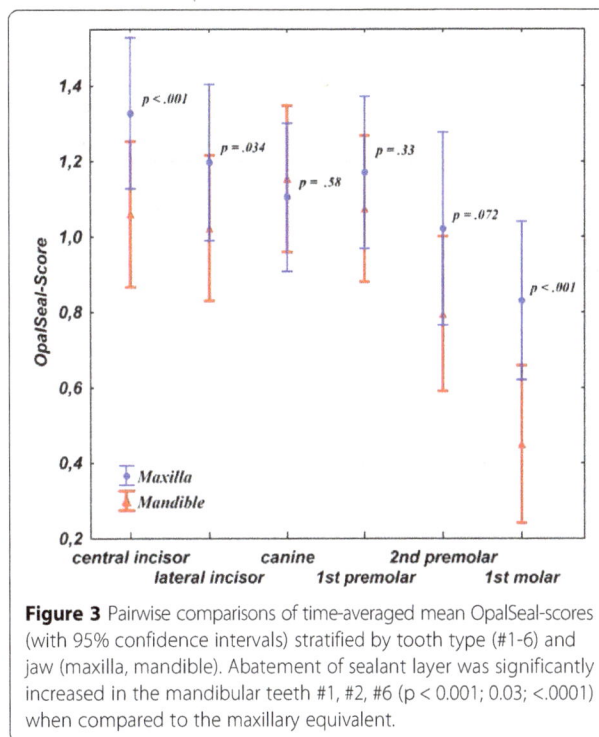

Figure 3 Pairwise comparisons of time-averaged mean OpalSeal-scores (with 95% confidence intervals) stratified by tooth type (#1-6) and jaw (maxilla, mandible). Abatement of sealant layer was significantly increased in the mandibular teeth #1, #2, #6 ($p < 0.001$; 0.03; <.0001) when compared to the maxillary equivalent.

necessary to achieve sealant retention after months in treatment: It is a fact that additional, surplus etching of enamel surfaces not covered by bracket bases may trigger WSL formation itself [15]. The data presented here add some evidence to the unanswered questions of recommended time intervals for a renewal of the sealant, and, second, the unclear role of individual intensities of oral hygiene and mechanical tooth brushing abrasion on sealant durability: The null-hypothesis (1) of no significant global abatement of the sealant after 26 weeks in treatment was rejected, while the null hypothesis (2) was accepted, as we did not find a significant global effect of the factor of oral hygiene on the abatement of the sealant. Nonetheless, there was an increase in the abatement of the sealant from front teeth 1–4 to posterior teeth #5 or #6, which is significant (Table 1) and was found to be more rapid in well brushed lower posterior teeth (teeth #5 and #6 with negative API; Figure 2a). One possible interpretation might be that sealant layers may be literally wiped off by tooth brushing, and it may be concluded that sealants offer a slightly better protection of those teeth that are not sufficiently brushed. Another possible explanation would be that this abatement in mandibular posterior teeth may also be attributed to enhanced attrition by chewing activities. This would explain reductions of varnish layers in the upper enamel third of lower first molars and premolars, as those areas are more exposed to daily mechanical wear during consumption of food.

Mean sealant scores indicate that in both the well brushed and non-brushed teeth anterior teeth undercut the score "1" (less than 50% sealer left) at T3 (week 14), while there seems overall a slightly better preservation of the sealer before and after T3 in positive API-teeth, especially in the case of second premolars (Figure 3c).

However, globally, these slightly better results are not significantly improved compared to the non-brushed teeth (Table 2). Re-application can therefore be expected to be necessary from week 14 in the average case treated with orthodontic fixed appliances. This result is in agreement with Tüfekçi et al. who reported a preservation of 50% of the same sealant following ninety days [7].

Sealant re-application: Time intervals and mode

According to the manufacturer, re-application of OpalSeal implies prior etching for 15-30s, and subsequent light-curing for 10 s. Previous research hints at a potential iatrogenic triggering of WSL especially in those cases with surplus orthodontic etching prior to bracket bonding, especially when those areas are subsequently neither covered by bracket bases nor by bonding material [15]: This has been shown to have a significant deteriorating effect on WSL formation. Subsequent covering of those etched areas by a sealant prevents WSL formation, however, the results of the current study show that the sealant abates on average in about 3.5 months, and it is unclear whether there is an increased susceptibility to WSL after disappearance of the sealant. According to previous reports, teeth are especially susceptible to decalcification during the first six months in fixed appliances orthodontic treatment [4]. If this was due to some type of intra-oral customization to the fixed orthodontic appliances, simple re-application of sealants without repeating the step of etching may also be viable.

Advantages and drawbacks of the study design

Integrity and condition of the OpalSeal layers was assessed chair-side by a clinician who was blinded to the patient's trial time schedule, while notes were made by a study nurse, similar to previous studies on the topic of WSL formation in orthodontic patients [4]. The assessment of photos would not have been feasible here, as every single tooth would have to be photographed while being illuminated by the black-light lamp. However, as an advantage, the trial sample size and numbers of performed assessments are remarkable.

To the best of our knowledge, this is the first in-vivo trial with a screening of the integrity and durability of a sealant at different time points with a consideration of oral hygiene as a co-factor. While in-vivo research offers a more realistic picture of the study subject, standardization is more difficult to achieve in comparison to using an in-vitro setup, where standardization is easy, but applicability and generalisability of results are rather poor. This study has a limitation in that there was no standardization of the brushing regimes other than providing standardized brushing instructions and handing out identical tooth brushes. There was no left-/right handed distinction. Also, oral hygiene was screened before placement of brackets,

and then again 14 days following incorporation of brackets. That is, subjects were allocated to the groups of adequate or inadequate oral hygiene based on these two assessments, not considering potential improvement or deterioration afterwards.

The results of this study provide some evidence on the abatement characteristics of the longevity of a typical sealant used in orthodontics, and they indicate that a renewal of the OpalSeal layer after an average elapse of 3.5 months may be beneficial or necessary for an enduring suppression of WSL formation and frequencies. Previous studies on WSL formation following sealant application may be revisited in terms of fixed appliances orthodontic treatment duration versus presence or absence of sealant re-application. However, in this trial on the effects of time elapse and oral hygiene measures on sealant abatement, there was no assessment of WSL formation, but of sealant preservation only. That is, no conclusion can be drawn on the basis of our data that renewal of sealants after 3.5 months does indeed result in a further reduction of WSL numbers: It may also be conceivable that sealing of the enamel surfaces during the first months in fixed appliances orthodontic treatment may suffice, as it has been reported that teeth are especially susceptible to white-spot formation during this time period. Also, the interaction of sealant renewal with potentially necessary additional etching intervals needs to be considered.

Future research

Further research is required on the subject of the mode of OpalSeal re-application (with or without additional etching) in terms of (1) reduction of frequencies of WSL, and (2) durability and abatement of sealants re-applied the one way, or the other: As it is known that excessive phosphoric-acid etching of enamel as required prior to sealant application may trigger WSL formation itself [15], it is e.g. not clear whether enamel surfaces should be etched again prior to re-application, or if OpalSeal application renewal should be performed without a second etching interval, or not at all.

Conclusions

The following conclusions can be drawn from the study presented here:

- Diligent screening of sealant preservation in patients treated with fixed orthodontic appliances is a necessity.
- One single sealant application is unlikely to last throughout the entire stage of orthodontic treatment with fixed appliances.
- On average, re-application of OpalSeal can be expected to be necessary after 3.5 months (week 14) in treatment. Further clinical trials should address

the question if a re-application of sealants would be beneficial in terms of reducing frequencies of WSL.

- As etching of enamel surfaces is known to potentially trigger WSL formation, future research should also clarify if re-application of sealants should include an additional etching interval for an improvement of sealant durability, or not.

Competing interests
All authors declare that they have no competing interests.

Authors' contributions
All authors contributed extensively to the work presented in this paper. MK provided the idea for the project, was responsible for the study design, treated the patients orthodontically, carried out the measurements with YG, interpreted the data together with DE, implemented the literature search, and wrote the manuscript. YG collected the data, and compiled all medical records. DE carried out the statistical analyses. PS and DW reviewed the paper, and contributed to the writing. All authors approved the manuscript prior to submission.

Acknowledgement
We thank Dr. J. Raiman (Hannover, Germany) for the permission to conduct this study in his orthodontic practice and to release these data, and also C. Jerchel for her help in organizing the data.

Author details
[1]Department of Orthodontics, University Medical Center Göttingen (UMG), 37099 Göttingen, Germany. [2]Department of Medical Statistics, University Medical Center Göttingen (UMG), 37099 Göttingen, Germany. [3]Private Practice, Hannover, Germany. [4]Department of Orthodontics, Universidad de la Frontera (UFRO), Temuco, Chile. [5]Orthodontic Practice, Lindenstrasse 44, 49152 Bad, Essen, Germany. [6]Department of Orthodontics, Hannover Medical School (MHH), 30625 Hannover, Germany.

References
1. Øgaard B, Rolla G, Arends J. Orthodontic appliances and enamel demineralization. Part 1. Lesion development. Am J Orthod Dentofacial Orthop. 1988;94:68–73.
2. Melrose CA, Appleton J, Lovius BB. A scanning electron microscopic study of early enamel caries formed in vivo beneath orthodontic bands. Br J Orthod. 1996;23:43–7.
3. Richter AE, Arruda AO, Peters MC, Sohn W. Incidence of caries lesions among patients treated with comprehensive orthodontics. Am J Orthod Dentofacial Orthop. 2011;139:657–64.
4. Tüfekçi E, Dixon JS, Gunsolley JC, Lindauer SJ. Prevalence of white spot lesions during orthodontic treatment with fixed appliances. Angle Orthod. 2011;81:206–10.
5. Geiger AM, Gorelick L, Gwinnett AJ, Benson BJ. Reducing white spot lesions in orthodontic populations with fluoride rinsing. Am J Orthod Dentofacial Orthop. 1992;101:403–7.
6. Benson PE, Parkin N, Dyer F, Millett DT, Furness S, Germain P. Fluorides for the prevention of early tooth decay (demineralised white lesions) during fixed brace treatment. Cochrane Database Syst Rev. 2013;12, CD003809.
7. Tüfekçi E, Pennella DR, Mitchell JC, Best AM, Lindauer SJ. Efficacy of a fluoride-releasing orthodontic primer in reducing demineralization around brackets: an in-vivo study. Am J Orthod Dentofacial Orthop. 2014;146:207–14.
8. Lange DE, Plagmann HC, Eenboom A, Promesberger A. Klinische Bewertungsverfahren zur Objektivierung der Mundhygiene [Clinical methods for the objective evaluation of oral hygiene]. Dtsch Zahnarztl Z. 1977;32:44–7.
9. Splieth CH, Treuner A, Gedrange T, Berndt C. Caries-preventive and remineralizing effect of fluoride gel in orthodontic patients after 2 years. Clin Oral Investig. 2012;16:1395–9.
10. Årtun J, Bergland S. Clinical trials with crystal growth conditioning as an alternative to acid-etch enamel pretreatment. Am J Orthod. 1984;85:333–40.
11. Hu W, Featherstone JDB. Prevention of enamel demineralization: an in-vitro study using light-cured filled sealant. Am J Orthod Dentofacial Orthop. 2005;128:592–600.
12. O'Reilly MT, De Jesús VJ, Hatch JP. Effectiveness of a sealant compared with no sealant in preventing enamel demineralization in patients with fixed orthodontic appliances: a prospective clinical trial. Am J Orthod Dentofacial Orthop. 2013;143:837–44.
13. Todd MA, Staley RN, Kanellis MJ, Donly KJ, Wefel JS. Effect of fluoride varnish on demineralization adjacent to orthodontic brackets. Am J Orthod Dentofacial Orthop. 1999;116:159–67.
14. Farhadian N, Miresmaeili A, Eslami B, Mehrabi S. Effect of fluoride varnish on enamel demineralization around brackets: an in-vivo study. Am J Orthod Dentofacial Orthop. 2008;133(4 Suppl):S95–8.
15. Knösel M, Bojes M, Jung K, Ziebolz D. Increased susceptibility for white spot lesions by surplus orthodontic etching exceeding bracket base area. Am J Orthod Dentofacial Orthop. 2012;141:574–82.

6

The relationship between the cranial base and jaw base in a Chinese population

Alice Chin[1†], Suzanne Perry[2†], Chongshan Liao[2] and Yanqi Yang[2*]

Abstract

Introduction: The cranial base plays an important role in determining how the mandible and maxilla relate to each other. This study assessed the relationship between the cranial base and jaw base in a Chinese population.

Methods: This study involved 83 subjects (male: 27; female: 56; age: 18.4 ± 4.2 SD years) from Hong Kong, who were classified into 3 sagittal discrepancy groups on the basis of their ANB angle. A cephalometric analysis of the angular and linear measurements of their cranial and jaw bases was carried out. The morphological characteristics of the cranial and jaw bases in the three groups were compared and assessments were made as to whether a relationship existed between the cranial base and the jaw base discrepancy.

Results: Significant differences were found in the cranial base angles of the three groups. Skeletal Class II cases presented with a larger NSBa, whereas skeletal Class III cases presented with a smaller NSBa ($P < 0.001$). In the linear measurement, skeletal Class III cases presented with a shorter NBa than skeletal Class I and II cases ($P < 0.01$). There was a correlation between the cranial base angle NSBa and the SNB for the whole sample, ($r = -0.523$, $P < 0.001$). Furthermore, correlations between SBaFH and Wits ($r = -0.594$, $P < 0.001$) and SBaFH and maxillary length ($r = -0.616$, $P < 0.001$) were more obvious in the skeletal Class III cases.

Conclusions: The cranial base appears to have a certain correlation with the jaw base relationship in a southern Chinese population. The correlation between cranial base and jaw base tends to be closer in skeletal Class III cases.

Keywords: Cranial base, Jaw base, Chinese

Introduction

The cranial base separates the delicate tissues of the brain from the rest of the face and has a major influence on growth. The main postnatal growth site is the spheno-occipital synchondrosis, which lengthens the base of the skull. The positioning of the maxilla anterior to the synchondrosis and the mandible, which articulates posteriorly, gives the synchondrosis the potential to be a factor in facial disharmony and consequently malocclusion. The synchondrosis influences growth in the region until shortly after puberty, when it fuses. Growth at the spheno-occipital synchondrosis increases the length of the cranial base, and as the maxillary complex lies beneath the anterior cranial fossa and the mandible articulates with the skull at the temporomandibular joint, which lies beneath the middle cranial fossa, the cranial base plays an important part in determining how the mandible and maxilla relate to each other. The cranial base can be split into two parts, the anterior and the posterior; the anterior is measured from the foramen caecum to the sella turcica (S) and the posterior from the sella turcica to the basion (Ba). The growth of the cranial base in very early years follows a neural pattern, with the most rapid rate of growth in the first 3 years [1]. As a result, variations in the cranial base angle and the anterior and posterior lengths can potentially be a cause of imbalances in facial growth, and consequently occlusion.

Moss' functional matrix theory believes that environmental demands mold the pattern of growth of the genetically predetermined facial bones to result in a final outcome [2]. Van Limborgh's Compromise Theory accepts functional matrix theory of Moss but also supports some aspects of Sutural theory of Sicher and acknowledges genetic involvement [3]. The growth of the cranial base appears to be more genetically controlled than environmentally

* Correspondence: yangyang@hku.hk
†Equal contributors
²Faculty of Dentistry, University of Hong Kong, Hong Kong SAR, China
Full list of author information is available at the end of the article

affected and it is the cranial base synchondroses that are the major growth centers of the cranial base [4]. Genetics appear to play such a big role in facial growth that genetic influence is more apparent in some malocclusions than others, as can be seen in skeletal Class III cases [5]. So how much influence does the cranial base have on the jaw relationship?

Some studies have linked a reduction in cranial base angle, that is a more acute angle, to a more relatively anterior articulation of the eminence of the mandible with the glenoid fossa, which is more likely to lead to a Class III type malocclusion [6]; however, a more obtuse cranial base angle may be a causative factor in a Class II situation [7-9]. Anderson and Popovich, in a serial sample of data from the Burlington Growth Centre, and others, have observed an increasing cranial base angle spanning Class III to Class I to Class II malocclusions [10-14]. However, some debate has arisen due to conflicting results from other studies, and the matter remains inconclusive. An interesting study by Rothstein and Phan looked at 335 boys and girls between 10 and 14 with Class II Division 1 malocclusions and compared them cephalometrically to controls; they found no correlation between cranial base angle and sagittal jaw relationship between the two groups [15]. A similar study by Wilhelm et al. comparing Class I subjects to Class II subjects found no relationship between the cranial base angle and the skeletal growth pattern [16]. Dhopatkhar et al. were also unable to find any influence of the cranial base angle in four types of malocclusion [17].

Given these inconclusive findings, we would like to raise one other issue—racial differences. Scientific awareness of variations in racial cranial morphology has existed since the mid-1700's, when the German scientist Johan F. Blumenbach described the different features of skulls from five world regions. He commented on the different characteristics of skulls and hypothesized that the variations were due to factors such as diet, geographical location, and even specific mannerisms [18]. Other studies have also noted variations in cranial base angles in different races and notable differences in general craniofacial forms between races [19,20]. Furthermore, the prevalence of intermaxillary jaw discrepancy also varies between races. Angle first described such jaw relationships in 1890. Using the molar relationship, he classified malocclusion in his sample of Caucasians; he found that 69% had a normal or Class I occlusion, 24% had a Class II and around 3% had a Class III malocclusion (other 4% were unclassified due to teeth missing) [21]. As the majority of studies have been carried out in Caucasian populations, it is unclear how much influence the cranial base has on the jaw base relationship in a Chinese population. The importance of acquiring data relevant to a particular subgroup cannot be underestimated. To avoid the heterology of China, we focus on a southern Chinese population. The aims of this investigation are to assess if there is any evidence that the cranial base angle predisposes the jaw base relationship in a southern Chinese population, and to gain data specific to a southern Chinese population with particular reference to the angular and linear cranial base morphology.

Materials and methods

Samples

The samples for this retrospective study which was ethically approved were obtained from patients attending the orthodontic clinic at the Faculty of Dentistry, the University of Hong Kong during the period of 2012–2013 in a consecutive series. Their consent to use their clinical records for research purposes was obtained. All of the subjects were Hong Kong residents, of southern Chinese origin, and healthy with no evidence or history of medical complications, craniofacial malformation, or syndromes. Any subject with a previous history of orthodontic treatment was excluded from the study. Subjects with severe crowding were also excluded.

Based on a pilot study that we conducted, variance within groups (skeletal Classes I, II, and III) in cranial base angle (NSBa) was 4.9 degrees. Each group required 26 patients to yield a 95% power for identifying a significant difference in a one-way ANOVA at a 5% level of significance (alpha = 0.05). The power analysis was undertaken by G*Power 3.1.7 (a program developed by Axel Buchner, Edgar Erdfelder, and Franz Faul; http://www.psycho.uni-duesseldorf.de/abteilungen/aap/gpower3).

The final sample was comprised of 83 patients (male: 27; female: 56; age: 18.4 ± 4.2 SD years).

Cephalometric analysis

Lateral cephalometric radiographs were taken in centric relation as part of a routine orthodontic diagnostic process using a GE1000 (General Electric, Milwaukee, Wisconsin) machine with subjects in a natural head posture position. It was estimated that the magnification for a mid-sagittal structure would be close to the value of 8.8%. Subjects were then allocated into three defined groups of Class I, Class II, and Class III on the basis of their ANB angulations with the Chinese norm as the reference [22]. The criteria for the three classes were as follows:

skeletal class I, ANB angle of 0.6°- 5° with a favorable overjet and overbite;

skeletal class II, ANB angle of ≥5° with an increased overjet; and

skeletal class III, ANB angle of < 0.6° with a reduced overjet.

The radiographs were first traced by hand in a darkened room by a trained and calibrated orthodontist and then digitized (CASSOS 2001, Soft Enable Technology Limited, Hong Kong). The average value was taken of any double features not present on the mid-sagittal plane. A cephalometric analysis of the cranial base including angular measurements (NSBa and SBaFH) and linear measurements (SN, SBa, NBa, Wits) was carried out [23]. Jaw base length and relationship was assessed in the sagittal and vertical dimensions. The cephalometric variables analyzed in this study are shown in Figure 1.

Statistical analysis

For each of the three morphological subtypes, the means and standard deviations were calculated for each cephalometric variable in each group. A One-way Analysis of Variance (ANOVA) was carried out to compare the characteristics of cranial bases and jaw bases between the three groups. A Pearson Correlation Coefficient was calculated between each cephalometric variable with particular emphasis on the relationships between the cranial base angle and the sagittal jaw discrepancy markers for the whole sample and the three groups. Significance for the tests was noted at three levels, $P < 0.05$ (*), $P < 0.01$ (**), and $P < 0.001$ (***). The correlation was regarded as meaningful when $r > =0.5$ in addition to the significance revealed by $P < 0.05$, whereas the correlation was regarded as weak when $r < 0.5$, even if there was some statistical significance ($P < 0.05$). All of the statistical analyses were performed using Statistical Package for Social

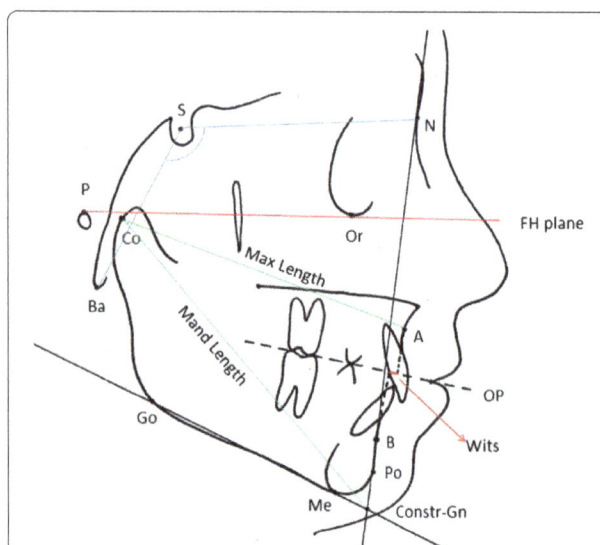

Figure 1 The cephalometric landmarks used in this study.
Reference point: cranial base: N (Nasion), S (Sella), P (Porion), Ba (Basion), Or (Orbitale); jaw base: Co (Condylion), Go (Gonion), Me (Menton), A (Supramentale), B (Supramentale), Po (Pogonion). Reference plane: FH (Frankfort plane), OP (Occlusal plane), Go-Me (Mandibular plane).

Sciences software package (SPSS for Windows, Version 10.0, Chicago, IL, USA).

Results

Cephalometric profile of the cranial base and jaw base of a southern Chinese sample

There were 27 subjects in the Class I group (18.1 ± 3.3 years old), 30 in the Class II group (19.1 ± 5.6 years old), and 26 in the Class III group (18 ± 3.2 years old). No significant difference was shown in the ages of the three groups ($P > 0.05$).

The cephalometric values for the whole sample and for each subgroup are presented in Table 1. For the cranial base, the angular measurement showed that there was a significant difference in the NSBa angle between the three groups ($P < 0.001$): the Class II group had a larger cranial base angle (NSBa) (131.9 ± 5.2), whereas the Class III cases had a smaller NSBa (127.0 ± 3.7). In the linear measurement, the Class III cases had a shorter NBa (105.0 ± 5.4) than the Class I (108.4 ± 5.8) and Class II cases (109.7 ± 4.0), ($P < 0.01$). For the jaw base relationship, the differences in the sagittal discrepancies among the three groups can be seen by the variation in SNB, ANB, Wits, maxillary length, and the mandibular length, all of which showed significance at $P < 0.001$. Vertically, the Class III cases had a lower maxillary-mandibular plane angle (MMPA) (24.1 ± 2.4) compared to the Class I (27.0 ± 2.3) ($P < 0.001$) and Class II cases (26.4 ± 2.4) ($P < 0.01$).

Correlation between the cranial base measurements

The two angular variables NSBa and SBaFH, which were based on different reference planes, showed significant correlation in the whole sample ($r = -0.706$; $P < 0.001$) (Table 2). The correlation between the angular measurement (i.e., NSBa) and linear measurement (i.e., SBa) existed in skeletal Class I cases ($r = -0.628$, $P < 0.001$), but not in Class II and III cases. Among the linear variables, it was found that NBa was correlated with both SBa ($r = 0.764$, $P < 0.001$) and SN ($r = 0.743$, $P < 0.01$), but SBa and SN did not have a strong correlation ($r = 0.461$, $P < 0.001$).

Correlation between the cranial base and jaw base

The analysis of the cranial base angle for the whole sample showed a noticeable correlation in the sagittal jaw base between NSBa and SNB ($r = 0.523$, $P < 0.001$), indicating that the SNB angle decreases as the cranial base angle increases (Table 3). The correlation of NSBa with ANB and Wits were weak ($r < 0.5$, $P < 0.01$), so were the correlation of SBaFH with Wits and maxillary length ($r < 0.5$, $P < 0.001$) for the whole sample. However, SBaFH had a stronger correlation with Wits ($r = -0.594$, $P < 0.001$) and maxillary length ($r = -0.616$, $P < 0.001$) for skeletal Class III cases.

Table 1 Cephalometric profile of the cranial base and jaw base in a Southern Chinese sample

			Class I (n=27)		Class II (n=30)		Class III (n=26)		Total (n=83)		P value (ANOVA)	
			Mean	SD	Mean	SD	Mean	SD	Mean	SD		
Cranial base	Angular measurements (°)	NSBa	130.0	4.4	131.9	5.2	127.0	3.7	130.0	4.9	0.001	***
		SBaFH	58.7	4.6	57.1	4.1	59.2	3.3	58.2	4.1	0.125	ns
	Linear measurements (mm)	SN	70.1	4.4	70.4	2.8	68.7	3.3	69.8	3.6	0.177	ns
		SBa	49.5	4.4	49.9	3.4	48.2	3.3	49.3	3.8	0.216	ns
		NBa	108.4	5.8	109.7	4.0	105.0	5.4	107.8	5.4	0.003	**
Jaw base	Angular measurements (°)	SNA	81.1	3.0	82.1	3.1	82.1	3.9	81.8	3.3	0.474	ns
		SNB	78.3	3.1	75.9	3.0	84.3	5.2	79.3	5.2	0.000	***
		ANB	2.8	1.2	6.2	1.3	-2.4	3.0	2.4	4.0	0.000	***
		MMPA	27.0	2.3	26.4	2.4	24.1	2.4	25.9	2.6	0.000	***
	Linear measurement (mm)	Wits	-3.5	3.5	1.6	2.6	-7.6	8.3	-2.9	6.4	0.000	***
		Max length	87.9	4.6	89.7	3.8	85.6	4.1	87.8	4.5	0.002	**
		M and length	122.0	7.1	117.4	7.0	126.4	9.0	121.7	8.4	0.000	***

*P < 0.05; **P < 0.01; ***P < 0.001; ns (no significance): P > 0.05.

For the cranial base length to jaw base relationship (Table 4), none of the linear variables of the cranial base correlated strongly with the sagittal jaw base relationship except for a negative correlation between NBa and SNA in skeletal Class III cases (r = −0.592, P < 0.001). NBa had the same correlated tendency to SNB (r = −0.486, P < 0.05), but not to ANB (P > 0.05) in skeletal Class III cases.

There was no correlation between any angular or linear measurement of the cranial base and MMPA, which defines the vertical skeletal pattern (P > 0.05) (Table 5).

In the relationship between cranial base length and jaw base length (Table 6), NBa was related to maxillary length in the whole sample (r = 0.665, P < 0.01), but not related to mandibular length in the Class III subgroup (P > 0.05), which means that the shorter NBa is, the shorter the maxillary length is; however, there was no influence on

mandibular length in the Class III cases. Similarly, SN was found to be correlated with maxillary length for the whole sample (r = 0.594, P < 0.001), but not mandibular length (P > 0.05). SBa showed low correlation with both maxillary length (r = 0.455, P < 0.001) and mandibular length (r = 0.261, P < 0.05) in the whole sample.

Discussion

Cranial base in relation to jaw base angle

In the choice of cranial base landmarks, debate has arisen over the use of the Articulare instead of the Basion (Ba)

Table 2 Correlation (r) between the cranial base measurements in a Southern Chinese sample

	Class I (n=27)	Class II (n=30)	Class III (n=26)	Total (n=83)
NSBa-SBaFH	**-0.692***	**-0.898***	-0.332 (ns)	**-0.706***
NSBa-NBa	-0.335 (ns)	0.209 (ns)	0.457*	0.211 (ns)
NSBa-SBa	**-0.628***	-0.216 (ns)	0.036 (ns)	-0.200 (ns)
NSBa-SN	-0.239 (ns)	-0.177 (ns)	0.248 (ns)	-0.001 (ns)
SBaFH-NBa	0.167 (ns)	-0.297 (ns)	-0.318 (ns)	-0.162 (ns)
SBaFH-SBa	0.290 (ns)	0.119 (ns)	-0.053 (ns)	0.111 (ns)
SBaFH-SN	0.039 (ns)	0.024 (ns)	-0.293 (ns)	-0.081 (ns)
NBa-SBa	**0.811***	**0.707***	**0.754***	**0.764***
NBa-SN	**0.728***	**0.595***	**0.851***	**0.743****
SBa-SN	**0.543***	0.240 (ns)	0.455*	**0.461***

*P < 0.05; **P < 0.01; ***P < 0.001; ns (no significance): P > 0.05.
Bolded: r > 0.5.

Table 3 Correlation (r) between the cranial base angle and jaw base in a Southern Chinese sample

	Class I (n=27)	Class II (n=30)	Class III (n=26)	Total (n=83)
NSBa-SNA	-0.423*	-0.449*	-0.372 (ns)	-0.372***
NSBa-SNB	-0.489**	-0.420*	-0.312 (ns)	**-0.523***
NSBa-ANB	0.219 (ns)	-0.100 (ns)	0.110 (ns)	0.384***
NSBa-wits	0.238 (ns)	0.031 (ns)	0.006 (ns)	0.280**
NSBa-MMPA	0.160 (ns)	-0.116 (ns)	-0.210 (ns)	0.110 (ns)
NSBa-Max length	-0.235 (ns)	0.001 (ns)	0.349 (ns)	0.161 (ns)
NSBa-Mand length	-0.447*	-0.097 (ns)	0.056 (ns)	-0.362***
SBaFH-SNA	0.116 (ns)	0.276 (ns)	-0.169 (ns)	0.071 (ns)
SBaFH-SNB	0.172 (ns)	0.226 (ns)	-0.236 (ns)	0.159 (ns)
SBaFH-ANB	-0.209 (ns)	0.136 (ns)	0.136 (ns)	-0.164 (ns)
SBaFH-wits	-0.249 (ns)	0.010 (ns)	**-0.594***	-0.363***
SBaFH-MMPA	0.005 (ns)	-0.009 (ns)	0.240 (ns)	-0.002 (ns)
SBaFH-Max length	-0.063 (ns)	-0.063 (ns)	**-0.616***	-0.262*
SBaFH-Mand length	0.142 (ns)	0.222 (ns)	-0.420*	0.093 (ns)

*P < 0.05; **P < 0.01; ***P < 0.001; ns (no significance): P > 0.05.
Bolded: r >0.5.

Table 4 Correlation (r) between the cranial base length and jaw base relationship in a Southern Chinese sample

	Class I (n=27)	Class II (n=30)	Class III (n=26)	Total (n=83)
NBa-SNA	0.007 (ns)	-0.040 (ns)	**-0.592*****	-0.231*
NBa-SNB	-0.016 (ns)	0.029 (ns)	-0.486*	-0.400***
NBa-ANB	0.063 (ns)	-0.168 (ns)	0.133 (ns)	0.345***
NBa-wits	0.213 (ns)	0.092 (ns)	0.317 (ns)	0.379***
SBa-SNA	0.259 (ns)	0.203 (ns)	-0.476*	-0.006 (ns)
SBa-SNB	0.320 (ns)	0.208 (ns)	-0.296 (ns)	-0.101 (ns)
SBa-ANB	-0.174 (ns)	-0.007 (ns)	-0.088 (ns)	0.132 (ns)
SBa-wits	0.169 (ns)	0.168 (ns)	0.239 (ns)	0.245*
SN-SNA	-0.163 (ns)	-0.044 (ns)	-0.443*	-0.222*
SN-SNB	-0.204 (ns)	-0.020 (ns)	-0.448*	-0.317**
SN-ANB	0.161 (ns)	-0.056 (ns)	0.267 (ns)	0.247*
SN-wits	0.294 (ns)	0.105 (ns)	0.285 (ns)	0.290**

*P < 0.05; **P < 0.01; ***P < 0.001; ns (no significance): P > 0.05.
Bolded: r > 0.5.

[24], suggesting that it is easier to identify. However, it can be argued that the Ba is closer to the cranial base and is more likely to be valid. Previous studies have shown that the correlation between the two points is high and the choice between them is unlikely to affect a study's results [25]. Therefore, based on the previous research [26], the Ba was chosen as the landmark point in this study. Previous studies have noted a possible improvement in validity using the Frankfurt (FH) plane in the measurements of the cranial base—they suggest that FH plane has less variation due to a balance in bone remodeling [27]. SBaFH is another variable that measures the cranial base angle using FH as the reference line. Hence, using SBaFH to assess the cranial base angle may reinforce the potential validity of the results.

We found an inverse correlation between the cranial base angle NSBa and the jaw base variable SNB (r = -0.523, P < 0.001) (Table 3), that is, an increased NSBa was accompanied by a reduced SNB, leading to a more Class II profile, and vice versa. This result would seem logical, as the mandible would be positioned more

Table 5 Correlation (r) between the cranial base and the MMPA in a Southern Chinese sample

	Class I (n=27)	Class II (n=30)	Class III (n=26)	Total (n=83)
NSBa-MMPA	0.160 (ns)	-0.116 (ns)	-0.210 (ns)	0.110 (ns)
SBaFH-MMPA	0.005 (ns)	-0.009 (ns)	0.240 (ns)	-0.002 (ns)
NBa-MMPA	0.057 (ns)	-0.204 (ns)	-0.258 (ns)	0.050 (ns)
SBa-MMPA	-0.093 (ns)	0.007 (ns)	-0.368 (ns)	-0.037 (ns)
SN-MMPA	0.005 (ns)	-0.085 (ns)	-0.033 (ns)	0.059 (ns)

ns (no significance): P > 0.05.

Table 6 Correlation (r) between the cranial base length and jaw length in a Southern Chinese sample

	Class I (n=27)	Class II (n=30)	Class III (n=26)	Total (n=83)
NBa-Max length	**0.685*****	**0.574*****	**0.560****	**0.665****
NBa-Mand length	**0.581*****	0.394*	0.243 (ns)	0.173 (ns)
SBa-Max length	**0.667*****	0.218 (ns)	0.264 (ns)	0.455***
SBa-Mand length	**0.703*****	0.267 (ns)	0.183 (ns)	0.261*
SN-Max length	**0.637*****	0.463**	**0.580****	**0.594*****
SN-Mand length	0.366 (ns)	0.320 (ns)	0.193 (ns)	0.165 (ns)

*P < 0.05; **P < 0.01; ***P < 0.001; ns (no significance): P > 0.05.
Bolded: r > 0.5.

posteriorly on the posterior cranial base leg, coinciding with previous studies [10-14,26]. However, this result was not repeated when the correlation of SBaFH to SNB was analyzed, nor to ANB (Table 3). These results perhaps are due to both NSBa and SNB share the same reference plane SN; but for SNB (with SN as the reference plane) and SBaFH (with FH as the reference plane), the individual variation of the SN-FH angle must be an interference factor.

For the interaction between the SBaFH angle and the linear variables (Table 3), it is helpful to use Wits analysis. The correlation between SBaFH and Wits was shown to be weak in the whole sample (r = -0.363, P < 0.001), but stronger in the skeletal Class III group (r = 0.594, P < 0.001). Similarly, the correlation between SBaFH and maxillary length was also stronger in skeletal Class III cases (r = -0.616, P < 0.001). The negative correlation of SBaFH to Wits and maxillary length indicated that a higher SBaFH was related to a lower Wits and maxillary length, which indicates that the correlation between cranial base and jaw base is closer in skeletal Class III cases than in the other malocclusions. Here we would like to clarify that SBaFH is an acute angle and an increase in SBaFH represented a reduced NSBa, which coincided with a significant correlation between NSBa and SBaFH (r = -0.706, P < 0.001) (Table 2). Hence, these results coincided with the results of NSBa and SNB.

The relationship between the cranial base and the maxilla was first noted by Jarvinen who published the link between SNA and the cranial base: an increased cranial base angle would lead to a smaller SNA [28], and this link was later explained with a detailed statistical analysis [13]. Further studies have shown that the correlation between the two values was probably high due to topographical factors, most likely the rotation of the SN plane [12,17]; thus the SN value was deemed an unreliable indicator. As a result, it has been suggested that the position of the maxilla is likely to be determined more by genetic or epigenetic factors rather than directly by the cranial base [29]. In our study, we did not find any correlation between SBaFH and SNA (P > 0.05) and only a weak correlation between NSBa and SNA (r = -0.372, P < 0.001) (Table 3). The linear variable NBa had a stronger correlation with SNA (r = -0.592, P < 0.001) in skeletal Class III samples (Table 4), possibly because both of the parameters share the same reference point N, which may lead to a closer correlation regardless of the individually varied positions of point N. However, the weak correlation between NBa and SNB (r = -0.486, P < 0.05) made the correlation between NBa and ANB insignificant (P > 0.05). Therefore, there is no obvious evidence supporting the relationship between cranial base and maxillary position.

Vertical discrepancies can affect the sagittal position due to a downward and backward rotation of the mandible. In this study, Class III cases had lower MMPA than Class I and Class II cases (Table 1), which confirmed the correlation in the sagittal and vertical dimensions. Jarvinen looked at the cranial base angle in relation to the vertical facial pattern, and found the low angle group had a larger cranial base angle, and the high angle group had a shorter cranial base [13]. This conflicts with the results of this study, specifically, that Class II cases had a higher MMPA than Class III cases (but not Class I cases) and a larger NSBa, whereas Class III cases had a lower MMPA and a smaller NSBa (Table 1). Furthermore, in this study, we did not find any significant correlation between any angular or linear measurements of the cranial base and MMPA (Table 5). Therefore, we are unable conclude that there is a correlation between the cranial base and the vertical skeletal pattern.

Cranial base in relation to jaw base length
The skeletal discrepancy can be caused by an abnormal jaw position or insufficient/overgrowth of the jaws, leading to an abnormal maxillary and/or mandibular length. In this study, the maxillary length was taken from the Condylion to Point A and the mandibular length was defined from the Condylion to the constructed Gnathion. The correlation between NSBa and mandibular length was extremely weak (r = -0.362, P < 0.001), but the correlation between SBaFH and maxillary length was stronger in skeletal Class III cases (r = -0.616, P < 0.001) (Table 3). Again, this supported the suggestion that an increased SBaFH (as with a decreased NSBa) was related to a reduced maxillary length, i.e., a Class III problem, which also supported the closer correlation between cranial base and jaw base in skeletal Class III cases.

The correlation between cranial base length and jaw length was also assessed. Geometrically, the length of the posterior cranial base in particular has a significant role to play in the sagittal presentations. Previous studies have suggested that a longer posterior cranial base can exacerbate a sagittal Class II situation and a shorter base

may increase the chance of a Class III relationship [6,7,27,30]. In contrast, other studies have not been able to confirm such findings regarding cranial base length, but still report some significance differences in angle [14]. In this study, the posterior cranial base length SBa was only found to be correlated to maxillary length and mandibular length in skeletal Class I cases, not in Class II or Class III cases (Table 6). This correlation to both maxillary and mandibular length showed the same change tendency (positive correlation) for skeletal Class I. The cranial base length NBa was strongly correlated to both maxillary and mandibular length in skeletal Class I cases, but only related to maxillary length in skeletal Class III cases. This suggested that the shorter the cranial base, the shorter the maxillary length, i.e., a Class III problem. These results further proved that the correlation between cranial base and jaw base was more obvious in skeletal Class III cases. The importance of considering the cranial base was also shown in a study by Andria et al. which suggested a shorter posterior cranial base in Class II patients may lead to an increased treatment time [27]. Combined with a more obtuse cranial base angle, a shorter posterior cranial base would lead to a higher level placement of the condyle and glenoid fossa, potentially leading to increased MMPA and a greater vertical component to mandibular growth.

Factors of age and gender
To hypothesize future changes from current patterns, and so produce effective and successful clinical results, it is important to have a good understanding of a process. The growth of the cranial base in the very early years follows a neural pattern, with the most rapid rate of growth in the first 3 years [1]. The cranial base angle is reasonably stable after the age of five [10,31]. Changes in angular and linear parameters during the observation period occurred mostly between the ages of 10 and 12 years [32]. The synchondrosis influences growth in the region until shortly after puberty when it fuses [4]. After puberty, the angle appears to remain stable [33]. In this study, we chose a sample comprised of young adults (mean age: 18.4 years old) to exclude the interference from unknown growth.

The pilot study revealed a similar correlation tendency among the cephalometric variables in males and females. Therefore, in this study, we analyzed the data for males and females together.

Racial differences
Craniofacial variation between different races has been well documented, with Africans typically having a more dolicocephalic shape and the Mongoloids a more brachycephalic shape than Caucasians [20]. A Finnish study related historical skulls to present-day populations,

and showed the differences in inter-racial craniofacial differences [34]. The cranial base angle can potentially influence the sagittal position of the jaws and therefore go some way to explaining the differences in races.

The prevalence of Class III malocclusion in a Chinese population is higher than Caucasian population (3-4%), which has been noted to be around 13% and has even been as high as 23% [21,35,36]. It is important when comparing such studies to remember that differing criteria for subject selection and differing indices may have been used. A previous comparison between Chinese and Caucasian Class III surgical cases found a difference in linear cranial base morphology, but not angular cranial base morphology [37]. A significant linear difference was noted in both anterior and posterior cranial bases, where the Chinese sample had a shorter anterior but longer posterior cranial base. Unfortunately, the sample size in that study was on the small side, with only 30 subjects overall (Caucasian = 14, Chinese = 16).

Our study had a sample size of 83 subjects with three different sagittal skeletal patterns and a more homogeneous original of southern China; it expanded the dataset for the cranial base-jaw base relationship in a Chinese population. The results reinforce the previous study of Chinese surgical Class III cases [37]. Class III is known to have a strong genetic element and in this study it was found that the correlation between cranial base and jaw base was closer in skeletal Class III cases.

In the future population study, a bigger sample size can be considered. Besides, 3-dimensional cone beam computer tomography (CBCT) is more viable than two dimension cephalometric radiographs and can also solve the problem of image overlapping. Further investigation can be carried out in the future to evaluate the relationship between cranial base and jaw base 3-dimensionally for a specific population.

Conclusions

This study looked into a southern Chinese population to investigate a possible link between sagittal jaw relationships and the cranial base angle. It is found that the SNB angle decreases as the cranial base angle increases; the short NBa is, the shorter the maxillary length is. The cranial base appeares to have a certain correlation with the jaw base relationship in a southern Chinese population, and the correlation tends to be closer in skeletal Class III cases.

Competing interests
The authors declare that they have no conflict of interests.

Authors' contributions
YY designed the study and calibrated the investigator who made the cephalogram measurements. AC measured the cephalograms and analyzed the data. SP analyzed and interpreted the data and drafted the manuscript. CL drafted the manuscript and drew the figure. All of the authors read and approved the final manuscript.

Acknowledgements
The study was supported by the Small Project Funding, the University of Hong Kong (201209176136). Thanks to Shadow Yeung for his assistance with the statistical analysis.

Author details
[1]Hong Kong SAR, China. [2]Faculty of Dentistry, University of Hong Kong, Hong Kong SAR, China.

References
1. Ohtsuki F, Mukherjee D, Lewis AB, Roche AF: **A factor analysis of cranial base and vault dimensions in children.** *Am J Phys Anthropol* 1982, **58**:271–279.
2. Moss ML, Salentijn L: **The primary role of functional matrices in facial growth.** *Am J Orthod* 1969, **55**:566–577.
3. Van Limborgh J: **The role of genetic and local environmental factors in the control of postnatal craniofacial morphogenesis.** *Acta Morphol Neerl Scand* 1972, **10**(1):37–47.
4. Nie X: **Cranial base in craniofacial development: developmental features, influence on facial growth, anomaly, and molecular basis.** *Acta Odontol Scand* 2005, **63**:127–135.
5. Xue F, Wong RWK, Rabie ABM: **Genes, genetics, and Class III malocclusion.** *Orthod Craniofac Res* 2010, **13**:69–74.
6. Björk A, Palling M: **Adolescent age changes in sagittal jaw relation, alveolar prognathy, and incisal inclination.** *Acta Odontol* 1955, **12**:201–232.
7. Hopkin GB, Houston WJ, James GA: **The cranial base as an aetiological factorin malocclusion.** *Angle Orthod* 1968, **38**:250–255.
8. Kerr WJ, Hirst D: **Craniofacial characteristics of subjects with normal and postnormal occlusions: a longitudinal study.** *Am J Orthod Dentofacial Orthod* 1987, **92**:207–212.
9. Kerr WJ, Adams CP: **Cranial base and jaw relationship.** *Am J Phys Anthropol* 1988, **77**:213–220.
10. Anderson DL, Popovich F: **Lower cranial height vs craniofacial dimensions in Angle Class II malocclusion.** *Angle Orthod* 1983, **53**:253–260.
11. Bacon W, Eiller V, Hildwein M, Dubois G: **The cranial base in subjects with dental and skeletal Class II.** *Eur J Orthod* 1992, **14**:224–228.
12. Klocke A, Nanda RS, Kahl-Nieke B: **Role of cranial base flexure in developing sagittal jaw discrepancies.** *Am J Orthod Dentofacial Orthop* 2002, **122**:386–391.
13. Jarvinen S: **Saddle angle and maxillary prognathism: a radiological analysis of the association between the NSAr and SNA angles.** *Brit J Orthod* 1984, **11**:209–213.
14. Proff P, Will F, Bokan I, Fanghanel J, Gedrange T: **Cranial base features in skeletal Class III patients.** *Angle Orthod* 2008, **78**:433–439.
15. Rothstein T, Phan XL: **Dental and facial skeletal characteristics and growth of females and males with Class II Division 1 malocclusion between the ages of 10 and 14 (revisited). Part II. Anteroposterior and vertical circumpubertal growth.** *Am J Orthod Dentofac Orthop* 2001, **120**:542–555.
16. Wilhelm BM, Beck FM, Lidral AC, Vig KW: **A comparison of cranial base growth in Class I and Class II skeletal patterns.** *Am J Orthod Dentofac Orthop* 2001, **119**:401–405.
17. Dhopatkar A, Bhatia S, Rock P: **An investigation into the relationship between the cranial base angle and malocclusion.** *Angle Orthod* 2002, **72**:456–463.
18. Blumenbach JF: *Decas Collectionis Suae Diversarum Gentium Illustrata.* Gottingen: Dietrich JC; 1790.
19. Kasai K, Richards LC, Brown T: **Comparative study of craniofacial morphology in Japanese and Australian aboriginal populations.** *Hum Biol* 1993, **65**:821–834.
20. Kavitha L, Karthik K: **Comparison of cephalometric norms of caucasians and non-caucasians: A forensic aid in ethnic determination.** *J Forensic Dent Sci* 2012, **4**:53–55.
21. Angle: *Malocclusion of the teeth.* 7th edition. Philadelphia: White Mfg.Co; 1907.
22. Zhou L, Mok CW, Hagg U, McGrath C, Bendeus M, Wu J: **Anteroposterior dental arch and jaw-base relationships in a population sample.** *Angle Orthod* 2008, **78**:1023–1029.

23. Jacobson A: The "Wits" appraisal of jaw disharmony. *Am J Orthod* 1975, **67:**125–138.

24. Rivera AJR, Jiménez JC, Ruidíaz VC: Relationship between cranial base flexure and skeletal class. *Rev Odont Mex* 2011, **15**(4):214–218.

25. Bathia SN, Leighton BC: *A manual of facial growth.* Oxford: Oxford University Press; 1993.

26. Perillo L, Padricelli G, Isola G, Femiano F, Chiodini P, Matarese G: Class II malocclusion division 1: a new classification method by cephalometric analysis. *Eur J Paediatr Dent* 2012, **13**(3):192–196.

27. Andria LM, Leite LP, Prevatte TM, King LB: Correlation of the cranial base angle and its components with other dental/skeletal variables and treatment time. *Angle Orthod* 2004, **74:**361–366.

28. Jarvinen S: Relation of the SNA angle to the saddle angle. *Am J Orthod* 1980, **78:**670–673.

29. Rana T, Khanna R, Tikku T, Sachan K: Relationship of maxilla to cranial base in different facial types–a cephalometric evaluation. *J Oral Biolo Craniofac Res* 2012, **2:**30–35.

30. Houston WJ: A cephalometric analysis of Angle class II, division II malocclusion in the mixed dentition. *Dent Pract Dent Rec* 1967, **17:**372–376.

31. Björk A: Cranial base development: a follow-up x-ray study of the individual variation in growth occurring between the ages of 12 and 20 years and its relation to brain case and face development. *Am J Orthod* 1955, **41:**198–225.

32. Perillo L, Isola G, Esercizio D, Iovane M, Triolo G, Matarese G: Differences in craniofacial characteristics in Southern Italian children from Naples: a retrospective study by cephalometric analysis. *Eur J Paediatr Dent* 2013, **14**(3):195–198.

33. Kerr WJ: A method of superimposing serial lateral cephalometric films for the purpose of comparison: a preliminary report. *Brit J Orthod* 1978, **5:**51–53.

34. Argyropoulos E, Sassouni V, Xeniotou A: A comparative cephalometric investigation of the Greek craniofacial pattern through 4,000 years. *Angle Orthod* 1989, **59:**195–204.

35. Johnson JS, Soetamat A, Winoto NS: A comparison of some features of the Indonesian occlusion with those of two other ethnic groups. *Brit J Orthod* 1978, **5:**183–188.

36. Lew KK, Foong WC, Loh E: Malocclusion prevalence in an ethnicChinese population. *Aust Dent J* 1993, **38:**442–449.

37. Ngan P, Hagg U, Yiu C, Merwin D, Wei SH: Cephalometric comparisons of Chinese and Caucasian surgical Class III patients. *Int J Adult Orthodon Orthognath Surg* 1997, **12:**177–188.

7

Does low level laser therapy relieve the pain caused by the placement of the orthodontic separators? —a meta-analysis

Quan Shi, Shuo Yang, Fangfang Jia and Juan Xu[*]

Abstract

Objective: Pain caused by orthodontic treatment can affect patient's compliance and even force them to terminate treatments. The aim of this meta-analysis is to evaluate of the analgesic effect of low level laser therapy (LLLT) after placement of the orthodontic separators.

Methods: Five databases: PubMed, Embase, Cochrane library, China Biology Medicine disc (SinoMed CBM), China National Knowledge Infrastructure (CNKI) were searched for all the appropriate studies in June, 2014. Two reviewers screened the research results under our inclusion criteria and evaluated the risk of bias independently. Then the data of the included studies was extracted for quantitative analysis by the Review Manager 5.1 software.

Results: Six studies were included in our meta-analysis finally. Comparing to the placebo group, the LLLT has good analgesic effect at 6 h, 1d, 2d, 3d after placement of separators which is of statistical significance. While at 2 h, 4d, 5d after the placement, the results tend to support LLLT, but not statistically significant.

Conclusion: Based on current included studies, LLLT can reduce the pain caused by the placement of separators effectively. However, because of the high heterogeneity, well designed RCTs are required in the future.

Keywords: Pain, Orthodontic separators, Low level laser therapy, Analgesic effect, Meta-analysis

Introduction

Pain is a subjective experience and a common clinical symptom in orthodontic patients. Research shows that as many as 95 % of orthodontic patients will feel pain and 8-30 % of patients discontinue treatment because of pain [1–3]. Sometimes pain can affect patient's compliance and therefore affect treatment effect. Despite the orthodontic technology has been great developed, the issue of pain has not been solved very well.

Many orthodontic operations can cause pain [2, 4–7]. As a common and necessary operation, placement of separators to create enough space for bands can cause mild to moderate pain [8]. It is generally believed that when periodontal ligament under pressure, the mediators of inflammation are released, such as prostaglandins, histamine, substance P ,which cause sensitivity to the free nerve terminations and pain or discomfort after

placement of archwires or separators [2, 9]. In several methods currently available, the medication is thought to be the most effective [10], especially the non-steroidal anti-inflammatory drugs (NSAIDs). Some articles [1, 9–11] proved that they can relieve orthodontic pain effectively. But the medication also has its side effects which cannot be ignored: allergy and inhibiting tooth movement [10, 12]. Therefore, the application of medication is limited.

There are no effective clinically proven non-invasive, non-pharmacological methods used to relieve the pain caused by orthodontic. But some studies showed that low level laser maybe have analgesic effect [5, 13–20]. Low level laser, or low level laser therapy(LLLT), is a new internationally accepted designation and defined as laser treatment in which the energy output is low enough so as not to cause a rise in the temperature of the treated tissue above 36.5 °C or normal body temperature[20]. LLLT can inhibit the development of inflammation [21, 22], accelerate of bone repair [23], increase the rate of teeth movement [24]. Besides, LLLT have been used to treat

* Correspondence: newxj@hotmail.com
Department of Stomatology, Chinese People's Liberation Army General Hospital, 28 Fuxing Road, 100853 Beijing, China

temporal-mandibular joint disorder [25], relive the pain after teeth extraction [26].

As a non-invasive method, with no report of serious adverse effect events [10], LLLT is better than drugs in clinical application prospect. But there is still a lack of reliable evidence to prove that LLLT can effectively reduce the orthodontic pain. So the aim of this systematic review is to collect the randomized controlled trials (RCTs) or controlled clinical trials (CCTs) about LLLT relive the pain of patients after placement of separators and evaluate of the analgesic effect of LLLT.

Material and methods

The methods for this review were based on the Cochrane Handbook for Systematic Reviews of Interventions [27]. In the whole process, the studies were assessed by 2 observers independently and any disagreement will resolved by discussion. The data was analyzed by the Review Manager 5.1 software.

Literature search and study selection

The following electronic databases were searched in June 2014 without time and language restricted: PubMed, Embase, Cochrane library, China Biology Medicine disc (SinoMed CBM), China National Knowledge Infrastructure (CNKI). The search strategies of PubMed, Embase and Cochrane library were showed in Table 1.

Inclusion criteria

The following selection criteria were applied.

1. Design: the studies should be designed as RCT or controlled clinical trial (CCT), including split-mouth design.
2. Participants: patients received elastomeric separators on the premolar or molar.
3. Interventions and comparators: low level laser therapy (LLLT) vs placebo. (For some studies, there are not only these two groups, if we can filter out the data we need from the studies, we will include them either.)

4. Outcome: measurement of the pain after placing the elastomeric separators.

Exclusion criteria

The exclusion criteria were as follows:

1. In vitro study (laboratory studies and animal studies), case report or letters.
2. Study without available data can not be used by our meta-analysis.
3. The pain was caused by other operations of orthodontic instead of placing the elastomeric separators.
4. The participants had systemic disease or chronic pain or histories of neurologic and psychiatric disorders and other characteristics which will have influence on the outcome.

Data extraction

We designed a table to collect the experimental information and data which include the author, country, year of publication, design type, number of participant, measure method, the pain value and standard deviation, and so on. Then use a new table to record the parameters of the laser and the treatment regimen.

Risk of bias evaluation

Totally seven items need to be taken into consideration: (1) allocation concealment, (2) random sequence generation,(3)blinding of participants and personnel, (4) blinding of outcome assessment, (5) incomplete outcome data, (6) selective reporting, (7) other bias. The risk of bias for each item was judged as low risk, high risk, or unclear risk. The overall risk of bias for the each study was evaluated by the following criteria:

If the risk of bias is low for all the items, the study is of low risk.

If one (or more than one) of the risk of bias is high for the key items, the study is of high risk.

Table 1 Search strategy and results for T pubmed, Embase and cochranme library

Database	Search strategy	Result
pubmed	#1: pain OR discomfort OR toothache	591803
	#2 :(low power laser) OR (low level laser) OR LLLTOR (low output laser) OR (low intensity laser)	10881
	#3: orthodontic*	52498
	#4 : #1 AND #2 AND #3	33
EMBASE	#1: pain OR discomfort OR toothache	1054689
	#2 : (low power laser) OR (low level laser) OR LLLTOR (low output laser) OR (low intensity laser)	19478
	#3: orthodontic*	61408
	#4: #1 AND #2 AND #3	49
The Cochrane library	#1: (pain OR discomfort OR toothache) AND laser AND orthodontic*	42

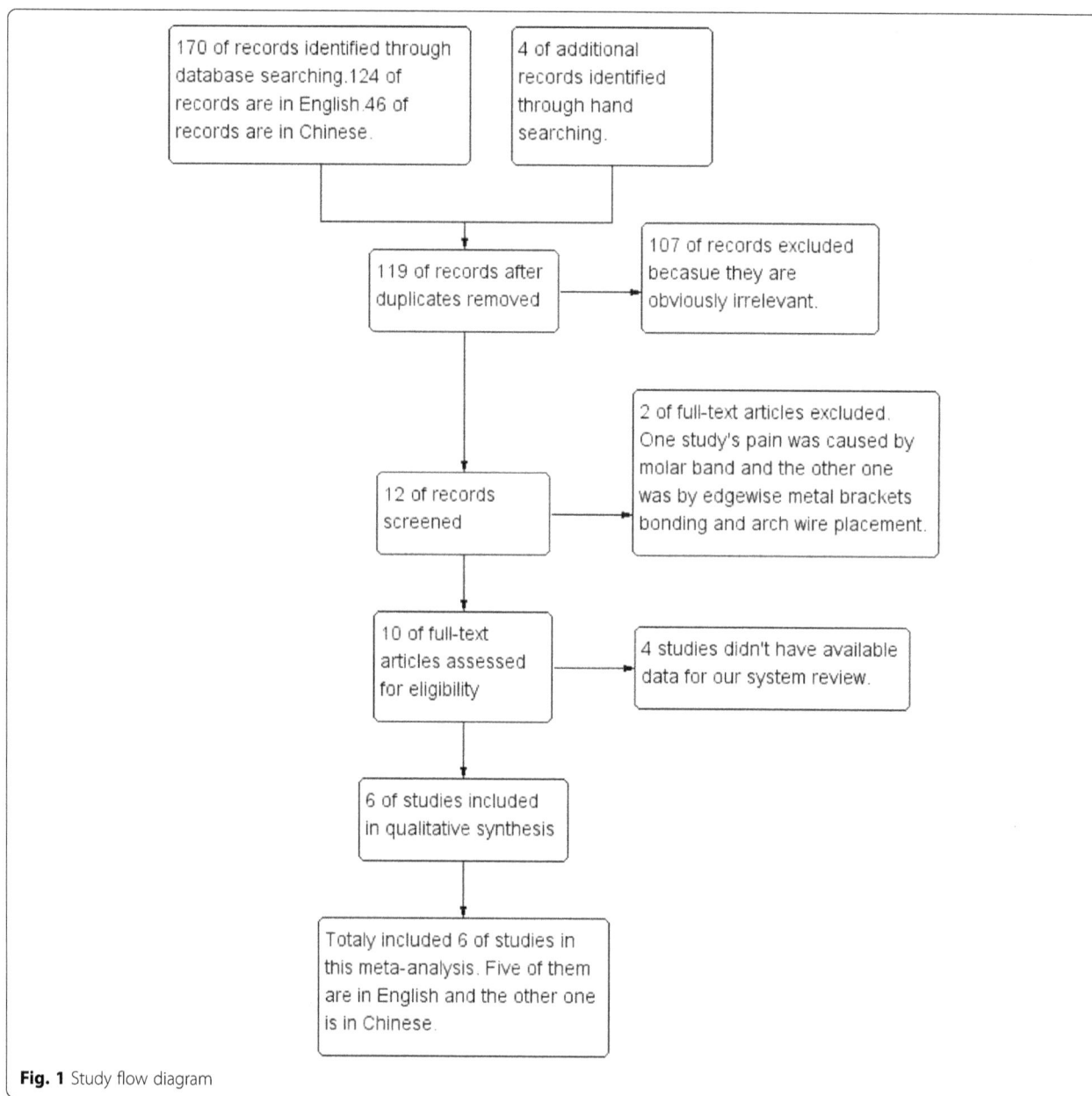

Fig. 1 Study flow diagram

Table 2 Characteristics of included studies

Study ID	Country	Design	Number (P/L)[a]	Average age	Separators
Celestino No´brega 2013	Brazil	RCT	60 (30/30)	17.5	3 M Unitek
Won Tae Kim 2012	Korea	RCT	58 (30/28)	21.52	Dentalastics Separators, Dentaurum, Ispringen, Germany,2.1 mm
Ladan Eslamian 2013	Iran	CCT (split mouth design)	37 (37/37)	24.97	Dentarum, Springen, Germany
Esper MA 2011	Brazil	RCT	38 (38/12)	23.4	Morelli, 4.0 mm, Ø 5/32"
Ida Marini 2013	Italy	RCT	80 (40/40)	23.0875	NR[b]
Zhang HY 2014	China	RCT	60 (30/30)	15.9	NR

[a]:P = placebo group; L = LLLT group
[b]:NR = not report

Table 3 Characteristics of included studies

Study ID	Teeth	Intervention method	Evaluation intervals	Pain measure method
Celestino No´brega 2013	mesial and distal sides of the first permanent lower molars on the left and right sides	each subject received irradiation one spot on the region of root apex, three points along the root axis on the buccal side	2 h,6 h,24 h,3 d,5 d	VAS ;The incidence of free of pain
Won Tae Kim 2012	mesially and distally on both of the maxillary first molars.	apply laser for 30 seconds on each area immediately then every 12 hours for 1 week with close contact between the tip and mucosa to irradiate the mesiobuccal, mesiolingual, distobuccal, and distolingual areas.	5 min,1 h,6 h,12 h,1 d, 2 d,3 d,4 d,5 d,6 d,7 d	VAS
Ladan Eslamian 2013	first permanent molars (distal and mesial), either on maxillary (22 patients) or mandibular (15 patients) arches	laser irradiation on the buccal side (at the cervical third of the roots), for distal and mesial of the second premolars and first permanent molars, as well as distal of second permanent molars (five doses) . The same procedure was repeated for the lingual or palatal side (five doses). After 24 h, patients returned to the clinic and received another 10 doses of laser irradiation on the same quadrant.	0 h,6 h,24 h,30 h, 3 d,4 d,5 d,6 d,7 d	VAS
Esper MA 2011	Placebo :mesial and distal of the first upper and lower molar on the right side while the Laser group on left side	Radiation was applied punctually, touching the gum perpendicularly on two points of the vestibular side and on the lingual side of the separated molars, both points were in the cervical and radicular region	pre-placement 2 h, 24 h,48 h,72 h,96 h	VAS
Ida Marini 2013	right first ,second premolar and first molar (upper arch or lower arch)	The laser probe was applied on the cervical third of buccal and lingual gingiva l covering of each root.	0 h,12 h,24 h,36 h,48 h,72 h,96 h	VAS,Questionnaire
Zhang HY 2014	First molar	the laser probe was 5 mm away from the mucosal ,Laser irradiation was applied on first molar root apical ,then Move up along the long axis of the tooth to the tooth neck (totally 4 points)	2 h,6 h,24 h,72 h,120 h	VAS

Table 4 Detail of the lasers and parameters

Study ID	Laser type	Wave length (nm)	Output power (mW)	Number of irradiated points or area (cm2)	Irradiation time	Frequency	Dose (J/cm2)	Field diameter
Celestino No´brega 2013	aluminum gallium arsenide diode laser	830	40.6	4 points	25 s per each 1 J/cm2, totally 125 s	after placing the separator	root apex 2 J/cm2,the other three points was 1 J/cm2, totally 5 J/cm2	2 mm
Won Tae Kim 2012	semiconductor laser device with an AlGaInP diode	635	6	4	30 seconds on each area	every 12 h for 1 week	NR[a]	5.6 mm
Ladan Eslamian 2013	Ga-Al-As laser	810	100	10	20 s	laser was applied immediately and 24 hours later after placing the separators	2	NR
Esper MA 2011	InGaAIP laser	660	30	4	25 s each point	after placing the separator	4 J/cm2 per point, totally 16 J/cm2 per tooth	5 mm
Ida Marini 2013	GaAs diode laser superpulsed wave	910	160	6	totally 340 s	The irradiation started immediately after placing orthodontic separators.	NR	8 mm
Zhang HY 2014	semiconductor laser	650 and 830	30	4	30S each point, totally 120 s per tooth	after placing the separator	NR	3-5 mm

[a]NR = not report

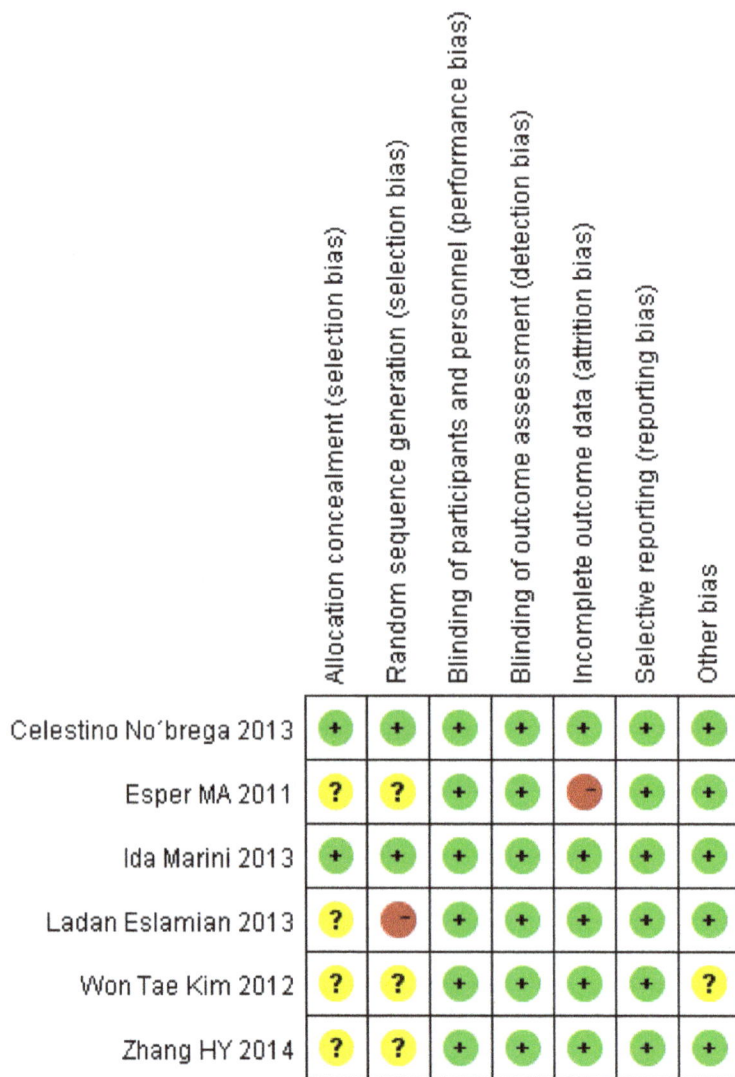

Fig. 2 Risk of bias for every study. Of the six included studies, two [13, 19] of them were judged to have a low risk of bias because all the items were of low risk of bias and one study [19] is a random, triple-blinding, placebo control clinic trail while the other one [13] is a random double-blinding, placebo control clinic trail. Two [14, 20] of the six studies were judged to have an unclear risk of bias, because the authors failed to describe the method of randomization and had no report of the allocation concealment. At the same time, the study of Won Tae Kim, et al. [14] was judged to have unclear bias on the item of "other bias" because the application of the laser was performed by the subjects at home, so there may be compliance bias. Two studies [15, 29] were judged to have a high risk of bias because one of the studies [15] used inappropriate method of randomization and there was a subject drop out without details description in the study of Esper MA, et al. [29]

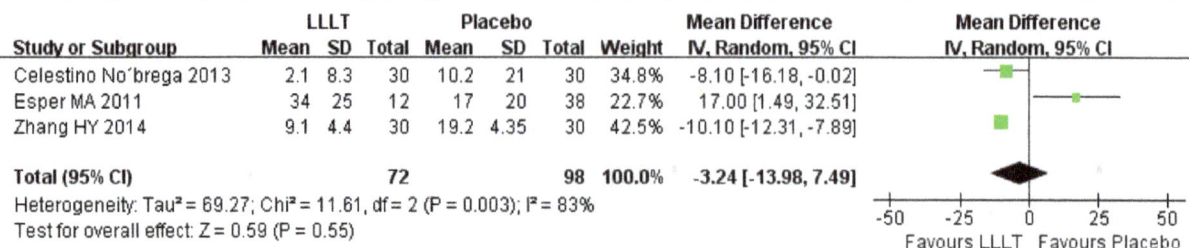

Study or Subgroup	LLLT			Placebo			Weight	Mean Difference IV, Random, 95% CI	Mean Difference IV, Random, 95% CI
	Mean	SD	Total	Mean	SD	Total			
Celestino No´brega 2013	2.1	8.3	30	10.2	21	30	34.8%	-8.10 [-16.18, -0.02]	
Esper MA 2011	34	25	12	17	20	38	22.7%	17.00 [1.49, 32.51]	
Zhang HY 2014	9.1	4.4	30	19.2	4.35	30	42.5%	-10.10 [-12.31, -7.89]	
Total (95% CI)			**72**			**98**	**100.0%**	**-3.24 [-13.98, 7.49]**	

Heterogeneity: Tau² = 69.27; Chi² = 11.61, df = 2 (P = 0.003); I² = 83%
Test for overall effect: Z = 0.59 (P = 0.55)

Favours LLLT   Favours Placebo

Fig. 3 Forest plot of pooled mean difference at 2 hours

Study or Subgroup	LLLT Mean	SD	Total	Placebo Mean	SD	Total	Weight	Mean Difference IV, Random, 95% CI	Mean Difference IV, Random, 95% CI
Celestino No´brega 2013	3.4	11	30	21.3	28.4	30	14.3%	-17.90 [-28.80, -7.00]	
Ladan Eslamian 2013	11	13.7	37	14.1	15.8	37	22.6%	-3.10 [-9.84, 3.64]	
Won Tae Kim 2012	19.59	5.53	28	25.32	5.33	30	32.2%	-5.73 [-8.53, -2.93]	
Zhang HY 2014	13.1	6.3	30	25.7	7	30	31.0%	-12.60 [-15.97, -9.23]	
Total (95% CI)			125			127	100.0%	-9.00 [-14.33, -3.67]	

Heterogeneity: Tau² = 20.94; Chi² = 14.76, df = 3 (P = 0.002); I² = 80%
Test for overall effect: Z = 3.31 (P = 0.0009)

Favours LLLT   Favours Placebo

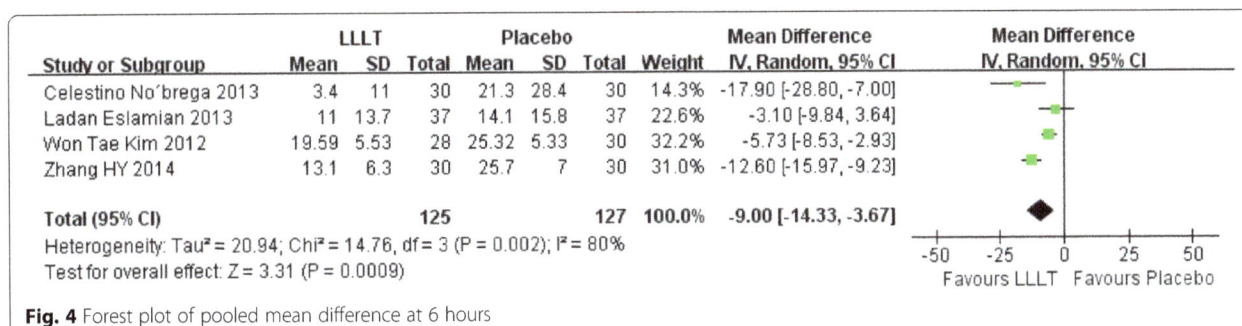

Fig. 4 Forest plot of pooled mean difference at 6 hours

If one (or more than one) of the risk of bias is unclear, the study is of unclear risk.

Data analysis

The meta-analysis was performed by combining the results of the included studies which had measured the pain at the same evaluation intervals for the continuous data. In addition, chi^2 and I^2 was used to estimate the degree of heterogeneity. Mean differences, standard deviations, and 95 % confidence intervals (CI) were to be calculated for individual trials and overall effect using a random effects model or a fixed effects model for continuous data.

Results

Searching and selection results

The selection progress is shown in Fig. 1. After reading the full-text of the 10 potential interests [13–17, 19, 20, 28–30], we found that five articles [13–15, 20, 29] have available data for our meta-analysis. For the rest studies, we contacted the authors of the articles by sending e-mail (except Lim HM et al. 1995 because there is no e-mail address in the article). But only one author [19] sent us the data we needed. Finally, we include six studies [13–15, 19, 20, 29] in our meta-analysis. Five of them [13–15, 19, 29] are in English and the other one [20] is in Chinese.

Characteristics of the included studies

The detailed descriptions of the characteristics about the six included studies are shown in Tables 2, 3 and Table 4.

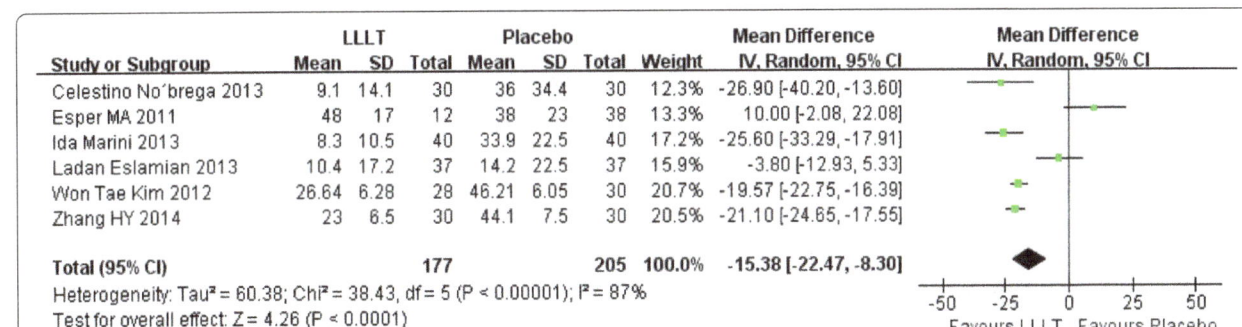

In the six studies we included, five of them are RCT [13, 14, 19, 20, 29], and one is CCT [15]. Six studies encompassing 295 subjects. One study [15] used a split mouth design method. Five studies [13–15, 20, 29] placed the separator on the mesial and distal of the first molar, and one [19] placed separator on the first, second premolar and the first molar at the same time (totally four separators per subjects).

The detail of the lasers and parameters are shown in Table 4. The wavelength of the laser ranged from 635 nm to 910 nm. One study [20] used a mix of 650 nm and 830 nm. All the studies used a semiconductor laser. The output power ranged from 6 mW to 160 mW.

All the included studies used VAS to evaluate the pain. The mean pain values and standard deviations of laser group and placebo group at each evaluation interval of the six studies are collected. In one study [19], the data was got from the author by sending e-mail. Although all of the studies used the VAS score to evaluate the pain, but the score ranged from 0 to 100 in two studies [14, 19]and the other four studies [13, 15, 20, 29] ranged from 0 to 10. However, all of them use the same method to evaluate the pain in each group. Therefore, the data of these two studies were converted to centesimal system.

Risk of bias evaluation

The risk of bias summary is shown in the Fig. 2. If there is inadequate information in the article, we will contact the author by e-mails or seek advice from statisticians. Of the

Study or Subgroup	LLLT Mean	SD	Total	Placebo Mean	SD	Total	Weight	Mean Difference IV, Random, 95% CI	Mean Difference IV, Random, 95% CI
Celestino No´brega 2013	9.1	14.1	30	36	34.4	30	12.3%	-26.90 [-40.20, -13.60]	
Esper MA 2011	48	17	12	38	23	38	13.3%	10.00 [-2.08, 22.08]	
Ida Marini 2013	8.3	10.5	40	33.9	22.5	40	17.2%	-25.60 [-33.29, -17.91]	
Ladan Eslamian 2013	10.4	17.2	37	14.2	22.5	37	15.9%	-3.80 [-12.93, 5.33]	
Won Tae Kim 2012	26.64	6.28	28	46.21	6.05	30	20.7%	-19.57 [-22.75, -16.39]	
Zhang HY 2014	23	6.5	30	44.1	7.5	30	20.5%	-21.10 [-24.65, -17.55]	
Total (95% CI)			177			205	100.0%	-15.38 [-22.47, -8.30]	

Heterogeneity: Tau² = 60.38; Chi² = 38.43, df = 5 (P < 0.00001); I² = 87%
Test for overall effect: Z = 4.26 (P < 0.0001)

Favours LLLT   Favours Placebo

Fig. 5 Forest plot of pooled mean difference at 1 day

Study or Subgroup	LLLT Mean	SD	Total	Placebo Mean	SD	Total	Weight	Mean Difference IV, Random, 95% CI	Mean Difference IV, Random, 95% CI
Esper MA 2011	40	19	12	37	20	38	24.8%	3.00 [-9.49, 15.49]	
Ida Marini 2013	7.7	10.4	40	25	20	40	34.7%	-17.30 [-24.29, -10.31]	
Won Tae Kim 2012	26.59	6.28	28	46.09	6.05	30	40.5%	-19.50 [-22.68, -16.32]	
Total (95% CI)			80			108	100.0%	-13.16 [-22.81, -3.51]	

Heterogeneity: Tau² = 57.19; Chi² = 11.75, df = 2 (P = 0.003); I² = 83%
Test for overall effect: Z = 2.67 (P = 0.008)

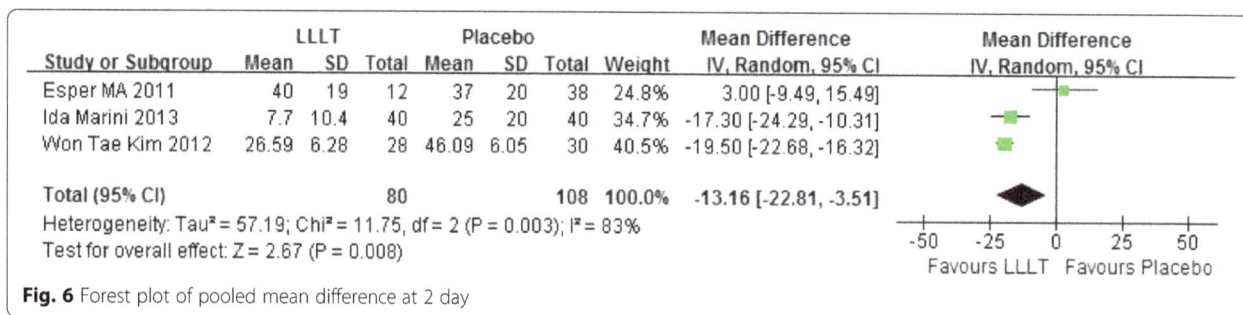

Fig. 6 Forest plot of pooled mean difference at 2 day

six included studies, two [13, 19] of them were judged to have a low risk of bias. Two studies [14, 20] were judged to have an unclear risk of bias. Two studies [15, 29] were judged to have a high risk of bias .

Meta-analysis for mean score of pain

In our included studies, if there were three or more studies measured the pain score at the same time point, we will make an analysis. Therefore, totally seven time points meet the requirements: 2 hours, 6 hours, 24 hours, 2 days, 3 days, 4 days, 5 days. Figs. 3, 4, 5, 6, 7, 8 and 9 showed the comparison between LLLT and Placebo on pain relief after placing the separators at each time point. Because of the high heterogeneity, a random effect was selected.

2 hours after the placement, the overall effect test showed no significant different between the LLLT and placebo (P = 0.55). The mean difference was –3.24 and 95 % CI(–13.98 , 7.49) (Fig. 3).

While for the time points of 6 h, 24 h, 2d, 3d, the overall effects favored the LLLT and showed a statistical difference between the LLLT and placebo, because all of the P values of the tests were less than 0.05 (Figs 4, 5, 6 and 7).

At 4th day and 5th day the overall effects showed there was no statistical difference between the LLLT and the placebo group (P = 0.06 at 4d and P = 0.15 at 5d).

The pain incidence

One of the included studies reported the rate of pain never appeared and never disappeared [19]. The result showed that 30 % of the LLLT group subjects did not feel pain while

the placebo group was 0 %. In another study [13], the proportion of subjects reporting the absence of pain was significantly higher in LLLT group at each time point. Meta-analysis is not feasible because of inadequate data.

Discussion

Pain caused by orthodontic treatment can affect patient's compliance and change their eating habits [8], even forcing them to terminate treatments [13]. Orthodontists have been working on the controlling of pain. Although the NSAIDs had been proved effective on pain control, the side effects limited its clinical application [9–12]. Some researches [5, 13–20] consider LLLT as an effective method to control orthodontic pain, therefore this system review is to confirm this analgesic effect after placement of separators. Because many orthodontic operations can induce pain, in order to reduce the heterogeneity of clinical, we select the studies of using LLLT to relief pain after placing the separators.

For the orthodontic treatment with fixed appliances, the separators were used to create enough space for the bands[8]. After placement, whether separators or arch wires, the periodontal ligament and the vessels were under pressure, causing the release of inflammatory mediators and inducing pain [2, 9].

However, it is difficult to measure the pain precisely because pain is a subjective experience, the individual variability of pain threshold and sensitivity can be influenced by physical and psychological effects [18, 19]. Besides, other factors, such as environmental, sociocultural, genetic

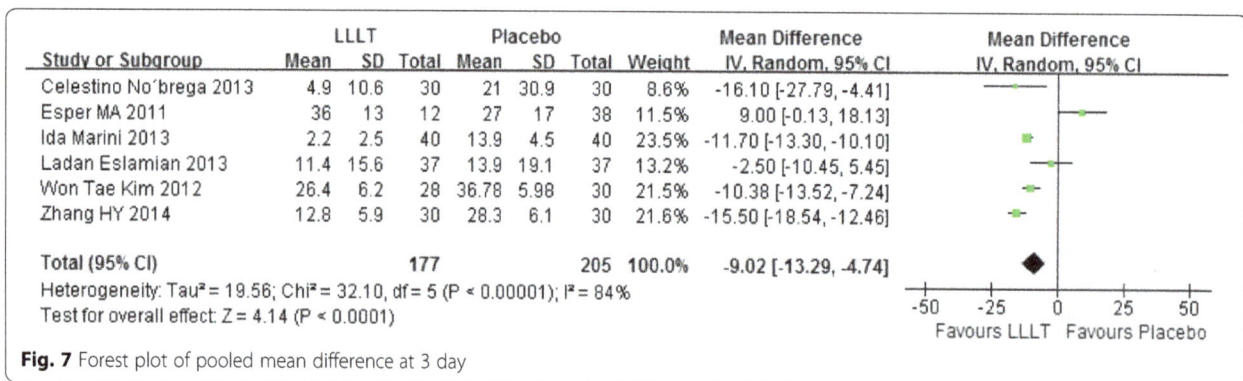

Study or Subgroup	LLLT Mean	SD	Total	Placebo Mean	SD	Total	Weight	Mean Difference IV, Random, 95% CI	Mean Difference IV, Random, 95% CI
Celestino No'brega 2013	4.9	10.6	30	21	30.9	30	8.6%	-16.10 [-27.79, -4.41]	
Esper MA 2011	36	13	12	27	17	38	11.5%	9.00 [-0.13, 18.13]	
Ida Marini 2013	2.2	2.5	40	13.9	4.5	40	23.5%	-11.70 [-13.30, -10.10]	
Ladan Eslamian 2013	11.4	15.6	37	13.9	19.1	37	13.2%	-2.50 [-10.45, 5.45]	
Won Tae Kim 2012	26.4	6.2	28	36.78	5.98	30	21.5%	-10.38 [-13.52, -7.24]	
Zhang HY 2014	12.8	5.9	30	28.3	6.1	30	21.6%	-15.50 [-18.54, -12.46]	
Total (95% CI)			177			205	100.0%	-9.02 [-13.29, -4.74]	

Heterogeneity: Tau² = 19.56; Chi² = 32.10, df = 5 (P < 0.00001); I² = 84%
Test for overall effect: Z = 4.14 (P < 0.0001)

Fig. 7 Forest plot of pooled mean difference at 3 day

Study or Subgroup	LLLT Mean	LLLT SD	LLLT Total	Placebo Mean	Placebo SD	Placebo Total	Weight	Mean Difference IV, Random, 95% CI
Esper MA 2011	24	10	12	18	13	38	18.4%	6.00 [-1.01, 13.01]
Ida Marini 2013	1.3	2.9	40	8.6	5.2	40	33.2%	-7.30 [-9.15, -5.45]
Ladan Eslamian 2013	8.5	13.1	37	10.9	17.7	37	18.2%	-2.40 [-9.50, 4.70]
Won Tae Kim 2012	22.5	5.87	28	30.3	5.65	30	30.3%	-7.80 [-10.77, -4.83]
Total (95% CI)			117			145	100.0%	-4.12 [-8.46, 0.22]

Heterogeneity: Tau² = 13.89; Chi² = 14.95, df = 3 (P = 0.002); I² = 80%
Test for overall effect: Z = 1.86 (P = 0.06)

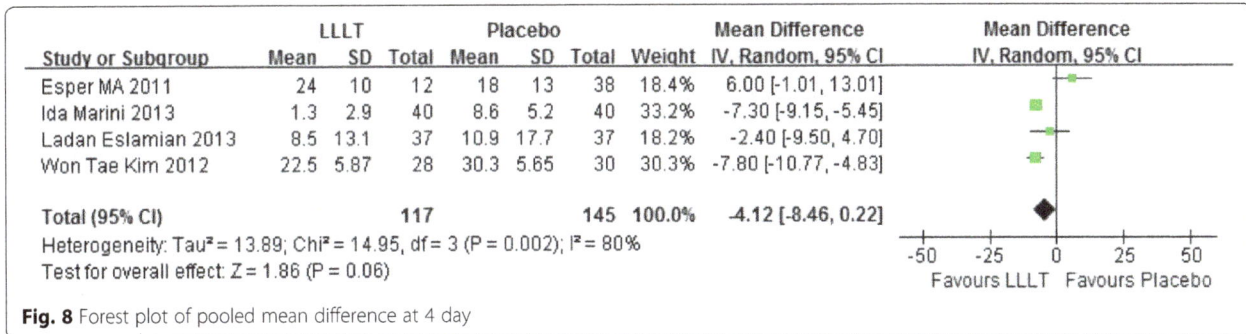

Fig. 8 Forest plot of pooled mean difference at 4 day

factors, and so on, can influence pain [15]. Therefore, from these viewpoints, the split-mouth design perhaps is the best choice. In our included studies, only one is split-mouth design. There are no objective measurements for pain. The VAS is one of the most common used tools to measure pain intensity at present [8, 16]. All of the six included studies in this review used this method. What's more, in order to avoid the psychological effect, we need well designed clinical trials to evaluate the pain. Using placebo is one of our included criteria, which would increase the reliability of the results and decrease the psychological effects. Two of the six included studies used red light [19] or light-emitting diode(LED) [14] whose intensity was very low compared to the laser. The other four studies used pseudo-laser as placebo. Only two studies [13, 19] reported the correct random sequence generation method and allocation concealment.

In our meta-analysis, compare to the placebo group, the LLLT has good analgesic effect and the results favored the LLLT at 6 h, 1d, 2d, 3d after placement of separators which is of statistical significance. While at 2 h, 4d, 5d, the results tend to support LLLT without statistically significant. A system review [26] concluded that LLLT modulates biochemical inflammatory markers and produces local anti-inflammatory effects in cells and soft tissue which contribute to relief acute pain in the short-term. Besides, the review found there were strong evidences that LLLT can improve angiogenesis. Because of high heterogeneity of different studies which may be caused by

different races, laser parameters, using methods and frequency, bias risk, we chose a random effect model. At present, the most commonly used non-surgical lasers are diode, with a wave length ranging from 600 to 1,000 nm, and potencies between 10 and 100 mW [29]. The wave length of laser used in the six included studies ranged from 635-910 nm and the output power between 6 and 160 mW. All the LLLT in the six studies used semiconductor laser. Besides, the frequency and use method were different in each study. According to some research [5, 13, 15], the laser does not inhibit the cell activity if the dose less than 20 J/cm². The laser doses of included studies were all less than 20 J/cm². At the same time, there were no adverse effects reported by these studies using the lasers under the current parameter ranges.

Two studies [13, 19] report the rate of free of pain (VAS = 0). One [19] report the rate of pain never appeared and the result showed that 30 % of the LLLT group subjects did not feel pain while the placebo group was 0 %. In the other one study [13], the proportion of subjects reporting the absence of pain was significantly higher in LLLT group at each time point. Although it is impossible to make a meta-analysis because of clinical heterogeneity and insufficient data, their results support the effective analgesic effect of LLLT.

According to the results of our meta-analysis, LLLT can reduce the pain caused by the placement of separators effectively without adverse effect under current evidence. Considering LLLT may increase the speed of tooth

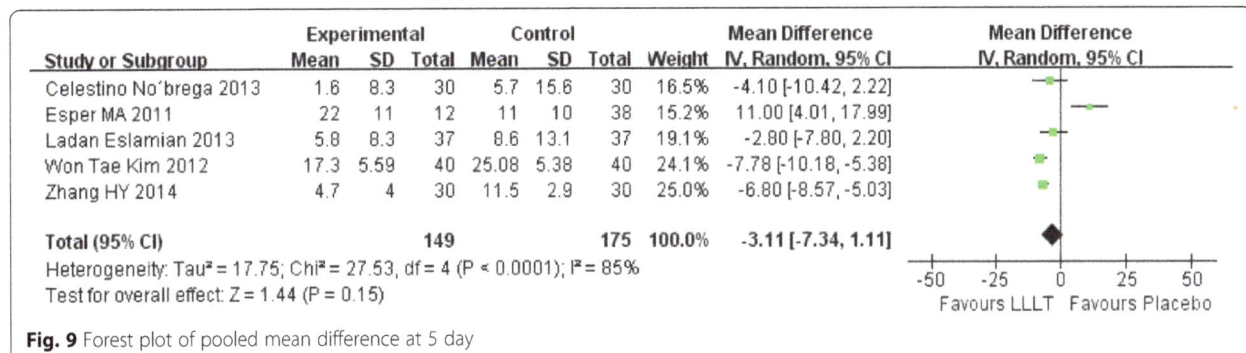

Study or Subgroup	Experimental Mean	Experimental SD	Experimental Total	Control Mean	Control SD	Control Total	Weight	Mean Difference IV, Random, 95% CI
Celestino No'brega 2013	1.6	8.3	30	5.7	15.6	30	16.5%	-4.10 [-10.42, 2.22]
Esper MA 2011	22	11	12	11	10	38	15.2%	11.00 [4.01, 17.99]
Ladan Eslamian 2013	5.8	8.3	37	8.6	13.1	37	19.1%	-2.80 [-7.80, 2.20]
Won Tae Kim 2012	17.3	5.59	40	25.08	5.38	40	24.1%	-7.78 [-10.18, -5.38]
Zhang HY 2014	4.7	4	30	11.5	2.9	30	25.0%	-6.80 [-8.57, -5.03]
Total (95% CI)			149			175	100.0%	-3.11 [-7.34, 1.11]

Heterogeneity: Tau² = 17.75; Chi² = 27.53, df = 4 (P < 0.0001); I² = 85%
Test for overall effect: Z = 1.44 (P = 0.15)

Fig. 9 Forest plot of pooled mean difference at 5 day

movement [22], in the field of orthodontics, LLLT may have broad application prospects. But different studies used different separators, different lasers and parameters, different method and frequency of laser, different test positions (mandible or maxilla or both), different design and different risk of bias, and these can lead to the high heterogeneity. Therefore, well designed RCTs are required to evaluate the analgesic effect of LLLT.

Conclusion

Under current studies and evidences, the results of our meta-analysis reveals that LLLT can reduce the pain caused by the placement of separators effectively at 6 h, 1d, 2d, 3d after the placement of the orthodontic separators without adverse effect reports. Besides, there is no evidence reveals that LLLT can bring forward the most painful day. These results indicate the good clinical application prospect. However, because of the high heterogeneity and the bias risk of included studies, well designed RCTs are required in the future.

Competing interests

This work was supported by Clinical scientific research fund (No.320.6750.15029) from Wu Jieping Medical Foundation.

Authors' contributions

SQ carried out the literature research and drafted the manuscript. The part of study selection, data extraction, risk of bias evaluation was finished by SQ and YS. For the part of data analysis, it was completed by SQ and JFF. XJ is the Corresponding author and she undertook the work of design of this meta-analysis, coordination and helped to draft the manuscript. All authors read and approved the final manuscript.

Acknowledgments

We are grateful to Dra. Maria Ângela L. R. Esper (Institute for Ortodontia e Ortopedia Especializada), Bortolotti F (Institute for Department of Neurosciences, Section of Orthodontics, University of Naples "Federico II", Italy, via Pansini), and A. Puigdollers (Department of Orthodontics and Dentofacial Orthopedics, Dental School, International University of Catalunya, Campus Sant Cugat, Josep Trueta s/n)), for giving us the data we need and answering our questions by E-mail.

References

1. Krishnan V. Orthodontic pain: from causes to management–a review. Eur J Orthod. 2007;29(2):170–9.
2. Bergius M, Kiliaridis S, Berggren U. Pain in orthodontics. A review and discussion of the literature. J Orofac Orthop. 2000;61(2):125–37.
3. Hoar S, Linnell KJ. Cognitive load eliminates the global perceptual bias for unlimited exposure durations. Atten Percept Psychophys. 2013;75(2):210–5.
4. Zawawi KH. Acceptance of orthodontic miniscrews as temporary anchorage devices. Patient Prefer Adherence. 2014 Jun 30;8:933–7.
5. Tortamano A, Lenzi DC, Haddad AC, Bottino MC, Dominguez GC, Vigorito JW. Low-level laser therapy for pain caused by placement of the first orthodontic archwire: a randomized clinical trial. Am J Orthod Dentofacial Orthop. 2009;136(5):662–7.
6. Youssef M, Ashkar S, Hamade E, Gutknecht N, Lampert F, Mir M. The effect of low-level laser therapy during orthodontic movement: a preliminary study. Lasers Med Sci. 2008;23(1):27–33.
7. Erdinç AM, Dinçer B. Perception of pain during orthodontic treatment with fixed appliances. Eur J Orthod. 2004;26(1):79–85.
8. Bondemark L, Fredriksson K, Ilros S. Separation effect and perception of pain and discomfort from two types of orthodontic separators. World J Orthod. 2004;5(2):172–6.

9. Polat O, Karaman AI. Pain control during fixed orthodontic appliance therapy. Angle Orthod. 2005;75(2):214–9.
10. Xiaoting L, Yin T, Yangxi C. Interventions for pain during fixed orthodontic appliance therapy. A systematic review. Angle Orthod. 2010;80(5):925–32.
11. Salmassian R, Oesterle LJ, Shellhart WC, Newman SM. Comparison of the efficacy of ibuprofen and acetaminophen in controlling pain after orthodontic tooth movement. Am J Orthod Dentofacial Orthop. 2009;135(4):516–21.
12. Kyrkanides S, O'Banion MK, Subtelny JD. Nonsteroidal anti-inflammatory drugs in orthodontic tooth movement: metalloproteinase activity and collagen synthesis by endothelial cells. Am J Orthod Dentofacial Orthop. 2000;118(2):203–9.
13. Nóbrega C, da Silva EM, de Macedo CR. Low-level laser therapy for treatment of pain associated with orthodontic elastomeric separator placement: a placebo-controlled randomized double-blind clinical trial. Photomed Laser Surg. 2013;31(1):10–6.
14. Kim WT, Bayome M, Park JB, Park JH, Baek SH, Kook YA. Effect of frequent laser irradiation on orthodontic pain. A single-blind randomized clinical trial. Angle Orthod. 2013;83(4):611–6.
15. Eslamian L, Borzabadi-Farahani A, Hassanzadeh-Azhiri A, Badiee MR, Fekrazad R. The effect of 810-nm low-level laser therapy on pain caused by orthodontic elastomeric separators. Lasers Med Sci. 2014;29(2):559–64.
16. Artés-Ribas M, Arnabat-Dominguez J, Puigdollers A. Analgesic effect of a low-level laser therapy (830 nm) in early orthodontic treatment. Lasers Med Sci. 2013;28(1):335–41.
17. Fujiyama K, Deguchi T, Murakami T, Fujii A, Kushima K, Takano-Yamamoto T. Clinical effect of CO_2 laser in reducing pain in orthodontics. Angle Orthod. 2008;78(2):299–303.
18. He WL, Li CJ, Liu ZP, Sun JF, Hu ZA, Yin X, et al. Efficacy of low-level laser therapy in the management of orthodontic pain: a systematic review and meta-analysis. Lasers Med Sci. 2013;28(6):1581–9.
19. Marini I, Bartolucci ML, Bortolotti F, Innocenti G, Gatto MR, Alessandri Bonetti G. The effect of diode superpulsed low-level laser therapy on experimental orthodontic pain caused by elastomeric separators: a randomized controlled clinical trial. Lasers Med Sci. 2013. [Epub ahead of print]
20. Zhang HY, Yan Y, Deng HY, Liu HX. Clinical therapeutic evaluation of low-level laser in alleviating pain during orthodontic elastomeric separator placement. Journal of Chinese Practical Diagnosis and Therapy. 2014;28(3):256–8.
21. Saygun I, Karacay S, Serdar M, Ural AU, Sencimen M, Kurtis B. Effects of laser irradiation on the release of basic fibroblast growth factor (bFGF), insulin like growth factor-1 (IGF-1), and receptor of IGF-1 (IGFBP3) from gingival fibroblasts. Lasers Med Sci. 2008;23(2):211–5.
22. Pallotta RC, Bjordal JM, Frigo L, Leal Junior EC, Teixeira S, Marcos RL, et al. Infrared (810-nm) low-level laser therapy on rat experimental knee inflammation. Lasers Med Sci. 2012;27(1):71–8.
23. Pinheiro AL, Gerbi ME. Photoengineering of bone repair processes. Photomed Laser Surg. 2006;24(2):169–78.
24. Sousa MV, Scavinini MA, Sannomiya EK, Velasco LG, Angelieri F. Influence of low-level laser on the speed of orthodontic movement. Photomed Laser Surg. 2011;29(3):191–6.
25. Fikáčková H, Dostálová T, Navrátil L, Klaschka J. Effectiveness of low-level laser therapy in temporomandibular joint disorders: a placebo-controlled study. Photomed Laser Surg. 2007;25(4):297–303.
26. Bjordal JM, Johnson MI, Iversen V, Aimbire F, Lopes-Martins RA. Low-level laser therapy in acute pain: a systematic review of possible mechanisms of action and clinical effects in randomized placebo-controlled trials. Photomed Laser Surg. 2006;24(2):158–68.
27. Higgins JPT, Green S, editors. Cochrane handbook for systematic reviews of interventions [version 5.1.0]. The Cochrane Collaboration. 2011.
28. Lim HM, Lew KK, Tay DK. A clinical investigation of the efficacy of low level laser therapy in reducing orthodontic postadjustment pain. Am J Orthod Dentofacial Orthop. 1995;108(6):614–22.
29. Esper MA, Nicolau RA, Arisawa EA. The effect of two phototherapy protocols on pain control in orthodontic procedure–a preliminary clinical study. Lasers Med Sci. 2011;26(5):657–63.
30. Abtahi SM, Mousavi SA, Shafaee H, Tanbakuchi B. Effect of low-level laser therapy on dental pain induced by separator force in orthodontic treatment. Dent Res J (Isfahan). 2013;10(5):647–51.

8

New regression equations for predicting human teeth sizes

Vanessa Paredes[1], Beatriz Tarazona[1*], Natalia Zamora[1], Rosa Cibrian[2] and Jose Luis Gandia[1]

Abstract

Introduction: The aims of the study were; to evaluate the applicability of the Moyers and Tanaka-Johnston Methods to individuals with a Spanish ancestry, to propose new regression equations using the lower four permanents incisors as predictors for the sum of the widths of the lower permanent canine and premolars, and to compare the new data to those from other populations.

Methods: A total of 359 Spanish ancestry adolescents were selected. Their dental casts were measured using a 2D computerized system. Real teeth measurements were compared with those predicted using Moyers probability tables and Tanaka and Johnston equations, and standard regression equations were then developed.

Results: Results showed that Upper and Lower Canine and Premolar (UCPM, LCPM) predictions are quite different depending on the used method. Moyers tables can only be validly applied to a 75% percentile for the mandible in both, males and females, 85% in males and 90-92% in females.

Conclusions: Moyers predictions tend to underestimate UCPM and LCPM whereas Tanaka-Johnston predictions tend to overestimate them. Equations for estimating the combined width of the unerupted canine and premolars were; Male: UCPM = 12.68 + 0.42 LI and LCPM = 11.71 + 0.44 LI. Female: UCPM = 12.06 + 0.43LI and LCPM = 10.71 + 0.46 LI.

Keywords: Moyers, Prediction, Regression equations, Tanaka-Johnston

Introduction

Predicting unerupted tooth size of Upper and Lower Canine and Premolars (UCPM, LCPM) in mixed dentition is important for a good diagnosis and for choosing a therapy [1]. To date, three basic groups have been used to determine the mesiodistal widths of unerupted canines and premolars.

1- Analyses based on correlation and regression equations, expressed as prediction tables. Both Moyers' regression scheme [2] and Tanaka and Johnston's equations [3] have achieved widespread clinical acceptance because of their simplicity and ease of application. 2- Analyses based on measurements taken from radiographs [4,5] of unerupted teeth. 3- Analyses based on a combination of correlations and regression equations and measurements on radiographs [6-8].

However, bearing in mind that these prediction methods are based on individuals of North American ancestry, it is not appropriate to use them on different populations of different biological origin. For this reason, several linear regression equations have been proposed for different populations [9-23].

Odontometric data from Spanish ancestry children are not so widely available and, to date, there is no study in the literature examining the accuracy of Moyers probability tables and Tanaka and Johnston equations in predicting the size of unerupted canines and premolars in a Spanish ancestry sample. The aims of the present study were, therefore, to evaluate the applicability of the Moyers and Tanaka-Johnston methods to Spanish ancestry individuals; to propose new regression equations using the lower four permanent incisors as predictors of the sum of the widths of the lower and upper permanent canine and premolars; and to compare the new data with those of other populations.

* Correspondence: beatriz.tarazona@hotmail.com
[1]Orthodontics Department, Faculty of Dentistry and Medicine, University of Valencia, Gasco Oliag nº1, 46010 Valencia, Spain
Full list of author information is available at the end of the article

Material and methods

500 patients attending the Orthodontics Department of the University of Valencia, Spain were chosen. Subjects presented to the orthodontic clinic in sequential order over a fixed period of time (January 2010-January 2012). A retrospective study was carried out and approved by the Ethics Committee of Research into Humans of the Experimental Research Ethics Committee at Valencia University, Spain. Reference number H1373014083626. All patients whose records were used in this work received detailed information about the study, reflected on an informed consent. There was also a confidentiality agreement stating that patients' personal data and their records would only be used for scientific purposes.

In order to predict unerupted teeth sizes under the best conditions, patient selection criteria were:

- Permanent dentition from first molar to first molar.
- Lower and upper first molar totally erupted and without the gingiva overlapping the distal surface of the tooth.
- Good quality casts.
- No tooth agenesis or extractions.
- No previous orthodontic treatment.
- No restorations or teeth with anomalous shapes that could change the mesiodistal diameter of the tooth or bruxism.
- Spanish ancestors from at least 1 previous generation (Spanish means people living in Spain, Europe with at least 1 previous generation of Spanish ancestors).
- Class I relationship with no arch discrepancy.

The Spanish ancestry sample finally included 359 patients (169 = 47.1% males and 190 = 52.9% females), with a mean age of 14.8 years (range 11.2-19.2) similar for both sex.

The power analysis showed that 359 patients were needed to achieve 90% power to detect clinically meaningful differences of the values. To compensate for possible dropouts during the study, more patients were we enrolled.

All the study casts were digitized with a conventional scanner and calibrated before any measurement was taken, using a simple method. In this calibration system, dental casts were surrounded by millimeter paper sheet. When the arches have been digitized, the magnification of the millimeter paper in the two axes is known and the dental cast magnification can be calculated [24]. A 2D digital software program designed by the University of Valencia, previously tested and found to be accurate and reliable [16], was used to determine dental sizes (in millimeters) of the lower four permanent incisors. With the aid of the mouse as a user interface, mesiodistal size of each permanent tooth on the image of the casts was marked. The software determines dental sizes in millimeters automatically.

The Tanaka and Johnston [3] equations used are as follow;

$$1/2 \text{MD Lower Incisors(LI)width} + 10.5\text{mm}$$
$$= \text{Estimated LCPM width} 1/2\text{MD Lower Incisors(LI)width}$$
$$+11.0\text{mm} = \text{Estimated UCPM width}$$

Statistical analysis

All statistical analyses were performed using the SPSS statistics package for Windows.

The descriptive analysis provides the relevant statistics for primary analysis variables: the mesiodistal sizes of the lower incisors (LI), the upper canine-premolars (UCPM) and lower canine-premolars (LCPM). The two latter ones are calculated as a mean of those recorded on both sides of each arch.

To evaluate the predictive power of the Moyers table, differences were calculated between the real values of those parameters (UCPM, LCPM) in the sample and those predicted by tables for percentiles in accordance with LI values. Likewise, the differences between the real values of the UCPM, LCPM and the values predicted by the Tanaka-Johnston [3] formula were calculated. For all of them, basic descriptive statistics and confidence levels of 95% are provided. All the mentioned information is segmented by sex, as sexual dimorphism is a key aspect of this investigation.

Regarding the inferential analysis undertaken, unpaired Student t-tests were applied to compare the mean equality hypothesis of UCPM and LCPM in males and females. The Student t-test for paired samples was applied to reach a conclusion over the equality of real mean values and estimated values, whether those of the Moyers' tables [2] or the Tanaka-Johnston equation [3]. Assumptions regarding normality of parameters and homogeneity of variances were checked by means of Kolmogorov-Smirnov and Levene's test respectively.

A simple linear regression analysis was developed to estimate, through least squares, the equation that relates the UCPM and LCPM to LI, in men and women. Correlation coefficients (r) and regression equations (y = a + bx) were formulated to evaluate the relationship between the summed widths of the 4 LI in millimeters (x, independent variable) and the canines and premolars (y, dependent variable), "a" the slope and "b" the intercept of each dental arch. Constants "a" and "b" in the standard linear regression equations (y = a + bx), determination coefficients (r^2), and the standard errors of the estimates (SEE) were calculated for combined sexes and for each sex separately. The r^2 value indicates the predictive accuracy of the regression equation for y based on values

Table 1 Mesiodistal Lower Incisor (LI), Upper Canine and Premolar (UCPM) and Lower Canine and Premolar (LCPM) tooth sizes per sex

			N	Mean ± SD(mm)	Minimum	Maximum	S. Error	CI 95%	P value
LI	Sex	T	359	23.04 ± 1.45	17.77	26.39	.08	22.89 – 23.19	
		M	169	23.04 ± 1.46	17.77	26.39	.11	22.82 – 23.26	n.s.
		F	190	23.03 ± 1.44	19.39	26.11	.10	22.83 – 23.24	
UCPM		T	359	22.11 ± 1.07	19.49	25.49	.06	21.99 – 22.22	
		M	169	22.31 ± 1.06	19.68	25.25	.08	22.15 – 22.47	**
		F	190	21.92 ± 1.04	19.49	25.49	.08	21.77 – 22.07	
LCPM		T	359	21.60 ± 1.12	18.37	24.62	.06	21.48 – 21.71	
		M	169	21.82 ± 1.11	19.35	24.62	.09	21.65 – 21.99	**
		F	190	21.40 ± 1.09	18.37	24.47	.08	21.25 – 21.56	

t-Test of independent samples for assessing homogeneity of measurements per sex. n.s = notsignificant; ** = $p < 0.01$. Male + Female(Total); Male(M) and Female(F).

of x. Hypothesis of normality; homoscedasticity and no autocorrelation of residuals were checked. Re-estimation of equations was carried up in 75% of the sample in order to check its acceptance at an independent sample (25% remaining).

Results

The reproducibility of the digital method was analysed by determining intra- and inter-examiner measurement errors, calculated by coefficients of variation (CVs = standard deviation- 100/mean) expressed as a percentage. Twenty dental casts from the present study were randomly selected. The measurements of the twenty dental casts were again determined by the same examiner (VP) (intra-examiner error) and by two different examiners (RC and JLG) (inter-examiner error) in order to obtain the CV. All CVs were very low (below 5.8 per cent) and similar between examiners. Digital methods CVs were 0.05 – 2.88

Table 2 The difference(mm) between the mean values of real Upper and Lower Canine and Premolar (UCPM, LCPM) tooth sizes and those predicted from Moyers' charts per sex

Percentile level %	Sex								
	T			M			F		
	N	Mean difference ± SD(mm)	P value	N	Mean difference ± SD	P	N	Mean difference ± SD	P
UCPM 5	348	2.65 ± 0.95	***	161	2.24 ± 0.87	***	187	3.00 ± 0.87	***
15		2.06 ± 0.92	***		1.73 ± 0.87	***		2.35 ± 0.87	***
25		1.73 ± 0.91	***		1.43 ± 0.87	***		1.98 ± 0.87	***
35		1.44 ± 0.90	***		1.16 ± 0.87	***		1.68 ± 0.87	***
50		1.08 ± 0.90	***		0.84 ± 0.87	***		1.28 ± 0.87	***
65		0.72 ± 0.89	***		0.53 ± 0.87	***		0.88 ± 0.87	***
75		0.43 ± 0.88	***		0.27 ± 0.87	***		0.57 ± 0.86	***
85		0.10 ± 0.87	*		−0.03 ± 0.87	n.s.		0.21 ± 0.86	**
95		−0.49 ± 0,.87	***		−0.55 ± 0.87	***		−0.44 ± 0.86	***
LCPM 5	348	2.74 ± 0.88	***	161	2.65 ± 0.90	***	187	2.81 ± 0.86	***
15		2.02 ± 0.88	***		1.95 ± 0.90	***		2.07 ± 0.86	***
25		1.58 ± 0.88	***		1.51 ± 0.90	***		1.64 ± 0.86	***
35		1.24 ± 0.88	***		1.16 ± 0.90	***		1.30 ± 0.86	***
50		0.79 ± 0.88	***		0.72 ± 0.90	***		0.84 ± 0.86	***
65		0.32 ± 0.88	***		0.26 ± 0.90	***		0.37 ± 0.86	***
75		−0.01 ± 0.88	n.s.		−0.06 ± 0.90	n.s.		0.03 ± 0.86	n.s.
85		−0.44 ± 0.88	***		−0.50 ± 0.90	***		−0.39 ± 0.86	***
95		−1.18 ± 0.88	***		−1.24 ± 0.90	***		−1.12 ± 0.86	***

t-Test of dependent samples for assessing homogeneity of measurements between the real values of the sample and those predicted by Moyers. n.s = not significant; * = $p < 0.05$; ** = $p < 0.01$; *** = $p < 0.001$. Male + Female(Total); Male(M) and Female(F).

Table 3 The difference (mm) between the mean values of real Upper and Lower Canine and Premolar(UCPM, LCPM) tooth sizes and those predicted from Tanaka-Johnston's equations per sex

	Sex								
	T			M			F		
	N	Mean difference ± SD(mm)	P	N	Mean ± SD	P	N	Mean ± SD	P
UCPM	359	−0.41 ± 0.88	***	169	−0.21 ± 0.88	**	190	−0.59 ± 0.85	***
LCPM		−0.42 ± 0.91	***		−0.20 ± 0.91	**		−0.61 ± 0.86	***

t-Test of dependent samples for assessing homogeneity of measurements between the realand predicted values of the sample. n.s = not significant; ** = p < 0.01; *** = p < 0.001.Male + Female(Total); Male(M) and Female(F).

and 0.16 – 5.70 per cent for intra- and inter-examiner calibrations, respectively.

Since right and left side values are highly correlated (and non-independent) within individuals, mean of right and left side values was chosen in these statistical comparisons. Table 1 presents descriptive information on LI, UCPM and LCPM, sizes segmented by sex.

The first method used for prediction was Moyers' tables. Table 2 provides the descriptive statistics for the difference in mm between the real values and those estimated by Moyers for the UCPM and LCPM, for the different percentile levels. For this analysis, those individuals whose LI values were either below or above the Moyers' limits (1 and 10 respectively) were excluded, a margin of 0.25 mm. being accepted. Hence the effective sample in this section consisted of 348 cases. Moyers' values systematically tend to underestimate the real values in the Spanish population.

The second method used was Tanaka-Johnston regression equations. For that, the difference between the real value and the predicted value was calculated using these equations for the UCPM and LCPM sizes (Table 3). In contrast to Moyers' tables, these equations tend to overestimate the real values of the UCPM and LCPM sizes in the Spanish population. Thirdly, estimation from an own regression equation was proposed. Table 4 summarises the results of the 6 regression models undertaken: total maxilla, male maxilla, female maxilla, total mandible, male mandible and female mandible. The equations for

estimating the combined width of the unerupted canine and premolars were:

$$\text{Males}: \text{UCPM} = 12.68 + 0.42\text{LI and LCPM}$$
$$= 11.71 + 0.44\text{LI}$$
$$\text{Females}: \text{UCPM} = 12.06 + 0.43\text{LI and LCPM}$$
$$= 10.71 + 0.46\text{LI}$$

These regression equations allow the construction of a basic table of predictions to be constructed according to arch and sex, as showed in Table 5.

Table 6 presents a comparison of regression constants among different populations including the own sample.

Finally, in Figure 1, predictions of the three methods are compared; estimated regression lines, Moyers tables at 50% and at 85%, and the Tanaka-Johnston Rule.

Table 4 Regression parameters for predictions of UCPM and LCPM tooth sizes in each arch and per sex

			Constants				
			r	a	b	SEE	r²
UCPM	T		0.574	12.34***	0.42***	0.87	0.330
	Sex	M	0.574	12.68***	0.42***	0.87	0.330
		F	0.592	12.06***	0.43***	0.84	0.351
LCPM	T		0.587	11.17***	0.45***	0.91	0.345
	Sex	M	0.577	11.71***	0.44***	0.91	0.333
		F	0.616	10.71***	0.46***	0.86	0.379

r (Pearson linear regression coefficients); a and b, regression equation coefficients y = a + bx; SEE (standard error of estimate); r2, coefficient of determination. n.s. not significant;*** p < 0.001. Male + Female(Total); Male(M) and Female(F).

Table 5 Prediction table for the Spanish population based on regression equations

LI (mm)	UCPM(mm)			LCPM(mm)		
	T	M	F	T	M	F
19	20.32	20.66	20.23	19.72	20.07	19.45
19.5	20.53	20.87	20.45	19.95	20.29	19.68
20	20.74	21.08	20.66	20.17	20.51	19.91
20.5	20.95	21.29	20.88	20.40	20.73	20.14
21	21.16	21.50	21.09	20.62	20.95	20.37
21.5	21.37	21.71	21.31	20.85	21.17	20.60
22	21.58	21.92	21.52	21.07	21.39	20.83
22.5	21.79	22.13	21.74	21.30	21.61	21.06
23	22.00	22.34	21.95	21.52	21.83	21.29
23.5	22.21	22.55	22.17	21.75	22.05	21.52
24	22.42	22.76	22.38	21.97	22.27	21.75
24.5	22.63	22.97	22.60	22.20	22.49	21.98
25	22.84	23.18	22.81	22.42	22.71	22.21
25.5	23.05	23.39	23.03	22.65	22.93	22.44
26	23.26	23.60	23.24	22.87	23.15	22.67
26.5	23.47	23.81	23.46	23.10	23.37	22.90

Lower Incisors (LI), Upper and Lower Canines and Premolars (UCPM, LCPM) tooth sizes. Male + Female(Total); Male(M) and Female(F).

Table 6 Regression parameters for predicting UCPM and LCPM tooth sizes in each arch and per sex

Study	Population	Sample (n)	Sex	Arch	Constants				
					r	a	b	SEE	r²
Tanaka and Jhonston [3]	North American Whites	T = 506	M + F	Mx	0.63	10.41	0.51	0.86	0.35
			M + F	Mb	0.65	9.18	0.54	0.85	0.42
Al khadra [9]	Saudi Arabian	T = 34	M + F	Mx	0.65	7.20	0.63	-	0.42
			M + F	Mb	-	8.60	0.55	-	0.40
Diagne et al [14]	Senegalese	25(M) + 25(F)	M + F	Mx	0.68	9.87	0.53	0.71	0.46
		=50	M + F	Mb	0.73	5.67	0.70	0.81	0.54
Frankel and Benz [21]	Black Americans	39(M) + 41(F)	M + F	Mx	0.65	10.18	0.52	0.87	0.42
		T = 80	M + F	Mb	0.70	8.30	0.64	0.94	0.49
Jaroontham and Godfrey [12]	Northeastern Thai	215(M) + 215(F)	M + F	Mx	0.60	11.87	0.47	0.84	0.36
		T = 430	M + F	Mb	0.64	10.30	0.50	0.82	0.41
Melgaco et al [15]	White Brazilians	240(M) + 223(F)	F	Mx	0.69	9.20	0.55	-	0.48
		=500	M	Mb	0.70	8.90	0.58	-	0.50
Nourallah et al [13]	Syrians	320(M) + 280(F)	M + F	Mx	0.67	9.87	0.50	0.79	0.45
		T = 600	M + F	Mb	0.68	9.32	0.55	0.83	0.46
Uysal et al [17]	Turkish	100(M) + 128(F)	M + F	Mx	0.99	4.07	0.76	0.01	0.98
		T = 228	M + F	Mb	0.99	3.74	0.75	0.01	0.98
Paredes et al. (this study)	Spanish	169(M) + 190(F)	M + F	Mx	0.574	12.34	0.42	0.87	0.330
		T = 359	M + F	Mb	0.587	11.17	0.45	0.91	0.345
Bherwani and Fida [19]	Pakistani	100(M) + 100(F)	M + F	Mx	0.65	8.56	0.54	0.79	0.42
		T =200	M + F	Mb	0.59	10.52	0.48	0.82	0.35
Yuen et al [10]	Hong Kong Chinese	61(M) + 51(F)	M + F	Mx	0.72	8.13	0.63	0.74	0.52
		T = 112	M + F	Mb	0.73	7.74	0.61	0.71	0.53
Abu Alhaija et al [23]	Jordanian	130(M) + 96(F)	M + F	Mx	0.57	10.55	0.53	0.99	0.32
		T = 226	M + F	Mb	0.59	9.41	0.56	0.99	0.35
Philip NI et al [18]	Indian	300(M) + 300(F)	M + F	Mx	0.65	7.29	0.65	0.43	0.76
		T = 600	M + F	Mb	0.67	5.85	0.69	0.45	0.75
Chan et al [11]	Asian Americans	T = 201	M + F	Mx	0.64	8.19	0.63	0.90	0.41
			M + F	Mb	0.66	7.46	0.62	0.85	0.44
Tahere et al [22]	Iranian	25(M) + 25 F)	M + F	Mx	0.53	11.06	0.45	0.80	0.28
		T = 50	M + F	Mb	0.70	6.42	0.64	0.70	0.49

r (Pearson linear regression coefficients); a and b, regression equation coefficients y = a + bx; SEE, r², coefficient of determination. Male + Female (Total); Male(M) and Female(F) of different populations. Mx (maxilla) and Mb (mandible).

Discussion

No statistically significant differences between males and females were found for LI mesiodistal size, unlike those of UCPM and LCPM, where males presented statistically higher mesiodistal sizes than females. These results for the LI agree with studies published on Chinese [10] and Indian [18] populations, but are contrary to studies on Brazilian [15], Pakistani [19], Turkish [17] or Thai [12] populations, where statistically significant differences were found in LI sizes, as well as in UCPM and LCPM sizes.

Moyers Tables [2] are classified from the 95th to 5th prediction level. The most practical level from the

clinical point of view is the 75th level, although in theory the 50th level of probability should be used, as any error will be evenly distributed in either direction.

Taking the prediction of upper arch at total level into account, as showed in Table 2, all differences are positive, indicating that the Moyer's Tables tend to underestimate the real values of the UCPM in the sample of Spanish individuals, apart from for the 95% level. Practically, statistically significant differences were found at all confidence levels apart from those for males at the 85% confidence level, where no statistically significant difference was found and thus, homogeneity can be accepted. In females, homogeneity

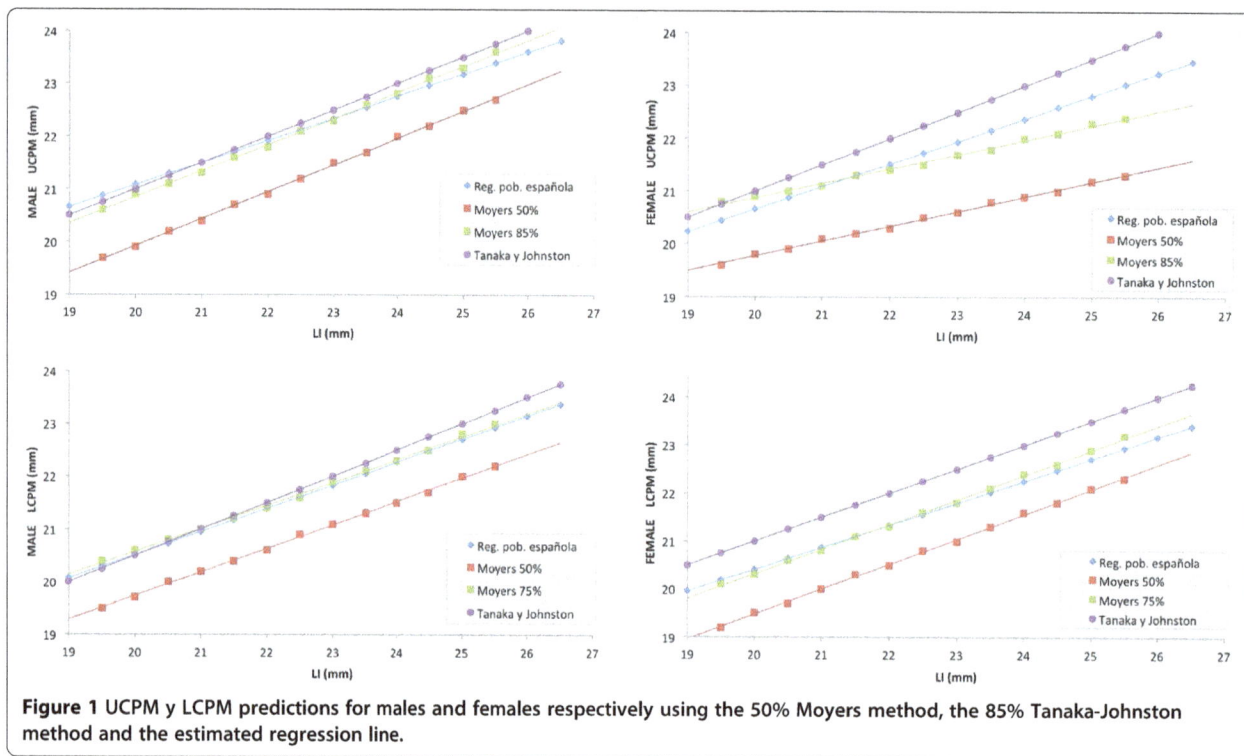

Figure 1 UCPM y LCPM predictions for males and females respectively using the 50% Moyers method, the 85% Tanaka-Johnston method and the estimated regression line.

may be verified for a slightly higher percentile of around 90%.

Regarding the lower arch, the applicability of Moyer's [2] tables is only useful for the 75th percentile, both at total level and for each sex where no statistically significant differences were found, contrary to all the other levels evaluated. Generally speaking, it can be stated that Moyer's values systematically tend to underestimate real values in the Spanish population. These results coincide with studies in a Brazilian population [15] at the 50th and 75th percentile levels and in a Jordanian population [23] except for the 65th and 75th percentile for female subjects and the 85th for male subjects, in a Pakistani population [19] and for South Indian children [18]. On the other hand, Saudi Arabian population [9] studies found that the recommended 75th percentile overestimated the mesiodistal sizes of canine and premolars.

Estimates obtained from the Tanaka-Johnston equation [3] produced several equally disputable results as both at the mandible and maxilla level, in both males and females, the predictions tended to overestimate the real UCPM and LCPM sizes of individuals, with all the discrepancies found being statistically significant. These results coincide with those of other authors on Iranian [22] and Pakistani [19] populations, whereas they differ from those on a Jordanian population [23], where the regression equations underestimated the real teeth value.

Finally, as it can be observed, adjustment for regression presents quite similar accuracy regardless of the arch and

sex of patients, even though it tends to be slightly greater among females, as showed in other studies.

Pearson's linear correlation coefficient (r) ranges from between 0.57 and 0.61 depending on combinations. Therefore, the proportion of total variance of the UCPM or LCPM variable explained by the LI, ranges from between 33.3% and 37.9%. SSE denotes the standard error in the predictions that were obtained with the corresponding regression equation. This fluctuates in the range of 0.84-0.91. The above mentioned equations presented a degree of accuracy similar to studies performed on Saudi-Arabians [9], Hong Kong Chinese [10], Asian Americans [11], North-Eastern Thais [12], Syrians [13], Senegalese [14], white Brazilians [15], Indian [18], Pakistani [19], black Americans [21], Iranian [22] and Jordanian [23] individuals, but lower than for the Turkish population [17] as can be seen in Table 6. The reason may lie in a greater dispersion of the CPM spaces belonging to the dental morphology of the individuals of the studied group. Likewise, it can be observed that the mandibular arch obtained higher "r" values than the maxillar in almost all of the studied populations. However, the validity of some data can be questioned due to the sample sizes of some studies.

Analysing Figure 1, the part corresponding to the UCPM for males, it can be observed that the line for the regression equation is the one better fitting the reality of the sample. It can be seen that up to LI values of around 23.5-24 mm, the predicted UCPM is greater than that estimated by Moyer's [2] at 85% and by Tanaka-Johnston [3]. However, from 24 mm upwards the trend is reversed. In contrast, predictions for females present a clearly different pattern from those of males. With the exception of the lowest LI values, the predictions obtained with the regression model are situated at an intermediate level between the underestimate of Moyers [2] at 85% and the overestimate of Tanaka and Johnston [3].

For predictions of LCPM in males, the different methods present similar estimation lines to those of the UCPM. For predictions of LCPM in females, the graphic is again very similar to that of the UCPM, with the exception of the Moyers predictions at 75% that graphically present a very homogenous line to that of the regression line drawn up for the Spanish population. It can also be observed in the four graphics that Tanaka-Johnston method tends to overestimate more than other methods, UCPM and LCPM values.

Teeth size differ among people of various biological origins, tooth sizes differ. Some of the most used methods to predict the size of unerupted posterior permanent teeth were developed for North Americans ancestry, so the applicability and the effectiveness of these methods in others populations are inadequate, hence the need to draw up tables for each population.

Conclusions

The conclusions of the study are:

1. Predictions of UCPM and LCPM sizes from LI for the Spanish ancestry population are evaluated quite differently depending on the used method.
2. Moyer's tables tend to underestimate UCPM and LCPM in Spanish ancestry subjects, only being of use at the 75% level percentile for the mandible, both in males and females, and for the maxilla at the 85% and 90% level percentile for males and females respectively.
3. Estimates obtained from the Tanaka-Johnston equation tend to overestimate UCPM and LCPM sizes in Spanish ancestry subjects.
4. The equations for estimating the combined width of the unerupted canine and premolars are:

$$\text{Males} : \text{UCPM} = 12.68 + 0.42\text{LI and LCPM}$$
$$= 11.71 + 0.44\text{LI}$$
$$\text{Females} : \text{UCPM} = 12.06 + 0.43\text{LI and LCPM}$$
$$= 10.71 + 0.46\text{LI}$$

Competing interests
All other authors declare that they have no competing interests.

Authors' contributions
All authors contributed extensively to the work presented in this paper. JLG provided the idea for the project. VP and BT treated the patients orthodontically and contributed to the writing. NZ recruited the participants, collected the data, and compiled all medical records and RC carried out the statistical analyses. All authors approved the manuscript prior to submission.

Author details
[1]Orthodontics Department, Faculty of Dentistry and Medicine, University of Valencia, Gasco Oliag nº1, 46010 Valencia, Spain. [2]Physiology Department, Faculty of Medicine and Dentistry, University of Valencia, Spain, Valencia, Spain.

References

1. Irwin RD, Herold JS, Richardson A. Mixed dentition analysis: a review of methods and their accuracy. Int J Pediatr Dent. 1995;5:137–42.
2. Moyers RE. Handbook of Orthodontics. 3rd ed. Chicago, IL: Mosby Year Book; 1973. p. 230–40.
3. Tanaka MM, Johnston LE. The prediction of the size of unerupted canines and premolars in a contemporary orthodontic population. J Am Dent Assoc. 1974;88:798–801.
4. Nance HN. The limitation of Orthodontic treatment I. Mixed dentition diagnosis and treatment. Am J Orthod Oral Surg. 1947;33:177–233.
5. De Paula S, Almeida de Oliveira MA, Lee PCF. Prediction of mesiodistal diameter of unerupted lower canines and premolars using 45° cephalometric radiography. Am J Orthod Dentofacial Orthop. 1995;107:309–14.
6. Hixon EH, Oldfather RE. Estimation of the sizes of unerupted cuspid and bicuspid teeth. Angle Orthod. 1958;28:236–40.
7. Bishara SE, Staley RN. Mixed dentition mandibular arch analysis. Am J Orthod. 1984;86:130–5.
8. Staley RN, Kerber RE. A review of the Hixon and Oldfather mixed dentition prediction Method. Am J Orthod Dentofacial Orthop. 1980;78:296–302.
9. Al-Khadra BH. Prediction of the size of unerupted canines and premolars in a Saudi Arab population. Am J Orthod Dentofacial Orthop. 1993;104:369–72.
10. Yuen KK, Tang EL, So LL. Mixed dentition analysis for Hong-Kong Chinese. Angle Orthod. 1998;68:21–8.
11. Lee-Chan S, Jacobson BN, Chwa KH, Jacobson RS. Mixed dentition analysis for Asian Americans. Am J Orthod Dentofacial Orthop. 1998;113:293–9.
12. Jaroontham J, Godfrey K. Mixed dentition space analysis in a Thai population. Eur J Orthod. 2000;22:127–34.
13. Nourallah AW, Gesch D, Khordaji MN, Splieth C. New regressions equations for predicting the size of unerupted canines and premolars in a contemporary population. Angle Orthod. 2002;72:216–21.
14. Diagne F, Diop-Ba K, Ngom PI, Mbow K. Mixed dentition analysis in Senegalese population: elaboration of prediction tables. Am J Orthod Dentofacial Orthop. 2003;124:178–83.
15. Melgaço CA, Araújo MT, Ruellas AC. Applicability of three tooth size prediction methods for white Brazilians. Angle Orthod. 2006;76:644–9.
16. Paredes V, Gandia JL, Cibrian R. A new, accurate and fast digital method to predict unerupted tooth size. Angle Orthod. 2006;76:14–9.
17. Uysal T, Bascifici FA, Goyenc Y. New regression equations for mixed-dentition arch analysis in a Turkish sample with no Bolton tooth-size discrepancy. Am J Orthod Dentofacial Orthop. 2009;135:343–8.
18. Philip NI, Prabhakar M, Arora D, Chopra S. Applicability of the Moyers mixed dentition probability tables and new prediction aids for a contemporary population in India. Am J Orthod Dentofacial Orthop. 2010;138:339–45.
19. Bherwani AK, Fida M. Development of a prediction equation for the mixed dentition in a Pakistani sample. Am J Orthod Dentofacial Orthop. 2011;14:626–32.
20. Paredes V, Williams FD, Cibrian R, Williams FE, Meneses A, Gandia JL. Mesiodistal sizes and intermaxillary tooth-size ratios of two populations; Spanish and Peruvian. A comparative study. Med Oral Patol Oral Cir Bucal. 2011;16:e593–9.
21. Frankel HH, Benz EM. Mixed dentition analysis for black Americans. Pediatr Dent. 1986;8:226–30.
22. Nik Tahere H, Majid S, Fateme M, Kharazi Fard K, Javad M. Predicting the size of unerupted canines and premolars of the maxillary quadrants in an Iranian population. J Clin Pediatr Dent. 2007;32:43–8.
23. Abu Alhaija ES, Qudeimat MA. Mixed dentition space analysis in a Jordanian population: comparison of two methods. Int J Paediatr Dent. 2006;16:104–10.

9

Effects of a novel magnetic orthopedic appliance (MOA-III) on the dentofacial complex in mild to moderate skeletal class III children

Ning Zhao[*], Jing Feng, Zheng Hu, Rongjing Chen and Gang Shen

Abstract

Introduction: The objective of this study was to evaluate the changes of skeletal and dental structures in mild to moderate skeletal Class III children following the use of a new magnetic orthopedic appliance (MOA-III).

Methods: A total of 36 patients (14 boys and 22 girls, mean age 9 years and 5 months) who presented with a mild to moderate skeletal Class III jaw discrepancy were treated with MOA-III. Another group of 20 untreated patients (9 boys and 11 girls, mean age 9 years and 2 months) with the same level of deformity served as the control group. The average treatment time was 6.6 months. Radiographs were taken at the same time intervals for both groups. A paired t test was used to determine the significant differences before and after treatment, and a two-sample t test was used to analyze the differences between the treatment and control groups.

Results: The anterior crossbite in all subjects was corrected after MOA-III therapy. The maxillomandibular relationship showed favorable changes (ANB, Wits, overjet increased significantly, $P < 0.001$). The maxilla was anteriorly positioned (SNA, ptm-A, ptm-S increased significantly, $P < 0.001$) with clockwise rotation (PP-FH increased, $P < 0.001$). The mandible showed a slight downward and backward rotation (SNB decreased, $P < 0.05$, MP-SN, Y-axis increased, $P < 0.05$). The length of the mandibular body showed no significant changes (Go-Pg, $P > 0.05$). Significant upper incisor proclination and lower incisor retroclination were observed (UI-NA increased, $P < 0.001$, LI-NB, FMIA decreased, $P < 0.001$). The upper lip moved forward, and the lower lip moved backward (UL-EP increased, $P < 0.001$, LL-EP decreased, $P < 0.05$). In the control group, most of the parameters showed normal growth, except for some unfavorable mandibular skeletal and soft tissue changes (Go-Pg, Go-Co, MP-SN, N'-SN-Pg' increased, $P < 0.001$). Significant positive changes were induced with the MOA-III appliance compared to the untreated group.

Conclusions: The MOA-III was effective for the early treatment of a mild to moderate Class III malocclusion in children.

Keywords: Magnetic, Twin-block, Angle Class III, Adolescent

Introduction

Skeletal Class III anomalies are associated with maxillary retrusion, mandibular protrusion, or both. In growing children, treatment may involve the stimulation of maxillary growth and restriction of mandibular growth by orthopedic forces.

Among the armamentarium for the early treatment of class III malocclusion, the chin cup, facemask, and reverse pull headgear are classical orthopedic appliances [1]. However, these appliances need an extraoral apparatus to create heavy orthopedic forces. These appliances are not convenient for patients to wear, and the patients cannot usually guarantee that they will wear them for a sufficient period of time because of their aesthetics. Therefore, the development of new types of intraoral orthopedic appliances to resolve these problems is necessary.

With the introduction of high energy rare earth permanent magnets in the late fifties and early sixties ($SmCO_5$, Sm_2Co_{17}) [2], the application of small magnets to create sufficiently high orthopedic forces in the limit-spaced oral cavity became possible. Neodymium iron boron ($Nd_2Fe_{14}B$) is a new generation high energy rare earth permanent magnet with a high magnetic flux density in relation to its small size. Because of the characteristics

* Correspondence: zhaon1995@126.com
Department of Orthodontics, Shanghai Key Laboratory of Stomatology, Shanghai No. 9 Hospital, ShanghaiJiaotong University School of Medicine, Shanghai, China

of magnetic forces, magnets became another choice to produce the predictive forces used in the field of orthodontics. Blechman and Smiley [3] first moved canines distally using magnetic forces in a cat model in 1978, and since then, magnets have been used in both research and clinical practice. Attractive magnetic forces have been used in closing the diastemas [4], dealing with unerupted or impacted teeth [5–7], intruding posterior teeth [8, 9], moving teeth [10], and manufacturing magnetic edgewise brackets [11]. They were also incorporated into several functional appliances [12–16] to produce orthopedic forces. Repulsive magnetic forces were used for molar distalization [17–19] and palatal expansion [20, 21], and some appliances were used for the treatment of an open bite [22–25] or Class III malocclusion [26].

In this study, we developed a new magnetic orthopedic appliance (MOA-III) using attractive forces at our University. The objective of this study was to examine the craniofacial and dentoalveolar changes in subjects with mild to moderate skeletal class III malocclusion after treatment with this appliance.

Methods
Appliance design
The MOA-III appliance was constructed from upper and lower removable appliances with two $7 \times 5 \times 4$ mm³ $Nd_2Fe_{14}B$ magnetic units bonded to each appliance (Fig. 1). The two magnetic units were in the attracting configuration. Figure 2 shows the relationship between the forces and distances with 5×4 mm² interfaces overlapped, with 1/3 offset and 2/3 offset. The upper magnets were located at the position of the first premolar and bonded to the appliance with two expansion screws,

and the lower magnets were positioned labially to the lower canine. The expansion screws were opened to maximum when the appliances were manufactured. After insertion of the MOA-III, the appliances were adjusted by closing the screws to maintain the distances between the paired magnets on both sides. The initial force was 300 g per side when the patients were at the maximal mouth closure position and the two opposing magnets were approximately 1.2 mm apart. The directions of forces were parallel to the occlusal plane. The magnets were conformal coated with Parylene C and encapsulated in dental acrylic, and the opposing poles were covered with a thin layer of acrylic (approximately 0.3-mm thickness). The patients were recalled for an examination two weeks after the first MOA-III delivery. The appointment intervals then were adjusted to four weeks, and screw reactivations were performed by parents one turn each week (0.25 mm/week).

Case selection
A total of 36 patients (14 boys and 22 girls) complaining of concave profiles or prominent lower jaws by their parents or themselves were included in this study. Their ages ranged from 7.9 to 11.6 years of age, and the average age was 9.5 years (the mean treatment period was 6.6 months). Another 20 patients (9 boys and 11 girls) without treatment served as the control group. Their ages ranged from 7.6 to 11.2 years of age, and the average age was 9.2 years. In most cases, the treatment was postponed for the control group due to the presence of primary molars. The patients in this group were informed that they would receive their treatment after six months. The selection of the cases (treatment and

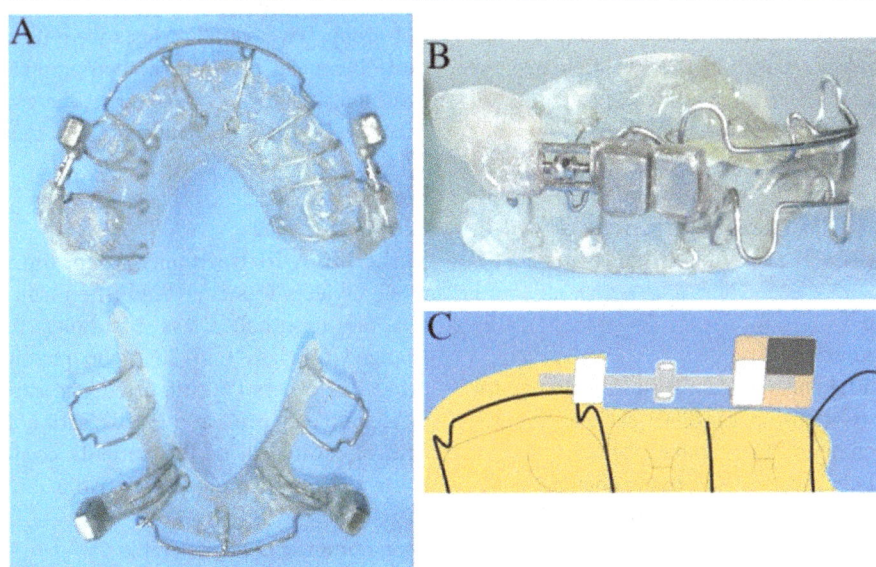

Fig. 1 Upper and lower appliance of MOA (**a**), Attractive configuration of magnets extraorally (**b**), Schematic view of appliance of MOA (**c**)

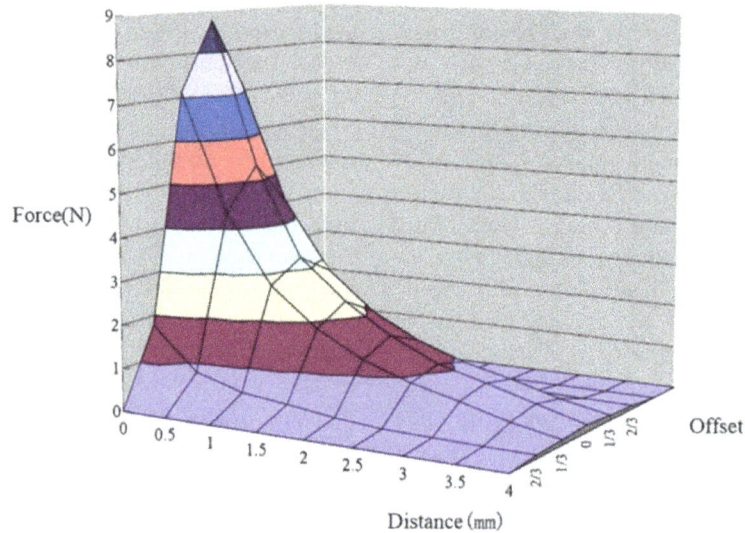

Fig. 2 Attractive forces produced between two $7 \times 5 \times 4$ mm^3 Nd$_2$Fe$_{14}$B magnets

control groups) was based on the following criteria: ①
0°›ANB›-3°; ②Wits distance‹0 mm; ③Angle`s class III
molar relationship with anterior cross-bite; ④ with some
anterior dental compensation, the upper incisor proclined labially and the lower incisor retroclined lingually,
but there were no obviously transverse discrepancies
and no need of maxillary expansion; ⑤ the patients
could not retrude to edge to edge; and ⑥ without cleft
palate or craniofacial syndrome.

Intraoral and extraoral pictures, model casts, and standardized panoramic and cephalometric radiographs were
taken at the same time intervals for both groups.

The ethics committee of Ninth People's Hospital affili-
ated to Shanghai Jiao Tong University, School of Medicine
(Reference No: HE25MAR2012-D03326) approved this
study. The treatment procedure in this research met the
WMA Declaration of Helsinki - Ethical Principles for
Medical Research Involving Human Subjects.

Written informed consent for all participants in this
study was obtained from the patients and their parents
or guardians. The photo release letters were signed by
the parents of the patients presented in this paper.

Radiograph method
Cephalometric measurement
We selected 40 sagittal and vertical measurements for the
maxillomandibular relationship, maxillary skeletal changes,
maxillary dental changes, mandibular dental changes,
mandibular skeletal changes and soft tissue changes to determine the dentofacial effects created by the MOA-III
treatment. The reference points and lines are shown in
Fig. 3, and the cephalometric measurements are shown in
Table 1.

Statistical methods and method error (ME) analysis
The error of the stated and calculated method values were
determined by retracing the radiographs with Dahlberg's
formula, $ME = \sqrt{\dfrac{\sum d^2}{2n}}$. The cephalometric radiographs were traced and evaluated twice by two independent orthodontists (N Z and Z H) on two separate
occasions approximately two months apart. There were
no significant differences between the two repeated measurements at the two assessment times ($P > 0.05$).

Paired t tests were performed with SPSS (Statistical Package for Social Sciences, Chicago, Illinois, USA) 15.0 for
Windows to evaluate the significant differences between the
pre- and the post-treatment groups and changes in the control group. Two-sample t tests were used to detect significant differences between the two groups by comparing the
treatment-induced changes versus the growth-only-induced
changes. The level of significance was set at $P < 0.05$.

Results
Occlusal changes
In the MOA-III treatment group, the anterior crossbite
in all subjects was corrected (the mean treatment period
was 6.6 months). Class III molar relationships were
changed to class I in 32 of 36 patients and were improved in others. We reported one case to show the effects between pre- and post-treatment (Fig. 4). In the
control group, all of the patients continued to demonstrate a Class III molar relationship.

Cephalometric changes (Table 1)
In the maxilla, sagittally, many measurements were
significantly increased as follows: ANB ($P < 0.001$),

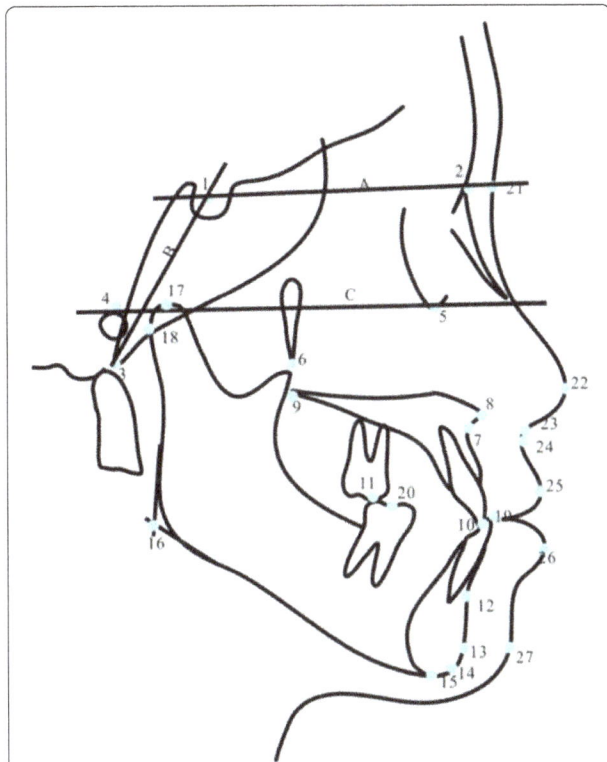

Fig. 3 Reference points and reference lines. Reference points: (1) Sella (S), (2) Nasion (N), (3) Basion (Ba), (4) Porion (P), (5) Orbitale (Or), (6) Pterygomaxillary fissure (Ptm), (7) Point A (A), (8) anterior nasal spine (ANS), (9) Posterior nasal spine (PNS), (10) Upper incisor (UI), (11) Upper first molar (U6), (12) Point B, (13) Pogonion (Pog), (14) Gnathion (Gn), (15) Menton (Me), (16) Gonion (Go), (17) Condylion (Co), (18) Articulare (Ar), (19) Lower incisor (LI), (20) Lower first molar (L6), (21) Nasion of soft tissue (N'), (22) Pronasale (Prn), (23) Subnasale (Sn), (24) Point A of soft tissue (A'), (25) Upper labrale (UL), (26) Lower labrale (LL), and (27) Pogonion of soft tissue (Pg'). Reference lines of hard the tissues: (A) Anterior cranial base plane (SN), (B) Cranial base plane (N-Ba), and (C) Frankfort horizontal plane (FH)

Wits ($P < 0.001$), overjet ($P < 0.001$). SNA ($P < 0.001$), Ptm-A ($P < 0.001$), Ptm-S ($P < 0.001$) and N-ANS ($P < 0.001$). Vertically, the FMA ($P < 0.001$) and Y-axis angle ($P < 0.001$) increased significantly. The overbite deepened significantly ($P < 0.01$), but the ANS-Me ($P > 0.05$), ANS-Me/N-Me ($P > 0.05$) and S-Go/N-Me ($P > 0.05$) showed no significant changes. The PP-FH ($P < 0.001$) and OP-SN ($P < 0.001$) were rotated clockwise significantly. The upper incisors and molars also showed some significant changes. The UI-NA ($P < 0.001$) and UI-AP ($P < 0.001$) increased significantly. The upper first molar moved forward significantly, with U6-PTM ($P < 0.01$). Vertically, the UI-PP ($P < 0.01$) increased significantly, but the U6-PP showed no significant difference ($P > 0.05$). For the lower, the SNB angle ($P < 0.001$) and Pcd-S ($P < 0.001$) significantly decreased. The length of the mandibular body showed no significant changes (Go-Pg, $P > 0.05$). However,

the length of the mandibular ramous showed a significant increase (Go-Co, $P < 0.001$). The LI-NB ($P < 0.001$), LI-AP ($P < 0.001$), and FMIA ($P < 0.001$) decreased significantly, although there were no significant changes in the LI-MP ($P > 0.05$) and L6-MP ($P > 0.05$). Much of the soft tissue also showed significant changes. The UL-EP ($P < 0.001$), LL-EP ($P < 0.01$), and UL-A'-FH ($P < 0.01$) increased significantly. The LL-EP ($P < 0.01$) and N'-Sn-Pg' ($P < 0.001$) decreased significantly. The Z-angle ($P > 0.05$) showed no significant difference.

In the control group, all of the patients continued to demonstrate a class III molar relationship, and most of the cephalometric measurements showed no significant difference. However, the mandibular skeletal measurements and soft tissue measurement showed significant changes. The SNB、Go-Pg、and Pcd-S showed a significant increase ($P < 0.05$). For the soft tissue measurement, the LL-EP, UL-A'-FH, N'-Pg'-FH, and N'-SN-Pg' increased ($P < 0.01$) and the UL-EP decreased ($P < 0.01$) (Table 2). Comparison of the treated and untreated control group showed that ANB, Wits, overjet, Ptm-A, N-ANS, PP-FH, UI-NA, LI-NB, LI-AP, FMIA, UL-EP, and N'-SN-Pg'changed significantly ($P < .001$) (Table 3).

Discussion

Rare-earth magnets, which generate static magnetic fields, have been advantageously used as a 'force source' in orthodontic treatments, such as molar distalization, palatal expansion, and impacted tooth movement [4–10]. There is little evidence regarding the biological safety of static magnetic field application. Some studies suggested that static magnetic fields may increase the rate of bone repair [35] and new bone deposition [33] and may also prevent decreases in bone mineral density caused by surgical invasion or implantation [36]. Bondemark demonstrated that there was no difference between test and control tissues in human buccal mucosa, except for some contact irritation. An overview of rare earth magnets used in orthodontics by Noar [37] suggested that neodymium-iron-boron magnets must be coated with a substance when they are used in the oral environment. In this study, the magnets were conformal coated with Parylene C and encapsulated in dental acrylic.

In our previous study, Xu [26] developed a type of magnetic twin-block appliance (TMA) using repelling magnetic forces for the treatment of early skeletal class III malocclusion. This pilot study presented favorable results in growing subjects. However, there were also several unfavorable effects, such as a counter clockwise rotation of the palatal plane and clockwise rotation of the mandibular plane. We also investigated the effects of repelling magnetic orthopedic forces in rhesus monkeys [27] and showed the same advantages and disadvantages as TMA treatment. This phenomenon may be because

Table 1 Cephalometric changes between pre- and posttreatment

			Differences	SD	Significance
Maxillomandibular relationship	Saggital	ANB(dg)	2.281	0.789	0.000***
		Wits(mm)	2.394	0.825	0.000***
		overjet(mm)	3.000	0.658	0.000***
	Vertical	FMA(dg)	1.156	1.468	0.007**
		Y-axis(dg)	1.243	1.162	0.001***
		ANS-Me(mm)	−0.518	1.587	0.308 NS
		S-Go(mm)	1.574	1.448	0.001***
		S-Go/N-Me	0.007	0.010	0.014*
		ANS-Me/N-Me	−0.007	0.010	0.014*
		overbite(mm)	0.600	0.572	0.001***
Maxillary skeletal changes	Saggital	SNA(dg)	1.887	0.840	0.000***
		ptm-A(mm)	1.356	0.765	0.000***
		ptm-S(mm)	1.012	0.637	0.000***
	Vertical	N-ANS(mm)	0.950	0.346	0.000***
		PP-FH(dg)	2.381	0.658	0.000***
		OP-SN(dg)	0.962	1.163	0.005***
Changes in maxillary dentition	Saggital	UI-NA(dg)	2.493	1.647	0.000***
		UI-NA(mm)	1.637	1.067	0.000***
		UI-AP(mm)	1.606	0.715	0.000***
		U6-PTM(mm)	1.100	1.130	0.001***
		UI-SN(dg)	3.123	1.569	0.000***
	Vertical	UI-PP(mm)	0.416	0.413	0.002**
		U6-PP(mm)	−0.412	0.923	0.094 NS
Changes in mandibular dentition	Saggital	LI-NB(dg)	−0.743	0.511	0.000***
		LI-NB(mm)	−0.975	0.425	0.000***
		LI-AP(mm)	−1.731	0.967	0.000***
		FMIA(dg)	−1.987	0.770	0.000***
	Vertical	LI-MP(mm)	0.506	1.021	0.066 NS
		L6-MP(mm)	0.075	1.096	0.788 NS
Mandibular skeletal changes	Saggital	SNB(dg)	−0.494	0.843	0.033*
		Go-Pg(mm)	0.781	1.957	0.131 NS
		Pcd-S(mm)	0.350	0.603	0.035*
	Vertical	Go-Co(mm)	0.762	0.396	0.000***
		MP-SN(dg)	1.175	1.064	0.001***
		Y-axis(dg)	1.256	1.400	0.003**
Soft tissue changes		UL-EP(mm)	1.312	0.602	0.000***
		LL-EP(mm)	−1.575	1.498	0.001***
		Z-angel(dg)	1.238	3.086	0.130 NS
		UL-A'-FH(dg)	1.875	2.513	0.009**
		N'-Pg'-FH(dg)	−2.056	2.134	0.002**
		N'-SN-Pg'(dg)	−4.586	1.333	0.000***

NS indicates nonsignificance
*P < .05. **P < .01. ***P < .001

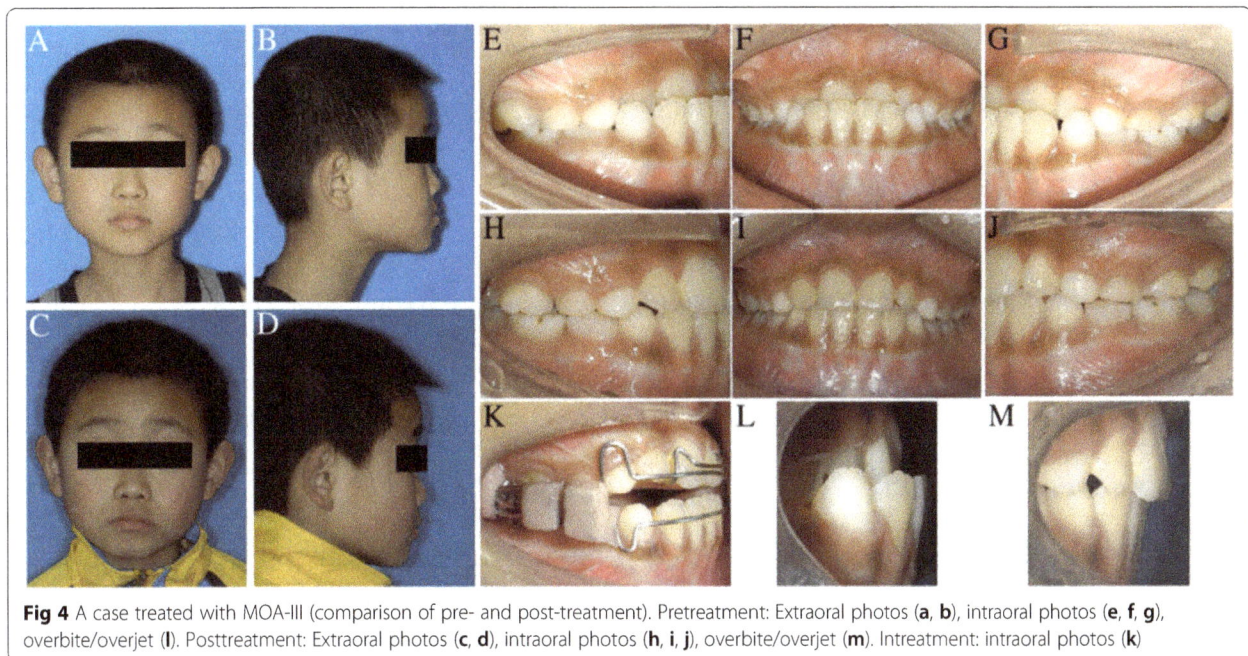

Fig 4 A case treated with MOA-III (comparison of pre- and post-treatment). Pretreatment: Extraoral photos (**a**, **b**), intraoral photos (**e**, **f**, **g**), overbite/overjet (**l**). Posttreatment: Extraoral photos (**c**, **d**), intraoral photos (**h**, **i**, **j**), overbite/overjet (**m**). Intreatment: intraoral photos (**k**)

the force vector in the maxillary magnets is divided into forward and upward components, whereas the forces in the lower magnets are divided into backward and downward components when the patient opens their mouth during masticating activities or at rest (Fig. 5a, c).

Therefore, in this study, we modified the MOA-III appliance to overcome these disadvantages by using attractive forces. When the patients open their mouth while they are speaking, masticating, or performing other oral activities, the attracting magnets create downward and forward force vectors in the upper area and backward and upward vectors in the lower area. The force applied on the maxilla passes near the maxillary center of resistance and may reduce some of the anticlockwise rotations caused by other orthopedic appliances because the center of resistance for a maxilla is slightly inferior to the orbital for the maxilla. By contrast, the force on the lower jaw passed near the center of the condyle, which led to the restraint of mandibular growth (Fig. 5b, d). This intermaxillary force system could be resolved into horizontal, vertical, and transverse components. The horizontal vector pushes the maxilla forward and constrains the lower jaw in an advanced sagittal posture. The vertical forces pull the appliances together and encourage the patients to actively occlude. The transverse components could restrain some lateral mandibular movements. A distinctive aspect of this appliance is the placement of reverse screw expansioners that secure constant magnetic forces by maintaining an adequate distance between the attractive magnets.

During the early treatment of Class III malocclusion, several types of magnetic appliances were developed in clinic and animal studies. Vardimon and co-workers [14, 15]

developed Functional Orthopedic Magnetic appliances (FOMA III) and found that the cumulative protraction of the maxillary complex was initiated at the pterygomaxillary fissure, with an additional contribution provided by other circumaxillary sutures, and that the inhibition of mandibular length was minimal in monkeys. Darendeliler [13] used a Magnetic Expansion Device (MED) in conjunction with the MAD III appliance for the early treatment of a Class III malocclusion. After removal of the appliances, the patient showed a Class I dental relationship, with an adequate overjet and overbite and no crossbite. Xu [26] developed a type of magnetic twin-block appliance (TMA) that corrected the Class III molar relationship to Class I in growing subjects with skeletal Class III malocclusion. Tuncer [28] used a magnetic appliance in the treatment of functional Class III patients. The results indicate that the primary effect of this magnetic appliance was an increase in the posterior rotation of the mandible. In our study, the changes in the maxilla were the most important factors contributing to the treatment effect. Maxillary skeletal and dental changes in the anteroposterior direction were evidenced by the forward movement of the A point together with increases of SNA, ptm-A, ptm-S, UI-NA, UI-AP, and U6-Ptm. This was similar to other studies using a protraction facemask with or without maxillary expansion [29]. In the vertical dimension, increasing the N-ANS and clockwise rotations of the palatal plane and occlusion plane may be caused by the downward and forward force components in the upper appliance. In the mandible, the restraint of the lengths of the mandibular body and mandibular ramous were not significant. The increased MP-SN and Y-axis indicated slight downward and backward mandibular rotations. This was

Table 2 Cephalometric changes in untreatment group

			Differences	SD	Significance
Maxillomandibular relationship	Saggital	ANB(dg)	−0.113	0.146	0.065 NS
		Wits(mm)	0.112	0.216	0.185 NS
		overjet(mm)	−0.107	0.189	0.152 NS
	Vertical	FMA(dg)	0.062	0.417	0.684 NS
		Y-axis(dg)	0.100	0.141	0.085 NS
		ANS-Me(mm)	0.200	0.634	0.402 NS
		S-Go(mm)	0.200	0.160	0.010*
		S-Go/N-Me	−0.001	0.002	0.906 NS
		ANS-Me/N-Me	0.000	0.002	0.906 NS
		overbite(mm)	−0.037	0.199	0.611 NS
Maxillary skeletal changes	Saggital	SNA(dg)	0.400	0.523	0.067 NS
		ptm-A(mm)	0.312	0.083	0.036*
		ptm-S(mm)	0.225	0.128	0.002**
	Vertical	N-ANS(mm)	0.337	0.856	0.302 NS
		PP-FH(dg)	0.087	0.339	0.490 NS
		OP-SN(dg)	0.100	0.277	0.342 NS
Changes in maxillary dentition	Saggital	UI-NA(dg)	0.137	0.388	0.350 NS
		UI-NA(mm)	0.037	0.272	0.708 NS
		UI-AP(mm)	−0.142	0.440	0.700 NS
		U6-PTM(mm)	0.312	0.318	0.027*
		UI-SN(dg)	0.200	0.325	0.125 NS
	Vertical	UI-PP(mm)	0.025	0.401	0.143 NS
		U6-PP(mm)	0.137	0.184	0.073 NS
Changes in mandibular dentition	Saggital	LI-NB(dg)	−0.087	0.294	0.429 NS
		LI-NB(mm)	−0.213	0.314	0.096 NS
		LI-AP(mm)	−0.163	0.272	0.135 NS
		FMIA(dg)	−0.25	0.239	0.021*
	Vertical	LI-MP(mm)	0.187	0.325	0.064 NS
		L6-MP(mm)	0.175	0.211	0.310 NS
Mandibular skeletal changes	Saggital	SNB(dg)	0.363	0.082	0.003**
		Go-Pg(mm)	0.462	0.106	0.001**
		Pcd-S(mm)	0.212	0.124	0.002**
	Vertical	Go-Co(mm)	0.400	0.220	0.001***
		MP-SN(dg)	0.237	0.106	0.000***
		Y-axis(dg)	0.150	0.277	0.170 NS
Soft tissue changes		UL-EP(mm)	−0.225	0.116	0.001***
		LL-EP(mm)	0.250	0.141	0.002**
		Z-angel(dg)	−0.225	0.128	0.002**
		UL-A'-FH(dg)	0.025	0.362	0.850 NS
		N'-Pg'-FH(dg)	0.375	0.183	0.001***
		N'-SN-Pg'(dg)	0.375	0.070	0.000***

NS indicates nonsignificance
*$P < .05$. **$P < .01$. ***$P < .001$

Table 3 Changes between treatment and control group

			Differences	SD	Significance
Maxillomandibular relationship	Saggital	ANB(dg)	2.394	0.843	0.000***
		Wits(mm)	2.282	0.925	0.000***
		overjet(mm)	3.107	0.798	0.000***
	Vertical	FMA(dg)	1.094	1.557	0.013*
		Y-axis(dg)	1.143	1.349	0.007**
		ANS-Me(mm)	−0.718	1.574	0.057 NS
		S-Go(mm)	1.374	1.727	0.003**
		S-Go/N-Me	0.008	0.017	0.352 NS
		ANS-Me/N-Me	−0.007	0.016	0.304 NS
		overbite(mm)	0.637	0.651	0.005**
Maxillary skeletal changes	Saggital	SNA(dg)	1.487	0.935	0.000***
		ptm-A(mm)	1.044	0.740	0.000***
		ptm-S(mm)	0.787	0.835	0.005**
	Vertical	N-ANS(mm)	0.613	0.366	0.000***
		PP-FH(dg)	2.294	0.662	0.000***
		OP-SN(dg)	0.862	1.219	0.012 NS
Changes in maxillary dentition	Saggital	UI-NA(dg)	2.356	1.631	0.000***
		UI-NA(mm)	1.6	1.039	0.000***
		UI-AP(mm)	1.748	0.697	0.000***
		U6-PTM(mm)	0.788	1.179	0.015**
		UI-SN(dg)	2.923	1.524	0.000***
	Vertical	UI-PP(mm)	0.391	0.359	0.002**
		U6-PP(mm)	−0.549	0.892	0.108 NS
Changes in mandibular dentition	Saggital	LI-NB(dg)	−0.656	0.522	0.000***
		LI-NB(mm)	−0.762	0.421	0.000***
		LI-AP(mm)	−1.568	0.964	0.000***
		FMIA(dg)	−1.737	0.841	0.000***
	Vertical	LI-MP(mm)	0.319	1.076	0.243 NS
		L6-MP(mm)	−0.1	1.226	0.854 NS
Mandibular skeletal changes	Saggital	SNB(dg)	−0.857	0.813	0.072 NS
		Go-Pg(mm)	0.319	2.265	0.188 NS
		Pcd-S(mm)	0.138	0.577	0.050 NS
	Vertical	Go-Co(mm)	0.362	0.843	0.057*
		MP-SN(dg)	0.938	1.095	0.005**
		Y-axis(dg)	1.106	1.349	0.007**
Soft tissue changes		UL-EP(mm)	1.537	0.657	0.000***
		LL-EP(mm)	−1.825	1.522	0.004**
		Z-angel(dg)	1.463	3.281	0.270 NS
		UL-A′-FH(dg)	1.85	2.640	0.016 NS
		N′-Pg′-FH(dg)	−2.431	2.000	0.005**
		N′-SN-Pg′(dg)	−4.961	1.303	0.000***

NS indicates nonsignificance
*$P < .05$. **$P < .01$. ***$P < .001$

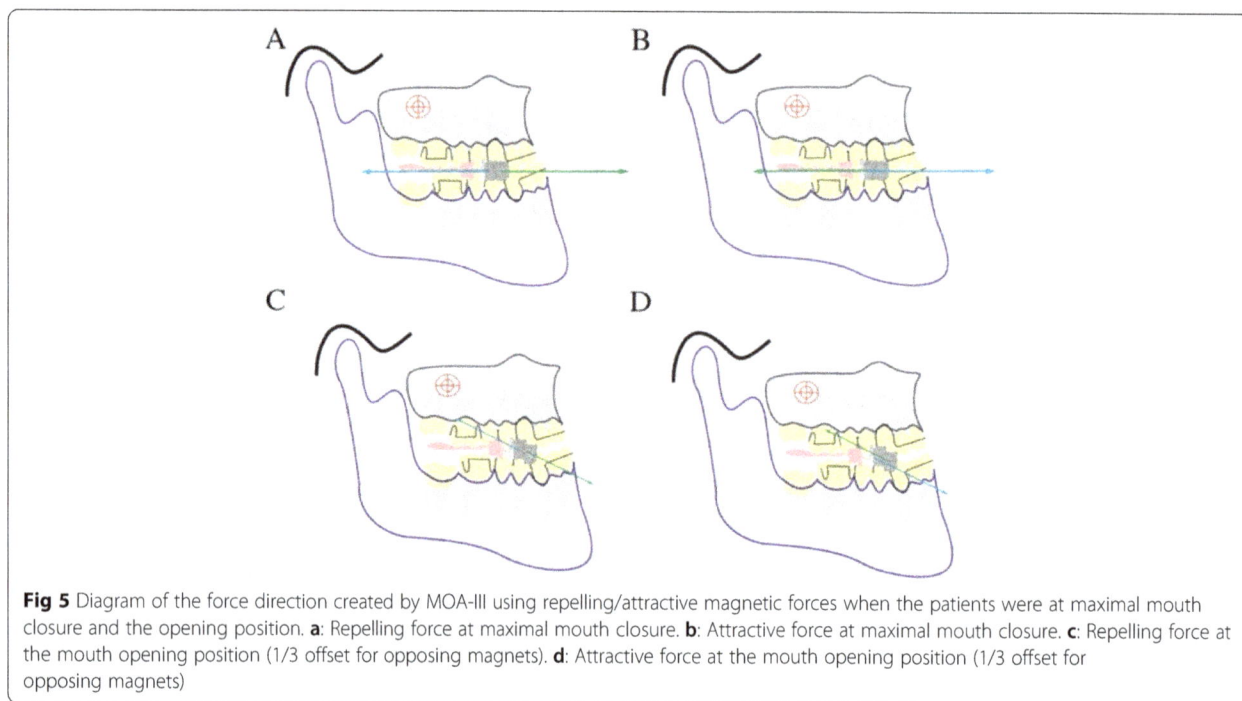

Fig 5 Diagram of the force direction created by MOA-III using repelling/attractive magnetic forces when the patients were at maximal mouth closure and the opening position. **a**: Repelling force at maximal mouth closure. **b**: Attractive force at maximal mouth closure. **c**: Repelling force at the mouth opening position (1/3 offset for opposing magnets). **d**: Attractive force at the mouth opening position (1/3 offset for opposing magnets)

similar to the treatment effects of using a chincap [30–32]. Significant changes were found in the lower incisors. The decrease of LI-NB, LI-AP, and FMIA indicated that the lower incisors tipped lingually under the backward forces in the lower appliance. Measurement of the soft tissue showed that the concave profile was improved and that the upper lip moved forward and the lower lip retruded backward. In a randomized controlled trial study using a removable mandibular retractor [34], the main significant findings were similar to our study. For example, there was an anterior morphogenetic rotation of the mandible, a significant increase in maxillary length, a significant increase in maxillary dentoalveolar protrusion, a significant decrease in mandibular dentoalveolar protrusion, a significant protrusion of the upper lip, a significant retrusion of the lower lip, and a significant reduction in the nasolabial angle.

In the untreated control group, the cephalometric measurements indicated that uncontrolled mandibular growth may exaggerate the Class III malocclusion and make the concave profiles worse.

By comparing the results of the MOA-III treatment with normal growth in the untreated Cl III subjects, we could conclude that MOA-III was effective for the treatment of mild skeletal Class III children.

Conclusion

- MOA-III was effective for the treatment of mild to moderate class III malocclusions in children.

- In the maxilla, both the skeleton and dentition moved forward in the anteroposterior direction. Simultaneously, the maxilla rotated forward and downward. In the mandible, the most significant changes were lingual compensation of the lower incisors. At the same time, the mandible rotated downward and backward, but the length of the mandible body showed no significant changes.

- For the soft tissue measurement, the upper lip moved forward and the lower lip retruded backward. The concave profiles were also improved.

Competing interests
The authors declare that they have no competing interests.

Authors' contributions
NZ and GS contributed to the conception and appliance design. NZ, JF, ZH, and RJC performed the clinical data collection, analysis and interpretation. NZ and GS drafted the manuscript. All authors read and approved the final manuscript.

References
1. Dermaut LR, Aelbers CM. Orthopedics in orthodontics: Fiction or reality. A review of the literature–Part II. Am J Orthod Dentofacial Orthop. 1996;110:667–71.
2. Chin GY. New Magnetic Alloys. Science. 1980;208(4446):888–94.
3. Blechman AM, Smiley H. Magnetic force in orthodontics. Am J Orthod. 1978;74:435–43.
4. Muller M. The use of magnets in orthodontics: an alternative means to produce tooth movement. Eur J Orthod. 1984;6:247–53.
5. Sandler JP. An attractive solution to unerupted teeth. Am J Orthod Dentofacial Orthop. 1991;100:489–93.
6. Mancini GP, Noar JH, Evans RD. The physical characteristics of neodymium iron boron magnets for tooth extrusion. Eur J Orthod. 1999;21:541–50.

7. Cole BO, Shaw AJ, Hobson RS, Nunn JH, Welbury RR, Meechan JG, et al. The role of magnets in the management of unerupted teeth in children and adolescents. Int J Paediatr Dent. 2003;13:204–7.

8. Woods MG, Nanda RS. Intrusion of posterior teeth with magnets: an experiment in nongrowing baboons. Am J Orthod Dentofacial Orthop. 1991;100:393–400.

9. Hwang HS, Lee KH. Intrusion of overerupted molars by corticotomy and magnets. Am J Orthod Dentofacial Orthop. 2001;120:209–16.

10. Blechman AM. Magnetic force systems in orthodontics. Clinical results of a pilot study. Am J Orthod. 1985;87:201–10.

11. Kawata T, Hirota K, Sumitani K, Umehara K, Yano K, Tzeng HJ, et al. A new orthodontic force system of magnetic brackets. Am J Orthod Dentofacial Orthop. 1987;92:241–8.

12. Bernhold M, Bondemark L. A magnetic appliance for treatment of snoring patients with and without obstructive sleep apnea. Am J Orthod Dentofacial Orthop. 1998;113:144–55.

13. Darendeliler MA, Chiarini M, Joho JP. Early class III treatment with magnetic appliances. J Clin Orthod. 1993;27:563–9.

14. Vardimon AD, Graber TM, Stutzmann J, Voss L, Petrovic AG. Reaction of the pterygomaxillary fissure and the condylar cartilage to intermaxillary Class III magnetic mechanics. Am J Orthod Dentofacial Orthop. 1994;105:401–13.

15. Vardimon AD, Graber TM, Voss LR, Muller TP. Functional orthopedic magnetic appliance (FOMA) III–modus operandi. Am J Orthod Dentofacial Orthop. 1990;97:135–48.

16. Vardimon AD, Stutzmann JJ, Graber TM, Voss LR, Petrovic AG. Functional orthopedic magnetic appliance (FOMA) II–modus operandi. Am J Orthod Dentofacial Orthop. 1989;95:371–87.

17. Bondemark L, Kurol J. Distalization of maxillary first and second molars simultaneously with repelling magnets. Eur J Orthod. 1992;14:264–72.

18. Itoh T, Tokuda T, Kiyosue S, Hirose T, Matsumoto M, Chaconas SJ. Molar distalization with repelling magnets. J Clin Orthod. 1991;25:611–7.

19. Gianelly AA, Vaitas AS, Thomas WM. The use of magnets to move molars distally. Am J Orthod Dentofacial Orthop. 1989;96:161–7.

20. Darendeliler MA, Strahm C, Joho JP. Light maxillary expansion forces with the magnetic expansion device. A preliminary investigation. Eur J Orthod. 1994;16:479–90.

21. Vardimon AD, Graber TM, Voss LR, Verrusio E. Magnetic versus mechanical expansion with different force thresholds and points of force application. Am J Orthod Dentofacial Orthop. 1987;92:455–66.

22. Dellinger EL. A clinical assessment of the Active Vertical Corrector–a nonsurgical alternative for skeletal open bite treatment. Am J Orthod. 1986;89:428–36.

23. Kiliaridis S, Egermark I, Thilander B. Anterior open bite treatment with magnets. Eur J Orthod. 1990;12:447–57.

24. Meral O, Yuksel S. Skeletal and dental effects during observation and treatment with a magnetic device. Angle Orthod. 2003;73:716–22.

25. Noar JH, Shell N, Hunt NP. The performance of bonded magnets used in the treatment of anterior open bite. Am J Orthod Dentofacial Orthop. 1996;109:549–56. discussion 557.

26. Xu Y, Hu J, Li P. The effects of twin-block magnetic appliance on the early skeletal Class III malocclusion. Zhonghua Kou Qiang Yi Xue Za Zhi. 1999;34:148–50.

27. Zhao N, Xu Y, Chen Y, Xu Y, Han X, Wang L. Effects of class III magnetic orthopedic forces on the craniofacial sutures of rhesus monkeys. Am J Orthod Dentofacial Orthop. 2008;133:401–9.

28. Tuncer C, Uner O. Effects of a magnetic appliance in functional Class III patients. Angle Orthod. 2005;75:768–77.

29. Kim JH, Viana MA, Graber TM, Omerza FF, BeGole EA. The effectiveness of protraction face mask therapy: a meta-analysis. Am J Orthod Dentofacial Orthop. 1999;115:675–85.

30. Mitani H. Early application of chincap therapy to skeletal Class III malocclusion. Am J Orthod Dentofacial Orthop. 2002;121:584–5.

31. Deguchi T, McNamara JA. Craniofacial adaptations induced by chincup therapy in Class III patients. Am J Orthod Dentofacial Orthop. 1999;115:175–82.

32. Abu Alhaija ES, Richardson A. Long-term effect of the chincap on hard and soft tissues. Eur J Orthod. 1999;21:291–8.

33. Darendeliler MA, Sinclair PM, Kusy RP. The effects of samarium-cobalt magnets and pulsed electromagnetic fields on tooth movement. Am J Orthod Dentofacial Orthop. 1995;107:578–88.

34. Saleh M, Hajeer MY, Al-Jundi A. Short-term soft- and hard-tissue changes following Class III treatment using a removable mandibular retractor: a randomized controlled trial. Orthod Craniofac Res. 2013;16:75–86.

35. Darendeliler MA, Darendeliler A, Sinclair PM. Effects of static magnetic and pulsed electromagnetic fields on bone healing. Int J Adult Orthod Orthognath Surg. 1997;12:43–53.

36. Yan QC, Tomita N, Ikada Y. Effects of static magnetic field on bone formation of rat femurs. Med Eng Phys. 1998;20:397–402.

37. Noar JH, Evans RD. Rare earth magnets in orthodontics: an overview. Br J Orthod. 1999;26:29–37.

10

Interradicular trabecular bone density of the lateral maxilla for temporary anchorage devices – a histomorphometric study

Elena Krieger[1*] and Heinrich Wehrbein[2]

Abstract

Objective: To analyze the interradicular trabecular bone density of the lateral maxilla regarding the insertion of temporary anchorage devices (TADs).

Material and methods: The material consisted of tissue blocks of autopsy material from 20 subjects (17 male, 3 female, 16 - 63y). The specimens comprised the dentated alveolar bone of the lateral maxilla. The interradicular areas (IRA) from canine to distally of the second molar (IRA 3–4, 4–5, 5–6, 6–7, 7d) were histomorphometrically measured with respect to the hard tissue fraction of the trabecular bone (HTFTB, %) and statistically analyzed.

Results: Histomorphometric measurements showed the following results: Mean HTFTB of IRA 3–4 was 44.08%, of IRA 4–5 31.07%, of IRA 5–6 33.96%, of IRA 6–7 36.33% and of IRA 7d 25.40%. Only the difference between the HTFTB of IRA 3–4 and the other IRAs was statistically significant ($p < 0.05$). Regarding the minimum and maximum HTFTB value of each IRA, there was a great amount of difference, especially for IRA 3–4: minimum HTFTB was 17.20% and maximum 67.03%.

Conclusion: Apart from the IRA between canine and first premolar, the HTFTB in the IRAs of the lateral maxilla have to be classified as low or even moderate. IRA 3–4 should also be considered cautious regarding its minimum values. Thus, it seems that the interradicular trabecular bone density of the lateral maxilla is unfavorable to achieve a good primary stability of TADs.

Keywords: Orthodontic, Anchorage, Implant, Insertion site, Failure rate, Bone density

Introduction

Temporary anchorage devices (TADs) are nowadays commonly used as anchorage for orthodontic tooth movement. They are temporarily inserted, and after accomplishing the treatment purposes removed. Several devices were developed and three types of TADs are usually applied: mini-plates (i.e. bone anchor), length-reduced mini-implants (i.e. palatal implant) and diameter-reduced mini-implants (i.e. mini-screw). Each type has its specific insertion area with individual failure rates, also including parameters of the individual patient [1].

The initial bone-implant-interface is highly important and influenced by the bone quality and quantity, the

implant geometry, and the site preparation technique [2]. Therefore, the bone quantity and quality of the specific insertion area is of major interest. Recently, several studies have been published investigating the bone density concerning orthodontic treatment and TADs by using computed tomography (CT) or cone beam computed tomography (CBCT) [3-7]: Samrit et al. [3] evaluated the bone density in interradicular bone between second premolars and first molars and its association with the clinical stability of mini-screws used for en masse retraction of anterior teeth in 10 extraction cases. A comparison between maxilla and mandible revealed higher values in mandibular cortical bone and no difference in cancellous bone values [3]. Kim and Park [4] measured the cortical bone thickness in the mandibular buccal and lingual areas in order to assess the suitability of these areas for application of TADs. Chugh et al. [5],

---
* Correspondence: elena.krieger@unimedizin-mainz.de
[1]Department of Orthodontics, Medical Centre of the
Johannes-Gutenberg-University Mainz, Augustusplatz 2, 55131 Mainz, Germany
Full list of author information is available at the end of the article

Chun and Lim [6], as well as Cassetta et al. [7] evaluated the alveolar cortical bone thickness and density differences between interradicular sites at different levels from the alveolar crest. All authors found differences in bone densities depending on the localization, anterior to posterior areas and from crest to base of the alveolar crest.

Marquezan et al. [8] compared with micro-CTs the primary stability of mini-screws inserted into bovine bone blocks of different densities with and without cortical bone, and investigated if trabecular properties could influence primary stability. They found that trabecular bone had an important role in primary stability in the presence or absence of cortical bone.

But evaluating the bone quantity histomorphometrically, only a few studies can be found: Wehrbein [9] assessed quantitatively the bone quality of the palatal bone of 22 human tissue blocks of autopsy material. He suggested a good primary stability of TADs inserted in this area [9]. Çehreli and Arman-Özçırpıcı [10] evaluated the primary stability and histomorphometric measurements of 72 mini-screws inserted in bovine iliac crest blocks. They found positive correlations between the bone-implant contact and cortical bone densities [10].

Thus, this is the first study assessing the interradicular trabecular bone density of the lateral maxilla regarding the insertion of temporary anchorage devices (TAD) histomorphometrically in humans.

Material and methods

The material consisted of tissue blocks of autopsy material from 20 subjects (17 male, 3 female), between 16 and 63 years of age. The specimens comprised tooth-bearing lateral segments of the maxilla from the canine to the second molar region. Inclusion criterion was that all observed teeth had to have an antagonist in the mandible; therefore, all teeth were functionally loaded during lifetime (i.e. mastication). Further inclusion criteria were the absence of crowns or bridges. The specimens were obtained from the Institute of pathology and the Institute of forensic medicine at the University of Aachen after the required authorization was given by the legally responsible person. According to the information given to us no diseases other medical conditions concerning the bone metabolism were present.

The following interradicular areas (IRA) were measured (Figure 1): between canine and first premolar (IRB 3–4); first and second premolar (IRB 4–5); second

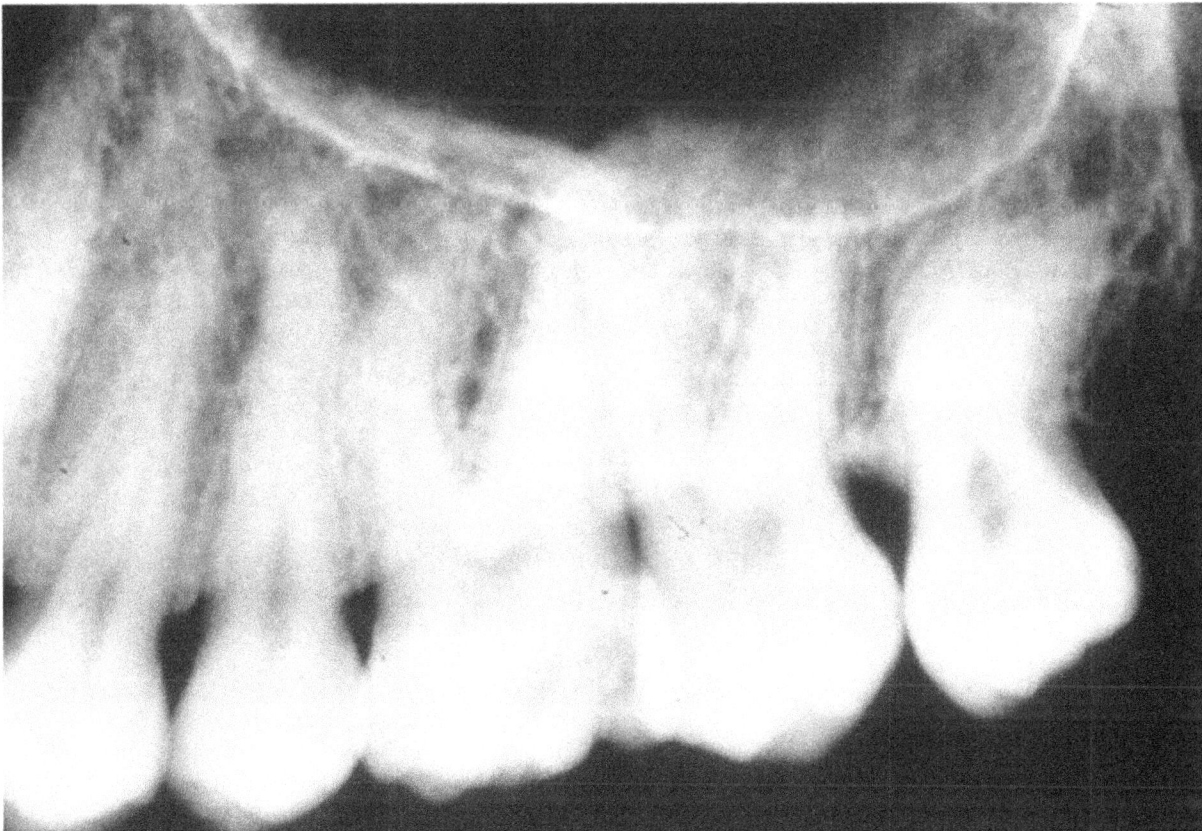

Figure 1 Radiographic of a specimen showing the interradicular areas.

premolar and first molar (IRB 5–6); first and second molar (IRB 6–7); distal end of the second molar (IRB 7d).

Histomorphometry

All specimens were assessed histomorphometrically. This procedure is by definition a quantitative study of the microscopic organization and structure of tissue (for example bone) particularly by means of computer-assisted analysis of images formed by a microscope.

The histological sections were prepared in the sagittal plane according to the ground-thin-section technology according to Donath 1988 [11] (Figure 2). Accordingly three series of slices from the middle section of the maxillary segments (5–20 µm thickness) were stained with toluidine blue (Figure 3). The evaluation of the specimen was performed by using the semiautomatic method for quantitative static and dynamic bone histology by Malluche et al. [12]: a microscope is equipped with a drawing tube through which the image of the digitizing platen is projected over the optical field; the investigator selects and traces all histologic structures to be measured by moving a cursor on the digitizing platen which is visible by its projection over the histologic field. Reliability and accuracy were shown by Malluche et al. [12].

The histomorphometry was carried out in our study with a computer (IBM, Armonk, USA), a SummaSketch digitizer and a digitizing tablet (Summagraphics Corporation, Lansdale, Pennsylvania USA) along with the appropriate software and a microscope (Leica Microsystems, Wetzlar, Germany). The magnification used was 390.6× . The microscope bearded a grid, which was subdivided into 25 squares. Each square had a side length of 435.89 µm. The grid was placed in each IRA and centered at the level of the apices. Of each specimen, ten of the 25 squares were analyzed and the trabecular bone

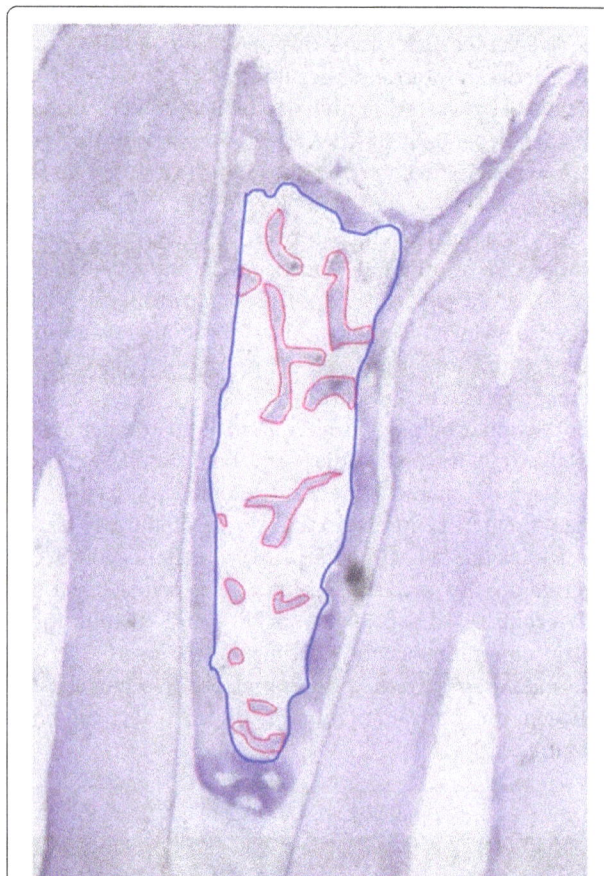

Figure 3 Magnification of the interradicular bone between first and second premolar of Figure 2: relatively low trabecular bone density (magnification × 2.5).

areas measured. The measured trabecular bone areas in relation to the total surface of the ten squares (i.e. total bone area = 1.900.000 µm^2) lead to the hard tissue fraction of the trabecular bone in percentage (HTFTB, %).

Statistics

Statistical analysis was performed by using the SAS program. Mean, minimum, maximum values and standard deviations were calculated for each IRA after computing the average value from the measurement of the three slices. Data of each IRA were compared using the Wilcoxon-test. A p-value was calculated and considered as statistically significant when $p < 0.05$.

Results

Location-specific bone quality

The histomorphometric measurements of the HTFTB of all interradicular areas are shown in Table 1. For example, The IRA 3–4 had a HBTFB of 44.08%, meaning a density of trabecular bone of 44.08% in relation to the total bone area (1.900.000 µm). The lowest mean

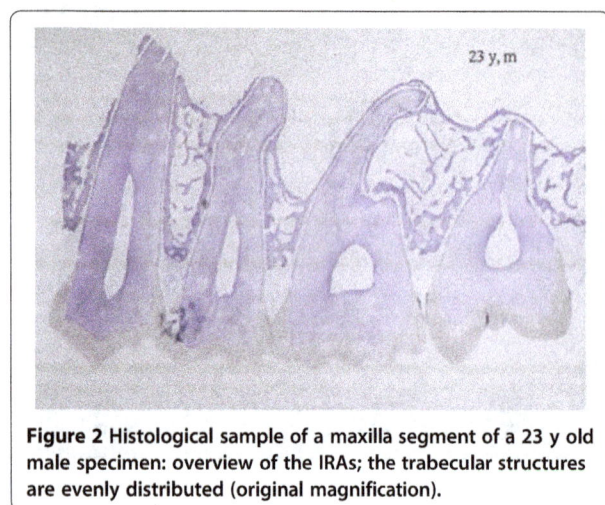

Figure 2 Histological sample of a maxilla segment of a 23 y old male specimen: overview of the IRAs; the trabecular structures are evenly distributed (original magnification).

Interradicular trabecular bone density of the lateral maxilla for temporary anchorage...

71

Table 1 Percentage of hard tissue fraction to total bone volume (HTFTB, %) of all interradicular areas: IRA 3–4, IRA 4–5, IRA 5–6, IRA 6–7 and IRA 7d; mean, standard deviation (SD), minimum (min), maximum (max) and variance

	IRA 3-4	IRA 4-5	IRA 5-6	IRA 6-7	IRA 7d
Mean	44.08%	31.07%	33.96%	36.33%	25.40%
SD	14.32%	12.18%	12.74%	8.12%	12.13%
Min	17.20%	16.82%	20.50%	27.20%	11.20%
Max	67.03%	52.20%	62.40%	53.90%	38.60%
Variance	202.198	164.229	162.554	67.998	147.244

HTFTB was found in the IRA 7d (25.40%), and the highest mean HTFTB in IRA 3–4 (44.08%).

Regarding the minimum and maximum value of each IRA, there was a great amount of difference, especially for the IRA 3–4: its minimum value was 17.20% and maximum 67.03%.

Regarding differences between the individual IRAs, only the difference between the HTFTB of the IRA 3–4 and the others was statistically significant ($p < 0.05$) (Wilcoxon-Test).

Discussion

Until now, investigations of the bone density of the alveolar bone taking into account to insert TADs for orthodontic treatment purposes, can only be found using CT or CBCTs for assessment [3-8,12-14]. The accordance between radiographic assessments and histomorphometric measurements was evaluated by González-García and Monje [15], but in terms of dental implants. They conducted a study to assess the reliability of CBCTs as a tool to pre-operatively determine radiographic bone density. Therefore, this is the first study assessing the interradicular trabecular bone density of the lateral maxilla regarding the insertion of TADs histomorphometrically in humans.

The primary stability of mini-screws is significantly influenced by the bone density of the cortical bone [13]. Marquezan et al. [8] reported in their micro-CT investigation of TADs in bovine bone that the presence of cortical bone increased the primary stability, and that the cortical bone had an important role when the trabecular bone had a lower bone density. We found mean HTFTB values of the lateral maxilla considering all IRAs from 25.40% (IRA 7d) up to 44.08% (IRA 3–4). The mean HTFTB values were similar from mesial to distal (between 25 and 44%). Nevertheless, the minimum values instead were between 11 and 27%. There was also a wide difference between the minimum and maximum values of each IRA, especially for IRA 3–4. The high standard deviations as well as differences between the minimal

and maximum values in the respective IRAs are probably due to different loading conditions (occlusal wear) in the respective individuals than to other medical conditions as to our information no diseases or other medical conditions concerning bone metabolism were known. Also, age and gender of the specimen might have been an influence factor. Accordingly, Wakimoto et al. [16], who investigated the bone quality and quantity of the anterior maxillary trabecular bone in dental implant sites, found that women had lower bone densities than men.

Therefore, we concluded that apart from IRA 3–4 the HTFTB in the IRAs of the lateral maxilla have to be classified as low (IRA 7d) or even moderate, but IRA 3–4 should also be considered cautious regarding its minimum values. Thus, the interradicular trabecular bone density of the lateral maxilla seems to be unfavorable to achieve a good primary stability of TADs. Therefore, the cortical bone thickness and density are still decisive factors for primary stability of TADs in the lateral maxilla.

Our findings are similar to Chugh et al. [5], who investigated the cortical bone density. They reported that the highest cortical bone density was observed between the second premolar and first molar at the alveolar bone level and between the first and second molars at the basal bone level in the maxilla [5]. The maxillary tuberosity presented the least bone density which is comparable to the IRA distally of the second molar (IRA 7d) in our investigation. Chun and Lim [6] evaluated bone density differences between interradicular sites. They suggested that mini-implants for orthodontic anchorage would more be effective when placed in areas with equivalent bone density up to 6 mm apical to the alveolar crest [6].

Comparing our results to the anterior palate, where a hard tissue fraction to total bone volume of 68% was found histomorphometrically [9], it is pointed out that this region is more appropriate for the insertion of TADs. The initial and possibly the subsequent hart tissue contact of TADs inserted in the anterior palate are twice as high as in the interradicular area of the maxilla [9]. The multicenter investigation by Jung et al. [17] reported about a failure rate of 4.6% (n = 239) when inserting a length-reduces implant in the anterior palate. Regarding all TADs, the meta-analysis of Schätzle et al. [1] demonstrated the following data: the failure rate for length-reduces palatal implants was 10.5%, for mini-screws inserted in the alveolar bone 16.4% and for mini-plates 7.3%. They reported that mini-plates and palatal implants together, representing torque-resisting TADs, showed a 1.92-fold lower clinical failure rate than mini-screws [1].

TADs are inserted to support orthodontic treatment purposes. Orthodontically induced tooth movement implies changes in the surrounding tissue (hard and soft).

Hsu et al. [18] assessed 2011 the bone density changes around the anterior teeth during orthodontic treatment by using CBCTs. The bone density around the teeth reduced significantly after the application of orthodontic forces [18]. This findings suggest, when inserting a TAD into alveolar bone, where recently orthodontic tooth movement was conducted, the primary stability could be even more reduced and therefore higher failure or migration rates might occur.

Conclusions

The following conclusions can be drawn:

- Apart from the interradicular area between canine and first premolar (IRA 3–4) the mean hard tissue fraction of the trabecular bone (HTFTB) in the interradicular areas of the lateral maxilla have to be classified as low (IRA 7d) or even moderate.
- There was a wide difference between the minimum and maximum values of each IRA, especially for IRA 3–4. Therefore, IRA 3–4 should also be considered cautious regarding its minimum values.
- Thus, it seems that the interradicular trabecular bone density of the lateral maxilla is unfavorable to achieve a good primary stability of TADs. Therefore, the cortical bone thickness and density are decisive factors for primary stability of TADs in the lateral maxilla.

Abbreviations

CBCT: Cone beam computed tomography; CT: Computed tomography; HTFTB: Hard tissue fraction of the trabecular bone; IRA: Interradicular area; TAD: Temporary anchorage device.

Competing interests

The authors declare that they have no competing interests.

Authors' contributions

EK and HW conceived the study design, assembled the data, conducted the analysis and interpretation of data, and drafted the manuscript. Both authors read and approved the final manuscript.

Author details

[1]Department of Orthodontics, Medical Centre of the Johannes-Gutenberg-University Mainz, Augustusplatz 2, 55131 Mainz, Germany. [2]Department of Orthodontics, Medical Centre of the Johannes-Gutenberg-University Mainz, Augustusplatz 2, 55131 Mainz, Germany.

References

1. Schätzle M, Männchen R, Zwahlen M, Lang NP. Survival and failure rates of orthodontic temporary anchorage devices: a systematic review. Clin Oral Implants Res. 2009;20:1351–9.
2. Misch CE. Density of bone: effect on treatment plans, surgical approach, healing, and progressive bone loading. Int J Oral Implantol. 1990;7:9.
3. Samrit V, Kharbanda OP, Duggal R, Seith A, Malhotra V. Bone density and miniscrew stability in orthodontic patients. Aust Orthod J. 2012;28:204–12.
4. Kim JH, Park YC. Evaluation of mandibular cortical bone thickness for placement of temporary anchorage devices (TADs). Korean J Orthod. 2012;42:110–7.
5. Chugh T, Ganeshkar SV, Revankar AV, Jain AK. Quantitative assessment of interradicular bone density in the maxilla and mandible: implications in clinical orthodontics. Prog Orthod. 2013;14:38.
6. Chun YS, Lim WH. Bone density at interradicular sites: implications for orthodontic mini-implant placement. Orthod Craniofac Res. 2009;12:25–32.
7. Cassetta M, Sofan AA, Altieri F, Barbato E. Evaluation of alveolar cortical bone thickness and density for orthodontic mini-implant placement. J Clin Exp Dent. 2013;5:245–52.
8. Marquezan M, Lima I, Lopes RT, Sant'Anna EF, de Souza MM. Is trabecular bone related to primary stability of miniscrews? Angle Orthod. 2014;84:500–7.
9. Wehrbein H. Bone quality in the midpalate for temporary anchorage devices. Clin Oral Implants Res. 2009;20:45–9.
10. Çehreli S, Arman-Özçırpıcı A. Primary stability and histomorphometric bone-implant contact of self-drilling and self-tapping orthodontic microimplants. Am J Orthod Dentofacial Orthop. 2012;141:187–95.
11. Donath K. Die Trenn-Dünnschliff-Technik zur Herstellung histologischer Präparate von nicht schneidbaren Geweben und Materialien. Der Präparator. 1988;34:197–206 (in German).
12. Malluche HH, Sherman D, Meyer W, Massry SG. A new semiautomatic method for quantitative static and dynamic bone histology. Calcif Tissue Int. 1982;34:439–48.
13. Cha JY, Kil JK, Yoon TM, Hwang CJ. Miniscrew stability evaluated with computerized tomography scanning. Am J Orthod Dentofacial Orthop. 2010;137:73–9.
14. Santiago RC, de Paula FO, Fraga MR, Assis NMSP, Vitral RWF. Correlation between miniscrew stability and bone mineral density in orthodontic patients. Am J Orthod Dentofacial Orthop. 2009;136:243–50.
15. González-García R, Monje F. The reliability of cone-beam computed tomography to assess bone density at dental implant recipient sites: a histomorphometric analysis by micro-CT. Clin Oral Implants Res. 2013;24:871–9.
16. Wakimoto M, Matsumura T, Ueno T, Mizukawa N, Yanagi Y, Iida S. Bone quality and quantity of the anterior maxillary trabecular bone in dental implant sites. Clin Oral Implants Res. 2012;23:1314–9.
17. Jung BA, Kunkel M, Göllner P, Liechti T, Wagner W, Wehrbein H. Prognostic parameters contributing to palatal implant failures: a long-term survival analysis of 239 patients. Clin Oral Implants Res. 2012;23:746–50.
18. Hsu JT, Chang HW, Huang HL, Yu JH, Li YF, Tu MG. Bone density changes around teeth during orthodontic treatment. Clin Oral Investig. 2011;15:511–9.

11

Comparison between rapid and slow palatal expansion: evaluation of selected periodontal indices

Stefano Mummolo[1], Enrico Marchetti[1], Francesca Albani[1], Vincenzo Campanella[2], Filippo Pugliese[1], Salvatore Di Martino[1], Simona Tecco[3*] and Giuseppe Marzo[1]

Abstract

Objectives: The aim of this pilot study was to evaluate the periodontal effects during rapid palatal expansion (RPE) or slow palatal expansion (SPE) and to compare them by means of some clinical indices, in order to establish the possible differences and advantages of one of these treatments in periodontal terms.

Methods: 10 patients (aged 6 to 7 years; average age 6.3 years) were submitted to RPE treatment and other 10 patients (aged 6 to 8 years, average age 6.3 years) to SPE treatment. They were treated with the Haas expander. The selected clinical indices (plaque index, PI; papillary bleeding index, PBI; probing pocket depth, PPD) were collected three times during the treatment (t_0, detected 7 days after the periodontal prophylaxis, at the beginning of the active orthodontic therapy; t_1, detected during the active therapy; t_2, detected after retention). All measurements were performed by the same examiner. The protocol was approved by the ethics committee.

Results: The effects of the prophylaxis were excellent to control inflammation and dental plaque before the beginning of the orthodontic-orthopaedic treatment, as in both the two groups, the PI and the PBI values were equal to 0.
In the group receiving slow expansion, the PPD remained unchanged from t_0 to t_1, while it significantly increased from t_0 to t_1 in the group of rapid expansion. At t_2 the values of the two groups returned to be overlapping.

Conclusions: Both rapid and slow expansion treatments present potential irritation effect (increase of PI index and PBI index) on the periodontium, suggested by the significant increase of PI and PBI from t_0 to t_1 in both the two groups; therefore prophylaxis and periodic controls are very important. There are no long-term benefits that might be referred unequivocally to one of the two treatments in terms of periodontal consequences, as demonstrated by the lack of significant differences between the two groups at t_2.

Keywords: Palatal expansion, Periodontal indices, Plaque index, Papillary bleeding index, Probing pocket depth

Introduction

Over the past years there has been an appreciable increase of the orthodontic treatments, but the clinicians must not forget that orthodontic therapies can cause side-effects affecting the periodontal tissues.

The oral cavity is a rich ecosystem with a plethora of microorganisms. Plaque bacteria are the major factor in the onset and progression of periodontal disease and caries, but these are really multifactorial diseases, and

there are situations which comprise what has been termed 'ecological stress', causing the shift of the microbiological balance, so creating conditions conducive to the growth, and appearance of cariogenic and/or periodontopathic bacteria [1]. The different components of a fixed orthodontic system may contribute to the shift in the balance of the oral ecology. Correlations have been observed between orthodontic treatment and its effects on periodontal tissues [2-4]. A periodontal interaction subsequent to rapid palatal expansion [5] has also been described in terms of fluctuation of the inflammatory mediators, such us interleukin-1β (IL-1β) e β-glucoronidase (βG) levels in the

* Correspondence: tecco.simona@hsr.it
[3]University Vita-Salute San Raffaele, Via Olgettina 60, 20132, Milano, Italy
Full list of author information is available at the end of the article

gingival crevicular fluid (GCF) of the first maxillary molars during rapid palatal expansion [6].

The effect of an orthodontic force also depends from the type of appliance [7].

Except for the type of the tested expansion therapy, none of the other examined orthodontic variables showed a statistically significant influence on the periodontal tissues [7].

Although the phenomenon of orthodontic movement is similar to inflammation, but relatively aseptic [8], additional inflammation, such as the one induced by plaque accumulation, should be avoided during orthodontic and orthopaedic treatment [6].

As the orthodontic appliances certainly facilitate the establishment of significant bacterial colonies that can alter the environment of oral cavity [9], the clinician must ensure that there are no active inflammatory processes in the periodontium before starting all orthodontic treatments. It is recommended to educate and motivate the patient to oral hygiene; to perform eventual periodontal prophylaxis; to carefully choose the typology of appliance; and to carry out periodic medical controls at shorts intervals [10].

The periodontal prophylaxis program depends on: patients age; clinical oral and systemic conditions; patients collaboration; and family and social environment.

This pilot study was aimed to evaluate the periodontal health clinical indices in patients subjected to rapid and slow palatal expansion (using the Haas expander), and compare them establishing the possible differences and advantages of one of these treatments.

Materials and methods

Due to the small cohort of this study, this can be considered only a pilot study.

It was performed at the Department of Oral Health, University of L'Aquila, Italy.

10 patients (5 males and 5 females) (Group I), aged 6 to 7 years (average age 6.3 years), were subjected to rapid palatal expansion (RPE) using the Haas expander. A second group included 10 patients (4 males and 6 females) (Group II), aged 6 to 8 years, average age 6.3 years, that were subjected to slow palatal expansion (SPE) with the same appliance activated in different times and ways.

The subjects were enrolled in the sample from april 2011 to november 2011. The parents of the participants agreed (informed) to partecipate to this study.

The following inclusion criteria were observed: no dental diseases (caries, fractures, granulomas, etc.), a constriction of the upper jaw, that needed the palatal expansion appliance mounted on bands in order to be treated; good general health; probing depth values not exceeding 3 mm in the whole dentition; no radiographic evidence of periodontal bone loss. In addition, patients showed normal gingival biotype [11,12].

The gingival biotype was objectively assessed using a metal periodontal probe in the sulcus to evaluate gingival tissue thickness: a thin biotype was recorded when the tip of the probe was visible through the gingiva; a normal biotype was assessed when the tip of the probe was not visible. See text for details [11,12].

Periodontal condition of the patients prior to starting the study was analyzed in detail and reported in Table 1.

Before the start of the expansion the patients received periodontal prophylaxis treatment, which included scaling, education and motivation to oral hygiene.

The patients were treated with the same appliance but using different clinical procedure. The Haas expander was anchored to the second deciduous molars with bands and bonded to the deciduous canines using acrylic resin [13,14].

After a week, in the group of patients receiving RPE (Group I), the jackscrew of the expander was activated once (0.25 mm) from the operator and once by the patient or his/her parent (total daily activation, 0.5 mm). Then the jackscrew was activated once in the morning and once in the evening (0.5 mm every 24 hours) for 20 days. After the active therapy, the appliance was stabilized by blocking the screw and there were 5 months of retention therapy [15].

At the same time, patients in Group II were subjected to slow palatal expansion. The jackscrew of the Haas expander was activated twice a week (total activation, 0.5 mm per week). After 3 months of active therapy, there was set a 3 months retention period with the same appliance [15].

The following periodontal clinical indices were used to assess the gingival and periodontal health:

– plaque index (PI, Silness e Löe) [16]: the measurement of the state of oral hygiene by Silness-Löe plaque index is based on recording both soft debris and mineralized deposits on the teeth. Each of the four surfaces of the teeth (buccal, lingual, mesial and distal) is given a score from 0–3. The scores from the four areas of the tooth are added and divided by four in order to give the plaque index for the tooth.
– papillary bleeding index (PBI, Saxer e Muhlemann) [17]: this index permits both immediate evaluation of the patient's gingival condition and his motivation, based upon the actual bleeding tendency of the gingival papillae. A periodontal probe is inserted into the gingival sulcus at the base of the papilla on the mesial aspect, and then moved coronally to the papilla tip. This is repeated on the distal aspect of the papilla. The intensity of any bleeding is recorded (0–4 scores).
– probing pocket depth (PPD).

Table 1 Periodontal conditions of the patients prior to starting the study

Group I	
(5 males and 5 females; average 6.3; range from 6 to 7 years old)	
Patient 1.	Probing depth values not exceeding 3 mm in the whole dentition; no radiographic evidence of periodontal bone loss; normal gingival biotype.
Patient 2.	Probing depth values not exceeding 3 mm in the whole dentition; no radiographic evidence of periodontal bone loss; normal gingival biotype.
Patient 3.	Probing depth values exceeding 3 mm only in two sites; no radiographic evidence of periodontal bone loss; normal/thin gingival biotype.
Patient 4.	Probing depth values exceeding 3 mm only one site in the whole dentition; no radiographic evidence of periodontal bone loss; normal gingival biotype.
Patient 5	Probing depth values not exceeding 3 mm in the whole dentition; no radiographic evidence of periodontal bone loss; normal gingival biotype.
Patient 6.	Probing depth values not exceeding 3 mm in the whole dentition; no radiographic evidence of periodontal bone loss; normal gingival biotype.
Patient 7.	Probing depth values exceeding 3 mm only in two sites; no radiographic evidence of periodontal bone loss; normal/thin gingival biotype.
Patient 8.	Probing depth values not exceeding 3 mm in the whole dentition; no radiographic evidence of periodontal bone loss; normal gingival biotype.
Patient 9.	Probing depth values not exceeding 3 mm in the whole dentition; no radiographic evidence of periodontal bone loss; normal gingival biotype.
Patient 10.	Probing depth values not exceeding 3 mm in the whole dentition; no radiographic evidence of periodontal bone loss; normal gingival biotype.
Group II	
(4 males and 6 females; average 6.3; range from 6 to 8 years old)	
Patient 1.	Probing depth values exceeding 3 mm only in one site; no radiographic evidence of periodontal bone loss; normal gingival biotype.
Patient 2.	Probing depth values exceeding 3 mm only in one siteno radiographic evidence of periodontal bone loss; normal gingival biotype.
Patient 3.	Probing depth values not exceeding 3 mm in the whole dentition; no radiographic evidence of periodontal bone loss; normal gingival biotype.
Patient 4.	Probing depth values not exceeding 3 mm in the whole dentition; no radiographic evidence of periodontal bone loss; normal gingival biotype.
Patient 5.	Probing depth values exceeding 3 mm only in two sites; no radiographic evidence of periodontal bone loss; normal/thin gingival biotype.
Patient 6.	Probing depth values not exceeding 3 mm in the whole dentition; no radiographic evidence of periodontal bone loss; normal/thin gingival biotype.
Patient 7.	Probing depth values not exceeding 3 mm in the whole dentition; no radiographic evidence of periodontal bone loss; normal gingival biotype.
Patient 8.	Probing depth values not exceeding 3 mm in the whole dentition; no radiographic evidence of periodontal bone loss; normal gingival biotype.
Patient 9.	Probing depth values exceeding 3 mm only in two sites; no radiographic evidence of periodontal bone loss; normal gingival biotype.
Patient 10.	Probing depth values not exceeding 3 mm in the whole dentition; no radiographic evidence of periodontal bone loss; normal gingival biotype.

The probing pocket depth was measured in 3 vestibular sites (mesio-buccal, buccal and disto-buccal) and 3 palatal sites (mesio-palatal, palatal and disto-palatal), at the level of the first upper molars, left and right. An standard WHO clinical periodontal probe was used. To standardize the procedure, the probe was inserted until its tip encountered the resistance of the junctional epithelium that forms the base of the sulcus. The pressure exerted with the probe tip against the junctional epithelium was between 10 and 20 grams. A sensitive scale that measures weight in grams was used to standardize the probing pressure. One author (SM) completed the experimental procedures.

The repeatability of the procedure was evaluated with the Intraclass Correlation Coefficient (ICC) applied to double measurements recorded from 5 subjects two times, at a distance of 30 minutes between the first and the second evaluations.

The ICC is the proportion of the total variance within the data that is explained by the variance between the two evaluations. The value of the ICC ranges from 0 to 1, where as the ICC approaches a value of one then we see a perfect agreement between the evaluations, and as the ICC approaches a value of zero then we see no agreement between the evaluations.

In the Group I (RPE), all these indices were detected in three stages:

- T_0, detected 7 days after the periodontal prophylaxis (at the beginning of the active orthodontic therapy);
- T_1, detected after 20 days of active therapy;
- T_2, detected after 5 months of retention therapy.

In the Group II, the collected data corresponded to:

- T_0, detected 7 days after the periodontal prophylaxis;
- T_1, detected during clinical control after 3 months of active therapy;
- T_2, detected after 3 months of restraint.

All measurements were performed by the same examiner.

Data analysis
A descriptive statistical analysis was conducted. The ANOVA evaluation and Tukey's post-hoc analyses were conducted to evaluate the intra-group differences among t_0, t_1 and t_2. The unpaired samples Student's T test was used to evaluate between groups differences at t_0, t_1 and t_2. The significance level was set at 95%.

Results
Demographic data and periodontal conditions prior to starting the study are reported in Table 1.

The Interclass Correlation Coefficient (ICC) is reported in Table 2.

As exposed in Table 3 at t_0, the effects of the periodontal prophylaxis were excellent in controlling periodontal inflammation and dental plaque before the beginning of the orthodontic and orthopaedic treatment, as in both the two groups, the PI and the PBI values were equal to 0.

Regarding the PPD of the first maxillary molars, for simplicity, the data detected in the palatal areas were assumed as reference values.

Table 2 Intra-observer method error calculated with Intraclass Correlation Coefficient (5 subjects)

	T0	T1	Intraclass Correlation Coefficient
PI	0	0.3	ICC: 0.9
PBI	0	0.2	ICC: 0.8
PPD (mm) 1.6	2.5	2.6	ICC: 0.9
PPD (mm) 2.6	2.5	2.5	ICC: 0.9

PI index
In the Group I, the average PI was 0 at t_0, 0.9 at t_1 and 0.5 at t_2.

In the Group II, the average PI was 0 at t_0, 0.7 at t_1 and 0.5 at t_2.

At t_2 the two groups overlapped the same value.

PBI index
In the Group I, the average PBI passed from 0 at t_0, to 0.9 at t_1, and to 0.3 at t_2.

In the Group II, the PBI passed from 0 at t_0 to 0.7 at t_1, and to 0.3 at t_2.

At t_2 the two groups overlapped the same value.

PPD index
In the Group I the average PPD in the right maxillary molar passed from 2.5 at t_0 to 2.9 (at t_1 and t_2); in the left maxillary molar it passed from 2.5 at t_0 to 2.9 at t_1, and 3 at t_2 (Table 3).

In the Group II, the PPD in the right maxillary molar was 2.4 at t_0 and t_1 and passed to 2.9 at t_2; the PPD of the left maxillary molar passed from 2.5 at t_0 to 2.4 at t_1 and 2.8 at t_2 (Table 3).

Discussion
In this study, the clinical indices of periodontal health were selected as they are easily assessable by an orthodontist for a regular periodic monitoring of periodontal health during the orthodontic treatment.

As exposed in Table 3, after 7 days of periodontal prophylaxis and before the beginning of the orthodontic-orthopaedic therapy (t_0), the values of the periodontal indices indicate an excellent state of periodontal health for the patients in both the groups. The PI and PBI were 0 in both the groups. The PPD values nearly overlap.

In both the groups there was an evident increase of the values of periodontal indices (PI and PBI) from t_0 e t_1.

These increases of PI and PBI indices were statistically significant with $p < 0.001$ in both the two Groups, suggesting that they were not due to chance, but to a real difference in periodontal conditions during the orthodontic treatment.

These observations suggest potential irritation effects of the palatal expander on clinical indices of periodontal health, as also demonstrated for fixed orthodontic brackets [18].

In particular, in Group I the increase of values from t_0 to t_1 regarding PI and PBI (0.9) was more pronounced than in Group II.

In addition, in the Group I, the differences between the averages of the PPD from t_0 to t_1 were both statistically significant for the left and the right molars (PPD: 2.9; $p < 0.05$) (Table 3).

Table 3 Main results of periodontal indices

	Group I				Group II				Difference between the 2 groups at T1	Difference between the 2 groups at T2
	T0	T1	Differences between T0 and T1	T2	T0	T1	Differences between T0 and T1	T2		
PI	0	0.9	t:9; p < 0.001	0.5	0	0.7	t:7; p < 0.001	0.5	NS	NS
PBI	0	0.9	t:9; p < 0.001	0.3	0	0.7	t:7; p < 0.001	0.3	NS	NS
PPD 1.6	2.5	2.9	t:2.6; p < 0.05	2.9	2.4	2.4	NS	2.9	NS	NS
PPD 2.6	2.5	2.9	t:2.6; p < 0.05	3	2.5	2.4	NS	2.8	NS	NS

PI: plaque index (Silness e Loe) [16] [13].
PBI: papillary bleeding index (Saxer e Muhlemann) [17] [14].
PPD: probing pocket depth (mm).
T0: 7 days after the periodontal prophylaxis (at the beginning of the active orthodontic therapy).
T1: after 20 days of active therapy.
T2: after 5 months of retention therapy.

On the contrary, in Group II, at t_1 the PPD did not increase in both the right and the left molars, and there was also a slight decrease of the relative average PPD value of the left molar, from 2.5 to 2.4.

Although these differences, the periodontal conditions remained in the periodontal health "range" at t_1 in both the Groups.

These observations seemed to suggest a potentially more dangerous effects of the rapid expansion (Group I) respect to slow expansion (Group II).

This is in accordance with studies about biological responses of these appliances, which suggested that the application of slow palatal expansion in areas of periosteal growth allows normal arch dimensions to develop at any age without undue tipping of the abutment teeth [19,20] potentially avoiding periodontal dangerous effects on the abutment teeth.

This has also been demonstrated for a tissue-borne, fixed, acrylic plate appliance used for RPE, respect to a quad-helix appliance used for SPE in another study [7], although the results of these two study are not directly comparable, because of the different employed appliances (acrylic or metal fixed plate used for RPE) and different recorded variables (clinical and radiographic variables).

In this study, the better state of periodontal health at t_1 observed in the Group II - emphasized by PPD of the left and right molars both equal to 2.4 – could be due to a greater number of controls during SPE, associated to the longer period of active therapy with SPE.

Results seem to mean that the SPE procedure provides for better monitoring of the clinical indices of periodontal health than the procedure of RPE. Therefore, during the RPE the clinician should pay more attention to the control of periodontal health through regular periodic monitoring, as also suggested in literature for other dental treatments [21].

At t_2 the data of periodontal indices (Table 3) of the two Groups nearly overlapped again, with slight differences,

and were in the periodontal health "range" because in both the Groups the PI was 0.5 and the PBI was 0.3.

At t_2 the PPD of the right molar was the same in both groups and equal to 2.9. The PPD of the left molar in Group I was slightly higher (value 3) than in Group II (value 2.8).

Thus in conclusion, there were not important differences in the periodontal health after the retention between RPE and SPE.

The results indicate that both RPE and SPE exhibit minimal differences in periodontal condition after retention (t_2), and the state of the periodontium is good in all groups, although a potential more dangerous effect of RPE during the active treatment. Although the average differences were clinically small, individual variations were evident among few patients subjected to a more pronounced periodontal breakdown in the central side of the first molars. Most of them in the group receiving RPE. Due to the small cohort of this study, it can be considered only a pilot study; thus certain clinical conclusions are not possible. In addition, as the attachment loss was not evaluated, it is not clear – on the base of these results - whether the appliance being in place for almost up to 3 months, would bring about gingival inflammation, potentially giving rise to a pseudo-pocket formation; this factor could have potentially affected the outcome of the study.

Finally, except for the type of the tested expansion therapy, none of the other examined orthodontic variables seemed to have an influence on the periodontal tissues.

Conclusions

According to the data discussed above, in view of the limits of the pilot study design, we can conclude that:

- periodontal prophylaxis appear successful in the control of periodontal health;
- the palatal expander seems to influence periodontal health: both rapid and slow expansion treatments present potential irritation effect (increase of plaque

and bleeding) on the periodontium, suggested by the significant increase of PI and PBI from t_0 to t_1 in both the two groups;

- the difference between the treatment of RPE and SPE during the active therapy (t_1), can be attributed with high probability to the greater number of clinical controls performed during the SPE treatment;
- there are no substantial differences in the long term (t_2) in the periodontal health, after the period of retention, between the treatment of RPE and SPE;
- there are no important advantages that can be unequivocally point to one of the two treatments in periodontal terms.
- PI, PBI and PPD can be used for measurement of periodontal status during the palatal expansion procedure;

The clinically relevant conclusion is that the palatal expansion procedure can affect periodontal health; therefore the clinician should pay more attention to the control of periodontal health through regular periodic monitoring.

Further related studies with a greater sample are recommended to better clarify these relationships.

Ethical approval

This protocol was approved by the Ethic Committee of the University of L'Aquila, in accordance with the principles of the D.Lgs. n. 200 del 6.11.2007, nel D.Lgs. n. 211 del 2003 e nel D.M. 12.5.2006 (Italian Law) with which the Legislator has regulated the establishment of ethics committees for clinical trials of medicinal products, and excluded from the scope of this legislation the so-called non-interventional drug trials (or observational studies), and the experimentation on the People that do not involve the use of drugs or involving human biological materials (tissues, cells, etc.). For protocols like this - non-interventional drug trials (or observational studies) - the Ethics Committee of the University of L'Aquila has recently instituted an apposite section called "Ethics Committee of the University for the evaluation of epidemiological and non-pharmacological observational studies" who gave positive think about the protocol (DR 206/2013, sit 16-7-2013).

Competing interests

The authors declare that they have no competing interests.

Authors' contribution

SM organized the protocol of research; EM coordinated the recording of data; FA helped in the recording of data; VC wrote and organized the manuscript; FP helped in the recording of data; SDM helped in the recording of data; ST organized the data, made the statistical analysis, the analysis of results and wrote the manuscript; and GM wrote and organized the manuscript and the interpretation of results. All the authors read and approved the final manuscript.

Acknowledgement

We acknowledge Miss. L. Rossi for the revision of the english language.

Author details

[1]Department MeSVA, University of L'Aquila, L'Aquila, Italy. [2]Unità Operativa Semplice Dipartimentale di Pronto Soccorso Odontoiatrico, con annessa Unità di Odontoiatria Conservativa, University of Tor Vergata, Roma, Italy. [3]University Vita-Salute San Raffaele, Via Olgettina 60, 20132, Milano, Italy.

References

1. Marsh PD: Are dental diseases examples of ecological catastrophes? *Microbiology* 2003, 149:279–294.
2. Bishara SE, Staley RN: Maxillary expansion: clinical implications. *Am J Orthod Dentofacial Orthop* 1987, 91:3–14.
3. Grieve WG 3rd, Johnson GK, Moore RN, Reinhardt RA, DuBois LM: Prostaglandin E (PGE) and interleukin-1 beta (IL-1 beta) levels in the gingival crevicular fluid during human orthodontic tooth movement. *Am J Orthod Dentofacial Orthop* 1994, 105:369–374.
4. Ousehal L, Lazrak L, Es-Said R, Hamdoune H, Elquars F, Khadija A: Evaluation of dental plaque control in patients wearing fixed orthodontic appliances: a clinical study. *Int Orthod* 2011, 9(1):140–155.
5. Rosa M, Cozzani M: *Espansione rapida del mascellare superiore nel rispetto del parodonto*. Milano, Italy: Schede di aggiornamento S.I.D.O; 1995.
6. Tzannetou S, Efstratiadis S, Nicolay O, Gribic J, Lamster I: Comparison of levels of inflammatory mediators IL-1 and G in gingival crevicular fluid from molars, premolars, and incisors during rapid palatal expansion. *Am J Orthod Dentofacial Orthop* 2008, 133(5):699–707.
7. Greenbaum KR, Zachrisson BU: The effect of palatal expansion therapy on the periodontal supporting tissues. *Am J Orthod* 1982, 81(1):12–21.
8. Garlet TP, Coelho U, Repeke CE, Silva JS, Cunha Fde Q, Garlet GP: Differential expression of osteoblast and osteoclast chemmoatractants in compression and tension sides during orthodontic movement. *Cytokine* 2008, 42(3):330–335.
9. Ro R, Oliveira CA, dos Santos-Pinto A, Jordan SF, Zambon JJ, Cirelli JA, Haraszthy VI: Clinical and microbiological studies of children and adolescents receiving orthodontic treatment. *Am J Dent* 2010, 23(6):317–323.
10. Zachrisson BU: Clinical Implications of recent orthodontic-periodontic research findings. *Semin Orthod* 1996, 2(1):4–12.
11. Kan JY, Rungcharassaeng K, Umezu K, Kois JC: Dimen- sions of peri-implant mucosa: an evaluation of maxillary anterior single implants in humans. *J Periodontol* 2003, 74(4):557–562.
12. Esfahrood ZR, Kadkhodazadeh M, Talebi Ardakani MR: *Gingival biotype: a review*. Gen Dent; 2013:14–17. www.agd.org.
13. Rosa M: Expansão rapida da maxila na dentizão mista sem incluir os dentes permanentes: indicazoes momento oportuno. *Rev Clin Ortod Dental Press* 2011, 10(5):106–118.
14. Cozzani M, Rosa M, Cozzani P, Siciliani G: Deciduous dentition-anchored rapid maxillary expansion in cross bite and non-cross bite mixed dentition patients: reaction of the permanent first molar. *Prog Orthod* 2003, 4(2):15–22.
15. Huynh T, Kennedy DB, Joondeph DR, Bollen AM: Treatment response and stability of slow maxillary expansion using Haas, hyrax, and quad-helix appliances: a retrospective study. *Am J Orthod Dentofacial Orthop* 2009, 136:331–339.
16. Silness J, Loe H: Periodontal disease in pregnancy. II. correlation between oral hygiene and periodontal condition. *Acta Odontol Scand* 1964, 22:121–135.
17. Saxer UP, Muhlemann HR: Motivation and Education. *SSO Schweiz Monatsschr Zahnheilkd* 1975, 85(9):905–919.
18. Mummolo S, Marchetti E, Giuca MR, Gallusi G, Tecco S, Gatto R, Marzo G: In-office bacteria test for a microbial monitoring during the conventional and self-ligating orthodontic treatment. *Head Face Med* 2013, 9:7.
19. McAndrew JR: *The continuous force control system*. Carlsbad, CA: Lancer Technical Report, Lancer Pacific; 1985.

12

The changes of oral health-related quality of life and satisfaction after surgery-first orthognathic approach: a longitudinal prospective study

Shengbin Huang[1], Weiting Chen[2], Zhenyu Ni[2] and Yu Zhou[2*]

Abstract

Background: To our best knowledge, there was little research to assess the changes of quality of life and satisfaction after orthognathic in one trial. The aim of this study was to evaluate the changes of oral health related quality of life and satisfaction between surgery-first and orthodontic-first orthognathic surgery.

Methods: Fifty Chinese orthognathic adluts patients completed two questionnaires: the Dental Impact on Daily Living questionnaire for assessment of his/her satisfaction and 14-item Oral Health Impact Profile for assessment of patient's quality of life. The subjects completed six sets of interviews and clinical evaluations at before treatment; 1 month after surgery (surgery-first); 6 months after treatment; 12 months after treatment ; and 18 month after treatment ; the finished treatment. The pre and post surgical orthodontic period was also recorded. Chi square tests and repeated-measures analysis of variance (ANOVA) were used to compare categorical variables and measure results. All analyses were carried out used Stata software.

Results: The quality of life was significant improved when finished treatment and the amounts of change did not show any significant difference in each domain and at 1, 6, 12 month after orthognathic surgery between two groups. However, in orthodontic-first group, the quality of life was deteriorated before orthognathic surgery. In surgery-first group, the quality of life was immediately improved which lead to better satisfaction.

Conclusions: Although the quality of life scores was no significant difference between two groups, surgery-first treatment could significant reduce treatment during and no deterioration stage of quality of life score which lead to better satisfactory compare to orthodontic-first group. However, some of limitations we need take caution. In future we still need conduct more study to assess the influence of surgery-first method on quality of life.

Keyword: Quality of life, Orthognathic surgery, Surgery-first, Orthodontic-first

Background

Dentofacial deformities are deformities that affect primarily the jaws and the dentition; therefore, they are extremely prominent, are not easily disguised, and affect one's quality of life immensely [1, 2]. Orthognathic surgery aims to correct these deformities via various osteotomies to achieve a desirable end result. Results deemed to be satisfactory from a clinician's aspect may not be so from the patient's aspect, because studies have shown that in patients with facial deformity, there is a close relationship between patient satisfaction and psychosocial functioning [3–6]. In recent years, research on quality of life assessment has been on the rise, and, more importantly, the area of focus has widened with greater emphasis placed on social well-being rather than disease mortality, tumor growth, etc., providing much-neglected subjective views of the treatment outcomes [7]. With increased relevance of health-related quality of life (HRQoL), it is now recognized that quality of life

* Correspondence: wzmczy@126.com
[2]Department of Orthodontics, Hospital of Stomatology, Wenzhou Medical University, 113 West College Road, 325000 Wenzhou, China
Full list of author information is available at the end of the article

(QoL) assessment is a key outcome measure in the management of dentofacial deformities [8–11].

However, the traditional orthognathic surgery treatment which included preoperative orthodontic treatment, orthognathic surgery, and postoperative orthodontic treatment have several disadvantage, such as long treatment during, worsen facial profile and dental function before received orthognathic surgery. Recently, a new surgery method was introduced to overcome the disadvantages of conventional surgical-orthodontic treatment procedures named surgery-first approach (SFA). Because this surgery did not need pre-operative orthodontic treatment, it can significant reduce total treatment time and improve facial profile immediately which may contribute to improving the satisfaction and quality of life in orthognathic surgery-patients [12–15].

Previous studies had showed that orthognathic surgery could improve dental esthetic and quality of life after treatment [16–18]. A recently systematic review [19] also showed that orthognathic surgery had a positive impact on the patient's facial appearance and oral function and found social advantages such as improved self confidence. However, the previous studies were concerning the changes of quality of life after traditional surgical-orthodontic treatment, it is also necessary to assess the influence of different surgery time on the quality of life. In additional, there was little research to investigate the improving patients' satisfaction after orthognathic surgery.

Thus, the aim of this study was to evaluate the changes of oral health related quality of life and satisfaction between surgery-first and orthodontic-first orthognathic surgery patients.

Methods
Ethical
Ethical approval was obtained from the Ethics Committee of the stomatology hospital of the WenZhou Medical University. (Ethics approval number: 201506352541) The participants were informed about the trail and given written consent.

Participants
A total of 50 patients who will receive orthognathic surgery at the Department of Orthodontic at the Stomatology Hospital of WenZhou Medical University were included in this study. The sample divided into 2 groups: the surgery-first group (female 12 , male13; 24.2 ± 5.8 years) and the orthodontic-first group (female 13, male 12; 25.2 ± 4.2 years).

The inclusion criteria were as follows: 1) severe Class III malocclusion need received orthognathic treatment; 2) patients receive either surgery-first or orthodontic-first orthognathic treatment plan;3) orthognathic surgery

consisted purely of bilateral sagittal split ramus osteotomy (BSSRO) to resolve mandibular setback. Subjects were excluded from the study if they had cleft lip and/or palate or other craniofacial anomaly; were taking medications; or had undergone previous orthognathic treatment.

Orthodontic treatment was carried out by one clinicians, and the surgical procedures also by one maxillofacial surgeons who familiar with orthodontist.

Instruments and measures
The patients were given two questionnaires, the Dental Impact on Daily Living (DIDL) questionnaire for assessment of his/her satisfaction after treatment and OHIP-14 for assessment of patient's quality of life.

During the interviews, we collected the baseline information of patients such as: gender, age, and social-economic status before treatment. For assessing the patient's satisfaction after treatment, the DIDL questionnaire has 36 items that are placed in five major categories and tackles five major dimensions of dental satisfaction, namely appearance, pain, oral comfort, general performance, and chewing and eating (Appendix 1), was used. The DIDL scale measures the effect and the proportional importance of each dimension to the patient. The scale has a score from 0 to 10 to show the relative importance of each dimension to the patients [20].

The Chinese version of the OHIP-14 which has shown good psychometric properties was used to assess the changes of oral health-related quality of life. The Chinese Version of the OHIP-14 including seven domains: functional limitation, physical pain, psychological discomfort, physical disability, psychological disability, social disability, and any handicaps. Each item was scored on a 5-point scale to rate the OHQOL. The higher scores indicating poorer OHQoL.

The subjects completed six sets of interviews and clinical evaluations at before treatment (T1); 1 month after surgery (T2); 6 months after treatment (T3); 12 months after treatment (T4); and 18 month after treatment (T5); the finished treatment (T6). The pre and post surgical orthodontic period was also recorded.

Data analysis
Chi square tests were used to compare categorical variables. Repeated-measures analysis of variance (ANOVA) was performed to statistically compare the measurements at each time to the baseline values (T1) in each group. ANOVA determined whether there were any significant overall differences among the groups at each time. Additionally, to identify the significance in each pair of groups, multiple comparison analysis was also performed for the time when the significant difference was noticed. One-way ANOVA and multiple comparison

analysis were performed to compare the amount of treatment during between two groups.

All analyses were carried out used Stata software (version 11.2; StataCorp, College Station, Tex). Significance levels were established at 0 .05.

Results

There was no significant difference between baseline between the surgery-first group and orthodontic-first group, see Table 1.

The mean treatment time was 16.6 + 2.4 month in surgery-first group and 25.3 + 2.4 month in orthodontic-first group. Treatment time was significantly longer in the orthodontic-first group compared to the surgery-first group.

Satisfaction with the DIDL questionnaire was shown in Table 2. There was no significant difference between two groups in each domain. However, the scores were relatively lower in surgery-first group than orthodontic-first group, though this difference did not reach a significant level. This result indicated that surgery-first may acquire better satisfaction compared to orthodontic-first group.

Quality of life level in surgery-first group was significantly improved after 1 month surgery (T2) when compared with baseline ($P < 0.000$). However, no statistical differences were observed between T4 (after 12 month) and T6 (end of treatment). In the orthodontic-first group, the quality of life was deteriorated until T3 (after 6 month treatment) though the difference was not significant. Following orthognathic surgery, a significant improved of quality of life levels was observed ($P < 0.05$). The changes in the quality of life levels are shown in detail in Tables 3 and 4.

Table 1 Demographic and clinical characteristics of surgery-first group and orthodontic-first group subjects

	Surgery-first group	Orthodontic-first group	P value
	n (mean ± SD or %)	n (mean ± SD or %)	
Sex			
Female	12(48)	13(52)	
Male	13(52)	12(48)	NS
Age			
18–25	5	4	
25–30	15	15	
30–35	5	6	NS
Social-economic class			
(high)	20(51)	19(49)	
(low)	5(45)	6(55)	NS

NS mean no significant

Though the quality of life scores were lower in surgery-first group, the difference did not come to a significant level between two groups at 1 month, 6 month and 12 month after received orhognhic surgery. The group comparisons are shown in Table 5.

Discussion

This is the first study to evaluate patient's satisfaction, treatment duration, and quality of life changes between SFA and conventional orthognathic method in Chinese, and we found some interesting results.

One of the most highlighted benefits of SFA is the reduction in treatment duration. The reason may be that, after surgery, orthodontic tooth movement can be easily achieved because the teeth are usually not occluded. Recently, a systematic review evaluated a few retrospective cohort studies and a larger number of case reports treated with SFA [21]. The results showed that the majority of cases were treated under a year. This agrees with our findings which show an average treatment duration of 10.5 months. This is a clear advantage over the conventional approach where treatment times have been reported in the realm of 7–12 months [22–29]. The different total treatment times for SFA depend on the severity of individual dento-skeletal problems,techniques of surgery, orthodontic mechanics, cooperation and biological response as well as desired results for each patient.

Assessment of patient satisfaction with their dentition after orthodontic treatment was carried out using the DIDL questionnaire. The DIDL questionnaire is a reliable, valid, and comprehensive test to measure patient satisfaction and effect of dental disease on patient daily living [30, 31]. The test has shown the ability to assess satisfaction with different aspects of oral cavity and dental status, and for these reasons, it was selected for this study. Orthodontic problems can affect many aspects of dental esthetics and function, and these aspects are well covered by the DIDL test.

Our results revealed that satisfaction after orthognathic surgery was high.

A total of 80 and 72 % of all patients rated postoperative outcomes after surgery in two group, respectively. There was no significant difference between two groups in each domain. However, the scores were relatively lower in surgery-first group than orthodontic-first group, though this difference did not reach a significant level. This result indicated that surgery-first may acquire better satisfaction compared to orthodontic-first group. The high patient satisfaction in SFA group may due to immediate improvement of facial profile at the beginning of the treatment14,29-30. The high satisfaction rate was in accordance with that reported in previous studies, which

Table 2 Frequency of Individual Satisfaction Dimensions in the Study Population

Dimension	Surgery-first group			Orthodontic-first group			P
	Dissatisfied	Relatively Satisfied	Satisfied	Dissatisfied	Relatively Satisfied	Satisfied	
Appearance	0(%)	1(4)	24(96)	0	2(8)	23(92)	NS
Pain	1(4)	7(28)	17(68)	2(8)	6(24)	14(68)	NS
Oral comfort	3(12)	4(16)	18(72)	2(8)	7(28)	16(64)	NS
General performance	0(0)	2(8)	23(92)	0(0)	3(12)	22(88)	NS
Eating and chewing	1(4)	2(8)	22(88)	2(8)	2(8)	21(84)	NS
Total	1(4)	4(16)	20(80)	2(8)	5(20)	18(72)	NS

NS Non-significant

Table 3 Comparison of quality of life scores at before treatment (T1); 1 month after surgery (T2); 6 months after treatment (T3); 12 months after treatment (T4); and 18 month after treatment (T5); the finished treatment(T6) with T1 (before treatment) in two group

Varies	Group	T1	T2	P (T2-T1)	T3	P (T3-T1)	T4	P (T4-T1)	T5	P (T5-T1)	T6	P (T6-T1)
functional limitation	Surgery-first group	8.42	5.22	0.034*	2.39	0.000***	1.99	0.000***	1.98	0.000***	1.89	0.000***
		(2.79)	(1.88)		(1.24)		(1.76)		(1.68)		(1.26)	
	Orthodontic-first group	8.45	8.30	0.867	8.79	0.758	5.42	0.000***	1.98	0.000***	1.92	0.000***
		(2.99)	(2.56)		(1.23)		(1.98)		(1.68)		(1.56)	
physical pain	Surgery-first group	5.26	3.22	0.045*	2.34	0.009**	1.59	0.000***	1.56	0.000***	1.34	0.000***
		(1.85)	(1.55)		(1.24)		(0.67)		(0.51)		(0.89)	
	Orthodontic-first group	5.46	5.30	0.920	6.02	0.052	3.51	0.000***	1.89	0.000***	1.75	0.000***
		(1.61)	(1.69)		(2.36)		(1.72)		(1.28)		(1.22)	
psychological discomfort	Surgery-first group	6.12	4.29	0.048*	2.22	0.000***	0.56	0.000***	0.52	0.000***	0.45	0.000***
		(2.12)	(1.22)		(1.12)		(1.10)		(0.18)		(0.13)	
	Orthodontic-first group	6.25	6.52	0.685	6.56	0.658	4.82	0.000***	2.82	0.000***	0.92	0.000***
		(2.09)	(2.23)		(2.85)		(2.29)		(1.31)		(1.26)	
physical disability	Surgery-first group	6.29	4.15	0.045*	1.64	0.000***	1.34	0.000***	0.12	0.000***	0.10	0.000***
		(2.64)	(1.72)		(1.08)		(1.22)		(0.11)		(0.03)	
	Orthodontic-first group	6.39	6.56	0.687	6.85	0.785	4.42	0.000***	2.41	0.000***	1.49(0.91)	0.000***
		(2.72)	(2.67)		(2.75)		(1.75)		(1.13)			
psychological disability	Surgery-first group	6.54	3.28	0.007**	1.64	0.000***	0.42	0.000***	0.20	0.000***	0.15	0.000***
		(2.52)	(1.76)		(1.08)		(0.21)		(0.12)		(0.12)	
	Orthodontic-first group	6.72	6.79	0.920	6.76	0.925	3.72	0.000***	1.83	0.000***	0.88	0.000***
		(2.42)	(3.41)		(3.06)		(1.58)		(1.15)		(1.13)	
social disability	Surgery-first group	6.03	4.26	0.042	1.24	0.000***	0.62	0.000***	0.19	0.000***	0.15	0.000***
		(2.32)	(1.98)		(1.08)		(0.35)		(0.22)		(0.15)	
	Orthodontic-first group	6.12	6.86	0.865	6.89	0.675	4.52	0.000***	1.64	0.000***	0.98	0.000***
		(2.68)	(2.88)		(2.29)		(2.56)		(1.18)		(1.12)	
handicaps	Surgery-first group	3.24	2.18	0.035	1.52	0.004**	0.38	0.000***	0.16	0.000***	0.12	0.000***
		(1.18)	(1.81)		(1.75)		(0.26)		(0.12)		(0.12)	
	Orthodontic-first group	5.66	6.34	0.901	6.61	0.921	2.42	0.000***	1.94	0.000***	0.78	0.000***
		(2.81)	(1.85)		(2.72)		(2.12)		(1.36)		(1.12)	
Total scores	Surgery-first group	38.68	27.72	0.031*	13.94	0.000***	6.90	0.000***	4.11	0.000***	3.89	0.000***
		(4.35)	(3.26)		(2.13)		(1.39)		(0.49)		(1.02)	
	Orthodontic-first group	39.55	41.67	0.654	48.48	0.124	28.86	0.000***	15.61	0.000***	8.68	0.000***
		(4.15)	(4.14)		(3.91)		(3.83)		(2.49)		(1.65)	

*P < 0.05; **P < 0.01; ***P < 0.001

Table 4 Statistical evaluation of quality of life scores between the surgery-first group and the orthodontic-first group at 1 month after surgery (T2); 6 months after treatment (T3); 12 months after treatment (T4); and 18 month after treatment (T5); the finished treatment (T6)

Varies	Varies	P(T2-T3)	P(T2-T4)	P(T2-T5)	P(T2-T6)	P(T3-T4)	P(T3-T5)	P(T3-T6)	P(T4-T5)	P(T4-T6)	P(T5-T6)
functional limitation	Surgery-first group	0.024*	0.000***	0.000***	0.000***	0.658	0.725	0.687	0.801	0.831	0.882
	Orthodontic-first group	0.824	0.000***	0.000***	0.000***	0.000***	0.000***	0.000***	0.654	0.702	0.783
physical pain	Surgery-first group	0.048*	0.004**	0.000***	0.000***	0.624	0.742	0.049*	0.903	0.921	0.920
	Orthodontic-first group	0.768	0.000***	0.000***	0.000***	0.000***	0.000***	0.000***	0.726	0.824	0.931
psychological discomfort	Surgery-first group	0.003**	0.000***	0.000***	0.000***	0.000***	0.000***	0.000***	0.869	0.902	0.965
	Orthodontic-first group	0.857	0.000***	0.000***	0.000***	0.000***	0.000***	0.000***	0.867	0.798	0.804
physical disability	Surgery-first group	0.003**	0.000***	0.000***	0.000***	0.687	0.000***	0.000***	0.145	0.263	0.687
	Orthodontic-first group	0.867	0.000***	0.000***	0.000***	0.000***	0.000***	0.000***	0.042*	0.032*	0.903
psychological disability	Surgery-first group	0.004**	0.000***	0.000***	0.000***	0.000***	0.000***	0.000***	0.035*	0.038*	0.867
	Orthodontic-first group	0.864	0.000***	0.000***	0.000***	0.000***	0.000***	0.000***	0.024*	0.034*	0.902
social disability	Surgery-first group	0.000***	0.000***	0.000***	0.000***	0.214	0.000***	0.000***	0.042*	0.038*	0.824
	Orthodontic-first group	0.875	0.000***	0.000***	0.000***	0.000***	0.000***	0.000***	0.042*	0.024*	0.897
handicaps	Surgery-first group	0.321	0.000***	0.000***	0.000***	0.000***	0.000***	0.000***	0.365	0.487	0.867
	Orthodontic-first group	0.806	0.000***	0.000***	0.000***	0.000***	0.000***	0.000***	0.035*	0.008**	0.421
Totalscores	Surgery-first group	0.000***	0.000***	0.000***	0.000***	0.000***	0.000***	0.000***	0.042*	0.031*	0.682
	Orthodontic-first group	0.654	0.000***	0.000***	0.000***	0.000***	0.000***	0.000***	0.000***	0.000***	0.725

*$P < 0.05$; ** $P < 0.01$; *** $P < 0.001$

Table 5 Comparisons of quality of life scores at the different time points for the surgery-first group and orthodontic-first group at 1 month, 6 month and 12 month after orthognathic surgery

Varies	Postoperative 1 month		P	Postoperative 6 month		P	Postoperative 12 month		P
	Surgery-first group(T2)	Orthodontic-first group(T4)		Surgery-first group(T3)	Orthodontic-first group(T5)		Surgery-first group(T4)	Orthodontic-first group(T6)	
functional limitation	5.22	5.42	NS	2.39	1.98	NS	1.99	1.92	NS
	(1.88)	(1.98)		(1.24)	(1.68)		(1.76)	(1.56)	
physical pain	3.22	3.51	NS	2.34	1.89	NS	1.59	1.75	NS
	(1.55)	(1.72)		(1.24)	(1.28)		(0.67)	(1.22)	
psychological discomfort	4.29	4.82	NS	2.22	2.82	NS	0.56	0.92	NS
	(1.22)	(2.29)		(1.12)	(1.31)		(1.10)	(1.26)	
physical disability	4.15	4.42	NS	1.64	2.41	NS	1.34	1.49	NS
	(1.72)	(1.75)		(1.08)	(1.13)		(1.22)	(0.91)	
psychological disability	3.28	3.72	NS	1.64	1.83	NS	0.42	0.88	NS
	(1.76)	(1.58)		(1.08)	(1.15)		(0.21)	(1.13)	
social disability	4.26	4.52	NS	1.24	1.64	NS	0.62	0.98	NS
	(1.98)	(2.56)		(1.08)	(1.18)		(0.35)	(1.12)	
handicaps	2.18	2.42	NS	1.52	1.94	NS	0.38	0.78	NS
	(1.81)	(2.12)		(1.75)	(1.36)		(0.26)	(1.12)	
Total scores	27.72	28.86	NS	13.94	15.61	NS	6.90	8.68	NS
	(3.26)	(3.83)		(2.13)	(2.49)		(1.39)	(1.65)	

NS Non-significant

ranged between 70 % [32] and 87 % [33], and which was also higher than that reported among pre-treatment and no-treatment control groups [34]. Hence, positive changes occurred in the personality profiles of patients. There was an obvious improvement in self-confidence in 67.5 % of patients as a result of an improved appearance and an improved chewing function.

The results of the present study showed a highly significant degree of overall improvement in patients'quality of life after orthognathic surgery in two group, others found the similar resluts [35–37]. However, we noticed that the quality of life scores was deteriorated before orthognathic in orthodontic-first group. This results indicated that the dental decompensation during pre-orthodontics could worsen the facial deformity, which has been perceived as the most stressful period of overall treatment by the patients [38] Esperao [39] found the similar results. It reminded us that we may need tell patients that he may experience short-term quality of life deterioration before orthognathic surgery.

We were very pleased to find that all the domain of quality of life scores were consistently lower in the surgery-first groups compared to the orthodontic-first group, although there were no significant statistical differences when patients received orthognathic surgery. The reason may be that surgery -first treatment could improve OHRQoL immediately and lead to better satisfactory compare to orthodontic-first group. It was important to doctors, because we not only gain perfect treatment results but also improve patients'quality of life and satisfaction.

The limitations of the study was small sample,we only included 50 patients which may weak the evidence of this study. Secondly, we did not objectively quantify the quality of orthodontic outcome. Although patient satisfaction is high, it has been noted by the orthodontists treating some of these patients that there is an urge to remove the orthodontic appliances very soon after orthognathic surgery. In future research we need including treatment results when assess the quality of life changes. Additionally, because of inclusion criteria of this article was limited to BSSRO, we think if two-jaw surgery was included in the study, the results will be different. In present, because of raised patient's requests, two-jaw surgery increases. Thus, future research need includ more two-jaw surgery patients.

Conclusions

Surgery-first treatment could significant reduce treatment during and no deterioration stage of quality of life score which lead to better satisfactory compare to orthodontic-first group. However, some of limitations we need take caution, such as small sample, no two-jaw surgery patients were included. In future we need

conduct a more larger sample randomized control trail to investigate the oral health-related quality of life in Chinese orthognathic surgery patients.

Competing interests

The authors declare that they have no competing interests.

Authors' contributions

ZY,SH and WC designed the study, gathered the information, performed the statistical analysis and wrote the first draft of the manuscript. ZN designed the form for data gathering and supervised the statistical analysis. All authors read and approved the final manuscript.

Author details

[1]Department of Prosthodontics, Hospital of Stomatology, Wenzhou Medical University, Wenzhou, China. [2]Department of Orthodontics, Hospital of Stomatology, Wenzhou Medical University, 113 West College Road, 325000 Wenzhou, China.

References

1. Ong MAH. Spectrum of dento-facial deformities: a retrospective survey. Ann Acad Med Singapore. 2004;33:239–42.
2. Cunningham SJ, Garratt AM, Hunt NP. Development of a condition-specific quality of life measure for patients with dentofacial deformity: II. Validity and responsiveness testing. Community Dent Oral Epidemiol. 2002;30:81–90.
3. Sarwer DB, Bartlett SP, Whitaker LA, Paige KT, Pertschuk MJ, Wadden TA. Adult psychological functioning of individuals born with craniofacial anomalies. Plast Reconstr Surg. 1999;103:412–8.
4. Versnel SL, Duivenvoorden HJ, Passchier J, Mathijssen IMJ. Satisfaction with facial appearance and its determinants in adults with severe congenital facial disfigurement: a case-referent study. J Plast Reconstr Aesthet Surg. In press.
5. Ahmed B, Gilthorpe MS, Bedi R. Agreement between normative and perceived orthodontic need amongst deprived multiethnic schoolchildren in London. Clin Orthod Res. 2001;4:65–71.
6. Hunt O, Hepper P, Johnston C, Stevenson M, Burden D. The aesthetic component of the index of orthodontic treatment need validated against lay opinion. Eur J Orthod. 2002;24:53–9.
7. Kiyak HA, Reichmuth M. Body image issues in dental medicine. In: Cash TF, Pruzinsky T, editors. Body image: a handbook of theory, research and clinical practice. New York: Guilford; 2002. p. 342–50.
8. Bellucci CC, Kapp-Simon KA. Psychological considerations in orthognathic surgery. Clin Plast Surg. 2007;34:e11–6.
9. Cunningham SJ, Hunt NP. Quality of life and its importance in orthodontics. J Orthod. 2001;28:152–8.
10. Bennett ME, Phillips CL. Assessment of health-related quality of life for patients with severe skeletal disharmony: a review of the issues. Int J Adult Orthod Orthognath Surg. 1999;14:65–75.
11. Han CW, Yajima Y, Nakajima K, Lee EJ, Meguro M, Kohzuki M. Construct validity of the Frenchay activities index for community-dwelling elderly in Japan. Tohoku J Exp Med. 2006;210:99–107.
12. Baek SH, Ahn HW, Kwon YH, Choi JY. Surgery-first approach in skeletal Class III malocclusion treated with 2- jaw surgery: evaluation of surgical movement and postoperative orthodontic treatment. J Craniofac Surg. 2010;21:332–8.
13. Ko EW, Hsu SS, Hsieh HY, Wang YC, Huang CS, Chen YR. Comparison of progressive cephalometric changes and postsurgical stability of skeletal Class III correction with and without presurgical orthodontic treatment. J Oral Maxillofac Surg. 2011;69:1469–77.
14. Liou EJ, Chen PH, Wang YC, Yu CC, Huang CS, Chen YR. Surgery-first accelerated orthognathic surgery: orthodontic guidelines and setup for model surgery. J Oral Maxillofac Surg. 2011;69:771–80.
15. Liao YF, Chiu YT, Huang CS, Ko EW, Chen YR. Presurgical orthodontics versus no presurgical orthodontics: treatment outcome of surgical-orthodontic correction for skeletal Class III open bite. Plast Reconstr Surg. 2010;126:2074–83.
16. Modig M, Andersson L, Wardh I. Patients' perception of improvement after orthognathic surgery: pilot study. Br J Oral Maxillofac Surg. 2006;44:24–7.

17. Motegi E, Hatch JP, Rugh JD. Health related quality of life and psychosocial function 5 years after orthognathic surgery. Am J Orthod Dentofacial Orthop. 2003;124:138–43.

18. NicodemoD, PereiraMD, FerreiraLM. Effect of orthognathic surgery for class III correction asmeasured by SF-36. Int Joral Maxillofac Surg 2007: 1231–1234.

19. Murphy C, Kearns G, Allen PF. The clinical relevance of orthognathic surgery on quality of life. Int J Oral Maxillofac Surg. 2011;40:926–30.

20. Leao A, Sheiham A. Relation between clinical dental status and subjective impacts on daily living. J Dent Res. 1995;74:1408–13.

21. Euro Qol Group. EuroQol—a new facility for the measurement of health-related quality of life. Health Policy. 1990;16:199–208.

22. Proffit WR, Miguel JA. The duration and sequencing of surgical-orthodontic treatment. Int J Adult Orthodon Orthognath Surg. 1995;10:35–42.

23. Slavnic S, Marcusson A. Duration of orthodontic treatment in conjunction with orthognathic surgery. Swed Dent J. 2010;34:159–66.

24. O'Brien K, Wright J, Conboy F, Appelbe P, Bearn D, Caldwell S, et al. Prospective, multi-center study of the effectiveness of orthodontic/orthognathic surgery care in the United Kingdom. Am J Orthod Dentofacial Orthop. 2009;135:709–14.

25. Diaz PM, Garcia RG, Gias LN, Aguirre-Jaime A, Perez JS, de la Plata MM, et al. Time used for orthodontic surgical treatment of dentofacial deformities in white patients. J Oral Maxillofac Surg. 2010;68:88–92.

26. Huang CS, Hsu SS, Chen YR. Systematic review of the surgery-first approach in orthognathic surgery. Biomed J. 2014;37:184–90.

27. Yu CC, Chen PH, Liou EJ, Huang CS, Chen YR. A Surgery-first approach in surgical-orthodontic treatment of mandibular prognathism—a case report. Chang Gung Med J. 2010;33:699–705.

28. Nagasaka H, Sugawara J, Kawamura H, Nanda R. "Surgery first" skeletal Class III correction using the skeletal anchorage system. J Clin Orthod. 2009;43:97–105.

29. Villegas C, Uribe F, Sugawara J, Nanda R. Expedited correction of significant dentofacial asymmetry using a "surgery first" approach. J Clin Orthod. 2010; 44:97–103.

30. Leao A. The Development of Measures of Dental Impacts on Daily Living [PhD thesis]. London, UK: London University; 1993.

31. Al-Omiri MK. Tooth Wear Impact on Daily Living [PhD thesis]. Belfast, UK: Queen's University Belfast; 2002.

32. Türker N, Varol A, Ogel K, Basa S. Perceptions of preoperative expectations and postoperative outcomes from orthognathic surgery: part I: Turkish female patients. Int J Oral Maxillofac Surg. 2008;37:710–5.

33. De Clercq CA, Neyt LF, Mommaerts MY, Abeloos JS. Orthognathic surgery: patients' subjective findings with focus on the temporomandibular joint. J Cranio-maxillo-facial Surg. 1998;26:29–34.

34. Lazaridou-Terzoudi T, Kiyak HA, Moore R, Athanasiou AE, Melsen B. Long-term assessment of psychologic outcomes of orthognathic surgery. J Oral Maxillofac Surg. 2003;61:545–52.

35. Tabrizi R, Rezaii A, Golkari A, Ahrari F. The impact of orthognathic surgery on oral health-related quality of life. J Dent Mater Technol. 2014;3:23–7.

36. Soh CL, Narayanan V. Quality of life assessment in patients with dentofacial deformity undergoing orthognathic surgery-a systematic review. Int J Oral Maxillofac Surg. 2013;42:974–80.

37. Kavin T, Jagadesan AG, Venkataraman SS. Changes in quality of life and impact on patients' perception of esthetics after orthognathic surgery. J Pharm Bioallied Sci. 2012;4:S290–3.

38. Hernndez-Alfaro F, Guijarro-Martnez R, Molina Coral A, Bada-Escriche C. "Surgery first" in bimaxillary orthognathic surgery. J Oral Maxillofac Surg. 2011;69:201–7.

39. Esperão PT, de Oliveira BH, de Oliveira Almeida MA, Kiyak HA, Miguel JA. Oral health-related quality of life in orthognathic surgery patients. Am J Orthod Dentofacial Orthop. 2010;137:790–5.

13

NCAM (CD56) Expression in keratin-producing odontogenic cysts: aberrant expression in KCOT

Beatriz Vera-Sirera[1], Leopoldo Forner-Navarro[1] and Francisco Vera-Sempere[2,3]*

Abstract

Objective: To investigate immunohistochemically the expression of neural cell adhesion molecule (NCAM), which has been identified as a signaling receptor with frequent reactivity in ameloblastomas (AB), in a series of keratin-producing odontogenic cysts (KPOCs).

Material and methods: Immunohistochemical expression of NCAM, using a monoclonal antibody, was determined in a series of 58 KPOCs comprising 12 orthokeratinized odontogenic cysts (OOCs) and 46 keratocystic odontogenic tumors (KCOTs), corresponding to 40 non-syndromic KCOT (NS-KCOTs) and 6 syndromic KCOT (S-KCOTs), associated with nevic basocellular syndrome (NBCS).

Results: NCAM expression was negative in all OOCs, but 36.45% of KCOTs exhibited focal and heterogeneous expression at the basal cell level, as well as in basal budding areas and the basal cells of daughter cysts. The latter two locations were especially applicable to S-KCOTs, with focal NCAM reactivity occurring in 66.66% of cases.

Conclusions: Aberrant NCAM expression, in KCOTs but especially in S-KCOTs, together with its immunomorphological location, suggests that this adhesion molecule and signaling receptor plays a role in the pathogenesis of KCOTs, with a probable impact on lesional recurrence.

Keywords: NCAM, Keratocysts, Keratocystic odontogenic tumor, Orthokeratinized odontogenic cyst, Immunohistochemistry

Introduction

Keratin-producing odontogenic cysts (KPOCs) form a heterogeneous group of cystic lesions that are often aggressive in character, with high rates of recurrence and multifocality [1]. The lesional spectrum of KPOCs includes odontogenic keratocysts, that according to last World Health Organization (WHO) guidelines [2] are also referred to as keratocystic odontogenic tumors (KCOTs), in accordance with the fact that KCOTs are true tumoral growths. Effective management of these cystic lesions is subject to frequent discussion [3] and malignant transformation is possible, albeit very rare [4].

NCAM (neural cell adhesion molecule), also known as CD56, was originally characterized as a cell-surface glycoprotein member of the immunoglobulin superfamily, implicated in calcium-independent intercellular adhesion [5]

and expressed in a wide variety of cells [6]. However, in the past decade the traditional view of NCAM has been challenged, such that it is now also considered a signaling receptor that impacts upon cellular migration, proliferation, differentiation, and survival, thereby playing a role in different models of tumor growth [7].

NCAM immunoreactivity in ameloblastomas within odontogenic tumors has been reported with very high frequency [8-11], and has also been observed in certain ameloblastic carcinomas [9]. In contrast, NCAM reactivity is indicated as relatively infrequent in KCOTs [10,11].

The aim of the present study was to assess the immunohistochemical expression of NCAM in a series of keratin-producing odontogenic cysts (KPOCs), and to evaluate the possible significance of adhesion molecule reactivity in this heterogeneous group of odontogenic cysts.

* Correspondence: fco.jose.vera@uv.es
[2]Departaments of Pathology, University of Valencia, Valencia, Spain
[3]Service of Pathology, Hospital Universitario y Politécnico La Fe, Avda Campanar 21, Valencia 46009, Spain
Full list of author information is available at the end of the article

Materials and methods

We studied 58 cases of KPOC diagnosed over a period of 10 years at the Department of Pathology of La Fe University Hospital, Valencia, Spain. Histological material was retrieved from storage. Our work formed part of a project previously approved by our Ethics Committee for Biomedical Research (protocol no. 2013/0045).

We selected KPOC cases using a pathological diagnosis database (Pat Win®, ver. 4.1.4), and performed a 10-year retrospective search employing the following search terms: "keratinized cyst", "keratocyst", "primordial cyst", "keratocystic odontogenic tumor (KCOT)", and "ortho-keratinized odontogenic cyst (OOC)". All of these terms have been used over time to describe various lesions, including KPOCs [4,12].

All original histological sections were reviewed microscopically by two observers, and were reclassified according to the WHO (2005) criteria [2], into 46 examples of KCOT and 12 of OOC. In all KCOT cases the presence or absence of daughter/satellite cysts in the cystic wall, and/or budding areas of the basal layer, was noted because the morphological features of these lesions have been implicated in their recurrence [13,14].

Clinical and radiological data of all patients were collected using the Mizar® (ver. 2.0) medical records platform, in conjunction with the viewfinder software package Luna® (ver. 3.0). Clinical/radiological follow-up findings, the number of recurrences, and any clinical, pathological, or genetic data suggesting syndromic association were retrieved. Following verification of the diagnostic criteria of Kimonis et al. [15] for nevic basocellular syndrome (NBCS), 6 of the 46 KCOT were considered syndromic KCOTs (S-KCOTs). The remaining 40 cases qualified as sporadic or non-syndromic KCOTs (NS-KCOTs). Therefore, the biopsy material finally included was as follows: 12 OOC; 40 NS-KCOT; and 6 S-KCOT.

Sections of 5-μm thickness were cut from the original paraffin-embedded blocks and mounted on poly-L-lysine-coated glass slides prior to immunohistochemical staining, performed using the lyophilized mouse monoclonal antibody NCL-CD56-504 (clone CD564; Novocastra™, Leica Biosystems, Newcastle upon Tyne, UK), at 1/50 dilution, and with a 60-min incubation time. Epitope retrieval proceeded at 97°C for 20 min, in a citrate buffer of pH 9. Immunostaining was visualized using the high-pH EnVision FLEX system (Dako®, Glostrup, Denmark): hematoxylin was used for counterstaining. Tonsil sections served as positive staining controls: the negative controls were mock-stained test sections (the primary antibody was replaced by PBS).

NCAM (CD56) immunostaining was semi-quantitatively assessed on a scale ranging between 0 and 3+ (0 = *absent*; 1+ = *weak*; 2+ = *moderate*; 3+ = *intense*), and also classified as diffuse (>50% of cells), extensive (10-50% of cells) or focal (<10% of cells expressing NCAM).

NCAM immunohistochemical results for the different KPOC subtypes expressed as categorical variables with numbers and percentages, as well as associations between NCAM expression and recurrence, were compared using Firth's logistic regression test. Statistical analyses were performed using the SPSS for Windows software package (ver. 14.0; SPSS Inc., Chicago, IL). A value of $p < 0.05$ was taken to indicate statistical significance.

Results

Of 58 KPCOs, only 16 cases (27,58%) dysplayed NCAM expresión at the of epithelial level and inmunoreactivity was in positive cases of focal character (<10% of cells expressing NCAM) with a weak (1+) to moderate (2+) intensity, and always demostrating a heterogeneous distribution within the structure of the cystic lesion.

NCAM expression was absent in all 12 OOC cases, with the epithelial lining of the cysts entirely negative for CD56. In contrast, focal NCAM reactivity was observed at the epithelial level in 16 of 46 KCOT cases (36.95%). There was a significant difference in NCAM expression in cases of OOC *vs.* KCOT ($p = 0.012$).

NCAM immunostaining was differentially expressed in NS- and S-KCOTs: four of the six cases of S-KCOT (66.66%) exhibited focal NCAM reactivity at the epithelial level, in contrast to only 12 of the 40 (30%) cases of NS-KCOT (Table 1). OOC did not recur in any case during clinical/radiological follow-up at 39.2 ± 26.01 m. In contrast, all cases of S-KCOT recurred at a mean follow-up of 112 ± 76.1 m. In NS-KCOT0 cases, the recurrence rate was 35% at a mean follow-up of 29.6 ± 31.04 m. When analyses were performed independent of lesional subtype, there was no association between recurrence and NCAM expression ($p = 0.52$).

In positive cases, NCAM expression was always epithelial, with weak (1+) to moderate (2+) intensity and a heterogeneous and focal distribution (Figures 1A and 1B). NCAM positivity (Table 2) was most frequent in the basal layer of cystic epithelium, followed by areas of basal budding (Figures 2A and 3A-D) and the basal portion of daughter cysts or satellite epithelial nests (Figures 2B and 4A-D). In NCAM-positive S-KCOT cases (four of six), NCAM positivity was discontinuous, weak or moderate, in the locations indicated above, although only 50% of satellite

Table 1 NCAM expression in KPOC

Lesional Type	No. cases	NCAM+ cases (%)	Recurrence
OOC	12	0/12 (0,00%)	0,00%
S- and NS-KCOT	46	16/46 (36,95%)	43,47%
NS-KCOT	40	12/40 (30,00%)	35,00%
S-KCOT	6	4/6 (66,66%)	100,00%

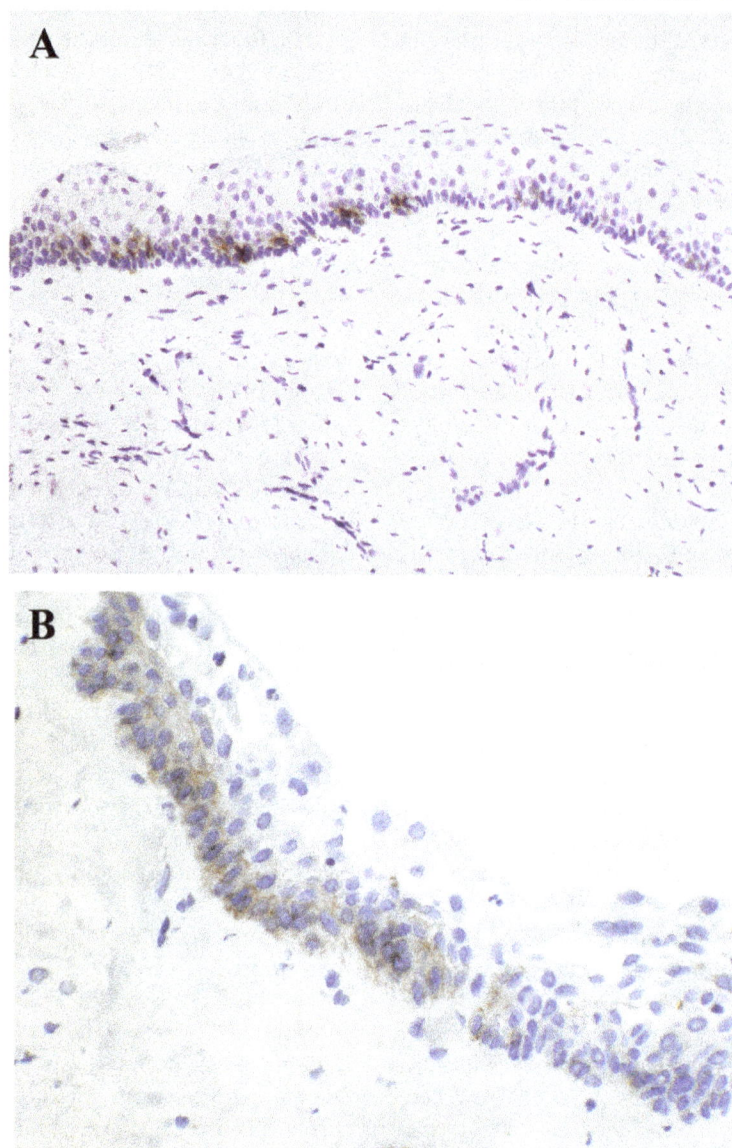

Figure 1 KCOT showing NCAM reactivity at basal cells with a discontinuous pattern (A) and occasional extension to suprabasal level (B). NCAM 200x.

epithelial nests or cysts demonstrated basal positivity. Similarly, in NS-KCOTs, the most frequent NCAM-positive location was the basal cell layer of the cystic lining (observed in all cases exhibiting NCAM positivity), followed by areas of basal budding ($n = 4$) and basal portions of daughter cysts ($n = 3$).

Discussion

Neural cell adhesion molecule (NCAM), a member of the immunoglobulin superfamily adhesion molecule, is expressed by a wide variety of neuroectodermal and mesenchymal cells [6]. Originally, NCAM was exclusively characterized as a mediator of cell-cell adhesion,

Table 2 NCAM $^+$ location in KPOC

Lesional Type	No. cases	NCAM$^+$ cases (%)		Basal cells		Basal budding		Daughter cysts	
OOC	12	0/12	(0,00%)	0/12	(0,00%)	0/12	(0,00%)	0/12	(0,00%)
S- and NS-KCOT	46	16/46	(36,95%)	16/46	(34,78%)	7/46	(15,21%)	6/46	(13,04%)
NS-KCOT	40	12/40	(30,00%)	12/40	(30,00%)	4/40	(10,00%)	3/40	(7,50%)
S-KCOT	6	4/6	(66,66%)	4/6	(66,66%)	3/6	(50,00%)	3/6	(50,00%)

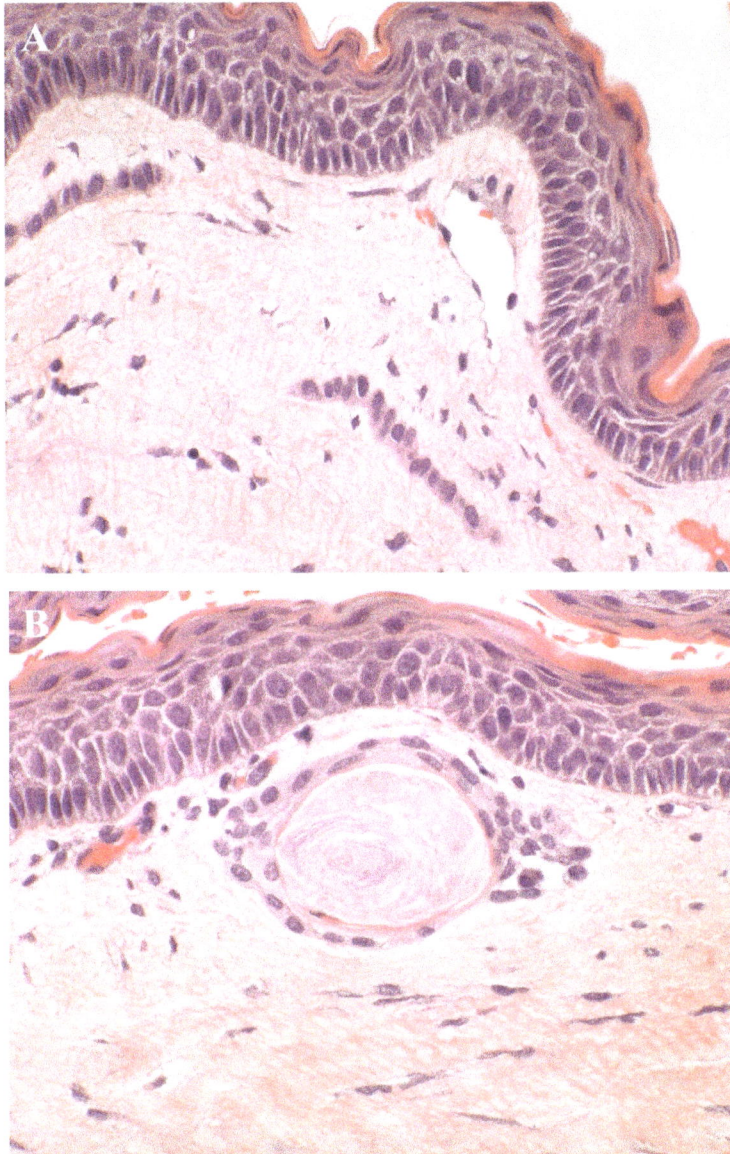

Figure 2 Epithelial budding (A) and daughter microcyst (B) in KCOT. HE 200 and 250x.

but is now also considered to be a signaling receptor that impacts upon cellular adhesion, migration, proliferation, apoptosis, differentiation, and survival. NCAM is involved in various models of tumorigenesis [7], including certain types of odontogenic tumor: NCAM expression has been reported in certain ameloblastic carcinomas [9], and especially in the outer columnar cells of ameloblastoma (AB) [8-11]. This expression could be indicative of neuroectodermal differentiation in AB [10], especially considering the fact that neural crest cells are associated with tooth development, particularly ectomesenchymal differentiation in tooth germs [15].

The purpose of the present study was to assess the presence and significance of NCAM reactivity in a series

of KPOCs. Our results highlight a total absence of NCAM expression in OOCs, a form of KPOCs characterized by orthokeratotic keratinization, reduced proliferative activity and non-recurrence [16,17]. Recurrence was not observed for any case of OOC, but in KCOTs, a form of KPOC now considered as a true odontogenic tumor [1,2,4], we observed focal and heterogeneous NCAM expression in 36.95% of cases, a significantly higher rate than OOC. Prior to our investigation, only two studies assessed NCAM expression in odontogenic cysts. Cairns et al. [11] reported NCAM expression in only 5.26% of KCOTs, with focal NCAM reactivity occurring at the basal cell level; in contrast, AB exhibited high levels of NCAM reactivity. More recently, Kusafuka et al. reported that 50% of KCOTs

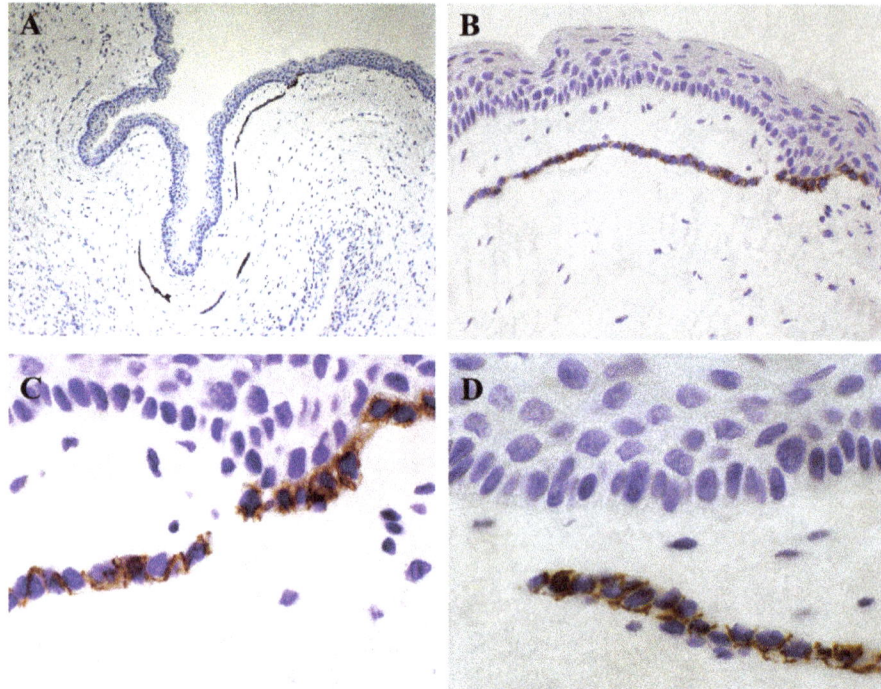

Figure 3 KCOT showing epithelial buds (A) arising of basal cells (B and C) displaying NCAM reactivity with a predominantly membranous pattern **(D).** (NCAM, 200 and 400x).

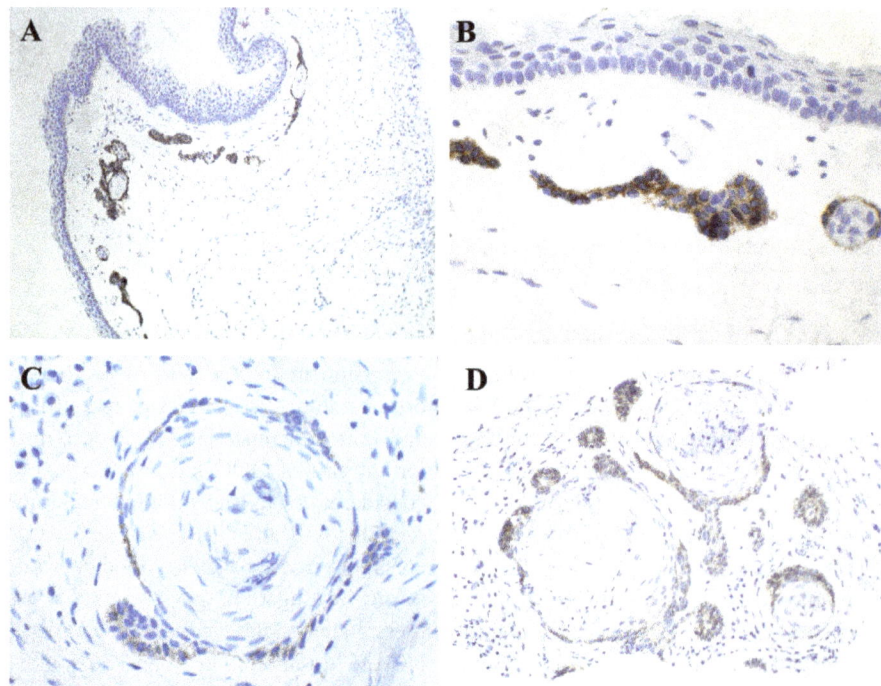

Figure 4 NCAM reactivity in satellite epithelial nests of small size (A and B) as well as in basal cells of daughter cysts (C and D) located in KCOT wall (NCAM, 200, 250 and 400x).

demonstrated NCAM reactivity, also with exclusive expression at the basal cell level [10]. Our series therefore represented an intermediate rate of positive observations.

In our KCOT cases, NCAM expression was exclusively focal and heterogeneous, with weak-to-moderate reactivity. Despite this limited, focal reactivity, our results demonstrate NCAM expression in locations not described previously: earlier studies noted NCAM reactivity only in the basal cell layer of KCOTs [10,11]. Furthermore, in one of these studies, which analyzed three cases of S-KCOT, there was no relationship between NCAM expression and this syndromic form of KCOT [11]. In contrast, we not only observed discontinuous positivity in the basal portion of cystic epithelium but also in areas of basal budding and in the basal portion of daughter cysts, both of which are occasionally detectable in KCOTs, and particularly in S-KCOTs.

Epithelial budding, arising from the basal layer of cystic lining, is a peculiar morphological aspect of KCOT that has been suggested as the source of daughter cysts; [18-20] influences lesional recurrence; [13,14,21] and is most frequently observed in S-KCOTs [22]. Aberrant NCAM expression in epithelial buds and the basal portion of daughter cysts of KCOTs was observed in 50% of S-KCOTs and represents a possible influence on NCAM expression in instances of lesion recurrence.

In our series, all S-KCOT cases recurred; in NS-KCOTs the recurrence rate was 35%. NCAM expression was detected in 66.66% and 32.50% of S- and NS-KCOTs, respectively. Systematic review of cases of NS-KCOT indicated an average recurrence rate of 28% [23], although rates were heavily influenced by the duration of follow-up, and especially by the type of treatment administered [3], indicating that adequate management of NS-KCOTs may prevent recurrence [2,24].

When we analyzed the relationship between NCAM expression and recurrence independent of KPOC subtype, there was no significant association. However, there was an important limitation: observations were not treated homogeneously due to the retrospective nature of the series. Nevertheless, the fact that NCAM expression was observed in morphological locations involved in recurrence [13,14,21] suggests a possible relationship between NCAM expression and lesional recurrence. Further studies pertaining to NCAM expression, in larger series of KCOTs treated with homogenous procedures or subjected to prospective randomized analysis [25], are required to obtain definitive conclusions. Likewise should be verify a possible association between increased expression of CD56 and others markers [26,27] and genes [28] overexpressed in KCOT.

A final interesting observation concerned NCAM expression in AB, another frequently recurring odontogenic tumor in which NCAM reactivity, in contrast to KCOTs, is virtually certain [11]. AB and KCOTs have been considered two morphologically distinct odontogenic tumors [29]. However, certain morphological and evolutionary data indicate a degree of overlap between these tumors; [30] this similarity is clearly reflected in so-called keratoameloblastoma [31,32], as well as in the solid variant of KCOT [33], characterized by hybrid AB and KCOT morphological features. Accordingly, aberrant NCAM expression in KCOTs could be indicative of foci of ameloblastic differentiation. As suggested previously [27,34], collaborative studies (given the scarcity of observations) concerning NCAM in keratoameloblastomas are required to confirm if this is the case.

Conclusions

The present study investigated the immunomorphological pattern of NCAM expression in KPOCs, and highlighted that NCAM expression in OOCs is entirely absent. In relation to KCOT our immunohistochemical analysis indicated NCAM reactivity in locations not reported previously (e.g., areas of basal budding and basal cells of daughter cysts), especially with respect to S-KCOTs. This suggests a possible role for this signaling molecule in lesional recurrence in KCOTs. Futures studies using homogeneously treated series of KCOT cases are required to confirm the influence of NCAM on lesion recurrence, as well as its potential utility as a marker of ameloblastic differentiation.

Competing interests
The authors declare that they have no competing interests.

Authors' contributions
BVS conceived of the study, participated in its design and coordination and as well as in reading immunohistochemical techniques. LFN participated in the design of the study and performed the statistical analysis. FVS carried out the immunohistochemical tests and participated reading immunohistochemical stains. All authors read and approved the final manuscript.

Author details
[1]Departaments of Stomatology, University of Valencia, Valencia, Spain.
[2]Departaments of Pathology, University of Valencia, Valencia, Spain. [3]Service of Pathology, Hospital Universitario y Politécnico La Fe, Avda Campanar 21, Valencia 46009, Spain.

References
1. Shear M. The aggressive nature of the odontogenic keratocyst: it is a benign cystic neoplasm? part 1. clinical and early experimental evidence of aggressive behaviour. Oral Oncol. 2002;38:219–26.
2. Barnes L, Eveson JW, Reichart P, Sidransky D. World health organization classification of tumours, Pathology and genetics of head and neck tumours. Lyon: IARC; 2005.
3. Johnson NR, Batstone MD, Savage NW. Management and recurrence of keratocystic odontogenic tumor: a systematic review. Oral Surg Oral Med Oral Pathol Oral Radiol. 2013;116:e271–6.
4. Barghava D, Deshpande A, Pogrel MA. Keratocystic odontogenic tumor (KCOT) - a cyst to a tumour. Oral Maxillofac Surg. 2012;16:163–70.
5. Lanier LL, Chang C, Azuma M, Ruitenberg JJ, Hemperly JJ, Phillips JH. Molecular and functional analysis of human natural killer cell-associated neural cell adhesion molecule (N-CAM / CD56). J Immunol. 1991;146:4421–6.

6. Kishimoto T, Kikutani H, von der Borne AEGK, Goyert SM, Mason DY, Miyasaka M, et al. Leukocyte typing VI: white cell differentiation antigens. New York: Garland; 1997. p. 271. 1155, 1211.

7. Gattenlöhner S, Stühmer T, Leich E, Reinhard M, Etschmann B, Völker HU, et al. Specific detection of CD56 (NCAM) isoforms for the identification of aggressive malignant neoplasms with progressive development. Am J Pathol. 2009;174:1160–71.

8. Er N, Dagdevirem A, Tasman F, Zeibek D. Neural cell adhesion molecule and neurothelin expression in human ameloblastoma. J Oral Maxillofac Surg. 2001;59:900–3.

9. Kawai S, Ito E, Yamaguchi A, Eishi E, Okada N. Immunohistochemical characteristics of odontogenic carcinomas: their use in diagnosing and elucidating histogenesis. Oral Med Pathol. 2009;13:55–63.

10. Kusafuka K, Hirobe K, Wato M, Tanaka A, Nakajima T. CD56 expression is associated with neuroectodermal differentiation in ameloblastomas: an immunohistochemical evaluation in comparison with odontogenic cystic lesions. Med Mol Morphol. 2011;44:79–85.

11. Cairns L, Naidu A, Robinson CM, Sloan P, Wright JM, Hunter KD. CD56 (NCAM) expression in ameloblastomas and other odontogenic lesions. Histopathology. 2010;57:544–8.

12. Nayak MT, Singh A, Singhvi A, Sharma R. Odontogenic keratocyst: what is the name? J Nat Sci Biol Med. 2013;4:282–5.

13. Woolgar JA, Rippin JW, Browne RM. A comparative study of the clinical and histological features of recurrent and non-recurrent odontogenic keratocysts. J Oral Pathol. 1987;16:124–8.

14. Kimonis VE, Goldstein AM, Pastakia B. Clinical manifestations in 105 persons with nevoid basal cell carcinoma syndrome. Am J Med Genet. 1997;69:299–308.

15. Obara N, Suzuki Y, Nagai Y, Nishiyama H, Mizoguchi I, Takeda M. Expression of neural cell-adhesion molecule mRNA during mouse molar tooth development. Arch Oral Biol. 2002;47:805–13.

16. Wright JM. The odontogenic keratocyst: orthokeratinized variant. Oral Surg. 1981;51:609–18.

17. Dong Q, Pan S, Sun LS, Li TJ. Orthokeratinized odontogenic cyst. a clinicopathological study of 61 cases. Arch Pathol Lab Med. 2010;134:271–5.

18. Regezi JA. Odontogenic cysts, odontogenic tumors, fibroosseous, and giant cell lesions of the jaws. Mod Pathol. 2002;15:331–41.

19. Kuroyanagi N, Sakuma H, Miyabe S, Machida J, Kaetsu A, Yokoi M, et al. Prognostic factors for keratocystic odontogenic tumor (odontogenic keratocyst): analysis of clinico-pathologic and immunohistochemical findings in cysts treated by enucleation. J Oral Pathol Med. 2009;38:386–92.

20. Mendes RA, Carvalho JFC, van der Waal I. Characterization and management of the keratocystic odontogenic tumor in relation to its histopathological and biological features. Oral Oncol. 2010;46:219–25.

21. Myoung H, Hong SP, Hong SD, Lee JI, Lim CY, Choung PH, et al. Odontogenic keratocyst: review of 256 cases for recurrence and clinicopathological parameters. Oral Surg Oral Med Oral Pathol. 2001;91:328–33.

22. Woolgar JA, Rippin JW, Browne RM. A comparative histological study of odontogenic keratocysts in basal cell naevus syndrome and control patients. J Oral Pathol. 1987;16:75–80.

23. MacDonal-Jankowsk DS. Keratocystic odontogenic tumor: systematic review. Dentomaxillofac Radiol. 2011;40:1–23.

24. Lo Muzio L, Staibano S, Pannone G, Bucci P, Nocini PF, Bucci E, et al. Expression of cell cycle and apoptosis-related proteins in sporadic odontogenic keratocysts and odontogenic keratocysts associated with the nevoid basal cell carcinoma syndrome. J Dent Res. 1999;78:1345–53.

25. Zecha JAEM, Mendes RA, Lindeboom VB, Van der Waal I. Recurrence rate of keratocystic odontogenic tumor after conservative surgical treatment without adjunctive therapies – A 35-year single institution experience. Oral Oncol. 2010;46:740–2.

26. Oliveira MG, Lauxen IS, Filho MSA. P53 protein reactivity in odontogenic lesions: an immunohistochemical study. R Fac Odonto Porto Alegre. 2005;46:31–5.

27. Vera-Sirera B, Forner-Navarro L, Vera-Sempere F. Differential expression of cyclin D1 in keratin-producing odontogenic cysts. Med Oral Patol Oral Cir Bucal. 2015;20:e59–65.

28. Heikinheimo K, Jee PR, Morgan N, Nagy S, Knuutila S, Leivo I. Genetic changes in sporadic keratocystic odontogenic tumors (odontogenic keratocysts). J Dent Res. 2007;86:544–9.

29. Eversole LR, Sabes WR, Rovin S. Aggressive growth and neoplastic potential of odontogenic cysts: with special reference to central epidermoid and mucoepidermoid carcinomas. Cancer. 1975;35:270–82.

30. Ide F, Ito Y, Muramatsu T, Saito I, Abiko Y, et al. Histogenetic relations between keratoameloblastoma and solid variant of odontogenic keratocyst. Oral Surg Oral Med Oral Pathol Oral Radiol Endod. 2012;114:812–3.

31. Whitt JC, Dunlap CL, Sheets JL, Thompson ML. Keratoameloblastoma: a tumor sui generis or a chimera? Oral Surg Oral Med Oral Pathol Oral Radiol Endod. 2007;104:368–76.

32. Geng N, Lv D, Chen QM, Zhu ZY, Wu RQ, He ZX. Solid variant of keratocystic odontogenic tumor with ameloblastomatous transformation: a case report and review of the literature. Oral Surg Oral Med Oral Pathol Oral Radiol Endod. 2012;114:223–9.

33. Ketabi MA, Dehghani N, Sadeghi HM, Shams MG, Mohajerani H, Azarsina M, et al. Keratoameloblastoma, a very rare variant of ameloblastoma. J Craniofac Surg. 2013;24:2182–6.

34. Geng N, Chem Q-M. Differentiating solid variants of keratocystic odontogenic tumors and keratoameloblastomas. Oral Surg Oral Med Oral Pathol Oral Radiol Endod. 2013;114:813–4.

14

Stability of treatment with self-ligating brackets and conventional brackets in adolescents: a long-term follow-up retrospective study

Zhou Yu[1], Lin Jiaqiang[1], Chen Weiting[1], Yi Wang[1], MinLing Zhen[1] and Zhenyu Ni[1,2*]

Abstract

Objectives: The aim of this study was to assess the long-term stability of treatment with self-ligating brackets compared with conventional brackets.

Materials and methods: The long-term follow-up retrospective study sample consisted of two groups of patients: group SL (including passive and interactive self ligating braces) comprised 30 subjects treated with self-ligating brackets at a mean pretreatment (T0) age of 13.56 years, with a mean follow up period for 7.24 years; group CL comprised 30 subjects treated with conventional brackets at a mean pretreatment age of 13.48 years, with a mean follow up period for 7.68 years. Relapse were evaluated by dental casts examination using the Peer Assessment Rating (PAR) index and the Little irregularity index. The two groups were evaluated for differences in the changing of PAR and Little irregularity index using paired-t tests. Inter-observer and intra-observer reliability was assessed by means of the Pearson's correlation coefficients method.

Results: There were no significant differences changed in PAR and the Little irregularity index between groups for the long-term follow-up period.

Conclusions: The study revealed that brackets type did not affect the long-term stability. Considering self-ligating brackets were expensive, given comprehensive consideration for the patients to choose suitable orthodontic bracket type was of critical importance.

Keyword: Self-ligating brackets, Conventional brackets, Stability

Introduction

The stability of aligned teeth is variable and unpredictable [1]. Therefore, the maintenance of dental alignment after orthodontic treatment is considered to be a challenge for the orthodontics. Follow-up studies of treated cases have shown that although improvement in the dentition can obviously be achieved, there is a tendency of relapse many years after treatment [2,3]. The reason is complex, several factors may account for this relapse, including inter-canine width [4], mandibular growth rotation [5], third molar eruption [6], influence of gingival tissues [7], or treatment modalities [8]. Some investigators claim that lower force produced by self ligating bracket systems might result in more physiological tooth movement, therefore, SLBs produce more stable treatment results [9].

Self-ligation bracket is not a new concept. This brace system has undergone a renaissance over the past 20 years with enhanced ingenuity and reliability [10]. According to the ligating mechanisms, self-ligating brackets can be divided into 2 main categories, active and passive self-ligating brackets. Active self-ligating brackets have a spring clip which press against the arch-wire for better control of rotation and torque. Conversely, passive self-ligating brackets usually have a slide that press no active force on the arch-wire.

Many advantages of self-ligating bracket system have been claimed, including reduced friction [11], more efficient tooth movement, less treatment time, increased patients acceptance, and superior treatment results [12,13].

* Correspondence: 156089794@qq.com
[1]DDS, Hospital of Stomatology, Wenzhou Medical University, Wenzhou, China
[2]Department of Orthodontics, Hospital of Stomatology, Wenzhou Medical University, Wenzhou,113 west college road, 325000 Wenzhou, China

Unfortunately, a systematic review [14] claimed that there was lack of significant overall effects apparent in this meta-analysis contradicts evidence-based statements on the advantages of self-ligating brackets over conventional ones regarding discomfort during initial orthodontic therapy, number of appointments, and total treatment time. Besides, a recent systematic review of self-ligating bracket stated [9] that, at this time, no studies comparing the stability of treatment result with self-ligating brackets to conventional brackets were identified.

Therefore, the objective of this study was to assess the long-term stability of treatment with self-ligating brackets compared with conventional brackets.

Materials and methods
Subjects
This research was approved by the Ethics Committee of the WenZhou Medical University.

The sample size for each group was calculated based on an alpha significance level of 0.05 and a beta of 0.1 to achieve 90% power to detect a clinically meaningful difference of two (PAR/IR) between the self-ligating group (SL) (including passive and interactive self ligating braces) and the conventional brackets group (CL). The power analysis showed that 16 patients should be recruited in each group.

The sample consisted of 60 subjects were randomly selected from three profession orthodontists who had the same concept of treatment philosophy and were familiar with each other (Table 1). Subjects included in the study satisfied the following selection criteria: patients must be

(1) older than 12 years; (2) Hawley retainer was used in both upper and lower dental arch approximately 2 years.; (3) A non-extraction treatment plan; (4) Class I molar relationship, (5) crowding less than 5 mm (6) follow-up at least more than 5 years (6) permanent dentition (7) treatment included 0.022-in slot brackets with similar wire sequences (SL brackets, Time, Adenta, Gilching/ Munich, Germany, or SmartClip,3 M Unitek, Monvoria, Calif; or CL brackets, 3 M Unitek, Monrovia, Calif,) (8) extract third molar if impacted.

Patients with hypodontia, oligodontia, hypothyroidism, cleft-lip/palate, syndromes were excluded. Participants who met these inclusion criteria were recruited. At the time of recruitment, it was routine practice to obtain written consent for participation in the trial.

Methods
Dental casts were routinely made at the following stages: pre-treatment (TP); post-treatment (T0); 2 years after T0 (T2); more than 5 years after T0 (T5). Five variables were measured, including the following: Irregularity Index [15]; Inter-canine width; Inter-molar width; PAR index [16]; arch length.

Three examiners were incorporated in this study. To determine the measurement error in the PAR and assess the intra-observer and inter-observer agreement, 18 randomly selected patients were evaluated by the three observers. The dental casts at TP and at T5 were re-measured for these patients. The time interval between two intra-observer assessments was at least 3 weeks.

Statistical analysis
Descriptive and analytically statistical analyses were performed with SPSS software (release 18.0, SPSS for Windows). Systematic differences between observers were tested by the paired t test. Inter-observer and intra-observer reliability was expressed as Pearson's correlation coefficients between re-measurements. The magnitude of the intra-observers and inter-observers measurement error in the PAR was calculated.

Statistical analysis was performed by using standard methods. Groups were compared by Student's t-test for independent group, and significance of changes across time was determined by the Student's t-test for paired data. The level of statistical significance was established at $P < 0.05$.

Results
No significantly systematic differences were found between examiners. The measurement errors were 0.9. The intra-observer correlation ranged over the two periods from 0.98 to 0.99 and the inter-observer correlation from 0.96 to 0.99, indicating a high level of reliability. No significant differences were detected in age, gender, follow up period, and PAR and Little index before treatment (Table 1).

Table 1 Demographics and clinical characteristics of sample

Variable	SL group		CL group		P value
	Mean	SD	Mean	SD	
Age	13.56	1.62	13.48	1.46	0.53
gender					
male	15		14		
female	15		16		0.34
Follow up period	7.24	1.32	7.68	1.6	0.46
Arch length Md	50.36	5.21	50.12	4.98	0.59
Arch length Max	59.32	4.68	59.12	4.96	0.35
Inter-canine width Md	27.36	1.40	28.12	1.34	0.36
Inter-canine width Max	34.23	1.68	34.26	1.59	0.33
Inter-molar width Md	36.26	2.13	36.59	2.36	0.48
Inter-molar width Max	42.32	2.36	41.89	2.29	0.67
II Md	11.26	4.56	11.89	5.36	0.24
II Max	10.38	3.89	9.87	4.12	0.18
PAR	28.48	10.23	27.68	10.98	0.34

Max indicates maxillary; Md indicates mandibular; II indicates Irregularity Index; P > 0.05 indicates no statistically significant change.

Three dimensions of the dental arch, including maxillary inter-canine width and the two inter-molar widths, did not change significantly over the long-term follow-up period for each group (Table 2).

Inter group comparison results showed that, at T (P) and T (0), both groups presented smaller PAR and Little indexes. In the follow up period, both groups showed minor increasing in PAR and Little maxillary indexes, but the changes in irregularity index and the PAR index were not significantly greater in SL group than in CL group (Table 3).

Discussion

The orthodontists' goal for the patients is to have a satisfactory occlusion and alignment of the teeth after many years post-retention [17]. However, relapse is an inevitable outcome of combined action of many factors, so how to

Table 2 Differences between Post-treatment and Post-retention Arch Dimensions (mm) of SL and CL group

Variable	SL group		Cl group		P
	Mean	SD	Mean	SD	
Arch length Max					
T(0)-T(P)	1.68	1.34	1.23	1.45	0.23
T(2)-T(0)	−2.09	1.21	−1.99	1.35	0.16
T(5)-T(2)	−0.71	0.35	−0.93	0.23	0.45
Arch length Md					
T(0)-T(P)	2.31	1.56	1.98	1.76	0.36
T(2)-T(0)	−1.23	0.83	−1.29	0.79	0.48
T(5)-T(2)	−1.08	0.79	1.10	0.86	0.38
Inter-canine width Max					
T(0)-T(P)	1.89	1.23	1.86	1.36	0.47
T(2)-T(0)	−2.79	1.45	−2.61	1.21	0.26
T(5)-T(2)	−0.34	0.78	−0.31	0.67	0.56
Inter-canine width Md					
T(0)-T(P)	0.68	1.46	0.56	1.56	0.35
T(2)-T(0)	−2.19	1.39	−1.98	1.36	0.47
T(5)-T(2)	−0.24	0.36	−0.54	0.52	0.12
Inter-molar width Max					
T(0)-T(P)	2.36	1.20	1.12	0.87	*
T(2)-T(0)	−2.13	1.35	−2.03	1.52	0.34
T(5)-T(2)	−0.78	0.32	−0.76	0.36	0.21
Inter-molar width Md					
T(0)-T(P)	2.14	1.56	2.06	1.68	0.32
T(2)-T(0)	−2.68	1.26	−2.55	1.36	0.26
T(5)-T(2)	−1.23	1.32	−1.34	1.36	0.18

Max indicates maxillary; Md indicates mandibular; T(P) = pretreatment; T(0) = post-treatment; T(2) = 2 years post-retention; T(5) = more than 5 years post-retention; P > 0.05 indicates no statistically significant change.

Table 3 Post-treatment and Post-retention Occlusal Dimensions (mm, except for PAR) of SL and CL group

Variable	SL group		Cl group		P
	Mean	SD	Mean	SD	
II Max					
T(0)-T(P)	−9.56	4.68	−8.96	5.12	0.25
T(2)-T(0)	0.89	1.26	0.79	1.45	0.12
T(5)-T(2)	0.68	1.11	0.56	1.34	0.09
II Md					
T(0)-T(P)	−10.68	5.23	−10.69	5.69	0.35
T(2)-T(0)	1.69	1.23	1.89	1.35	0.25
T(5)-T(2)	0.26	0.78	0.34	0.66	0.39
PAR					
T(0)-T(P)	−26.68	10.26	−25.88	10.98	0.78
T(2)-T(0)	1.64	1.98	1.56	1.68	0.35
T(5)-T(2)	0.98	1.25	1.23	1.39	0.37

Max indicates maxillary; Md indicates mandibular; II indicates Irregularity Index; T(P) = pretreatment; T(0) = post-treatment; T(2) = 2 years post-retention; T(5) = more than 5 years post-retention; P > 0.05 indicates no statistically significant change;* indicates statistically significant change.

maintain the stability of teeth become urgent problems to orthodontists.

The results of this study indicate a satisfactory long-term post-retention stability, as defined by Little's irregularity index of <3.5 mm, which is achievable in both groups. These findings agree with previous studies which indicated a satisfactory post-retention stability (irregularity index <3.5 mm) for their samples or subsamples [18-21].

It is generally agreed that dental arch form and width should be maintained during orthodontic treatment [22,23]. Several studies showed that inter-canine and inter-molar widths decreased during the post-retention period, especially if it had been expanded during treatment [24-27]. For this reason, the maintenance of arch form is generally recommended.

This study found that the dental arch had a certain degree expansion in both groups and that there was no statistically significant increases in inter-canine width; but SL brackets resulted in statistically greater increase in inter-molar width than conventional appliances. However SL did not show greater post-retention decrease in their molar width than CL, which may be related to the fact that the two groups existed statistically significant differences, but the difference was only 1 mm, which was not clinically different. A systematic review [28] found the similar result that arch dimensional changes arising with SLBs and conventional systems appeared to be similar: identical levels of incisor proclination and inter-canine expansion developed in both systems.

In this study, the mean reduction in the PAR at the end of active treatment was 26.68 ± 10.26 in SL group, while 25.88 ± 10.98 for CL group. It means that PAR score reductions were unaffected by the choice of appliances. After more than 5 years post-retention, PAR score slightly increased in both groups, but the increase was still no significantly different. This indicated that most of the achieved orthodontic treatment results had been maintained in both groups after more than 5 years post-retention. This revealed that small amount of relapse is not only the result of orthodontic treatment, but also due to the physiological and pathological changes in the dentition and surrounding tissues during those years. It had been shown by Behrents [29] and Schols et.al [30] that considerable craniofacial alteration occurred beyond the age of 17 years old in human beings. This process was accompanied by compensatory changes in the dentition. The orthodontist has little control over these biological processes.

The claim of reduced friction with self-ligating brackets was often cited as a primary advantage over conventional brackets [31]. With reduced friction and hence less force was needed to produce tooth movement [32], self-ligating brackets are proposed to have the potential advantages of producing more physiologically harmonious tooth movement not by overpowering the musculature and interrupting the periodontal vascular supply [33].

Previous studies also stated that moderate crowding was alleviated about 2.7 times faster with Damon 2 brackets than with conventional appliances [34]. Therefore, it may made CL group easier to recurrence, but the results found in our study indicated that there was no statically significant increases of irregular index in both groups. The reason of recurrence may be the result of comprehensive factors work together. As previously reported, post-retention increases in irregularity were not correlated with crowding before treatment or amount of treatment change [35]. There was a tendency for the mandibular incisor to rebound, These findings could be interpreted to support Blake's [36] contention that the initial position of the mandibular incisors is the best guide for their lab-lingual stable position and many investigators who had noted a rebound effect for displaced incisors [37-39].

A limitation of this study was designed as a longitudinal retrospective study. Generally speaking, it is very difficult to avoid confounding factors. But, we can reduce the effects of bias by making strict inclusion criteria. AS shown in Table 1, we can see the baseline levels of two groups are in consistency. And malocclusion type might affect the results, therefore, in this study only patients with Angle Class I were included so as to minimize the impact of confounding factors on the experimental results. Another problem related to longitudinal retrospective studies might be the information bias. We had gone through repeated trials, and surveyors and final statistics do not know the group of data. Therefore, this study was relatively real, which may reflect the actual results accurately.

PAR, Little irregularity index, dental arch length and width index measured in our study can comprehensively reflect the statues of relapse, because relapse not only included the change of overbite/overjet, but also the change of dental arch length and width. Some researches [1,17] used only PAR or irregular index to evaluate long term stability, which has certain one-sidedness.

In a word, in terms of long term stability between SL and CL brackets, no significant differences were found in our study. Due to the fact that self-ligating braces are expensive, the advantages of saving time and reducing root absorption still need stronger evidence to be proven, meanwhile, given that cost-effectiveness, orthodontists should consider multiple factors in choosing suitable orthodontic bracket type for the patients.

Conclusions

- There were no statistical differences in long-term stability of treatment between self-ligating brackets and conventional brackets.

Competing interests

The authors declare that they have no competing interests. There is no support and funding source for conducting the review.

Authors' contributions

ZY and ZYN designed the study, gathered the information, Jiaqiang Lin and WC performed the statistical analysis and wrote the first draft of the manuscript. YW and MZ designed the form for data gathering and supervised the statistical analysis. All authors read and approved the final manuscript.

References

1. Al Yami EA, Kuijpers-Jagtman AM, Van't Hof MA: **Stability of orthodontic treatment outcome: follow-up until 10 years post-retention.** *Am J Orthod Dentofacial Orthop* 1999, **115:**300–304.
2. Elms TN, Buschang PH, Alexander RG: **Long-term stability of Class II, Division 1, nonextraction cervical face bow therapy: I. model analysis.** *Am J Orthod Dentofacial Orthop* 1996, **109:**271–276.
3. Elms TN, Buschang PH, Alexander RG: **Long-term stability of Class II, Division 1, nonextraction cervical face bow therapy: II. cephalometric analysis.** *Am J Orthod Dentofacial Orthop* 1996, **109:**386–392.
4. Rossouw PE, Preston CB, Lombard CJ, Truter JW: **A longitudinal evaluation of the anterior border of the dentition.** *Am J Orthod Dentofacial Orthop* 1993, **104:**146–152.
5. Fudalej P, Artun J: **Mandibular Growth Rotation Effects on Postretention Stability of Mandibular Incisor Alignment.** *Angle Orthod* 2007, **77:**199–205.
6. Harradine NW, Pearson MH, Toth B: **The effect of extraction of third molars on late lower incisor crowding: a randomized controlled trial.** *Br J Orthod* 1998, **25:**117–122.
7. Edwards JG: **A long-term prospective evaluation of the circumferential supracrestal fiberotomy in alleviating orthodontic relapse.** *Am J Orthod Dentofacial Orthop* 1988, **93:**380–387.
8. Little RM, Riedel RA, Engst ED: **Serial extraction of first premolars—postretention evaluation of stability and relapse.** *Angle Orthod* 1990, **60:**255–262.
9. Chen SS, Greenlee GM, Kim JE, Smith CL, Huang GJ: **Systematic review of self-ligating brackets.** *Am J Orthod Dentofacial Orthop* 2010, **137(726):**e1–e726. e18.
10. Harradine NW: **Self-ligating brackets: where are we now?** *J orthod* 2003, **30:**262–273.

Stability of treatment with self-ligating brackets and conventional brackets...

97

11. Henao SP, Kusy RP: Evaluation of the frictional resistance of conventional and self-ligating bracket designs using standardized archwires and dental typodonts. *Angle Orthod* 2004, **74**:202–211.

12. Turnbull NR, Birnie DJ: Treatment efficiency of conventional vs self-ligating brackets: effects of archwire size and material. *Am J Orthod Dentofacial Orthop* 2007, **131**:395–399.

13. Eberting JJ, Straja SR, Tuncay OC: Treatment time, outcome, and patient satisfaction comparisons of Damon and conventional brackets. *Clin Orthod Res* 2001, **4**:228–234.

14. Čelar A, Schedlberger M, Dörfler P, Bertl M: Systematic review on self-ligating vs. conventional brackets: initial pain, number of visits, treatment time. *J Orofac Orthop* 2013, **74**:40–51.

15. Little RM: The irregularity index: a quantitative score of mandibular anterior alignment. *Am J Orthod* 1975, **68**:554–563.

16. Richmond S, Shaw WC, Roberts CT, Andrews M: The PAR index (Peer Assessment Rating): methods to determine outcome of orthodontic treatments in terms of improvement and standards. *Eur J Orthod* 1992, **14**:180–187.

17. Boley JC, Mark JA, Sachdeva RC, Buschang PH: Long-term stability of Class I premolar extraction treatment. *Am J Orthod Dentofacial Orthop* 2003, **124**:277–287.

18. Dugoni SA, Lee JS, Varela J, Dugoni AA: Early mixed dentition treatment: postretention evaluation of stability and relapse. *Angle Orthod* 1995, **65**:311–320.

19. Sadowsky C, Schneider BJ, BeGole EA, Tahir E: Long-term stability after orthodontic treatment: nonextraction with prolonged retention. *Am J Orthod Dentofacial Orthop* 1994, **106**:243–249.

20. Vaden JL, Harris EF, Gardner RL: Relapse revisited. *Am J Orthod Dentofacial Orthop* 1997, **111**:543–553.

21. Glenn G, Sinclair PM, Alexander RG: Nonextraction orthodontic therapy: posttreatment dental and skeletal stability. *Am J Orthod Dentofacial Orthop* 1987, **92**:321–328.

22. McCauley DR: The cuspid and its function in retention. *Am J Orthod* 1944, **30**:196–205.

23. Riedel RA: A review of the retention problem. *Angle Orthod* 1960, **30**:179–199.

24. Welch KN: *A study of treatment and postretention dimensional changes in mandibular dental arches [MSD Thesis]*. Seattle: University of Washington; 1956.

25. Amott RD: *A serial study of dental arch measurements on orthodontic subjects: 55 cases at least 4 years postretention [MSD Thesis]*. Chicago: Northwestern University Dental School; 1962.

26. Arnold ML: *A study of the changes of the mandibular intercanine and intermolar widths during orthodontic treatment and following postretention period of five or more years [MSD Thesis]*. University of Washington: Seattle; 1963.

27. Kahl-Nieke B, Fischbach H, Schwarze CW: Post-retention crowding and incisor irregularity: a long-term follow-up evaluation of stability and relapse. *Br J Orthod* 1995, **22**:249–257.

28. Fleming PS, Johal A: Self-ligating brackets in orthodontics. A systematic review. *Angle Orthod* 2010, **80**:575–584.

29. Behrents RG: *Growth in the aging craniofacial skeleton. Monograph 17. Craniofacial Growth Series*. Ann Arbor: Center for Human Growth and Development; 1985.

30. Schols JGJH: Van der Linden FPGM:Development of the dentition and facial growth during adolescence. *Inform Orthod Kieferorthop* 1988, **68**:439–444.

31. Kim TK, Kim KD, Baek SH: Comparison of frictional forces during the initial leveling stage in various combinations of self-ligating brackets and archwires with a custom-designed typodont system. *Am J Orthod Dentofacial Orthop* 2008, **133**(187):e15–e24.

32. Berger JL: The influence of the SPEED bracket's self-ligating design on force levels in tooth movement: a comparative in vitro study. *Am J Orthod Dentofacial Orthop* 1990, **97**:219–228.

33. Damon DH: The rationale, evolution and clinical application of the self-ligating bracket. *Clin Orthod Res* 1998, **1**:52–61.

34. Pandis N, Polychronopoulou A, Eliades T: Self-ligating vs conventional brackets in the treatment of mandibular crowding: A prospective clinical trial of treatment duration and dental effects. *Am J Orthod Dentofacial Orthop* 2007, **132**:208–215.

35. Little RM, Riedel RA, Stein A: Mandibular arch length increase in the mixed dentition: postretention evaluation of stability and relapse. *Am J Orthod Dentofacial Orthop* 1990, **97**:393–404.

36. Blake M, Bibby K: Retention and stability: a review of the literature. *Am J Orthod Dentofacial Orthop* 1998, **114**:299–306.

37. Weinstein S, Haack DC, Morris LY, Snyder BB, Attaway HE: On an equilibrium theory of tooth position. *Angle Orthod* 1963, **33**:1–26.

38. Brodie AG: Does scientific investigation support the extraction of teeth in orthodontic therapy? *Am J Orthod Oral Surg* 1944–1945, **42**:61–77.

39. Litowitz R: A study of the movements of certain teeth during and following orthodontic treatment. *Angle Orthod* 1948, **18**:113–131.

15

Influence of maxillary advancement surgery on skeletal and soft-tissue changes in the nose — a retrospective cone-beam computed tomography study

Andreas F. Hellak[1]*, Bernhard Kirsten[2], Michael Schauseil[1], Rolf Davids[2], Wolfgang M. Kater[2] and Heike M. Korbmacher-Steiner[1]

Abstract

Objectives: Surgical correction of skeletal maxillary retroposition is often associated with changes in the morphology of the nose. Unwanted alar flaring of the nose is observed in many cases. The aim of the present study was therefore to investigate the influence of surgical advancement of the maxilla on changes in the soft-tissue morphology of the nose. Having a coefficient that allows prediction of change in the nasal width in Caucasian patients after surgery would be helpful for treatment planning.

Materials and methods: All 33 patients included in this retrospective study were of Caucasian descent and had skeletal Class III with maxillary retrognathia. They were all treated with maxillary advancement using a combination of orthodontic and maxillofacial surgery methods. Two cone-beam computed tomography (CBCT) datasets were available for all of the study's participants (16 female, 17 male; age 24.3 ± 10.4 years): the first CBCT imaging was obtained before the planned procedure (T0) and the second 14.1 ± 6.4 months postoperatively (T1). Morphological changes were recorded three-dimensionally using computer-aided methods (Mimics (Materialise NV, Leuven/Belgium), Geomagic (Geomagics, Morrisville/USA)). Statistical analysis was carried out using SPSS 21 for Mac.

Results: The mean sagittal advancement of the maxilla was 5.58 mm. The width of the nose at the alar base (Alb) changed by a mean of + 2.59 mm (±1.26 mm) and at the ala (Al) by a mean of + 3.17 mm (±1.32 mm). Both of these changes were statistically highly significant ($P = 0.000$). The increase in the width of the nose corresponded to approximately half of the maxillary advancement distance in over 80 % of the patients. The nasolabial angle declined by an average of −6.65° (±7.71°).

Conclusions: Maxillary advancement correlates with a distinct morphological change in nasal width. This should be taken into account in the treatment approach and in the information provided to patients.

Keywords: Nasal changes, Orthognathic surgery, Retrognathia, CBCT superimposition, Three-dimensional analysis

Introduction

Changes in the position of the maxilla and/or mandible are associated with corresponding changes in the soft tissue overlying the bone [1]. After surgical correction of maxillary retrognathia with maxillary advancement or bimaxillary surgery, with maxillary advancement and mandibular setback, undesirable changes in the nose have been observed in some cases. For many patients, a disturbing aesthetic appearance is the reason for undergoing surgery, in addition to functional problems [2]. It has been clinically and scientifically proven that the external nose undergoes changes in the context of surgical relocation of the maxilla [3]. This aspect should be examined in greater detail, and it would be of interest to know in what way advancement of the maxilla leads to alar flaring. Measurement of a coefficient capable of

* Correspondence: hellak@med.uni-marburg.de
[1]Department of Orthodontics, University Hospital, Georg-Voigt-Strasse 3, Marburg 35039, Germany
Full list of author information is available at the end of the article

Table 1 All patients (n = 33) underwent maxillary advancement

Mandibular setback	Mandibular advancement	Maxillary dorsal impaction	Maxillary impaction	Maxillary repositioning as two-piece maxilla	Rotation of the maxilla	n	%
✓	✗	✗	✓	✗	✗	14	42 %
✓	✗	✗	✗	✗	✗	7	21 %
✓	✗	✓	✗	✗	✗	3	9 %
✗	✗	✗	✗	✗	✗	3	9 %
✓	✗	✓	✗	✓	✗	2	6 %
✗	✗	✓	✗	✗	✗	2	6 %
✗	✓	✗	✗	✗	✓	1	3 %
✗	✗	✗	✓	✗	✗	1	3 %

The table shows the distribution of additional surgical procedures (in numbers and percentage distribution)

relating the skeletal displacement to nasal changes might be helpful for surgical planning and patient education.

The effect of maxillofacial surgery on the facial soft tissue has been investigated in many studies in the past [1, 4–16]. However, there is a lack of research on the relationship between the advancement distance and the amount of alteration measured [10, 17, 16]. A wide variety of analyses have been used for the purpose. The methods most often used in the past have included photography and two-dimensional lateral cephalography [18–21]. Recently, various optical procedures such as laser projection, glancing-light projection, and stereophotogrammetry have made it possible to capture spatial, three-dimensional parameters [18, 22, 23]. In radiography, computed tomography (CT) and cone-beam computed tomography (CBCT) can be used [18, 22–24]. In contrast to optical procedures, radiographic methods are not limited to depicting only the surface of the body; deeper bone structures can also be captured. Three-dimensional changes in the osseous structures and the resulting changes in the soft tissues can be analyzed using CBCT.

Only patients of Asian descent have previously been investigated in connection with this topic [8, 11, 13, 15, 16, 25–27, 14]. Due to ethnic differences in facial structure, it is not possible to transfer the findings to Caucasian patients [26]. It is regarded as clinically and scientifically proven that the external nose is subject to flattening and widening when surgical repositioning is carried out in the maxilla.

The aim of the present study was therefore to use three-dimensional CBCT data to detect dependencies between skeletal advancement of the maxilla and alterations in the morphology of the nose. In the case of a confirmed association, the aim was to evaluate whether any dependency on the extent of the advancement could be identified.

Materials and methods

Two CBCT datasets for each of 33 patients (16 female, 17 male) — i.e., a total of 66 CBCTs — were examined retrospectively. The patients' mean age was 24.3 ± 10.4 years. All of the patients had an Angle class III anomaly with maxillary retrognathia preoperatively. They were examined clinically and radiographically in the Department of Oral and Maxillofacial Surgery in Bad Homburg, Germany, and were of Caucasian descent.

Weight variations of more than 5 kg were not permitted during the study period. This information was obtained from the anesthesia protocol. The following inclusion and exclusion criteria were set. The criteria for inclusion in the patient group were:

- Caucasian descent
- Maxillary retrognathia (SNA < 80°)
- Surgical advancement of the maxilla
- During the preoperatively conducted model operation, available current plaster jaw models had to allow stable occlusion in Angle class I

Table 2 Relevant points, distances, planes and angles

Variable	Explanation
Al	Alar width
Alb	Alar base width
Albl	Deepest point at the transition between the left ala to the cheek to air at the sagittal level (left alar base)
Albr	Deepest point at the transition between the right ala to the cheek to air at the sagittal level (right alar base)
All	Furthest transverse extent of the left ala
Alr	Furthest transverse extent of the right ala
Co	Columella tangent point, bridge of the nose
FH	Frankfurt horizontal plane, two poria and an infraorbital point
Ls	Labrale superius, edge of the upper lip (transition from vermilion border to white portion)
Sn	Subnasal point, transition from the bridge of the nose to the upper lip
Sn–Ls–Co	Nasolabial angle

The criteria for exclusion from the patient group were:

- No maxillary retrognathia (SNA > 80°)
- Not of Caucasian descent
- Additional intraoperative augmentation of the midface
- Craniofacial anomalies or syndromes, or any form of cheilognathouranoschisis

Surgically, a Le Fort I osteotomy of the maxilla in combination with bridle sutures for the bases of the two ala was used [16, 17, 28, 29]. The Le Fort I osteotomy method used by the surgeon (exclusively W.K.) is based on the fracture line described by René Le Fort in 1901 [30]. The osteotomy starts at the piriform aperture cranial to the anterior nasal spine and passes through the facial maxillary sinus wall, the zygomaticoalveolar crest, and the maxillary tuberosity to the dorsal surface of the maxillary sinus, separates the caudal tip of the pterygoid process of the sphenoid bone, bends forward to the nasal cavity, runs through the lateral nasal wall in its basal portion, and from there returns to the piriform aperture [30]. After repositioning of the maxilla using the face-bow and glabella support, or with a surgical splint prepared in advance to determine the occlusal relationship of the maxilla to the mandible, the maxilla is fixed in its final position using an adapted titanium mini-plate and accompanying screws. In addition, alar cinch sutures are created for the bases of the two

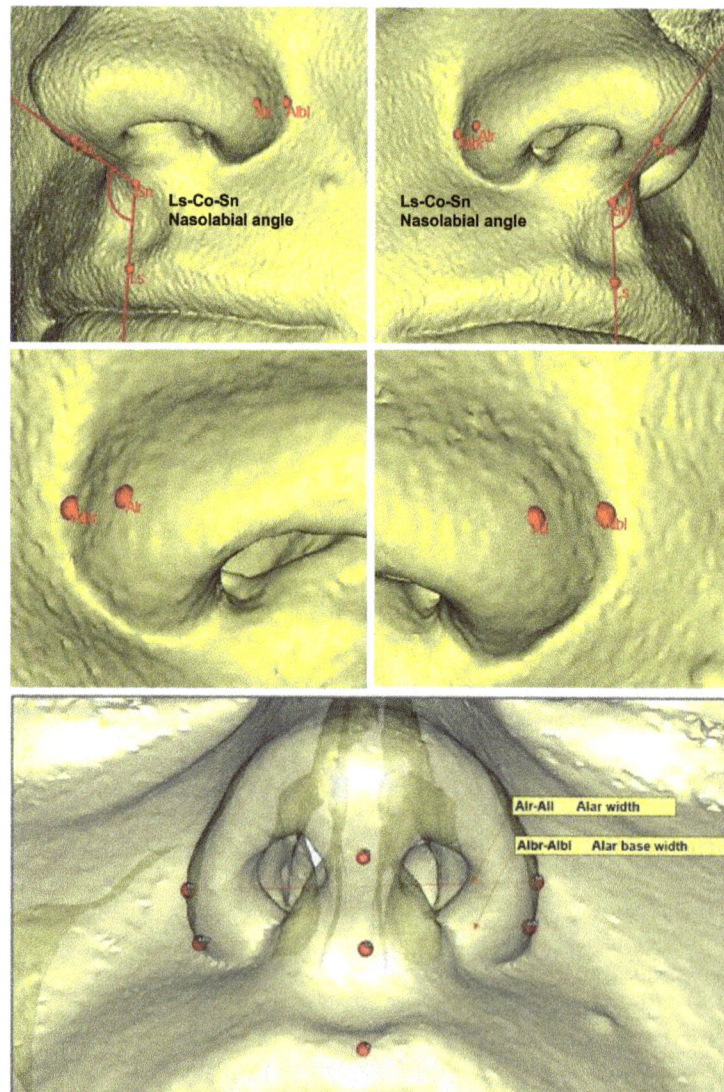

Fig. 1 Soft-tissue points and distances. The nasolabial angle (NLA) is the angle between the labrale superius (Ls), the columellar tangential point (Co), and the subnasal point (Sn). The alar base width (Alb) is the distance from the alar base on the right (Albr) to the alar base on the left (Albl). The alar width (Al) is the distance from the right ala (Alr) to the left ala (All)

nostrils and attached with this technique at the anterior nasal spine [17, 3, 29, 28]

All 33 patients underwent maxillary advancement. A bimaxillary operation with maxillary advancement and mandibular setback was carried out in the majority of the patients. Table 1 presents an overview of the additional surgical procedures used and their frequencies.

The first CBCT imaging procedure was carried out 2–3 weeks before the planned procedure (T0). The second images were obtained after surgery (T1; 14.1 ± 6.4 months postoperatively), but not before the completion of soft-tissue healing. Completion of soft-tissue healing was defined as 6 months after surgery, based on the results of earlier studies [31, 32].

Identical parameters were used for all CBCT imaging procedures. All of the CBCT images were taken with a KaVo 3D eXam device (KaVo Dental Ltd., Bieberach/Riss, Germany). This CBCT device has a high-frequency X-ray source with a constant potential of 120 kVp (kilovolt peak) and pulsed 3–8 mA. The settings used for all of the CBCT imaging procedures were identical, with a scanning time of 26.9 s, a voxel size of $0.25 \times 0.25 \times 0.25$ mm, an effective irradiation period of 7 s, anode voltage of 120 kV, and tube current of 5 mA (for details, see KaVo). The maximum field of view (FOV) of the device was 16×13 cm. Depending on the issue and indication, the height of the FOV was 6, 8, or 11 cm and the image had to include all relevant points.

All of the patients provided written informed consent to the inclusion of their data in the study. The data were pseudonymized. The CBCT datasets were given identifiers numbered 1–66 and the underlying names of the patients were deleted. Deallocation was only permissible for the director of the study (HKS).

Collection and analysis of the soft-tissue datasets were carried out using the Mimics 15.0 (Materialise NV, Leuven/Belgium) computer program. Table 2 shows all of the relevant points, distances, planes, and angles.

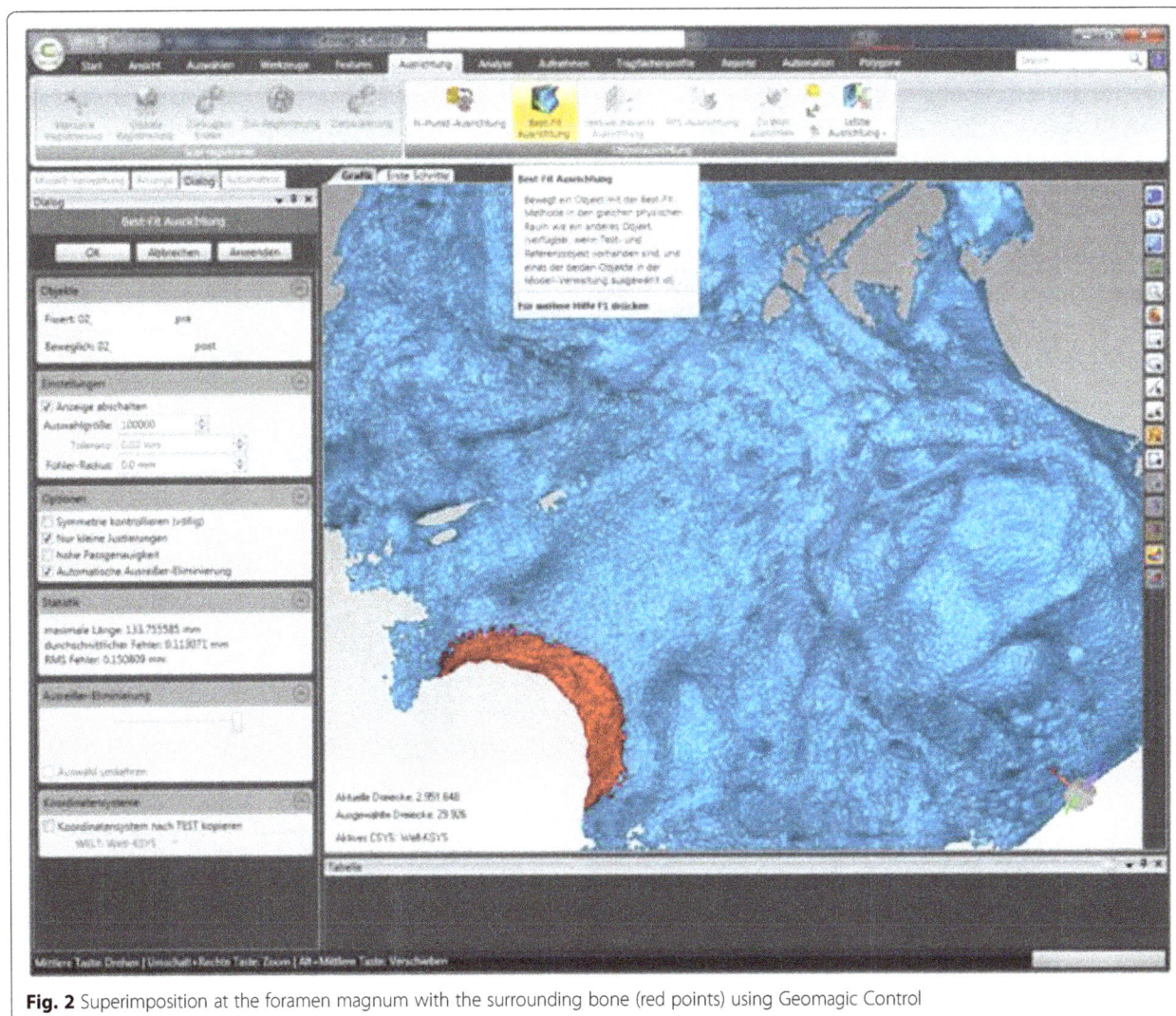

Fig. 2 Superimposition at the foramen magnum with the surrounding bone (red points) using Geomagic Control

The nasolabial angle (NLA [33]), alar base width (Alb), and alar width (Al) were measured to assess changes in the nasal soft tissues. The soft-tissue points shown in Fig. 1 were used for measurements. The following distances and angles were formed from the measurement points:

- Alar base width (Alb): from Albr to Albl: Alb distance
- Alar width (Al): from All to Alr: Al distance
- Nasolabial angle (NLA): angle between Ls to Co and Sn

For measurement of the skeletal repositioning of the maxilla, the CBCT for T0 and T1 were superimposed using Geomagic Control 2014.0 (Geomagics, Morrisville, USA). Superimposition was carried out at the foramen magnum with surrounding bone and at the anterior skull base at 100,000 polygons [34, 35] (Fig. 2). Figure 3

shows the user interface in Geomagic Control after completion of the superimposition. A level parallel with the Frankfurt plane was placed through the A point (Fig. 4). At this level, individual measurement values were collected in regions 13, 11, 21, and 23 in the needle view, and a mean was calculated (Fig. 5). The calculated repositioning of these points represents the skeletal advancement of the maxilla. All of the measurements were repeated by the same operator after an interval of 2 weeks.

Statistics

Statistical analysis was performed using IBM SPSS Statistics for Mac, version 21.0 (IBM Corporation, Armonk, New York, USA). Methodological error was estimated using Spearman rank correlation. As the Shapiro-Wilk test showed significant deviations from the normal distribution, Student's t-test and the Wilcoxon

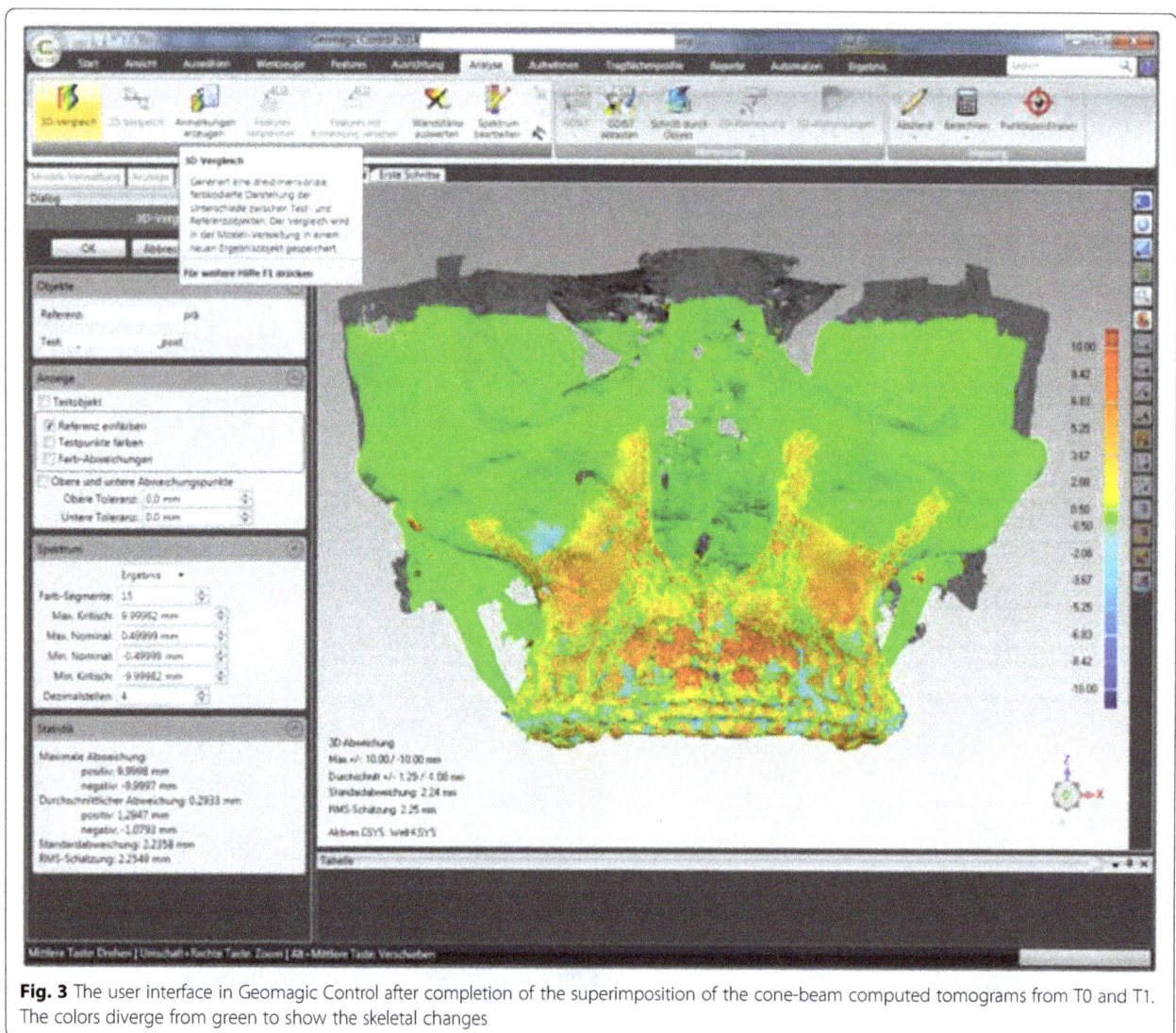

Fig. 3 The user interface in Geomagic Control after completion of the superimposition of the cone-beam computed tomograms from T0 and T1. The colors diverge from green to show the skeletal changes

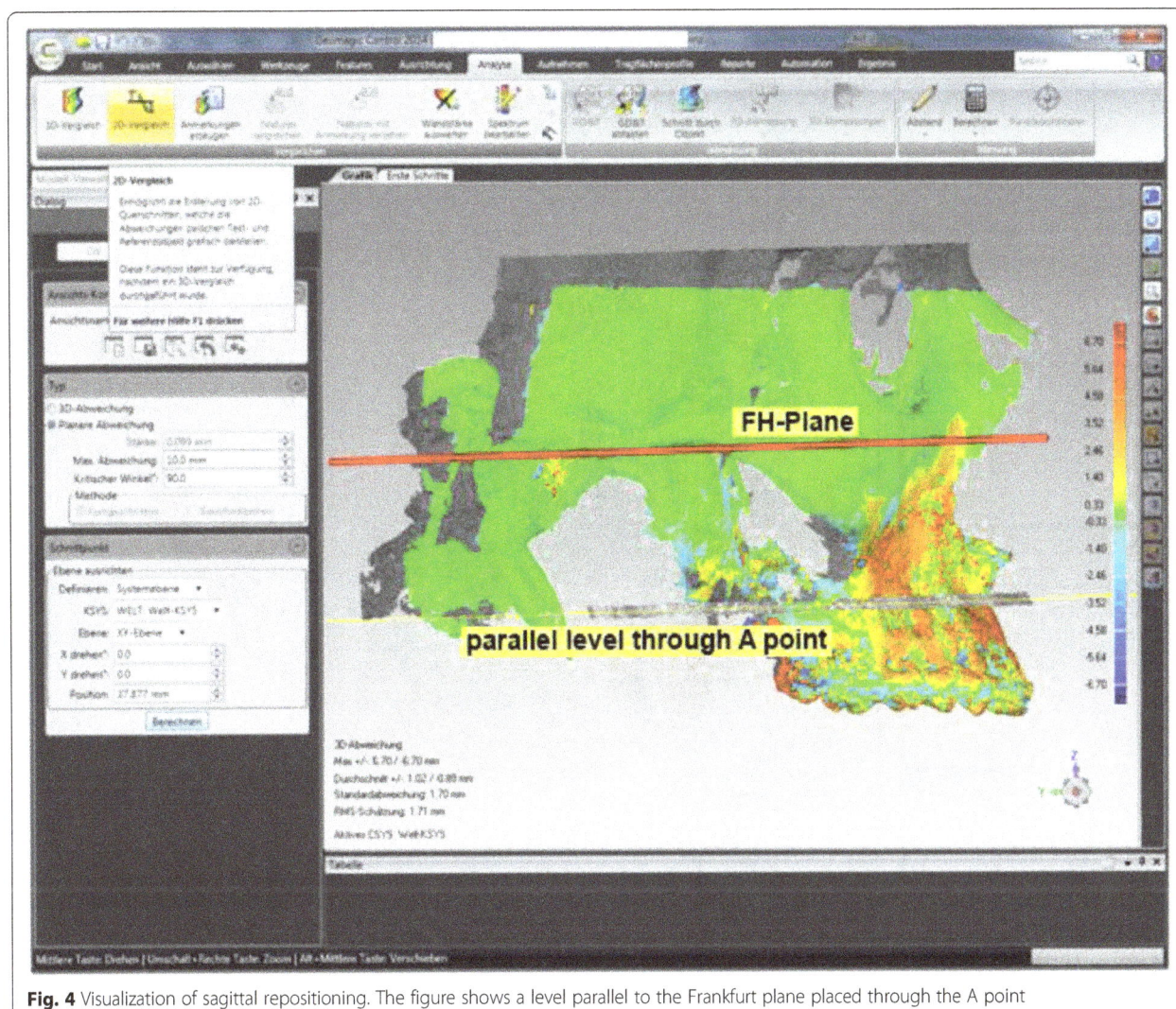

Fig. 4 Visualization of sagittal repositioning. The figure shows a level parallel to the Frankfurt plane placed through the A point

test were carried out. The significance level was set at $P < 0.05$.

Using SPSS, a formula was generated to calculate the amount of change in the width of the nose. A regression between the amount of maxillary advancement and the widening of the ala and alar base was prepared by transformation of the sagittal displacement distance with the square root and soft-tissue enlargement with the logarithm. The transformed variables followed a sufficiently Gaussian normal distribution. The relation of the transformed values was not purely linear, but curved. A second-degree polynomial was used to calculate the regression.

Results

The reproducibility of the measurement values represented by Spearman rank correlation showed highly significant correlations ($P = 0.000$) (Tables 3). The mean

sagittal repositioning of the maxilla was 5.58 mm. The calculated smallest repositioning distance was 2.02 mm and the largest distance was 10.84 mm (Table 4).

The width of the nose increased highly significantly between T0 and T1 as a result of the maxillary advancement ($P = 0.000$). As Table 5 shows, highly significant changes in the alae (Al), alar base (Alb), and nasolabial angle (NLA) were observed ($P = 0.000$). The alar width Al (mean + 3.17 ± 1.32 mm) increased in all 33 patients. The alar base width Alb (mean + 2.59 ± 1.26 mm) also increased. The nasolabial angle declined in 28 patients and increased in five patients (mean −6.65° ± 7.71°). As Table 6 shows, the increases in the width of the alar base and alar width correlated highly significantly with the skeletal advancement of the maxilla ($P = 0.000$).

The change in the nasolabial angle was not entirely independent of the sagittal repositioning, but this was not statistically significant ($P > 0.05$).

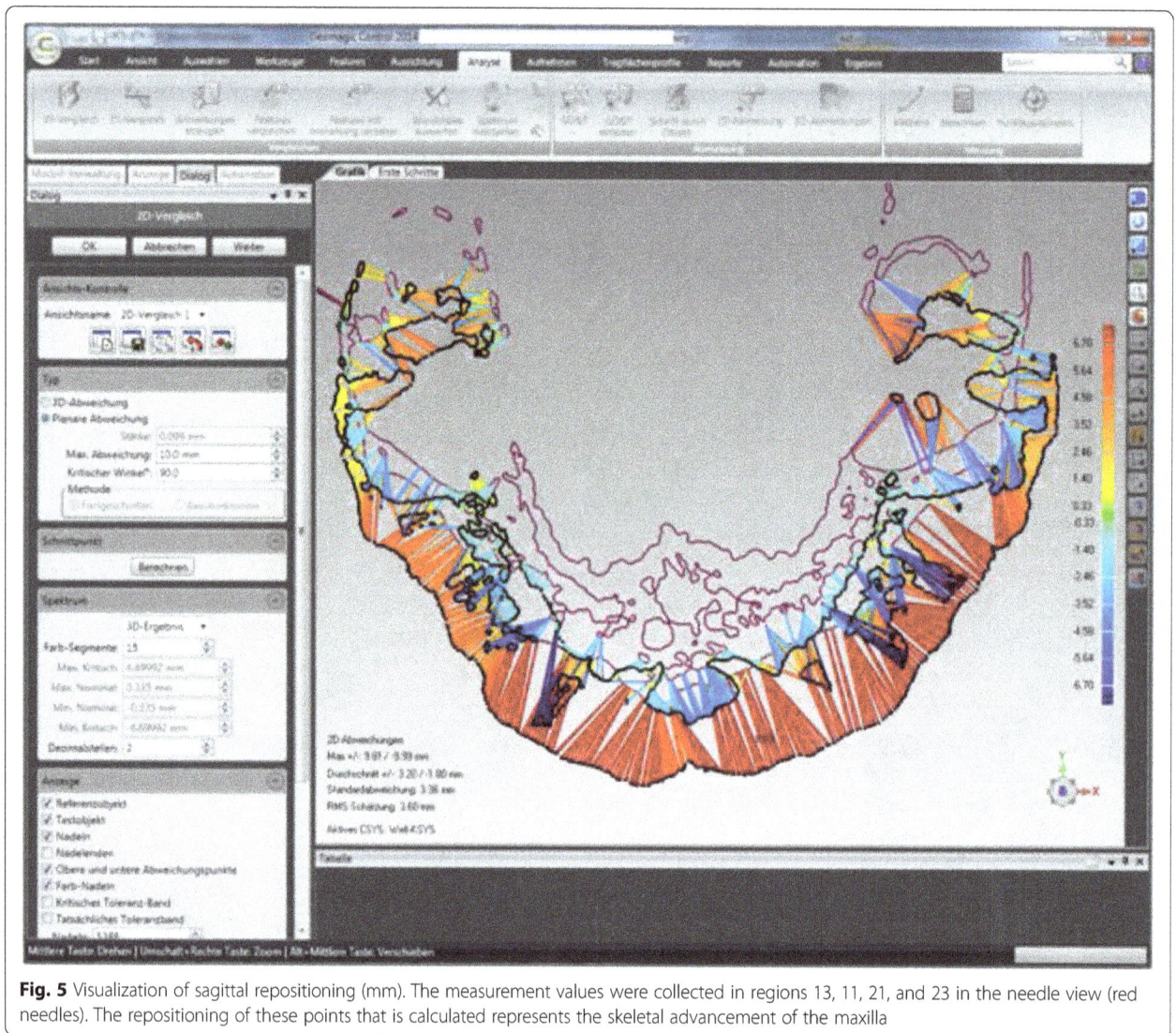

Fig. 5 Visualization of sagittal repositioning (mm). The measurement values were collected in regions 13, 11, 21, and 23 in the needle view (red needles). The repositioning of these points that is calculated represents the skeletal advancement of the maxilla

Table 3 Measurement error represented by correlation between the first measurement and follow-up measurement of nasal soft-tissue changes (Alb, Al, Sn–Ls–Co) and maxillary advancement (M–A); intraoperator correlation

		r	P
Nasal soft-tissue changes before treatment	Alb	0.9987	<0.000005***
	Al	0.9980	<0.000005***
	Sn–Ls–Co	0.9766$_{Sp}$	<0.000005***
Nasal soft-tissue changes after treatment	Alb	0.9978	<0.000005***
	Al	0.9976	<0.000005***
	Sn–Ls–Co	0.9729$_{Sp}$	<0.000005***
Maxillary advancement	M–A	0.9566	<0.000005***

r and P from the product–moment correlation or from Spearman rank correlation (Sp) ($n = 33$) for alar base, alar width, and nasolabial angle
***p< 0.001

Based on the results, the following formulas were developed to allow prediction of soft-tissue changes relative to skeletal advancement:

Alar base width:

- Patients ($n = 33$), regression coefficient $R^2 = 0.4764$, standard deviation $s = 0.1338959$

Table 4 Skeletal maxillary advancement (M–A) on the Frankfurt plane (mm)

Region	n	Mean	SD	Maxillary advancement (mm)		Minimum	Maximum
				Mean	68 % CI		
Front	33	5.580	2.412	5.728	2.820 8.159	2.0163	10.841

CI confidence intervals, *SD* standard deviation

Table 5 Comparison of values at T0 and T1; *P* with Student's *t*-test and the Wilcoxon test (W) (*n* = 33)

		Mean	SD	Increase		*P*
				Mean	SD	
Alb	Before treatment	33.665	2.632	3.171	1.322	<0.000005***
	After treatment	36.837	2.651			
Al	Before treatment	35.459	2.912	2.588	1.255	<0.000005***
	After treatment	38.047	2.851			
Sn–Ls–Co	Before treatment	102.992	14.388	−6.652	7.712	0.00002***W
	After treatment	96.339	12.748			

***p< 0.001

- Formula for y = ΔAlb in the course of x = maxillary advancement:
  $\log(\Delta Alb) = 0.4558889 + 0.124167 \times z + 0.010571 \times z^2$, where $z = (\sqrt{\text{(maxillary advancement)}} - 2.305)/0.5255$

Alar width:

- Patients (*n* = 33), regression coefficient $R^2 = 0.5281$, standard deviation *s* = 0.1403169
- Formula for y = ΔAl in the course of x = maxillary advancement:
  $\log(\Delta Al) = 0.3704371 + 0.1435941 \times z - 0.001474 \times z^2$, where $z = (\sqrt{\text{(maxillary advancement)}} - 2.305) / 0.5255$

Advancement by 5 mm would thus lead to a mean widening of the alar base of ≈ 2.8 mm. Ninety percent of the patients would have widening of between ≈ 1.7 mm and ≈ 4.6 mm (Table 7). As Table 8 shows, advancement of 5 mm would lead to a mean widening of the ala of ≈ 2.2 mm. Ninety percent of the patients could expect widening of between ≈ 1.3 mm and ≈ 3.8 mm.

Discussion

Investigations have been carried out since the 1980s to analyze associations between changes occurring in the facial soft tissue in connection with Le Fort I osteotomies in dysgnathia surgery. A correlation between sagittal repositioning of the maxilla and the amount of alar

Table 6 Correlations of changes in the external nose (alar base width, alar width, nasolabial angle) relative to skeletal advancement of the maxilla

Increase in	Region	n	rho	*P*
Alar base width	Front	33	0.6949	0.00001***
Alar width	Front	33	0.7688	<0.000005***
Nasolabial angle	Front	33	−0.3102	0.079

Soft-tissue parameters as the difference in means from T0 to T1; skeletal measurements as means from T1 to T0 for maxillary advancement. *P* from Spearman's rank correlation
***p< 0.001

flaring was not identified at that time [36]. Preoperative and postoperative lateral cephalograms or photographs were used for measurements in the early studies [10]. However, these techniques did not allow any conclusions to be drawn regarding correlations with the changing width of the nose [11].

Three-dimensional measurement of hard-tissue models obtained from CBCT and CT imaging is now increasingly being used, mainly for the planning of dental implants in dental medicine [37]. The amount of correlation between the initial measurements and control measurements of the soft tissue after 2 weeks is highly significant. Discussion is needed on mistakes during the reproducibility of these measurements. The reproducibility and reliability of different measurement points on lateral cephalograms has been frequently investigated in the past and has also been classified [38–40]. Similar findings were obtained with measurement points derived from lateral cephalograms created with CBCT [41]. The measurement points created on three-dimensional surfaces using CBCT scans are thus regarded as being highly reliable [42–44].

The sagittal movement of the maxilla was registered on a plane parallel to the Frankfurt plane. In 2012, Daboul et al. reported that the reproducibility and reliability of the Frankfurt plane on 3D multiplanar reformatting (MPR) images was excellent [45]. Similar

Table 7 Prediction of changes in alar base width

Maxillary advancement	Percentiles for increase in Alb (mm)				
	5.0 %	10.0 %	50.0 %	90.0 %	95.0 %
2 mm	1.13653	1.26409	1.88730	2.81777	3.13401
3 mm	1.29681	1.44235	2.15346	3.21515	3.57598
4 mm	1.46956	1.63449	2.44031	3.64343	4.05233
5 mm	1.65802	1.84409	**2.75326**	4.11066	4.57200
6 mm	1.86481	2.07410	3.09666	4.62337	5.14224
7 mm	2.09245	2.32728	3.47467	5.18774	5.76995
8 mm	2.34348	2.60649	3.89153	5.81012	6.46218
9 mm	2.62062	2.91473	4.35173	6.49721	7.22638
10 mm	2.92678	3.25524	4.86013	7.25626	8.07062

Approximate percentiles for Alb relative to maxillary advancement. A advancement of 5mm would lead to a mean widening of the alar base width of 2.8 mm

Table 8 Prediction of changes in alar width

Maxillary advancement	Percentiles for increase in Al (mm)				
	5.0 %	10.0 %	50.0 %	90.0 %	95.0 %
2 mm	0.77994	0.87191	1.32704	2.01974	2.25791
3 mm	0.95805	1.07102	1.63009	2.48098	2.77353
4 mm	1.13726	1.27136	1.93499	2.94504	3.29231
5 mm	1.32078	1.47652	**2.24725**	3.42030	3.82361
6 mm	1.51028	1.68837	2.56968	3.91103	4.37221
7 mm	1.70677	1.90802	2.90400	4.41985	4.94103
8 mm	1.91093	2.13626	3.25137	4.94855	5.53207
9 mm	2.12328	2.37365	3.61268	5.49846	6.14682
10 mm	2.34424	2.62067	3.98863	6.07066	6.78649

Approximate percentiles for Al relative to maxillary advancement. A advancement of 5mm would lead to a mean widening of the alar width of 2.2 mm

results were described by Ludlow et al. in 2009, who found amongst other things that identification of cephalometric landmarks is significantly more precise with MPR views of CBCT landmarks [46].

The first analysis of soft-tissue areas on the basis of three-dimensional CBCT reconstructions was reported by Han et al. in 2005. However, the patients included in the study were all of Asian descent [25]. In 2010, Kim et al. also investigated 3D reconstructions from CBCT images after repositioning of the maxilla at the Le Fort I level [47]. However, transverse changes in the size of the nose were not investigated. In 2012, the topic was again addressed by Park et al. using a new method, and transverse changes in the size of the nose were measured. The study also only included patients of Asian descent [14]. Farkas et al. noted that Asian individuals tend to have a nasal morphology that is very different from that in Caucasians [26, 48]. Direct comparison thus does not appear useful. In contrast to other publications, the present study therefore only includes patients of Caucasian descent and exclusively patients with maxillary retrognathic position. The results of the measurements of the width of the nose before surgical intervention were also compared with the results presented by Farkas. The T0 results were very similar to those of Farkas et al. in relation to the anthropometric measurements of Caucasian noses.

Measurement of soft-tissue models obtained from CBCT or CT imaging using Mimics has been confirmed as a valid method in various studies [49, 50]. Correlation of the initial measurements and follow-up measurements in the present study also showed that the measurement method is extremely accurate.

Using 3D radiographic evaluation, the present study shows that the transverse size of the nose increases when the maxilla is advanced during Class III surgical correction of occlusion anomalies. This result is also supported by the 3D photographic studies reported by

Honrado et al. in 2006 [5]. A considerable disadvantage with the use of methods based on conventional light is that only the skin is detected as a surface, with no information about the underlying structures. In addition, the undercutting ("shadow") that is produced by conventional light during detection of a three-dimensional surface can make evaluation impossible in some areas [23, 24]. These problems can be avoided with three-dimensional radiographic methods such as CBCT. Thanks to the different physical properties of skin and bone, the skin remains in the field of view when the underlying bone is being examined. In addition, CBCT produces an image that is true to scale, and undercutting does not occur.

The use of ionizing radiation for evaluation of a problem that is primarily aesthetic in nature may be questioned. It should be noted here that there is no indication for CBCT in the evaluation of soft tissue. Instead, when CBCT is required in any case for another indication, its findings can be enhanced using the techniques described here.

Overall, the results appear to be of major importance for everyday clinical purposes, since according to Göz et al., a poor aesthetic appearance is the most important reason why patients decide to undergo surgery for dysgnathia [2]. Subsequent widening of the nose is often regarded as an undesirable aesthetic change [2, 51]. If functional aspects allow it, the initial shape of the nose and the amount of maxillary advancement should be taken into account during the planning of the operation [27, 52, 28].

In addition to the usual information provided before surgery, it should therefore also be drawn to the patient's attention that the morphology of the external nose changes postoperatively and that surgical correction of the nose may become necessary later on [27, 52, 53]. The three-dimensional alteration coefficient of approximately 50 % calculated in the present study (with 1 mm of sagittal advancement of the maxilla equaling an increase in the width of the nose by 0.5 mm) could be used for preoperative assessment of the potential change.

The nasolabial angle decreases in most cases after sagittal repositioning, but there was no statistically significant correlation.

Conclusions

Maxillary advancement has effects on nasal morphology in individuals of Caucasian descent. The widening of the nose and narrowing of the nasolabial angle demonstrated in the present study may have a negative influence on the postoperative aesthetic result and should therefore be taken into account both in treatment planning and also in the information provided to patients.

The correlation coefficient calculated between sagittal advancement and soft-tissue changes in the nose may make prediction easier.

Ethical considerations

The study was compiled with the rules laid down by the Declaration of Helsinki. It was explained to the patients that inclusion of their data in the study was voluntary and that confidentiality and anonymity were guaranteed. They were also able to withdraw from the study at any time before publication without needing to give any reason. Written informed consent was obtained from all of the participants.

Abbreviations

Al: Alar width; Alb: Alar base width; Albl: Alar base on the left; Albr: Alar base on the right; All: Left ala; Alr: Right ala; CBCT: Cone-beam computed tomography; Co: Columellar tangential point; CT: Computed tomography; FOV: Field of view; Ls: Labrale superius; MPR: Multiplanar reformatting; NLA: Nasolabial angle; Sn: Subnasal point; SNA: Sella-nasion-A point angle.

Competing interests

The authors declare that they have no competing interests.

Authors' contributions

AH carried out the design and drafted the first manuscript. BK, MS, and RD carried out the measurements and helped with the design and coordination of the study and the drafting of the manuscript. WK performed the surgery and helped with the coordination of the study. HKS helped with the study design, the translation into English and the illustrations. All of the authors read and approved the final manuscript.

Author details

[1]Department of Orthodontics, University Hospital, Georg-Voigt-Strasse 3, Marburg 35039, Germany. [2]Private Practice, Bad Homburg, Germany.

References

1. Baik HS, Kim SY. Facial soft-tissue changes in skeletal Class III orthognathic surgery patients analyzed with 3-dimensional laser scanning. Am J Orthod Dentofacial Orthop. 2010;138(2):167–78. doi:10.1016/j.ajodo.2010.02.022.
2. Göz G. Die Motivation bei kieferorthopädischen Operationen. Freiburg i. Br: Albert-Ludwigs-Universität Freiburg i. Br; 1981.
3. Guymon M, Crosby DR, Wolford LM. The alar base cinch suture to control nasal width in maxillary osteotomies. Int J Adult Orthodon Orthognath Surg. 1988;3(2):89–95.
4. Choi JW, Lee JY, Oh TS, Kwon SM, Yang SJ, Koh KS. Frontal soft tissue analysis using a 3 dimensional camera following two-jaw rotational orthognathic surgery in skeletal class III patients. J Craniomaxillofac Surg. 2013. doi:10.1016/j.jcms.2013.05.004.
5. Honrado CP, Lee S, Bloomquist DS, Larrabee Jr WF. Quantitative assessment of nasal changes after maxillomandibular surgery using a 3-dimensional digital imaging system. Arch Facial Plast Surg. 2006;8(1):26–35. doi:10.1001/archfaci.8.1.26.
6. Hwang DS, Kim YI, Park SB, Lee JY. Midfacial soft tissue changes after leveling Le Fort I osteotomy with differential reduction. Cone-beam computed tomography volume superimposition. Angle Orthod. 2012;82(3):424–31. doi:10.2319/052411-342.1.
7. Johnson BM, McNamara JA, Bandeen RL, Baccetti T. Changes in soft tissue nasal widths associated with rapid maxillary expansion in prepubertal and postpubertal subjects. Angle Orthod. 2010;80(6):995–1001. doi:10.2319/033110-179.1.
8. Kim YI, Park SB, Son WS, Hwang DS. Midfacial soft-tissue changes after advancement of maxilla with Le Fort I osteotomy and mandibular setback surgery: comparison of conventional and high Le Fort I osteotomies by

9. Lee JY, Kim YI, Hwang DS, Park SB. Effect of setback Le Fort I osteotomy on midfacial soft-tissue changes as evaluated by cone-beam computed tomography superimposition for cases of skeletal Class III malocclusion. Int J Oral Maxillofac Surg. 2013;42(6):790–5. doi:10.1016/j.ijom.2012.11.012.
10. Radney LJ, Jacobs JD. Soft-tissue changes associated with surgical total maxillary intrusion. Am J Orthod. 1981;80(2):191–212.
11. Mansour S, Burstone C, Legan H. An evaluation of soft-tissue changes resulting from Le Fort I maxillary surgery. Am J Orthod. 1983;84(1):37–47.
12. McCance AM, Moss JP, Fright WR, James DR, Linney AD. A three dimensional analysis of soft and hard tissue changes following bimaxillary orthognathic surgery in skeletal III patients. Br J Oral Maxillofac Surg. 1992;30(5):305–12.
13. Mommaerts MY, Lippens F, Abeloos JV, Neyt LF. Nasal profile changes after maxillary impaction and advancement surgery. J Oral Maxillofac Surg. 2000;58(5):470–5. discussion 5–6.
14. Park SB, Yoon JK, Kim YI, Hwang DS, Cho BH, Son WS. The evaluation of the nasal morphologic changes after bimaxillary surgery in skeletal class III malocclusion by using the superimposition of cone-beam computed tomography (CBCT) volumes. J Craniomaxillofac Surg. 2012;40(4):e87–92. doi:10.1016/j.jcms.2011.05.008.
15. Ryckman MS, Harrison S, Oliver D, Sander C, Boryor AA, Hohmann AA, et al. Soft-tissue changes after maxillomandibular advancement surgery assessed with cone-beam computed tomography. Am J Orthod Dentofacial Orthop. 2010;137(4 Suppl):S86–93. doi:10.1016/j.ajodo.2009.03.041.
16. Westermark AH, Bystedt H, Von Konow L, Sallstrom KO. Nasolabial morphology after Le Fort I osteotomies. Effect of alar base suture. Int J Oral Maxillofac Surg. 1991;20(1):25–30.
17. Collins PC, Epker BN. The alar base cinch: a technique for prevention of alar base flaring secondary to maxillary surgery. Oral Surg Oral Med Oral Pathol. 1982;53(6):549–53.
18. Rustemeyer J, Martin A. Soft tissue response in orthognathic surgery patients treated by bimaxillary osteotomy: cephalometry compared with 2-D photogrammetry. Oral Maxillofac Surg. 2013;17(1):33–41. doi:10.1007/s10006-012-0330-0.
19. Kajikawa Y. Changes in soft tissue profile after surgical correction of skeletal class III malocclusion. J Oral Surg. 1979;37(3):167–74.
20. Lin SS, Kerr WJ. Soft and hard tissue changes in Class III patients treated by bimaxillary surgery. Eur J Orthod. 1998;20(1):25–33.
21. Kinzinger G, Frye L, Diedrich P. Class II treatment in adults: comparing camouflage orthodontics, dentofacial orthopedics and orthognathic surgery–a cephalometric study to evaluate various therapeutic effects. J Orofac Orthop. 2009;70(1):63–91. doi:10.1007/s00056-009-0821-2.
22. Verze L, Bianchi FA, Schellino E, Ramieri G. Soft tissue changes after orthodontic surgical correction of jaws asymmetry evaluated by three-dimensional surface laser scanner. J Craniofac Surg. 2012;23(5):1448–52. doi:10.1097/SCS.0b013e31824e25fc.
23. Holberg C, Heine AK, Geis P, Schwenzer K, Rudzki-Janson I. Three-dimensional soft tissue prediction using finite elements. Part II: Clinical application. J Orofac Orthop. 2005;66(2):122–34. doi:10.1007/s00056-005-0422-7.
24. Holberg C, Schwenzer K, Rudzki-Janson I. Three-dimensional soft tissue prediction using finite elements. Part I: Implementation of a new procedure. J Orofac Orthop. 2005;66(2):110–21. doi:10.1007/s00056-005-0421-8.
25. Han SY, Baik HS, Kim KD, Yu HS. Facial soft tissue measuring analysis of normal occlusion using three-dimensional CT imaging. Korean J Orthod. 2005;35(6):409–19.
26. Farkas LG, Katic MJ, Forrest CR, Alt KW, Bagic I, Baltadjiev G, et al. International anthropometric study of facial morphology in various ethnic groups/races. J Craniofac Surg. 2005;16(4):615–46.
27. Altman JI, Oeltjen JC. Nasal deformities associated with orthognathic surgery: analysis, prevention, and correction. J Craniofac Surg. 2007;18(4):734–9. doi:10.1097/SCS.0b013e3180684328.
28. Rauso R, Freda N, Curinga G, Del Pero C, Tartaro G. An alternative alar cinch suture. Eplasty. 2010;10, e69.
29. Millard Jr DR. The alar cinch in the flat, flaring nose. Plast Reconstr Surg. 1980;65(5):669–72.
30. Tessier P. The classic reprint: experimental study of fractures of the upper jaw. 3. Rene Le Fort, M.D., Lille, France. Plast Reconstr Surg. 1972;50(6):600–7.
31. Kau CH, Cronin A, Durning P, Zhurov AI, Sandham A, Richmond S. A new method for the 3D measurement of postoperative swelling following

superimposition of cone-beam computed tomography volumes. J Oral Maxillofac Surg. 2011;69(6):e225–33. doi:10.1016/j.joms.2010.12.035.

orthognathic surgery. Orthod Craniofac Res. 2006;9(1):31–7. doi:10.1111/j.1601-6343.2006.00341.x.

32. Oh KM, Seo SK, Park JE, Sim HS, Cevidanes LH, Kim YJ, et al. Post-operative soft tissue changes in patients with mandibular prognathism after bimaxillary surgery. J Craniomaxillofac Surg. 2013;41(3):204–11. doi:10.1016/j.jcms.2012.09.001.

33. Legan HL, Burstone CJ. Soft tissue cephalometric analysis for orthognathic surgery. J Oral Surg. 1980;38(10):744–51.

34. Cevidanes LH, Motta A, Proffit WR, Ackerman JL, Styner M. Cranial base superimposition for 3-dimensional evaluation of soft-tissue changes. Am J Orthod Dentofacial Orthop. 2010;137(4 Suppl):S120–9. doi:10.1016/j.ajodo.2009.04.021.

35. Gkantidis N, Halazonetis DJ. Morphological integration between the cranial base and the face in children and adults. J Anat. 2011;218(4):426–38. doi:10.1111/j.1469-7580.2011.01346.x.

36. O'Ryan F, Schendel S. Nasal anatomy and maxillary surgery. I. Esthetic and anatomic principles. Int J Adult Orthodon Orthognath Surg. 1989;4(1):27–37.

37. Neugebauer J, Ritter L, Mischkowski R, Zoller JE. Three-dimensional diagnostics, planning and implementation in implantology. Int J Comput Dent. 2006;9(4):307–19.

38. Baumrind S, Frantz RC. The reliability of head film measurements. 1. Landmark identification. Am J Orthod. 1971;60(2):111–27.

39. Miethke RR. Zur Lokalisationsgenauigkeit kephalometrischer Referenzpunkte. Prakt Kieferorthop. 1989;3:107–22.

40. Stabrun AE, Danielsen K. Precision in cephalometric landmark identification. Eur J Orthod. 1982;4(3):185–96.

41. Navarro Rde L, Oltramari-Navarro PV, Fernandes TM, Oliveira GF, Conti AC, Almeida MR, et al. Comparison of manual, digital and lateral CBCT cephalometric analyses. J Appl Oral Sci. 2013;21(2):167–76. doi:10.1590/1678-7757201302326.

42. Fourie Z, Damstra J, Gerrits PO, Ren Y. Accuracy and repeatability of anthropometric facial measurements using cone beam computed tomography. Cleft Palate Craniofac J. 2011;48(5):623–30. doi:10.1597/10-076.

43. Naji P, Alsufyani NA, Lagravere MO. Reliability of anatomic structures as landmarks in three-dimensional cephalometric analysis using CBCT. Angle Orthod. 2013. doi:10.2319/090413-652.1.

44. Oz U, Orhan K, Abe N. Comparison of linear and angular measurements using two-dimensional conventional methods and three-dimensional cone beam CT images reconstructed from a volumetric rendering program in vivo. Dentomaxillofac Radiol. 2011;40(8):492–500. doi:10.1259/dmfr/15644321.

45. Daboul A, Schwahn C, Schaffner G, Soehnel S, Samietz S, Aljaghsi A, et al. Reproducibility of Frankfort horizontal plane on 3D multi-planar reconstructed MR images. PLoS One. 2012;7(10), e48281. doi:10.1371/journal.pone.0048281.

46. Ludlow JB, Gubler M, Cevidanes L, Mol A. Precision of cephalometric landmark identification: cone-beam computed tomography vs conventional cephalometric views. Am J Orthod Dentofacial Orthop. 2009;136(3):312 e1–10. doi:10.1016/j.ajodo.2008.12.018. discussion −3.

47. Kim YI, Kim JR, Park SB. Three-dimensional analysis of midfacial soft tissue changes according to maxillary superior movement after horizontal osteotomy of the maxilla. J Craniofac Surg. 2010;21(5):1587–90. doi:10.1097/SCS.0b013e3181edc5c9.

48. Farkas LG, Phillips JH, Katic M. Anthropometric anatomical and morphological nose widths in Canadian Caucasian adults. Can J Plast Surg. 1998;6(3):149–51.

49. Gorgulu S, Gokce SM, Olmez H, Sagdic D, Ors F. Nasal cavity volume changes after rapid maxillary expansion in adolescents evaluated with 3-dimensional simulation and modeling programs. Am J Orthod Dentofacial Orthop. 2011;140(5):633–40. doi:10.1016/j.ajodo.2010.12.020.

50. Shaw K, McIntyre G, Mossey P, Menhinick A, Thomson D. Validation of conventional 2D lateral cephalometry using 3D cone beam CT. J Orthod. 2013;40(1):22–8. doi:10.1179/1465313312Y.0000000009.

51. Honn M, Goz G. The ideal of facial beauty: a review. J Orofac Orthop. 2007;68(1):6–16. doi:10.1007/s00056-007-0604-6.

52. Mitchell C, Oeltjen J, Panthaki Z, Thaller SR. Nasolabial aesthetics. J Craniofac Surg. 2007;18(4):756–65. doi:10.1097/scs.0b013e3180684360.

53. Rauso R, Tartaro G, Tozzi U, Colella G, Santagata M. Nasolabial changes after maxillary advancement. J Craniofac Surg. 2011;22(3):809–12. doi:10.1097/SCS.0b013e31820f3663.

16

Efficiency of pivot splints as jaw exercise apparatus in combination with stabilization splints in anterior disc displacement without reduction: a retrospective study

Mehmet Muhtarogullari[1], Mehmet Avci[2] and Bulem Yuzugullu[3*]

Abstract

Objective: To evaluate efficiency of pivot splints in jaw exercises, in combination with stabilization splints, in cases of anterior disc displacement without reduction of temporomandibular joint.

Subjects and methods: Twenty-three patients who referred to the prosthodontics clinic in 1995–1997 were included in the study, where anterior disc displacement without reduction of temporomandibular joint was diagnosed using magnetic resonance imaging and clinical examination. Pivot splints were used for jaw exercises for five minutes long; five times/day and stabilization splints were used at all other times. The patients were followed for 24 weeks. Lateral and protrusive excursions along with maximum mouth opening and were evaluated at each control. Bilateral palpation of temporal, masseter, sternocleidomastoid muscles and TMJ was assessed for pain perception before and after treatment. Data were statistically analyzed using Paired sample t-test and Independent Samples t-test ($p < .05$).

Results: Mean mandibular range of motion measurements increased from 28.74 mm prior to 49.17 mm on maximum opening; right/left lateral excursion from 7.61 mm to 12.04 mm and 4.09 mm to 7.3 mm on protrusion after treatment. All changes observed before and after treatment were found to be statistically significant. ($p < .001$) Pain symptoms were eliminated at the end of 24 weeks of treatment in all patients.

Conclusion: Using pivot splints as an exercise regimen along with a stabilization splint may be a viable treatment option for patients with anterior disc displacement without reduction; as normal mandibular range of motion was established and pain was eliminated.

Keywords: Temporomandibular joint, Internal derangement, Anterior disc displacement without reduction, Magnetic resonance imaging, Pivot splint, Stabilization splint

Introduction

Anterior disc displacement without reduction (ADDWoR) of the temporomandibular joint (TMJ), 'closed lock' is a widespread disorder that clinically presents itself with restriction in jaw movements, in which the morphology of the disc is altered while the discal ligaments have become elongated [1,2]. The longer the disc is displaced anteriorly and medially, the greater the thinning of its posterior border and the more the lateral discal ligament and inferior retrodiscal lamina will be elongated. Also, protracted anterior displacement of the disc will lead to a greater loss of elasticity in the superior retrodiscal lamina. The disc can be forced through the discal space, eventually collapsing the joint space behind it, trapping the disc in the forward position [3]. During mouth opening the effected joint exhibits rotation, but translation is limited or non-existent [4,5]. In these circumstances, providing function by re-establishing the ideal disc-condyle relationship or more often by reducing restriction in movement should be the goal of the treatment to eliminate pain [5]. When patients

* Correspondence: bulemy@gmail.com
[3]Department of Prosthodontics, Faculty of Dentistry, Baskent University, Ankara, Turkey
Full list of author information is available at the end of the article

complain about being locked for a week or less, manipulation to recapture the disc could be attempted. However, if recapturing cannot be accomplished, different approaches such as splint therapies, arthroscopic and/or open joint surgeries might be considered to reduce functional limitations along with pain control [3,6,7]. Nonsurgical therapy should be the first treatment choice to prevent risk of postoperative surgical complications although there were instances where surgical interventions may be successful. The splints may be classified into three major groups with respect to their hypothesized function: relaxation/stabilization splints, distraction/pivot splints and repositioning splints. The latter have been described for the therapy of painful disc displacement with reduction [8].

The purpose of this retrospective study was to investigate the efficiency of a treatment approach that consists of using pivot splints for jaw exercises in combination with stabilization splints in cases of ADDwoR with former unsuccessful manual reduction attempts history.

Methods
Study population
Twenty-three patients (3 male, 20 female) in an age range of 24 and 48 (mean age 27.1), referred to the Department of Prosthodontics in Hacettepe University, Faculty of Dentistry with the chief complaint of symptoms in the temporomandibular joint (TMJ) between the years of 1995–1997 were screened from the archives. The study was approved by the Ethics Committee of Hacettepe University (GO 14/97).

The inclusion criteria were: patients over 18 years old; previous history of limited mouth opening for more than 2 weeks; pain in the TMJ area aggravated by jaw movement and function; a positive diagnosis of unilateral or bilateral ADDwoR by means of magnetic resonance imaging (MRI); maximum mouth opening of <40 mm; and previous attempts of unsuccessful manual reduction. Patients who were unwilling or unable to receive splint and/or exercise therapy; had previously been treated for temporomandibular joint (TMJ) disorders (TMD); had extensive restorations, missing teeth, fixed or removable partial dentures; had systemic rheumatic disease, generalized joint pain or swelling, neurologic disorders, had concurrent use of steroids, anti-inflammatories, muscle relaxants or narcotics, major psychiatric disease and prior TMJ surgery were excluded.

The same operator performed all clinical examination, splint therapy and control in the follow-up appointments of all patients.

Baseline measurements
Mouth opening
The patients were asked to open their mouth as wide as possible to measure the incisal edge clearance in millimeters

(mm), The distance between the first right incisor of the maxilla and mandibula was measured with a millimetric ruler.

Lateral excursions
The patients were asked to open their mouth slightly (physiological rest position) and move their mandible as far as possible towards right or left (maximum lateral position). The midline labioincisal embrasure of the mandibular incisor was measured with a millimetric ruler.

Protrusion
The initial position was the physiological rest position from which the patient moved the mandible anteriorly without contacting the teeth. The distance from the incisal edge of the maxillary central incisor to the incisor edge of the mandibular incisor was measured in the maximum protruded position.

Pain assessment
The temporal, masseter, sternocleidomastoid muscles and TMJ were palpated bilaterally for pain perception.

Magnetic resonance imaging
Magnetic resonance imaging had been performed at Hacettepe University, Faculty of Medicine, Department of Radiology, with 0,5 Tesla MR scanner (Gyroscan, Phillips, Netherland) prior to treatment. T1 weighted oblique-sagittal images of both joints were obtained in 3 mm thick slices for each patient by using surface coil attachments with an internal diameter of 11 cm and an external diameter of 14 cm. Sequential bilateral images were obtained of the closed mouth and the maximal open mouth positions. Normal disc position was defined as the posterior band of the disk located superior of the head of the mandibular condyle. Disk displacement was defined as having the posterior band of the disk located anterior to the mandibular condyle.

Treatment protocol
Each patient received two maxillary splints made of clear auto polymerizing acrylic resin. Pivot splints were fabricated from acrylic resin and adjusted intraorally as described by Sears [9], with a bilateral pivot in the region of the second molar teeth.

Full arch maxillary stabilization splints were adjusted to have uniform and simultaneous contacts with the buccal cusp tips of posterior and incisor edges of the anterior teeth of the opposing arch. Eccentric guidance was established with acrylic prominences labial to the mandibular canines to have disclusion in the posterior teeth.

An exercise regimen of five minutes long, five times/day, with a minimum of three hours between each exercise, was recommended. In the exercise period, patients were asked to lie on a hard flat surface and exert force under the chin with one hand in an upward direction with the pivot splint in place (Figure 1). The patients were only allowed to remove the stabilization splints during mealtimes, oral hygiene procedures and daily exercises with the pivot splint. No muscle relaxants, analgesics or anti-inflammatory agents were prescribed during the course of the treatment. Clinical examinations were performed on a weekly basis for 24 weeks.

At all evaluation days, all patients were extensively informed about that overuse, misuse or parafunction could enhance or provoke their complaints. They received instructions to keep the jaw muscles relaxed, and avoid non-functional tooth contacts and excessive mouth opening.

During each evaluation appointment; maximum interincisal opening, protrusive and lateral excursions were recorded as assessed for the baseline measurements, TMJ, sternocleidomastoid, masseter, temporal and lateral pterygoid muscles were palpated and stabilization splints were adjusted if necessary. Treatment procedures were continued for 24 weeks. Magnetic resonance imaging had been performed at the end of the treatment period as described previously.

Statistical analysis

Paired sample t-test was used to determine the changes in the range of motion before and after treatment. Mean values of the range of motion (mm) of patient groups with change or no change in disc positions after treatment; related to age, locking duration, maximum mouth opening, lateral and protrusive eccentric movements were compared using the Independent Samples t-test.

Results

The mean average time from the onset of limited mouth opening was 13,74 ± 9,99 weeks. Mean mandibular range of movement measurements are shown on Table 1. All changes observed before and after treatment were found to be statistically significant (p < .001) (Table 1).

Differences in mean values of the range of motion (mm) of patient groups with change or no change in disc positions after treatment; related to age, locking duration, maximum

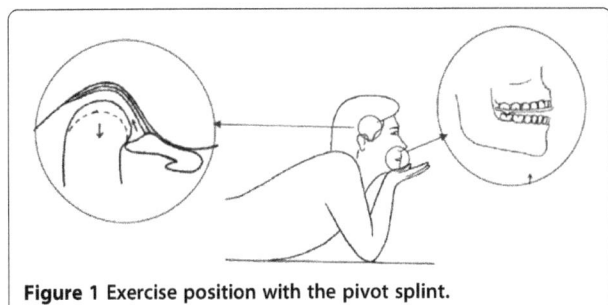

Figure 1 Exercise position with the pivot splint.

maximum mouth opening, lateral and protrusive eccentric movements are seen on Table 2. There was no statistically significant difference between changed and no-changed disc positioned groups related to age, locking duration and change in the disc location (Table 2).

While the bilateral palpation of the temporal, masseter, sternocleidomastoidmuscles and/or TMJ in patients revealed pain perception prior to treatment; the pain symptoms were eliminated at the end of 24 weeks of treatment in all patients.

Side effects of splint therapy, such as tooth intrusion, tooth loosening or sensitivity on biting, were not present in any of the patients.

Discussion

Standard treatment protocol for patients with acute ADDWoR mostly starts with manipulation of the mandible to recapture the dislocated disc. If this procedure is successful, an anterior repositioning splint is made. However, when the disc has lost its normal morphology, the chances of maintaining the disc in place become remote [3,10].

In the authors' experience, early intervention to treat ADDWoR, yields to good prognosis, particularly in young patients. Thus, it is well worth attempting to reduce the dislocated disc manually several times. However, for chronic cases the prognosis of using these stabilization splints alone has not been predictable, a new treatment protocol using jaw exercises with a pivot splint to mobilize the joint was devised.

A comparative study between jaw-stretch self-exercise and control groups in patients with ADDWoR demonstrated that the exercise group showed significant improvement in both maximum mouth opening and interference with life scores [11]. Another controlled evaluation of non-surgical treatment protocols results suggested that mouth-opening exercise has potential therapeutic effects although gradual reduction of signs and symptoms of ADDWoR was non-specific and was not related to the type of treatment [12]. Also in accordance with the present study results, Haketa et al [13] concluded that, the mouth opening range significantly increased in the exercise group in the 8-week follow-up period.

Any splint may cause an increase in the joint space and stress reduction at articulating surfaces. Stabilization splints have been used in treatment of a large variety of symptoms of TMDs of muscular and/or structural origin [14]. A pivot splint has been thought of having the additional benefit of mobilizing the condyle through the action of jaw-closing muscles over the force vectors created by jaw closing muscles have been found to position the condyle in anterosuperior position, decreasing the stress on the articulating surfaces. Use of elastic bandages from chin to head has been advocated as a mean to apply extraoral forces to cause distraction in the joint [15].

Table 1 Changes in the range of movements (mm) before and after treatment

Movements	Before treatment*	After treatment*	t	p-value
Right/Left lateral movement	7,61 ± 1,69	12,04 ± 1,41	12,990	<0.001
Protrusive movement	4,09 ± 1,41	7,3 ± 1,43	7,990	<0.001
Maximum interincisal opening	28,74 ± 5,51	49,17 ± 6,37	14,470	<0.001

*Results are expressed as mean ± standard deviation.

In the present study, exercises were preferred over the use of elastic bandages. These exercises are similar to those recommended in cervical vertebrae problem cases, where soft tissue and joint mobilization is aimed by traction [16]. Traction of the TMJ in a vertical direction may cause an increase in space between bony structures of the joint, creating an environment for the reduction of the dislocated disk and reducing interarticular pressure. Bilateral pivot points at the molar region of splints and extra oral force application provide the desired direction of force. Since constant use of the pivot splint has been associated with intrusion of the teeth under the pivot points, patients in the presented study were instructed to limit the use of the splint to exercise only. With the exception of hygiene, eating and exercise procedures, all patients were asked to wear stabilization splints at all times.

Most patients seek for treatment when pain interferes with daily activities and ADDWoR has been reported to be a painful disorder [17]. Reduction or elimination of pain is an important parameter in evaluation of a therapeutic approach. With similar cases Lundh et al [18] reported a 33%, Okeson et al [19] 50% and Carraro and Cafesse [20] 100% elimination of pain symptoms. However, the Visual Analogue Scale was not used to assess pain as in literature [8]. Pain was determined at the first examination and throughout the follow-up period by bilateral palpation of the TMJ and muscles and asking the patient if they perceived any pain. In our study, clinical assessment at the end of the 24-week treatment period, revealed absence of any joint or muscular pain; thus a 100% success was obtained.

In a study regarding the outcome of arthroscopic surgery, Davis et al [21] reported a mean maximum opening increase of 14.6 mm for unilateral, and 8.9 mm for bilateral ADDWoR cases 6 months after surgery. Eminectomy via open joint surgery has been reported to result in a mean increase of 17.9 mm in maximum opening among 18 closed lock patients [22]. Sodium hyaluronate injection to the superior compartment of the TMJ has resulted in 17.1 mm increase for an ADDWoR cases [23]. Dimitroulis [24] reported an increase in mean maximum opening from 24.6 mm to 42.3 mm when closed lock cases were treated with arthrosynthesis and lavage followed by manipulation to reduce the discs. Murakami et al [25] compared the outcome of arthrosynthesis, arthroscopy and nonsurgical treatment approaches for ADDWoR cases. The nonsurgical treatment consisted of non-steroidal anti-inflammatory drugs and muscle relaxants for the first two weeks, followed by manipulation to reduce the discs. Pivot splints were used for up to 12 weeks for cases that showed no improvement in this group. When success criteria were defined as absence or significant reduction of pain maximum opening beyond 38 mm and 6 mm minimum lateral and protrusive movements, 55.6% of the nonsurgical group, 70% of the arthrosynthesis and 91% of the arthroscopic surgery groups were found to be successful.

Another approach to evaluate the outcome of TMD treatment involves measurement of mandibular range of motion including not only maximum interincisal opening but left and right lateral and protrusive movements as well. 40–58 mm has been reported as average amount of maximum interincisal opening and 8–10 mm as lateral and protrusive movements [26]. In the presented study,

Table 2 Differences in mean values of the range of motion (mm) of patient groups with change or no change in disc positions after treatment; related to age, locking duration, maximum mouth opening, lateral and protrusive eccentric movements

Variables	Change in disc position (n = 11)	No change in disc position (n = 12)	Overall (n = 23)	t	p-value
Age	25,64 ± 11,01	28,58 ± 10,33	27,17 ± 10,52	0,660	*NS
Locking duration	12,91 ± 10,25	14,5 ± 10,13	13,74 ± 9,99	0,370	*NS
Right/Left lateral movement after treatment	12,33 ± 1,53	11,79 ± 1,28	12,04 ± 1,41	−1,290	*NS
Protrusive movement after treatment	7,64 ± 1,8	7 ± 0,95	7,3 ± 1,43	−1,070	*NS
Maximum mouth opening after treatment	50,73 ± 6,65	47,75 ± 6,03	49,17 ± 6,37	−1,130	*NS

*NS: Not significant.

significant increase of 20.43 mm in maximum opening, 4.43 mm in right/left lateral movement and 3.21 mm in protrusive movements were observed, when comparing the baseline measurements with post-treatment outcomes. These results are well within the normal range reported by previous studies [21-24]. The results also indicated that the most dramatic improvement in the range of motion was within the first 4 weeks of treatment. During the treatment, the progress of improvement gradually decreased but continued until the twenty forth week when the study was concluded.

Choi et al. [27] reported that, conservative treatment procedures that were used at ADDWoR cases were beneficial not because they change the position of displaced disk, instead they increase the mobility of condyle and an adaptation of posterior attachments occurs. Kirk [28] reported that the clinical success of treatment did not mean a change of anatomic relationships of TMJ. McNeill [29] reported that without recapturing the displaced disk, normal function could be obtained by the adaptation of retrodiscal tissue. The results of the presented study agree with previous studies.

This study have not compared the efficacy of pivot splint with any other treatment procedure, however, the symptoms of TMD have improved after 24-week treatment protocol. Since normal mandibular range of motion was reestablished and pain was absent after treatment among all patients, the treatment concept investigated seemed effective for cases diagnosed as having ADDWoR.

Competing interests
The authors declare that they have no competing interests.

Authors' contributions
MM carried out the clinical examination, treatment sequences and controls for all patients, MA participated in the design of the study and coordination, BY participated in the design of the study, interpretation of the data and drafted the manuscript. All authors read and approved the final manuscript.

Acknowledgements
The authors wish to thank Pınar Ozdemir for statistical consulting, Barış Guncu for helping revise and Prof Neslihan Arhun for English editing of the manuscript. This research was carried out without funding.

Author details
[1]Department of Prosthodontics, Faculty of Dentistry, Hacettepe University, Ankara, Turkey. [2]Private practice, Istanbul, Turkey. [3]Department of Prosthodontics, Faculty of Dentistry, Baskent University, Ankara, Turkey.

References
1. Kaplan A, Assel LA: Temporomandibular Disorders: Diagnosis and Treatment. First edition. Philadelphia: W.B. Saunders Company; 1991.
2. Vichaichalermvong S, Nilner M, Panmekiate S, Petersson A: Clinical follow-up of patients with different disc positions. J Orofacial Pain 1993, 7:61–67.
3. Okeson JP: 'Signs and symptoms of temporomandibular disorders' in: Management of Temporomandibular Disorders and Occlusion. 7th edition. St Louis: Elsevier; 2013:138–143. 325.
4. Mongini F: A modified extraoral technique of mandibular manipulation in disk displacement without reduction. J Craniomandib Pract 1995, 13:22–25.
5. Chung SC, Kim HS: The effect of the stabilization splint on the tmj closed lock. J Craniomandib Pract 1993, 11:95–101.
6. Yustin D, Kryshtalsky JB, Galea A: Use of hylan G-F 20 for viscosupplementation of the temporomandibular joint for the management of osteoarthritis: a case report. J Orofacial Pain 1995, 9:375–379.
7. Tallents RH, Katzberg RW, Miler TL, Manzione J, Macher DJ, Roberts C: Arthrographically assisted splint therapy: Painful clicking with a non-reducing meniscus. Oral Surg Oral Med Oral Pathol 1986, 61:2–7.
8. Stiesch-Scholz M, Kempert S, Wolter H, Tschernitschek H: Comparitave prospective study on splint therapy of anterior disc displacement without reduction. J Oral Rehabil 2005, 32:474–479.
9. Sears VH: Occlusal pivots. J Prosthet Dent 1956, 6:332–336.
10. Sarnat BG, Laskin DM: The Temporomandibular Joint: A Biological Basis for Clinical Practice. Fourth edition. Philadelphia: W.B. Saunders Company; 1992.
11. Yuasa H, Kurita K: Randomized clinical trial of primary treatment for temporomandibular joint disc displacement without reduction and without osseous changes: A combination of NSAISs and mouth-openning exercise versus no treatment. Oral Surg Oral Med Oral Pathol Oral Radiol Endod 2001, 91:671–675.
12. Minakuchi H, Kuboki T, Matsuka Y, Maekawa K, Yatani H, Yamashita A: Randomized controlled evaluation of non-surgical treatments for temporomandibular joint anterior disc displacement without reduction. J Dent Res 2001, 80:924–928.
13. Haketa T, Kino K, Sugisaki M, Takaoka M, Ohta T: Randomized clinical trial of treatment for TMJ disc displacement. J Dent Res 2010, 89:1259–1263.
14. Clark GT, Townsend GC, Carey SE: Bruxing Patterns in man during sleep. J Oral Rehabil 1984, 11:123–128.
15. Moncayo S: Biomechanics of pivoting appliances. J Orofacial Pain 1994, 8:190–196.
16. Boero RP: The physiology of splint therapy: a literature review. Angle Orthodontist 1989, 59:165–177.
17. McNeill C: Craniomandibular Disorders Guidelines for Evaluation Diagnosis and management: The American Academy of Craniomandibular Disorders. In 2nd printing. Chicago: Quintessence Publishing Co. Inc; 1990.
18. Lundh H, Westesson PL, Eriksson L, Brooks SL: Temporomandibular joint disk displacement without reduction. Treatment with flat occlusal splint versus no treatment. Oral Surg Oral Med Oral Pathol 1992, 73:655–658.
19. Okeson JP, Kemper JT, Moody PM: A study of the use of occlusion splints in the treatment of acute and chronic patients with craniomandibular disorders. J Prosthet Dent 1982, 48:708–712.
20. Carraro JJ, Caffesse RG: Effect of occlusal splints on TMJ symptomatology. J Prosthet Dent 1978, 40:563–566.
21. Davis CL, Kaminishi RM, Marshall MW: Arthroscopic surgery for treatment of closed lock. J Oral Maxillofac Surg 1991, 49:704–707.
22. Stassen LFA, Currie WJR: A pilot study of the use of eminectomy in the treatment of closed lock. Br J Oral Maxillofac Surg 1994, 32:138–141.
23. Fader KW, Grummons DC, Maijer R, Christensen LV: Pressurized infusion of sodium hyaluronate for closed lock of the temporomandibular joint. Part I: A Case Study. J Craniomandib Pract 1993, 11:68–72.
24. Dimitroulis G, Dolwick MF, Martinez A: Temproromandibular joint arthrocentesis and lavage for the treatment of closed lock: a follow-up study. Br J Oral Maxillofac Surg 1995, 33:23–27.
25. Murakami KI, Hosako H, Moriya Y, Segami N, Iizuka T: Short-term out come study for the management of temporomandibular joint closed-lock. A comparison of arthrocentesis to nonsurgical therapy and arthroscopic lysis and lavage. Oral Surg Oral Med Oral Pathol Oral Radiol Endod 1995, 80:253–257.
26. McCarty WL, Darnell MW: Rehabilitation of the temporomandibular joint through the application of motion. J Craniomandib Pract 1993, 11:298–307.
27. Choi BH, Yoo JH, Lee WY, Do K: Comparison of magnetic resonance imaging before and after nonsurgical treatment of closed lock. Oral Surg Oral Med Oral Pathol 1994, 78:301.
28. Kirk W: Magnetic resonance imaging and tomographic evaluation of occlusal appliance treatment for advanced internal derangement of the temporomandibular joint. J Oral Maxillofac Surg 1991, 49:9–12.
29. McNeill C: The optimum temporomandibular joint condyle position in clinical practice. Int J Perio Restor Dent 1985, 5:71–72.

17

Sinusitis and oroantral fistula in patients with bisphosphonate-associated necrosis of the maxilla

Pit Jacob Voss[1*], Gustavo Vargas Soto[2], Rainer Schmelzeisen[1], Kiwako Izumi[3], Andres Stricker[1], Gido Bittermann[1] and Philipp Poxleitner[1]

Abstract

Background: The management of bisphosphonate related necrosis of the jaw has become clinical routine. While approximately two thirds of the lesions are in the mandible, one third is located in the maxilla. In 40–50 % of maxillary necrosis the maxillary sinus is involved, leading to maxillary sinusitis and oro-antral communications.

Methods: This retrospective single center study includes all patients with diagnosis of BP-ONJ of the maxilla and concomitant maxillary sinusitis. The information collected includes age, gender, primary disease, bisphosphonate intake, involving type of bisphosphonate, route of administration and duration of BP treatment previous to surgical treatment and treatment outcome.

Results: A total of 12 patients fulfill the criteria of the diagnosis of maxillary sinusitis associated to maxillary necrosis, of which 6 Patients showed purulent sinusitis. All patients underwent surgical treatment with complete resection of the affected bone and a multilayer wound closure. A recurrence appeared in one patient with open bone and no sign of sinusitis and was treated conservatively.

Conclusions: Purulent maxillary Sinusitis is a common complication of bisphosphonate-related necrosis of the maxilla. The surgical technique described can be suggested for the treatment of these patients.

Keywords: Nose and paranasal sinuses, Medication-associated necrosis of the jaws, Zoledronate, Purulent sinusitis

Background

Since its first description in 2003, reports of bisphosphonate related osteonecrosis of the jaw (BP-ONJ) accumulate. With the ability to reduce bone turnover through selective inhibition of osteoclasts, Bisphosphonates are used widespread in treatment of osteoporosis and bony metastases of malignant diseases. They are administered orally or intravenously, whereat the bioavailability of oral bisphosphonates is below 1 % [1]. Once circulating in the blood, 70 % are covalently bound to hydroxyapatite in bony tissues, the remainder is secreted via the kidneys. BPs bound to the bone are biologically inert, however, when absorbed by osteoclasts they lead to concentration dependent apoptosis

via inhibition of Farnesyl-Pyrophosphate-synthase [2]. Being integrated only during bone turnover, concentration is suspected to be higher in areas of high turnover such as the alveolar processes [3]. Due to local factors like chewing forces, oral bacteria, the periodontal gap and a thin mucosa, the alveolar bone necessitates an elevated osteoclast-dependent bone turnover to maintain integrity [4]. When osteoclasts are diminished by a high local concentration of BPs, the bone is not capable to react to these local factors what may end in necrosis [5]. The prominent role of osteoclast inhibition in the pathogenesis of BP-ONJ is underlined by recent reports of osteonecrosis of the jaw following the treatment with Denosumab, a selective antibody against RANK-L and thus potent inhibitor of osteoclasts and its precursors, which have a similar incidence like BP-ONJ after the treatment with Zoledronate (ZOL), the BP with the highest antiresorptive potency [6].

* Correspondence: pit.voss@uniklinik-freiburg.de
[1]Department of Oral and Maxillofacial Surgery, Regional Plastic Surgery, Medical Center - University of Freiburg , Hugstetter Str. 55, 79106 Freiburg im Breisgau, Germany
Full list of author information is available at the end of the article

The incidence of BP-ONJ is dependent on bisphosphonate type, route of administration and cumulative dose, underlying disease, gender, co-medication and oral health. It is lowest for oral treatment of primary osteoporosis (0.05-0.2 %) and highest for intravenous treatment of malignant diseases with bone metastases, intravenous administration of ZOL and additional treatment with inhibitors of angiogenesis or tyrosine-kinase (up to 20.5 %) [7].

Treatment suggestions of BP-ONJ differ. In the 2014 update on Medication related osteonecrosis of the jaws the American Association of Oral and Maxillofacial Surgeons (AAOMS) recommends surgical debridement or resection only in stage 2 and 3. Their approach has the major treatment goals to enable continued oncological therapy and preserve quality of life [8]. However, the favored treatment with antibacterial mouth rinse and antibiotic therapy only leads to freedom of symptoms in 53 % of the patients [9]. After promising results of a surgical approach, that can lead to a closed oral mucosa and absence of inflammation signs in 80-100 % of the cases, other national associations favor a complete necrosectomy with primary wound closure when the patients general condition allows it [10].

Roughly two thirds of the lesions occur in the mandible, only one third arises in the maxilla. While a plethora of articles present different perspectives of BP-ONJ, only few studies explicitly highlight the manifestation in the maxilla and only a case series of three patients exists for a defined treatment regime [11–15].

The aim of this study was to review our cases with maxillary BP-ONJ and concomitant sinusitis and to introduce a technique for their management.

Method

This retrospective study includes all the patients with the diagnosis of bisphosphonates-related osteonecrosis of the maxilla and maxillary sinusitis that were operated in our department between 2007 and 2011. Patients without maxillary sinusitis, without a diagnosis consistent with BP-ONJ or with history of radiation therapy to the jaws were excluded. Data was collected using the hospital information system.

All patients underwent surgery in general anesthesia after two days of preoperative intravenous antibiotic therapy with penicillin and metronidazole. Microbiological samples are taken at the time of initial contact with the patient and at the time of surgery when purulent drainage was visible. After elevating a mucoperiosteal flap using a crestal incision including areas of exposed bone, all the affected bone was removed with Luehr forceps and round burrs. Teeth in contact with the affected bone were removed, sharp bony edges rounded. After removal of the necrotic bone and thus

opening of the maxillary sinus, polypoid mucosa was removed and the sinus was rinsed with iodine solution and xylometazoline. The sinus was endoscopically inspected. If the natural osteum was obstructed, it was widened with Weil's forceps. The wound was closed using a multilayer technique previously described for the mandible and adapted for the maxilla [16]. In this technique, after slitting of the vestibular periosteum, its mobile part is quilted under the palatinal mucosa with absorbable backstitches. A second layer of absorbable backstitches is used to align the wound edges to one level and tighten the closure. A running suture brings the mucosal edges together and closes the wound (Figs. 1 and 2).

Postoperatively, patients were fed via a nasogastric feeding tube for five days. Intravenous antibiotic treatment was continued until discharging the patient after 6 days. Until removal of sutures 18–21 days postoperatively, patients were asked to only eat soft food, avoid blowing their noses and use xylometazoline nasal spray and inhalation with natural brine and chlorhexidine mouthwash frequently.

Postoperative controls were carried out for removal of sutures and then every six months. When recall in our unit was not feasible (e.g. distant place of residence) controls were carried out by the local dentist.

Results

Twelve Patients met the inclusion criteria (10 female, 2 male) with a mean age of 67 years (range 55–82). Mean follow up time was 25 months (range 19 – 58). Mean duration of BP-treatment was 71 months (range 24–144 months), five patients received Zoledronate (mean 50 months, range 36–70), three patients were treated with Pamidronate (mean 117 months, 66–144 months), two with Ibandronate (mean 72 months, 48 and 96) and one with Alendronate (24 months) and Clodronate (84 months) each. Except for Alendronate and Clodronate, the route of administration was intravenously. The underlying diseases were breast cancer and multiple myeloma in five patients, and lung cancer and osteoporosis in one case respectively. BP-ONJ arose after tooth extraction in 6 patients. In 3 patients periodontitis was noted as initiating factor, which could not be clearly defined in the remaining three patients.

All patients were clinically classified BP-ONJ stage 3 [8]. Nine patients showed open bone lesions in the region of the second premolar or the first molar of one side of the maxilla, in two patients the incisor region was also involved. One Patient had intact mucosa of the toothless maxilla and no open bone intraorally but a sequestrum at the floor of the sinus with a purulent sinusitis (Fig. 3). In total, in six of the twelve patients the maxillary sinus was filled with ichor. Regarding the size of the defect three extensive defects with complete

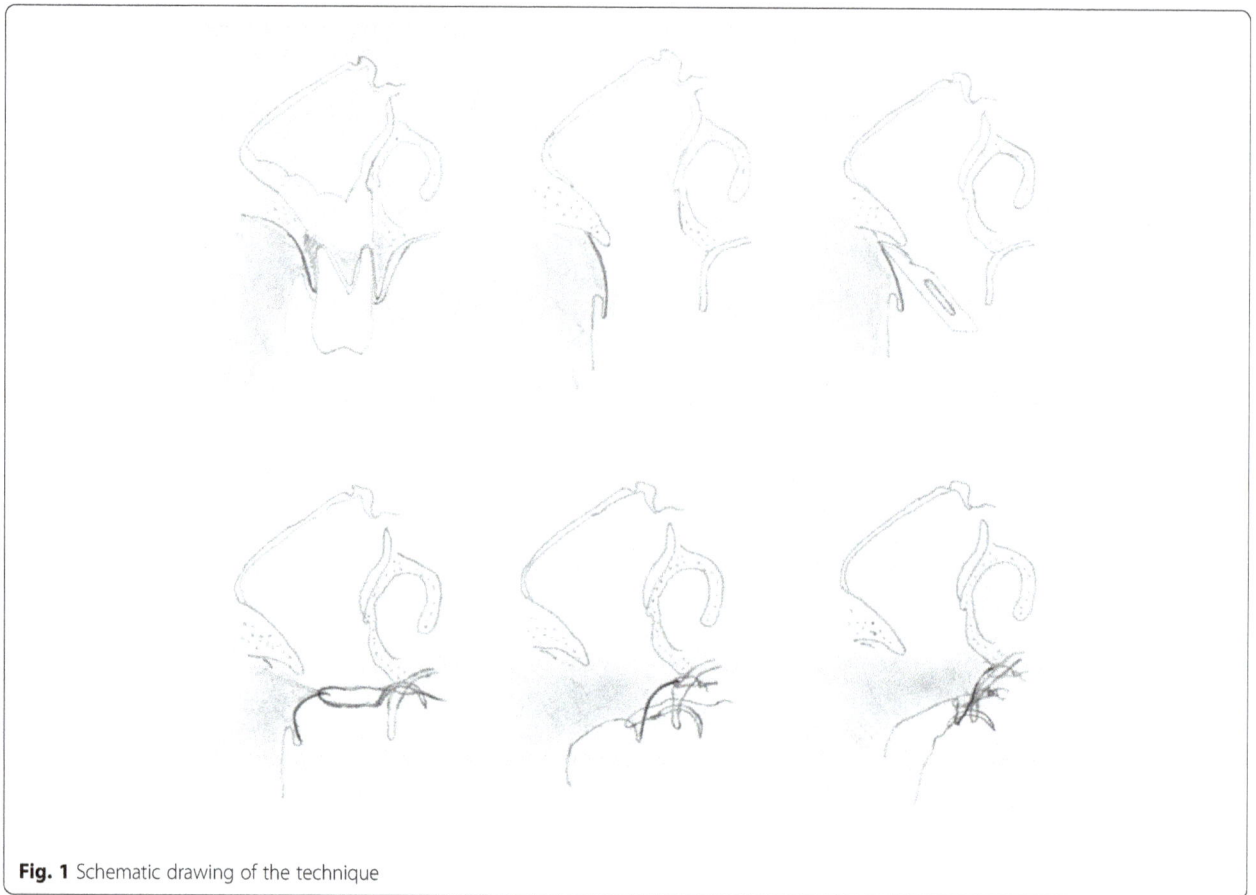

Fig. 1 Schematic drawing of the technique

opening of the basal alveolar crest, seven large defects ranging from 15–30 mm and two small defects ranging von 5 to 15 mm were seen.

Eleven of twelve patients had an uneventful wound healing. One patient had a relapse of open bone 18 months after the surgery. However, the sinus was obstructed with a thick soft tissue scar. It was decided only to remove

bony edges and sequestra not to endanger the delineation of the sinus. Two years later the patient showed up with an abscess of the ipsilateral cheek that was incised. Short time later she succumbed to the metastasizing breast cancer.

In all cases it was noticeable, that the Schneiderian membrane was easy to detach from the underlying bone.

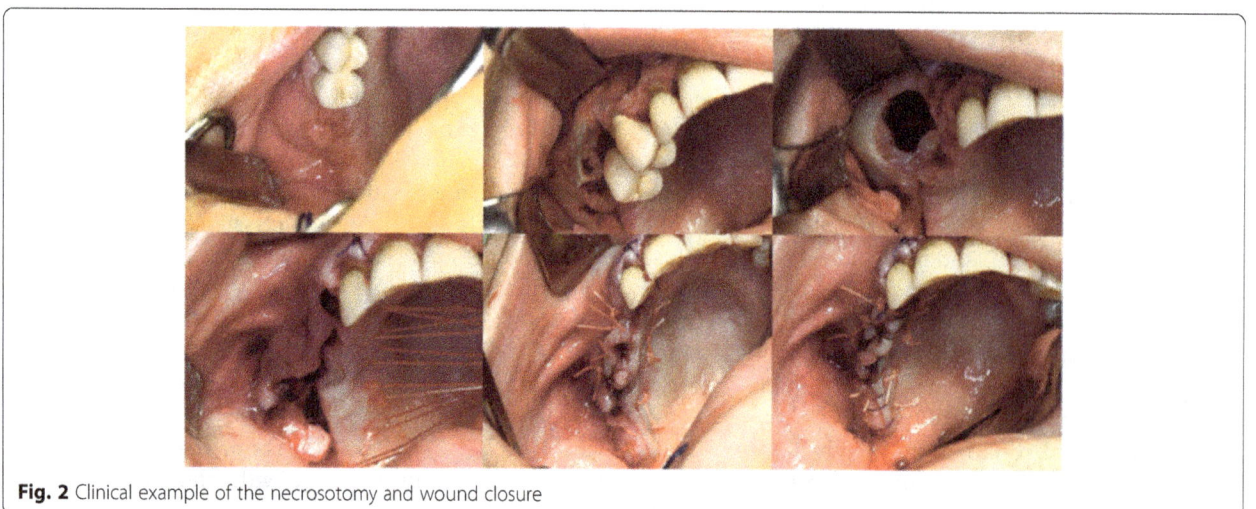

Fig. 2 Clinical example of the necrosotomy and wound closure

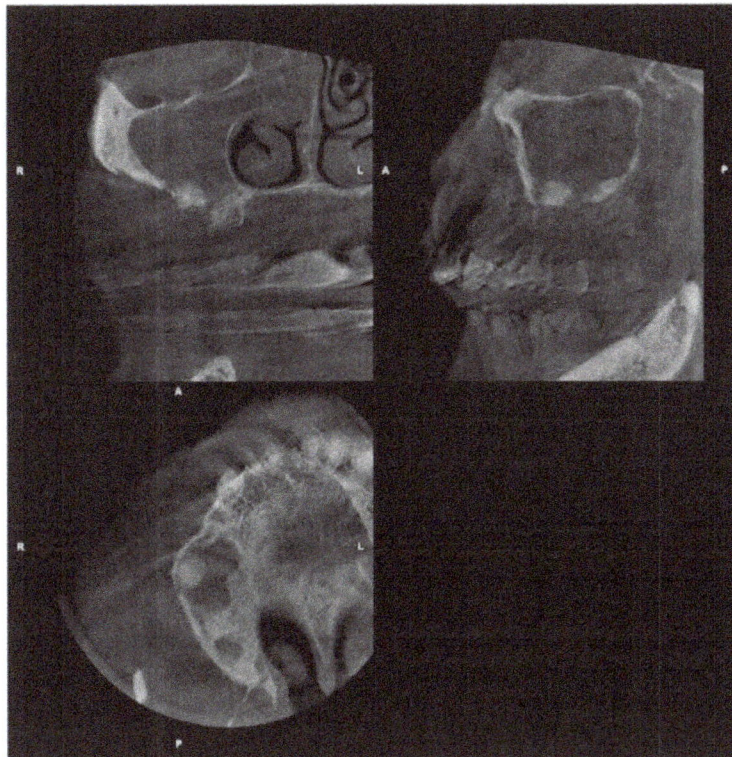

Fig. 3 Cone beam CT showing a sequestrum and sinusitis in a patient without intraoral bone exposure

Endoscopic examination revealed whitish reticular lines of the sinus mucosa consistently (Fig. 4). Histology of the mucosa and the underlying bone was taken in selected cases and resulted in regionally circumscribed necrotic and partially demineralized bone under a broadened mucosa (Fig. 5). The antibiotic testing of the microbiological samples revealed no resistances against the antibiotic regimen used.

Discussion

BP-ONJ is a side effect of antiresorptive treatment with growing importance that arises more frequently in the mandible than in the maxilla. The difference in bone architecture with its reduced blood supply might be an explanation, on the other hand, saliva and food particles accumulate in the mandible and might support local infections. Because of the good vascularization of

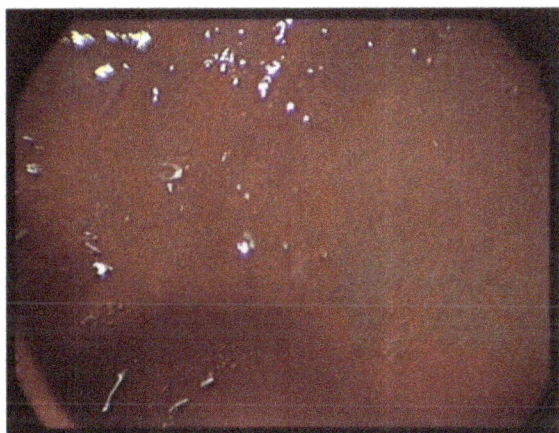

Fig. 4 Remarkable whitish lines in the endoscopic view of an involved maxillary sinus

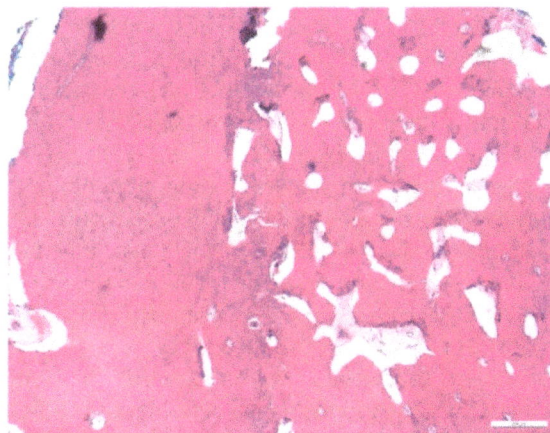

Fig. 5 Histology of an antral wall showing regionally circumscribed necrotic and partially demineralized bone under a broadened mucosa

the maxilla, osteomyelitis is rare in contrast to the mandible, where the thick cortical bone is nutritioned as an endartery system. Due to expansion of the maxillary sinus, the bony volume of the dorsal maxillary alveolar crest is mostly small, just reaching the root apices. Infections of the maxillary bone are likely to affect the maxillary sinus. The maxillary sinus itself is lined with a thin mucosa that early reacts to dental infections [17]. When periodontal infections or dental extractions lead to BP-ONJ of the dorsal maxilla, an involvement of the maxillary sinus is not unlikely: 40–50 % of the patients with a maxillary BP-ONJ show an ipsilateral maxillary sinusitis [12] and oro-antral fistulas occur in one third of the cases with maxillary BP-ONJ, and their management is demanding [15].

Triggering factors for BP-ONJ are tooth extractions and other dental surgical procedures, sharp bony edges and pressure marks. Other regions than the jaws are extremely rarely involved in Bisphosphonate-associated osteonecrosis. Some authors mention cutaneous manifestation such as dental sinus tracts [18], and only few case reports with Bisphosphonate-associated osteonecrosis of the external auditory canal (BPECO) are available [19]. The similarity of thin soft tissue coverage of the bone may explain a pathogenesis by minor self-inflicted trauma by regular aural toilet with cotton buds or fingers in the outer ear. Also secondary osteomyelitis can arise after otitis, mastoiditis or sinusitis and may lead to osteonecrosis.

Remarkably, the sinus mucosa in all patients of the present study was altered. Similarly to the oral mucoperiosteum, which can be very easily detached from the bone in patients treated with BPs, it could be removed from the underlying sinus bone without significant force. This supports the theory that soft tissue adjacent to bone is more affected by BPs than soft tissue that is not in connection with bone [20]. It is discussed that BPs are released from the bone by osteoclasts and low pH-values and then internalized by fibroblasts and epithelial cells [21]. Zoledronate inhibits proliferation and elevates apoptosis of these soft tissue cells, and inhibits expression of type-1-collagen [22]. As the periosteal membrane is connected to the bony surface by collagenous fibers, and type-1-collagen expression needs to be increased in maxillary mucosa healing, inhibition of fibroblasts and epithelial cells might explain the easier detachment of the periost and Schneiderian membrane [23]. Because vascular remodeling and neovascular formation is delayed, soft tissue regeneration may also be impaired in patients with BP-ONJ [24].

Treatment suggestions of manifest BP-ONJ differ. Whereas the first reports on management of BP-ONJ preferred a conservative approach, recent publications favor a surgical approach. While many authors describe treatment results between 84 and 100 % of mucosal

healing after complete necrosectomy and thorough wound closure [16, 25, 26] healing of the necrosis occurs in only 25 % after strictly conservative measures and 28–58 % after partial resections or debridement without soft tissue closure [27, 28]. The more advanced regimes also reflect the argument that in most patients a continued treatment with BPs is necessary. This leads to higher concentrations in the jawbones resulting in even worse healing of bone and soft tissue wounds when surgery is done at a subsequent date. However, in its 2014 update of the position paper the AAOMS still recommends management with antibacterial mouth rinses and antibiotics in most patients [8]. In the experience of our group the conservative treatment of maxillary sinusitis did not lead to healing but to purulent discharge [13]. Persisting oro-antral communications can be covered with obturators, albeit ill-fitting dentures my lead to new osteonecrosis [11].

The technique proposed is adapted from a report of our group published in 2012 where five of the 21 lesions implicated the maxilla [16]. One of the patients in this current paper with multiple myeloma and Zoledronate treatment was already reported in the previous paper. In contrast to the technique described by Gallego et al. we tried not to use the pedicled buccal fat pad in the first surgical intervention in order to have more options in a possible later operation [14]. While the buccal fat pad provides a mechanic protection and a rich vascularization in the BRONJ site, in the technique used, the periosteum that is quilted under the palatal mucosa serves as a second layer for a reliable wound closure and helps to develop a thick scar that seals off the bone from the oral flora.

Interestingly, one of our patients who had a purulent sinusitis with a 9 × 8 mm measuring sequestrum did not show any exposed bone intra- or extraorally, and tooth extractions in the right maxilla had been carried out more than one year before. In the last years, the non-exposed variant has led to a discussion concerning the staging of BP-ONJ [29]. In most reports however, sites with the absence of a clear mucosal breakdown were declared as non-exposed BP-ONJ even though sinus tracts or periodontitis lesions existed. To our best knowledge a purulent maxillary sinusitis caused by a BP-ONJ sequestrum with completely bland oral mucosa has not been described before. As they may lead to pansinusitis, and orbital or intracranial implication, purulent sinusitis has the potential of life threatening complications and need to be treated early [30]. In our case low dose cone beam CT helped to assess the sequestrum and a complete unilateral opacification of the sinus, and the patient had no remaining symptoms after sequester removal, sinus surgery, and meticulous wound closure.

Conclusions

Maxillary sinusitis and oro-antral communication associated to maxillary osteonecrosis is a severe complication of BP therapy. Cone beam computer tomography and endoscopy are helpful diagnostic and intraoperative tools. In combination with antibiotic treatment, the technique described can be suggested for the management of BP-ONJ and concomitant maxillary sinusitis.

Competing interests

The authors declare no conflict of interest.

Authors' contribution

PV, KI and GV conceived of the study. PV, KI and AS performed the operations and the postoperative follow up. PP and GB drafted the manuscript and participated in the design of the study. RS revised the final version of the manuscript. All authors read and approved the manuscript.

Acknowledgements

Consent from the local Ethics Committee was obtained prior to the study. All patients gave informed consent to publish clinical photographs. The article processing charge was funded by the German Research Foundation (DFG) and the Albert Ludwigs University Freiburg in the funding programme Open Access Publishing. There was no additional funding for this study.

Author details

[1]Department of Oral and Maxillofacial Surgery, Regional Plastic Surgery, Medical Center - University of Freiburg , Hugstetter Str. 55, 79106 Freiburg im Breisgau, Germany. [2]Department of Oral and Maxillofacial Surgery, Hospital San Juan de Dios, Universidad Latina, San José, Costa Rica. [3]Department of Oral and Maxillofacial Surgery, Fukuoka Dental College, Fukuoka, Japan.

References

1. Lin JH. Bisphosphonates: a review of their pharmacokinetic properties. Bone. 1996;18:75–85.
2. Kimmel DB. Mechanism of action, pharmacokinetic and pharmacodynamic profile, and clinical applications of nitrogen-containing bisphosphonates. J Dent Res. 2007;86:1022–33.
3. Dixon RB, Tricker ND, Garetto LP. Bone turnover in elderly canine mandible and tibia. J Dent Res. 1997;76:336.
4. Shibutani T, Murahashi Y, Tsukada E, Iwayama Y, Heersche JN. Experimentally induced periodontitis in beagle dogs causes rapid increases in osteoclastic resorption of alveolar bone. J Periodontol. 1997;68:385–91.
5. Cheong S, Sun S, Kang B, Bezouglaia O, Elashoff D, McKenna CE, et al. Bisphosphonate uptake in areas of tooth extraction or periapical disease. J Oral Maxillofac Surg. 2014;72(12):2461–8.
6. Lipton A, Fizazi K, Stopeck AT, Henry DH, Brown JE, Yardley DA, et al. Superiority of denosumab to zoledronic acid for prevention of skeletal-related events: a combined analysis of 3 pivotal, randomised, phase 3 trials. Eur J Cancer. 2012;48:3082–92.
7. Walter C, Al-Nawas B, Frickhofen N, Gamm H, Beck J, Reinsch L, et al. Prevalence of bisphosphonate associated osteonecrosis of the jaws in multiple myeloma patients. Head Face Med. 2010;6:11.
8. Ruggiero SL, Dodson TB, American Association of Oral and Maxillofacial Surgeons. Position paper on medication-related osteonecrosis of the jaws-2014 update. J Oral Maxillofac Surg. 2014;72(10):1938–56.
9. Van den Wyngaert T, Claeys T, Huizing MT, Vermorken JB, Fossion E. Initial experience with conservative treatment in cancer patients with osteonecrosis of the jaw (ONJ) and predictors of outcome. Ann Oncol. 2009;20:331–6.
10. Grötz KA, Piesold J-U, Kopp I, Follmann M, Berlin DKG, Marron M, et al. Bisphosphonat-assoziierte Kiefernekrose (BP-ONJ) und andere Medikamenten-assoziierte Kiefernekrosen. AWMF online. 2012;4:2012.
11. Infante-Cossio P, Lopez-Martin JC, Gonzalez-Cardero E, Martinez-de-Fuentes R, Casas-Fernandez-Tejerina A. Osteonecrosis of the maxilla associated with cancer chemotherapy in patients wearing dentures. J Oral Maxillofac Surg. 2012;70:1587–92.
12. Maurer P, Sandulescu T, Kriwalsky MS, Rashad A, Hollstein S, Stricker I, et al. Bisphosphonate-related osteonecrosis of the maxilla and sinusitis maxillaris. Int J Oral Maxillofac Surg. 2011;40:285–91.
13. Koulocheris P, Weyer N, Liebehenschel N, Otten JE, Gutwald R, Schmelzeisen R. Suppurative maxillary sinusitis in patients with bisphosphonate-associated osteonecrosis of the maxilla: report of 2 cases. J Oral Maxillofac Surg. 2008;66:539–42.
14. Gallego L, Junquera L, Pelaz A, Hernando J, Megias J. The use of pedicled buccal fat pad combined with sequestrectomy in bisphosphonate-related osteonecrosis of the maxilla. Med Oral Patol Oral Cir Bucal. 2012;17:e236–41.
15. Mast G, Otto S, Mucke T, Schreyer C, Bissinger O, Kolk A, et al. Incidence of maxillary sinusitis and oro-antral fistulae in bisphosphonate-related osteonecrosis of the jaw. J Craniomaxillofac Surg. 2012;40:568–71.
16. Voss PJ, Joshi Oshero J, Kovalova-Muller A, Veigel Merino EA, Sauerbier S, Al-Jamali J, et al. Surgical treatment of bisphosphonate-associated osteonecrosis of the jaw: technical report and follow up of 21 patients. J Craniomaxillofac Surg. 2012;40:719–25.
17. Connor SE, Chavda SV, Pahor AL. Computed tomography evidence of dental restoration as aetiological factor for maxillary sinusitis. J Laryngol Otol. 2000;114:510–3.
18. Fedele S, Porter SR, D'Aiuto F, Aljohani S, Vescovi P, Manfredi M, et al. Nonexposed variant of bisphosphonate-associated osteonecrosis of the jaw: a case series. Am J Med. 2010;123:1060–4.
19. Kharazmi M, Hallberg P, Persson U, Warfvinge G. Bisphosphonate-associated osteonecrosis of the auditory canal. Br J Oral Maxillofac Surg. 2013;51:e285–7.
20. Coxon FP, Thompson K, Roelofs AJ, Ebetino FH, Rogers MJ. Visualizing mineral binding and uptake of bisphosphonate by osteoclasts and non-resorbing cells. Bone. 2008;42:848–60.
21. Reid IR. Osteonecrosis of the jaw: who gets it, and why? Bone. 2009;44:4–10.
22. Ravosa MJ, Ning J, Liu Y, Stack MS. Bisphosphonate effects on the behaviour of oral epithelial cells and oral fibroblasts. Arch Oral Biol. 2011;56:491–8.
23. Sun X, Wang D, Yu H, Hu L. Serial cytokine levels during wound healing in rabbit maxillary sinus mucosa. Acta Otolaryngol. 2010;130:607–13.
24. Wehrhan F, Stockmann P, Nkenke E, Schlegel KA, Guentsch A, Wehrhan T, et al. Differential impairment of vascularization and angiogenesis in bisphosphonate-associated osteonecrosis of the jaw-related mucoperiosteal tissue. Oral Surg Oral Med Oral Pathol Oral Radiol Endod. 2011;112:216–21.
25. Markose G, Mackenzie FR, Currie WJ, Hislop WS. Bisphosphonate osteonecrosis: a protocol for surgical management. Br J Oral Maxillofac Surg. 2009;47:294–7.
26. Lemound J, Eckardt A, Kokemuller H, von See C, Voss PJ, Tavassol F, et al. Bisphosphonate-associated osteonecrosis of the mandible: reliable soft tissue reconstruction using a local myofascial flap. Clin Oral Investig. 2012; 16:1143–52.
27. Hoff AO, Toth BB, Altundag K, Johnson MM, Warneke CL, Hu M, et al. Frequency and risk factors associated with osteonecrosis of the jaw in cancer patients treated with intravenous bisphosphonates. J Bone Miner Res. 2008;23:826–36.
28. Boonyapakorn T, Schirmer I, Reichart PA, Sturm I, Massenkeil G. Bisphosphonate-induced osteonecrosis of the jaws: prospective study of 80 patients with multiple myeloma and other malignancies. Oral Oncol. 2008;44:857–69.
29. Patel S, Choyee S, Uyanne J, Nguyen AL, Lee P, Sedghizadeh PP, et al. Non-exposed bisphosphonate-related osteonecrosis of the jaw: a critical assessment of current definition, staging, and treatment guidelines. Oral Dis. 2012;18:625–32.
30. Sakkas N, Schoen R, Schmelzeisen R. Orbital abscess after extraction of a maxillary wisdom tooth. Br J Oral Maxillofac Surg. 2007;45:245–6.

18

Effect of aging and curing mode on the compressive and indirect tensile strength of resin composite cements

Nadja Rohr[*] ⓘ and Jens Fischer

Abstract

Background: Resin composite cements are used in dentistry to bond ceramic restorations to the tooth structure. In the oral cavity these cements are subjected to aging induced by masticatory and thermal stresses. Thermal cycling between 5 and 55 °C simulates the effect of varying temperatures in vitro. Purpose of this study was to compare indirect tensile to compressive strength of different cements before and after thermal cycling. The effect of the curing mode was additionally assessed.

Methods: Indirect tensile strength and compressive strength of 7 dual-curing resin composite cements (Multilink Automix, Multilink SpeedCem, RelyX Ultimate, RelyX Unicem 2 Automix, Panavia V5, Panavia SA Plus, Harvard Implant semi-permanent) was measured. The specimens were either autopolymerized or light-cured ($n = 10$). The mechanical properties were assessed after 24 h water storage at 37 °C and after aging (20,000 thermo cycles) with previous 24 h water storage at 37 °C.

Results: Indirect tensile strength ranged from 5.2 ± 0.8 to 55.3 ± 4.2 MPa, compressive strength from 35.8 ± 1.8 MPa to 343.8 ± 19.6 MPa.

Conclusions: Thermocyclic aging of 20,000 cycles can be considered a suitable method to simulate the degradation of indirect tensile strength but not compressive strength of resin composite cements. The effect of thermocycling and the curing mode on the resin composite cements is material dependent and cannot be generalized.

Keywords: Resin composite cement, Indirect tensile strength, Compressive strength, Thermocycling, Self-adhesive cement

Background

The use of esthetic ceramic materials in dentistry requires the application of resin composite cement to bond a restoration to the tooth structure. Resin composite materials are generally superior to conventional cements in providing higher strength, lower cement wear and improved esthetics [1–4]. Resin composite cements consist of three components: a polymer matrix, fillers and silanes that connect organic and inorganic phase [5–8]. These single components and their respective microstructure define the properties of the resin composite cement such as elasticity, hardness, strength and thermal as well as chemical stability [6, 9, 10]. To bond to the tooth substance, adhesive resin composite cements require the application of an acidic agent plus a priming system. Self-adhesive resin composite cements were thus designed to adhere to the tooth structure by themselves, while eliminating the need for additional pre-treatments of tooth structures. The polymer matrix of these self-adhesive resin cements is generally composed of phosphoric and/or carboxylic acid methacrylate monomers [3]. Self-adhesive cements interact only superficially with mineralized tissues hence they do not form a dentin hybrid layer nor resin tags [11, 12], resulting in lower bond strengths to both, dentin and enamel when compared to adhesive resin composite cements where an additional tooth conditioning system is applied [13]. Superior vickers hardness, modulus of elasticity, compressive and flexural strength were measured

---
* Correspondence: nadja.rohr@unibas.ch
Division of Materials Science and Engineering, Clinic for Reconstructive Dentistry and Temporomandibular Disorders, University Center for Dental Medicine, Hebelstrasse 3, CH-4056 Basel, Switzerland

for adhesive cements in comparison to self-adhesive cements [3, 14].

The polymerization of dual-curing resin composite cements is catalyzed by a chemically (autopolymerization) and a photo (light-curing) activated initiator. The polymerization reaction starts with the mixing of base and catalyst paste, thus activating the chemical initiator. Hence the processing time is limited. Photo initiation allows to advance the polymerization reaction at the time a restoration is correctly placed and cement excess is removed. However, areas under an opaque restoration that are not reached by the light may not polymerize as much as dual-cured areas. Most cement materials reveal a higher degree of conversion by dual-curing compared to autopolymerization [15–17]. The degree of conversion of autopolymerized cements is influenced by the concentration of monomer and catalyst as well as the ambient temperature [18–20]. Cements with a high degree of conversion also provide better mechanical properties [5, 16, 21].

Resin composite cements are brittle materials and therefore more susceptible to tensile loading than to compressive stress [22, 23]. Although, compressive strength of a cement is an important factor to predict a restoration's resistance against masticatory forces [24–26]. Cements in an aqueous medium such as saliva are exposed to a long-term aging process, which might significantly compromise their mechanical properties [27, 28]. The effects are wide-ranging but generally include the leaching of unreacted compounds and the degradation of the polymer network [27, 29]. To artificially age dental materials, several methods such as cyclic loading, water storage, or thermal cycling are commonly used. Thermal cycling between 5 and 55 °C simulates the effect of varying temperatures present in the oral cavity due to hot or cold beverages [30, 31]. The suggested duration of thermal cycling ranges from 3000 to 100,000 cycles [32–37]. It is proposed that 10,000 cycles may represent 1 year of service [38]. After the placement of a restoration, the cement is setting at 37 °C and polymerizes for up to 24 h, hence during this time, thermal stress is rare. Therefore, to imitate the clinical situation, prior to artificial aging the specimens should be stored at 37 °C for 24 h [22].

The impact of thermal cycling on indirect tensile strength and compressive strength has been systematically assessed for only one cement and should be verified with additional cements [22]. Purpose of this study was therefore to compare indirect tensile to compressive strength of a temporary, three self-adhesive and three adhesive cements before and after thermal cycling. The effect of the curing mode was additionally assessed. Hypotheses were that adhesive cements achieve higher indirect tensile and compressive strength than self-adhesive cements and that thermocyclic aging significantly decreases indirect tensile and compressive strength of the cements.

Methods

Indirect tensile strength (ITS) and compressive strength (CS) of 7 dual-curing resin composite cements were measured (Table 1). The specimens were either autopolymerized or light-cured. ITS and CS were measured after 24 h water storage at 37 °C and after 24 h water storage at 37 °C followed by thermocyclic loading. Cylindrical test specimens 3 mm in height and diameter ($n = 10$) were produced using a customized Teflon mold. The cement was filled into the respective cavities of the mold and kept in place with a plastic foil and a glass plate on each side. 10 specimens were produced for each group and either autopolymerized or light cured for 20 s from both sides (Elipar S10, 3 M ESPE, Seefeld, Germany). All specimens were then stored in 37 °C water for 24 h. Aging was performed for the respective specimens using a thermocycler (Thermocycler THE-1100, SD Mechatronik, Feldkirchen-Westerham, Germany). The specimens were immersed alternately in water baths of 5 and 55 °C, using a sieve for storage and transportation. The cycle duration was 1 min with a dwell time in each water bath of 20 s and a transfer time between baths of 10 s. 20,000 cycles within 14 days were performed to age the specimens.

Specimens were loaded until fracture either after 24 h of water storage or after thermal cycling using a universal testing machine (Z020, Zwick/Roell, Ulm, Germany) (Fig. 1). Cross-head speed was set to 1 mm/min. Prior to the measurements, the specimens were sized in diameter and height using a digital caliper (Cal IP 67, Tesa, Ingersheim, Germany). For compressive strength the load was applied axially, for indirect tensile strength radially. Strength values were calculated using the following equations:

$$Compressive strength : \sigma_c = F/\pi(d/2)^2$$

$$Indirect\ tensile\ strength\ \sigma_t = 2F/\pi dh$$

F is the fracture load; d the specimen diameter and h the specimen height. All data was tested for normal distribution using Shapiro-Wilk test. Since data was normal distributed, one-way ANOVA was applied followed by a Tukey HSD test to check for differences between the cement groups of ITS and ($p < 0.05$). Three-way ANOVA was performed with all ITS and CS values to test the effect of cement, curing mode and aging procedure (statplus pro V6.1.25, Analystsoft).

Results

Values for ITS and CS are listed in Table 2. Values of ITS or CS with no statistical difference within one cement are marked with identical superscript letters. To visualize the effect of aging and curing mode on the different cements, the mean values are correlated in Figs. 2 for ITS and Fig. 3 for CS. A grey line in each graphic indicates

Table 1 Cement material composition provided by the manufacturer

	Name	Manufacturer	Type	Monomers	Fillers	Initiators
MLA	Multilink Automix	Ivoclar Vivadent	Adhesive resin composite	Base paste: Bis-GMA, HEMA, 2-dimethylaminoethyl methacrylate Catalyst paste: ethyoxylated bisphenol A dimethacrylate, UDMA, HEMA	40 vol% - Barium glass - Ytterbium trifluoride - Spheroid mixed oxide Particle size: 0.25–3.0 µm	Dibenzoyl peroxide
MSC	Multilink Speed CEM	Ivoclar Vivadent	Self-adhesive resin composite	Base paste: UDMA, TEGDMA, polyethylene glycol dimethacrylate Catalyst paste: polyethylene glycol dimethacrylate, TEGDMA, Methacrylated phosphoric acid ester, UDMA	40 vol% - Barium glass - Ytterbium trifluoride Particle size: 0.1–7 µm	Dibenzoyl peroxide
RUL	RelyX Ultimate	3 M ESPE	Adhesive resin composite	Base paste: methacrylate monomers containing phosphoric acid groups, methacrylate monomers Catalyst paste: methacrylate monomers	43 vol% - Silanated fillers - Alkaline (basic) fillers Particle size: 13 µm	Sodium toluene-4-sulphinate, Disodium peroxodisulphate, Tert-butyl 3,5,5-trimethylperoxyhexanoate
RUN	RelyX Unicem 2 Automix	3 M ESPE	Self-adhesive resin composite	Base paste: phosphoric acid modified methacrylate monomers, bi-functional methacrylate Catalyst paste: methacrylate monomers	43 vol% - Alkaline (basic) fillers - Silanated fillers Particle size: 12.5 µm	Sodium toluene-4-sulphinate, Sodium Persulfate, Tert-butyl 3,5,5-trimethylperoxyhexanoate
PV5	Panavia V5	Kuraray	Adhesive resin composite	Paste A: Bis-GMA, TEGDMA, Hydrophobic aromatic dimethacrylate, Hydrophilic aliphatic dimethacrylate Paste B: Bis-GMA, Hydrophobic aromatic dimethacrylate, Hydrophilic aliphatic dimethacrylate	38 vol% - Silanated barium glass filler - Silanated fluoroalminosilicate glass filler - Colloidal silica - Silanated alminium oxide filler Particle size: 0.01–12 µm	dl-Camphorquinone
PSA	Panavia SA plus	Kuraray	Self-adhesive resin composite	Paste A: 10-MDP, Bis-GMA, TEGDMA, Hydrophobic aromatic dimethacrylate, HEMA Paste B: Hydrophobic aromatic dimethacrylate, hydrophobic aliphatic dimethacrylate	40 vol% - Silanated barium glass filler - Silanated colloidal silica Particle size: 0.02–20 µm	dl-Camphorquinone
HIS	Harvard Implant semi-permanent	Harvard Dental International	temporary resin cement	Methacrylates, zinc oxide	–	–

10-MDP 10-Methacryloyloxydecyl dihydrogen phosphate, *Bis-GMA* bisphenol A-glycidyl methacrylate, *HEMA* 2-hydroxyethyl methacrylate, *TEGDMA* triethyleneglycol dimethacrylate, *UDMA* urethane dimethacrylate

similar values on x-and y-axis meaning that if the dot of a material is close to the grey line, there is no effect of either a) curing-mode after 24 h, b) curing-mode after thermal cycling c) aging of light-cured specimens or d) aging of autopolymerized specimens.

Indirect tensile strength

ITS after 24 h water storage ranged within all groups between 5.2 ± 0.8 MPa for the autopolymerized temporary cement (HIS) and 55.3 ± 4.2 MPa for a light-cured adhesive resin composite cement (MLA). Effects of aging and light-

curing mode on ITS are visualized in Fig. 2. Statistical higher (MLA, RUL, PSA and HIS) or values with no statistical difference (MSC, RUN, PV5) were obtained for light-cured specimens compared to autopolymerized specimens after 24 h water storage (Fig. 2a). When light-cured specimens were compared to autopolymerized specimens after thermo-cycling, values of RUN were significantly lower ($p = 0.038$) and of PV5 significantly higher ($p < 0.001$) (Fig. 2b). For autopolymerized specimens, aging in the thermocycler significantly decreased values of MLA, MSC and PV5 (Fig. 2c). No statistical different values were found

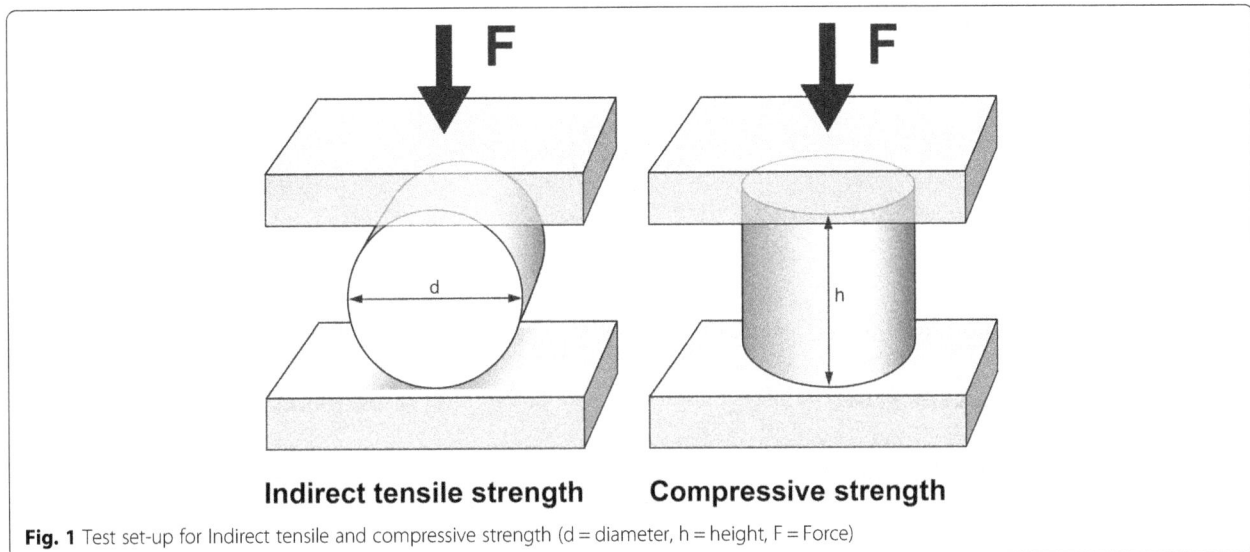

Fig. 1 Test set-up for Indirect tensile and compressive strength (d = diameter, h = height, F = Force)

for the other cements before and after aging of autopolymerized specimens. Aging of light-cured specimens significantly decreased ITS of MLA, MSC, RUL, RUN and PSA (Fig. 2d). Values for PV5, and HIS remained constant. Of all cements, highest values in all groups were obtained by either MLA or PV5. The ranking between MSC, RUL, RUN and PSA changed, depending on the curing or aging mode applied. HIS achieved statistically lowest values of all cements in all groups ($p < 0.001$). Three-way ANOVA revealed a significant effect on the ITS values of the cement, curing mode as well as the aging procedure ($p < 0.001$).

Compressive strength

CS ranged between 35.8 ± 1.8 MPa for autopolymerized and aged HIS and 343.8 ± 19.6 MPa for light-cured MLA after 24 h water storage. Effects of aging and light-curing mode on CS are visualized in Fig. 3. For specimens after 24 h water storage, light-curing increased CS values significantly for MLA, MSC, RUL and PSA (Fig. 3a).

After thermo-cycling, CS of light-cured specimens was significantly higher for MLA, PV5 and PSA (Fig. 2b). Autopolymerized specimens of RUN achieved significantly higher CS after aging than light-cured specimens ($p = 0.006$) (Fig. 3b). For autopolymerized specimens, aging significantly decreased CS for MLA and PV5 and increased CS of RUN and RUL. CS of all other cements (MSC, PSA, HIS) remained constant (Fig. 3c). Aging of light-cured specimens did not affect CS for all cements except MLA and MSC where the CS significantly dropped after aging. A linear correlation ($y = 1.038 \times / R^2 = 0.992$) was found for CS before and after aging for light-cured specimens (Fig. 3d).

For light cured specimens cements ranked as follows before and after aging: MLA > PV5 > PSA > RUL > RUN > MSC > HIS. For autopolymerized specimens before aging ranking was similar to the light-cured except for RUL and RUN switching places. After aging the cements ranked: RUN > RUL > MLA > PV5 > PSA > MSC > HIS. Three-way

Table 2 Indirect tensile strength and compressive strength mean values with standard deviations of the cements for light-cured and autopolymerized specimens after 24 h water storage at 37 °C (24 h) and aging (TC: 24 h water storage at 37 °C followed by 20,000 thermocycles)

(MPa)	Indirect tensile strength				Compressive strength			
	light-curing		autopolymerization		light-curing		autopolymerization	
cement	24 h	TC	24 h	TC	24 h	TC	24 h	TC
MLA	55.3 (4.2)[A]	43.9 (4.4)[B]	51.3 (1.7)[C]	41.1 (1.7)[B]	343.8 (19.6)[A]	326.3 (13.5)[B]	321.0 (9.3)[B]	300.5 (10.6)[C]
MSC	41.0 (2.2)[A]	36.0 (3.0)[B]	39.8 (2.9)[A]	33.9 (3.2)[B]	244.3 (11.0)[A]	220.9 (8.9)[B]	228.6 (12.7)[B]	222.9 (13.5)[B]
RUL	46.0 (4.8)[A]	38.0 (2.7)[B]	33.7 (3.7)[B]	39.2 (7.1)[B]	293.5 (10.5)[A]	286.6 (14.5)[A]	238.8 (28.8)[B]	301.7 (13.3)[A]
RUN	44.4 (4.7)[A]	33.3 (5.1)[B]	39.1 (3.6)[A,B]	40.2 (7.6)[A]	283.2 (17.3)[A,B]	273.1 (28.2)[A]	259.9 (20.8)[A]	305.2 (11.5)[B]
PV5	54.0 (3.2)[A]	52.2 (4.6)[A]	52.5 (5.0)[A]	43.7 (4.2)[B]	325.8 (12.3)[A]	312.3 (6.6)[A,B]	310.5 (15.2)[B]	283.8 (13.2)[C]
PSA	49.5 (2.5)[A]	37.4 (6.8)[B]	38.2 (1.9)[B]	40.9 (4.7)[B]	297.8 (7.1)[A]	300.8 (10.1)[A]	263.9 (13.8)[B]	267.3 (15.8)[B]
HIS	7.5 (1.4)[A]	6.9 (1.0)[A,B]	5.2 (0.8)[C]	6.1 (1.0)[B,C]	37.7 (3.3)[A]	39.8 (1.8)[A]	37.1 (7.0)[A]	35.8 (1.8)[A]

Values of ITS or CS with no statistical difference within one cement are marked with superscript letters (horizontal comparison)

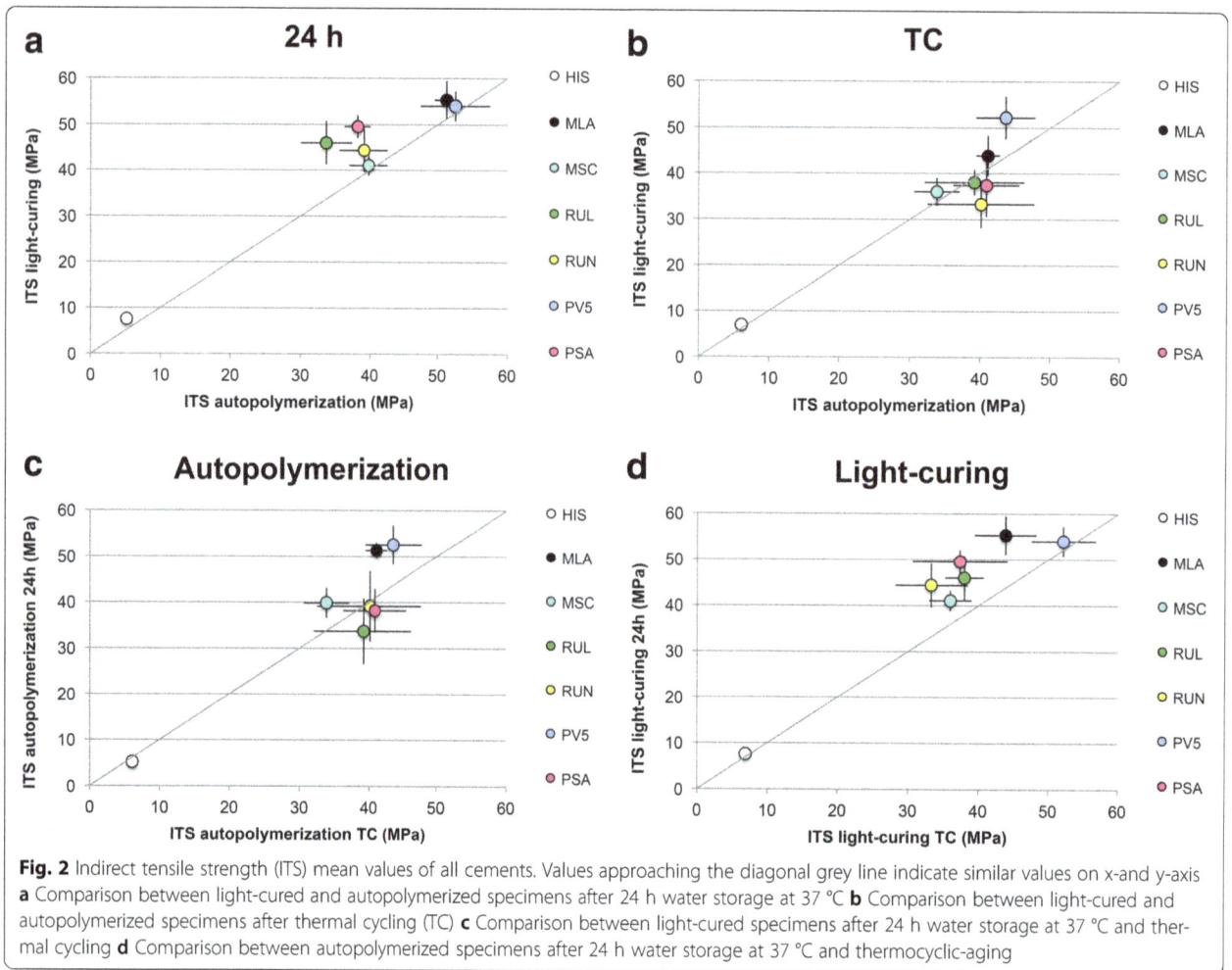

Fig. 2 Indirect tensile strength (ITS) mean values of all cements. Values approaching the diagonal grey line indicate similar values on x-and y-axis **a** Comparison between light-cured and autopolymerized specimens after 24 h water storage at 37 °C **b** Comparison between light-cured and autopolymerized specimens after thermal cycling (TC) **c** Comparison between light-cured specimens after 24 h water storage at 37 °C and thermal cycling **d** Comparison between autopolymerized specimens after 24 h water storage at 37 °C and thermocyclic-aging

ANOVA revealed a significant effect on the CS values of the cement and curing mode ($p < 0.001$), but not of the aging procedure ($p = 0.709$).

Correlation between indirect tensile and compressive strength

A linear correlation ($y = 0.160 \times /R^2 = 0.983$) was found between ITS and CS for light-cured ($y = 0.162 \times /R^2 = 0.992$) and autopolymerized ($y = 0.158 \times /R^2 = 0.960$) specimens after 24 h of water storage (Fig. 4). After thermo-cycling cements were affected differently by the aging process as described above, hence ITS and CS did not correlate likewise.

Discussion

Indirect tensile strength of a temporary, three self-adhesive and three adhesive cements was compared to compressive strength before and after thermal cycling. The effect of the curing mode was additionally assessed. The hypotheses that adhesive cements achieve higher indirect tensile and compressive strength than self-adhesive cements was rejected because the mechanical properties depended

rather on the cement's individual composition and filler types. That thermocyclic aging significantly decreases indirect tensile and compressive strength of the cements was verified for indirect tensile strength but not for compresssive strength.

Indirect tensile strength

After 24 h water storage higher ITS values were recorded for all light-cured cements than for autopolymerized, although the difference was only significant for MLA, RUL, PSA and HIS. This difference was probably due to a higher degree of polymerisation of the light-cured specimens, as it was previously reported [17, 20–22, 36].

After thermo-cycling ITS value of light-cured RUN was significantly lower and of PV5 significantly higher than the values obtained after autopolymerization. Aging affected each cement differently, hence no distinct effect of the curing mechanism could be observed when autopolymerized and light-cured specimens were compared after aging.

Aging of autopolymerized specimens significantly decreased values of MLA, MSC and PV5. ITS of the

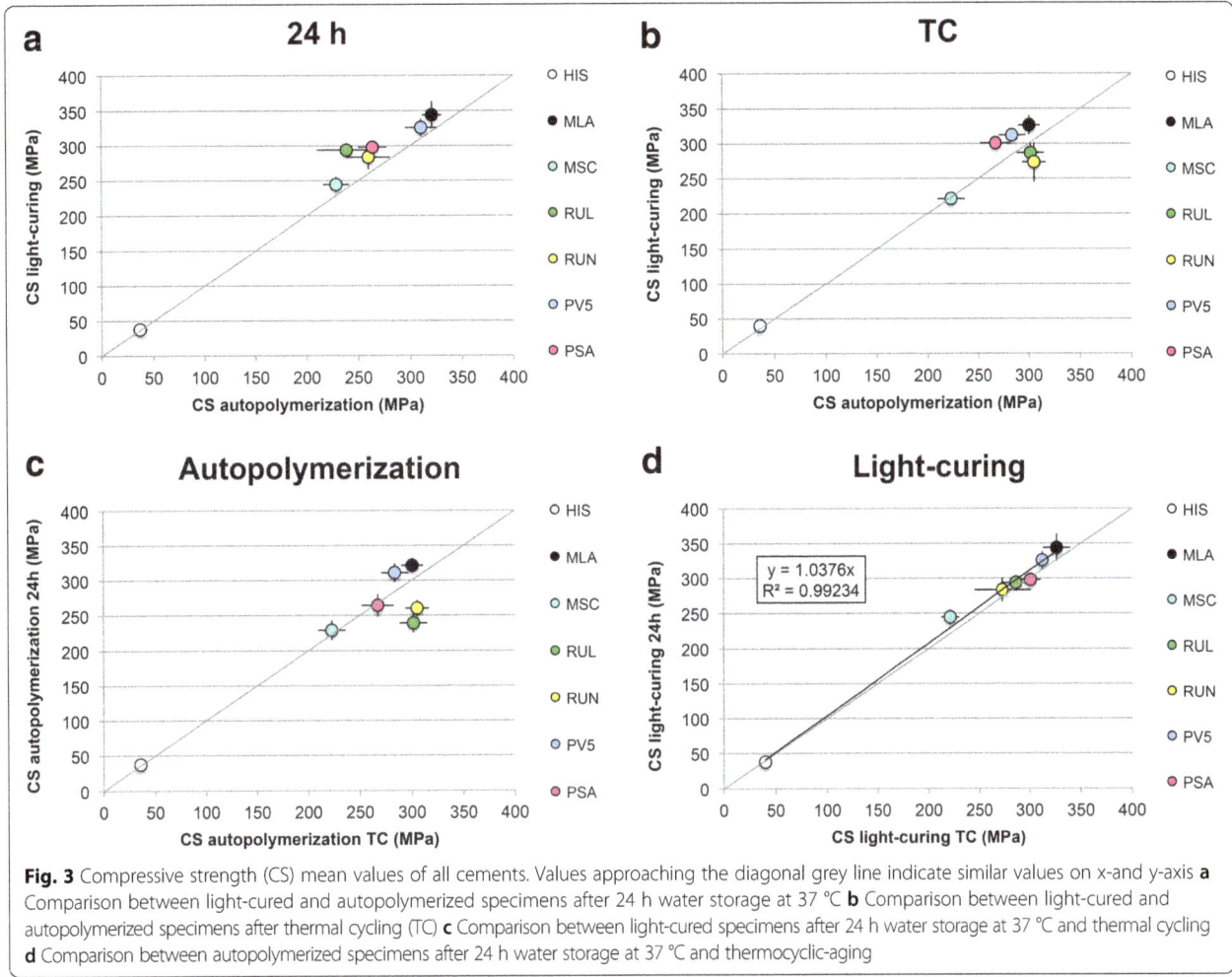

Fig. 3 Compressive strength (CS) mean values of all cements. Values approaching the diagonal grey line indicate similar values on x-and y-axis **a** Comparison between light-cured and autopolymerized specimens after 24 h water storage at 37 °C **b** Comparison between light-cured and autopolymerized specimens after thermal cycling (TC) **c** Comparison between light-cured specimens after 24 h water storage at 37 °C and thermal cycling **d** Comparison between autopolymerized specimens after 24 h water storage at 37 °C and thermocyclic-aging

other cements remained constant. The decrease of ITS of autopolymerized MLA, MSC and PV5 specimens indicates that these materials are more susceptible to temperature changes at the surface which may have induced the formation of superficial micro-cracks favored by the degradation of the polymer matrix and the absorption of water. An insufficient polymerization due to autopolymerization may have also resulted in a higher rate of unreacted and potentially leaching components inducing an increased surface inhomogeneity.

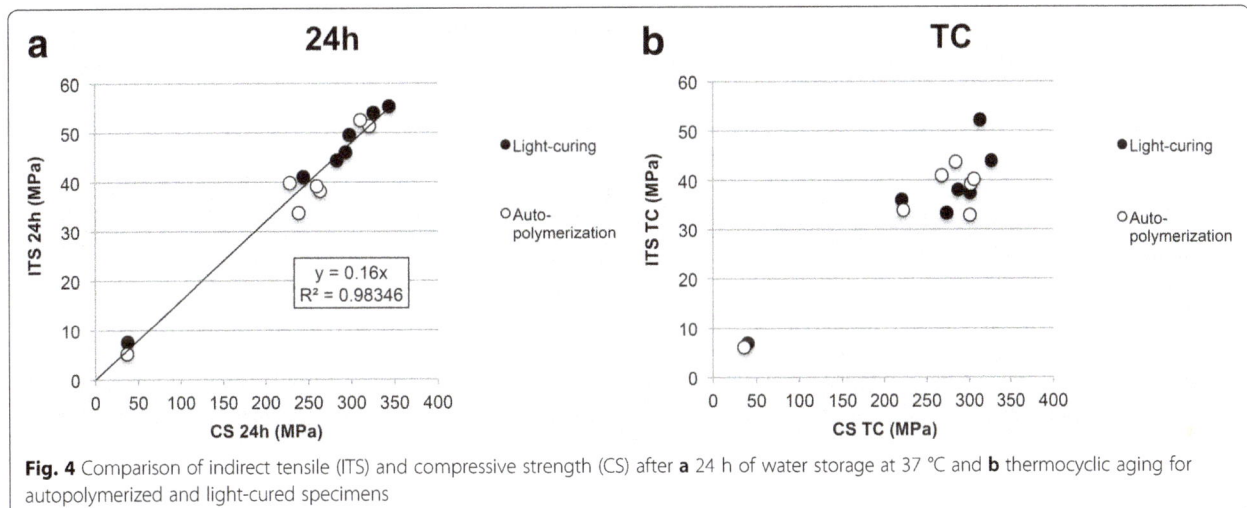

Fig. 4 Comparison of indirect tensile (ITS) and compressive strength (CS) after **a** 24 h of water storage at 37 °C and **b** thermocyclic aging for autopolymerized and light-cured specimens

Aging of light-cured specimens significantly decreased ITS of MLA, MSC, RUL, RUN and PSA. Due to the high ITS of the light-cured specimens after 24 h, these specimens may also be more susceptive to aging than the autopolymerized specimens.

Compressive strength

Higher CS values were obtained for light-cured specimens compared to autopolymerized specimens after 24 h water storage, although the difference was only statistically significant for MLA, MSC, RUL and PSA. These findings are consistent with the ones for ITS and due to the increased degree of conversion of the light-cured specimens. In comparison to the other cements, MLA, RUL and PSA revealed a stronger dependence on light-curing to achieve highest strength values. PSA contains 10-Methacryloyloxydecyl dihydrogen phosphate (MDP) inhibiting the polymerization reaction [39]. Significantly lower values were found for autopolymerized CS values of PSA compared to light-cured specimens after 24 h indicating that the polymerization reaction might have still been proceeding.

After thermo-cycling, CS of light-cured specimens was significantly higher for MLA, PV5 and PSA but lower for RUN compared to autopolymerized specimens. For RUN results were inverse, which might be explained by a higher amount of unreacted phosphoric acid ester groups, resulting in a higher degree of water up-take and thus an increased CS. Higher sorption was previously recorded for RUN for autopolymerized specimens [9]. Aging of autopolymerized specimens significantly decreased CS for MLA and PV5 due to a degradation of the material that might be due to a lower degree of polymerization than for the light-cured specimens. Values of RUN and RUL were increased after aging. RUL and RUN previously presented high sorption that might have been responsible for increasing their strength after thermal cycling [9]. Light-cured specimens correlated linearly before and after aging and were therefore less susceptible to aging than autoplymerized specimens. Since three-way ANOVA revealed no significant effect of the aging with 20,000 thermocycles on the CS values, the applied aging protocol does not seem suitable for this test method. Effects of a prolonged cycling should be further investigated.

Correlation between indirect tensile and compressive strength

The filler content [7], the degree of conversion [23] and the monomer type [8] are factors affecting the mechanical strength of resin composite cements. Autopolymerized specimens revealed a stronger variability in CS and ITS than dual-cured specimens [15, 17, 22]. As previously reported the effect of the curing mode varied among the cements and cannot be generalized [36]. According

to the linear correlation between CS of light-cured specimens before and after aging CS was less affected by aging than ITS indicating that the mechanical properties measured with a CS test are less susceptible to thermocyclic aging and for light-cured specimens the material properties are more stable, which findings are in accordance with previous results [22]. CS and ITS correlate linearly after 24 h water storage but not after aging because the cements age differently depending on their components.

Test method

Previously it was reported that a compressive strength test is a rather insensitive test method compared to indirect tensile strength [22] or flexural strength [28]. In the present study it was found that both ITS and CS tests have their eligibility since aging of the cements resulted in different effects for either ITS or CS. The ITS test is more sensitive to surface defects than the CS test [22]. CS test may depend mainly on the filler size and distribution and the quality of silanization. It is probably also affected by the mode of polymerization. The effect of the degradation mechanism on the ITS and CS should be further investigated.

Thermocyclic aging has been evaluated as the most efficient aging procedure and was recommended to perform for at least 4 days for resin composite cement [22]. Thermal cycling has a considerable effect on the cements' strength and the degree of the effect varied according to the cement's composition. It is suggested that the temperature change and the associated dimensional changes of the two phases – polymer matrix and fillers – generate internal stress [22, 35, 37] due to different coefficients of thermal expansion of organic and inorganic fillers [22].

Thermocyclic aging has been previously applied to ITS and CS specimens of different resin composite cements but only for 2000 cycles within 20 h [36]. In that study no statistically significant differences between the values after aging were found. Therefore, a thermocycling duration of 2000 cycles within 20 h can be considered insufficient to successfully age resin composite cements. In the present study 20,000 cycles were performed within 14 days, providing measurable aging effects on ITS values.

Clinical implications

CS test predicts the resistance against the masticatory force and therefore allows to estimate the cements clinical performance [24]. Materials with low intrinsic strengths such as silicate ceramics achieve a higher loading capacity when cemented with adhesive cement than with glass-ionomer [25]. A cement with a compressive strength above 320 MPa is ideal for cementing silicate ceramics on zirconia implants since the cement optimally supports the

Effect of aging and curing mode on the compressive and indirect tensile strength of resin...

127

restorative material [26]. Since these 320 MPa were measured for autopolymerized cements after 24 h 37 °C water storage, in the present investigation PV5 and MLA can be considered best cements applying to this requirement with mean autopolymerized CS values of 312 and 326 MPa. Although after aging of the autopolymerized specimens, the cements do not exceed the 320 MPa.

According to ISO 9917–1:2007 for water based dental cements, CS of dental cements should be over 70 MPa. All cements except HIS fulfill this requirement. HIS is not indicated for permanent cementation but for a long-term temporary cementation on implants. When covered by bulky restorations cements might be insufficiently light-cured [21], which can also affect the mechanical strength of the cements. For most cements light-curing was beneficial to increase the mechanical strength. Only RUN and RUL revealed better or similar mechanical properties after thermocyclic aging of autopolymerized specimens than of light-cured ones, which may be explained by more intense water uptake.

Conclusions

Within the limitations imposed by the current study, the following conclusions were drawn:

- Indirect tensile and compressive strength of the cements after 24 h water storage correlate linearly.
- Thermocyclic aging of 20,000 cycles can be considered a suitable method to simulate the degradation of indirect tensile strength but not compressive strength of resin composite cements.
- The effect of thermocycling on the resin composite cements is material dependent and cannot be generalized.

Abbreviations
CS: Compressive strength; HIS: Harvard Implant semi-permanent; ITS: Indirect tensile strength; MLA: Multilink Automix; MSC: Multilink SpeedCem; PSA: Panavia SA plus; PV5: Panavia V5; RUL: RelyX Ultimate; RUN: RelyX Unicem 2 Automix; TC: Thermal cycling

Acknowledgements
This study was kindly supported with materials by VITA Zahnfabrik, Bad Säckingen.

Funding
This research did not receive any specific grant from funding agencies in the public, commercial, or not-for-profit sectors.

Authors, contributions
NR designed the concept, collected and interpreted the data and wrote the manuscript. JF helped designing the concept, interpreted the data and proofread the manuscript. Both authors read and approved the final manuscript.

Competing interests
The authors declare that they have no competing interests.

References
1. Ban S, Hasegawa J, Anusavice KJ. Effect of loading conditions on bi-axial flexure strength of dental cements. Dent Mater. 1992;8:100–4.
2. Peutzfeldt A. Dual-cure resin cements: in vitro wear and effect of quantity of remaining double bonds, filler volume, and light curing. Acta Odontol Scand. 1995;53:29–34.
3. Ilie N, Simon A. Effect of curing mode on the micro-mechanical properties of dual-cured self-adhesive resin cements. Clin Oral Investig. 2012;16:505–12.
4. Attar N, Tam LE, McComb D. Mechanical and physical properties of contemporary dental luting agents. J Prosthet Dent. 2003;89:127–34.
5. Diaz-Arnold AM, Vargas MA, Haselton DR. Current status of luting agents for fixed prosthodontics. J Prosthet Dent. 1999;81:135–41.
6. Zandinejad AA, Atai M, Pahlevan A. The effect of ceramic and porous fillers on the mechanical properties of experimental dental composites. Dent Mater. 2006;22:382–7.
7. White SN, Yu Z. Physical properties of fixed prosthodontic, resin composite luting agents. Int J Prosthodont. 1993;6:384–9.
8. Asmussen E, Peutzfeldt A. Influence of UEDMA BisGMA and TEGDMA on selected mechanical properties of experimental resin composites. Dent Mater. 1998;14:51–6.
9. Müller JA, Rohr N, Fischer J. Evaluation of ISO 4049: water sorption and water solubility of resin cements. Eur J Oral Sci. 2017;125:141–50.
10. Peutzfeldt A. Resin composites in dentistry: the monomer systems. Eur J Oral Sci. 1997;105:97–116.
11. De Munck J, Vargas M, Van Landuyt K, Hikita K, Lambrechts P, Van Meerbeek B. Bonding of an auto-adhesive luting material to enamel and dentin. Dent Mater. 2004;20:963–71.
12. Monticelli F, Osorio R, Mazzitelli C, Ferrari M, Toledano M. Limited decalcification/diffusion of self-adhesive cements into dentin. J Dent Res. 2008;87:974–9.
13. Rohr N, Fischer J. An evaluation of tooth surface treatment strategies for adhesive cementation - an elaborated primer supersedes tooth etching. J Adv Prosthodont. 2017;9:85–92.
14. Piwowarczyk A, Lauer HC. Mechanical properties of luting cements after water storage. Oper Dent. 2003;28:535–42.
15. Caughman WF, Chan DC, Rueggeberg FA. Curing potential of dual-polymerizable resin cements in simulated clinical situations. J Prosthet Dent. 2001;85:479–84.
16. Braga RR, Condon JR, Ferracane JL. Vitro wear simulation measurements of composite versus resin-modified glass ionomer luting cements for all-ceramic restorations. J Esthet Restor Dent. 2002;14:368–76.
17. Fonseca RG, Santos JG, Adabo GL. Influence of activation modes on diametral tensile strength of dual-curing resin cements. Braz Oral Res. 2005; 19:267–71.
18. Cantoro A, Goracci C, Papacchini F, Mazzitelli C, Fadda GM, Ferrari M. Effect of pre-cure temperature on the bonding potential of self-etch and self-adhesive resin cements. Dent Mater. 2008;24:577–83.
19. Cantoro A, Goracci C, Carvalho CA, Coniglio I, Ferrari M. Bonding potential of self-adhesive luting agents used at different temperatures to lute composite onlays. J Dent. 2009;37:454–61.
20. Spinell T, Schedle A, Watts DC. Polymerization shrinkage kinetics of dimethacrylate resin-cements. Dent Mater. 2009;25:1058–66.
21. De Souza G, Braga RR, Cesar PF, Lopes GC. Correlation between clinical performance and degree of conversion of resin cements: a literature review. J Appl Oral Sci. 2015;23:358–68.
22. Blumer L, Schmidli F, Weiger R, Fischer JA. Systematic approach to standardize artificial aging of resin composite cements. Dent Mater. 2015;31:855–63.
23. Fonseca RG, Artusi TP, dos Santos JG, Adabo GL. Diametral tensile strength of dual-curing resin cements submitted exclusively to autopolymerization. Quintessence Int. 2007;38:e527–31.
24. White SN, Yu Z. Compressive and diametral tensile strengths of current adhesive luting agents. J Prosthet Dent. 1993;69:568–72.
25. Stawarczyk B, Beuer F, Ender A, Roos M, Edelhoff D, Wimmer T. Influence of cementation and cement type on the fracture load testing methodology of anterior crowns made of different materials. Dent Mater J. 2013;32:888–95.

26. Rohr N, Märtin S, Fischer J. Correlations between fracture load of zirconia implant supported single crowns and mechanical properties of restorative material and cement. Dent Mater J. 2017. In press.

27. Medeiros IS, Gomes MN, Loguercio AD, Filho LE. Diametral tensile strength and Vickers hardness of a composite after storage in different solutions. J Oral Sci. 2007;49:61–6.

28. Cassina G, Fischer J, Rohr N. Correlation between flexural and indirect tensile strength of resin composite cements. Head Face Med. 2016;12:29.

29. Ferracane JL. Hygroscopic and hydrolytic effects in dental polymer networks. Dent Mater. 2006;22:211–22.

30. Barclay CW, Spence D, Laird WR. Intra-oral temperatures during function. J Oral Rehabil. 2005;32:886–94.

31. Ernst CP, Canbek K, Euler T, Willershausen B. In vivo validation of the historical in vitro thermocycling temperature range for dental materials testing. Clin Oral Investig. 2004;8:130–8.

32. Hahnel S, Henrich A, Bürgers R, Handel G, Rosentritt M. Investigation of mechanical properties of modern dental composites after artificial aging for one year. Oper Dent. 2010;35:412–9.

33. Assunção WG, Gomes EA, Barão VA, Barbosa DB, Delben JA, Tabata LF. Effect of storage in artificial saliva and thermal cycling on Knoop hardness of resin denture teeth. J Prosthodont Res. 2010;54:123–7.

34. Weir MD, Moreau JL, Levine ED, Strassler HE, Chow LC, Xu HH. Nanocomposite containing CaF(2) nanoparticles: thermal cycling, wear and long-term water-aging. Dent Mater. 2012;28:642–52.

35. Kawano F, Ohguri T, Ichikawa T, Matsumoto N. Influence of thermal cycles in water on flexural strength of laboratory-processed composite resin. J Oral Rehabil. 2001;28:703–7.

36. Kim AR, Jeon YC, Jeong CM, Yun MJ, Choi JW, Kwon YH, Huh JB. Effect of activation modes on the compressive strength, diametral tensile strength and microhardness of dual-cured self-adhesive resin cements. Dent Mater J. 2016;35:298–308.

37. Versluis A, Douglas WH, Sakaguchi RL. Thermal expansion coefficient of dental composites measured with strain gauges. Dent Mater. 1996;12:290–4.

38. Morresi AL, D'Amario M, Capogreco M, Gatto R, Marzo G, D'Arcangelo C, Monaco A. Thermal cycling for restorative materials: does a standardized protocol exist in laboratory testing? A literature review. J Mech Behav Biomed Mater. 2014;29:295–308.

39. Nakamura T, Wakabayashi K, Kinuta S, Nishida H, Miyamae M, Yatani H. Mechanical properties of new self-adhesive resin-based cement. J Prosthodont Res. 2010;54:59–64.

19

Thorough documentation of the accidental aspiration and ingestion of foreign objects during dental procedure is necessary: review and analysis of 617 cases

Rui Hou[1*], Hongzhi Zhou[1], Kaijin Hu[1], Yuxiang Ding[1], Xia Yang[1], Guangjie Xu[1], Peng Xue[1], Chun Shan[1], Sen Jia[1] and Yuanyuan Ma[2]

Abstract

Objectives: To review the cases of accidental aspiration and ingestion of foreign objects during dental procedure, and to emphasize the importance of thorough documentation of the accidents.

Methods: A comprehensive search on (dental procedure/treatment/practice), (aspiration/inhalation), and (ingestion/ swallow) was performed for all years before 1st October 2014 available. The statistic analysis was made on the variables including journals and reported year, patients' age, gender, general conditions, dental procedure and location for procedure, foreign objects, site of involvement, possible causes, anesthesia during procedure and treatment, symptoms, treatment time and treatment modality, follow-up, and so on.

Results: A total of 617 cases reported by 45 articles from 37 kinds of journals were included and analyzed. Most reports made detailed record. While some important variables were recorded incompletely, including patient's general conditions, location for procedure, clinical experience of the involving dentists, tooth position of procedure, possible causes, and anesthesia during procedure and treatment for the accident.

Conclusions: Aspiration and ingestion of foreign objects are rare and risky complication during dental procedure. Each accident should have thorough documentation so as to provide enough information for the treatment and prevention.

Keywords: Aspiration, Ingestion, Foreign objects, Dental procedure, Documentation

Background

Aspiration and ingestion of foreign objects are potential complications that can occur during dental procedure, such as root canal therapy, implantation, extraction, and even routine examination. The foreign object included endodontic instruments, implant components, burs, posts, teeth, orthodontic brackets, restorations and even dental mirror and irrigation needle [1–5].

The incidences of aspiration and ingestion in dental procedure have been reported by many articles and reviews. As early as 1971, Grossman [6] determined that 87 % of foreign bodies entered the alimentary tract, whereas 13 % aspirated into the respiratory tract. Susini G et al. [7] reported that the incidences of aspiration and ingestion in root canal treatment were 0.001 per 100 000 and 0.12 per 100 000, respectively. From different dental college hospitals in Japan, the ingestion of foreign objects was reported 0.0041 and 0.0044 % [8, 9]. Moreover, the occurrence (cases/dentists) per year was 0.018, which was very close to the figure of 0.021 reported from two French insurance companies representing 24,651 French general dental practitioners over an 11-year period [7].

The literature also showed that although 90 % of ingested foreign objects could pass through the

* Correspondence: denthr@sina.com; hourui@fmmu.edu.cn
[1]State Key Laboratory of Military Stomatology & National Clinical Research Center for Oral Diseases & Shaanxi Clinical Research Center for Oral Diseases, Department of Oral Surgery, School of Stomatology, the Fourth Military Medical University, Xi'an City, Shaanxi Province 710032, China
Full list of author information is available at the end of the article

gastrointestinal tract uneventfully, there are roughly 10 % require endoscopic removal, while still 1 % will ever require operation [6, 8, 10, 11]. Although bronchoscopy has been reported 99 % effective on retrieve the aspirated foreign objects, the complication rate is between 2.4 and 5 % [12].

Many factors are reported related to the aspiration and ingestion. For example, patients' medical and mental condition, use of local anesthesia or intravenous sedation, difficulty of access, compromised direct view, and so on [2–5]. However, these factors are still in controversy. There were also some important variables recorded incompletely from the literature, such as tooth position of procedure, clinical experience of the involving dentists, and anesthesia during procedure. In addition, many articles even did not report the necessary information of the cases. Moreover, there were hardly any review on making comprehensive record and discussion of accidental aspirated and ingested cases.

Therefore, it has necessity to strengthen the thorough documentation so as to arouse the dental personnel's attention, and further to facilitate analysis of the reasons, accumulation of the experience and lessons, and summary of the prevention and treatment measures on accidental aspiration and ingestion.

Methods
Literature search
An extensive literature search was conducted in four electronic databases: PubMed, Cochrane Library, ScienceDirect, and Embase databases. The following filters were used in the search strategy: date (1970/01/01 to 2014/10/01) and species (humans) filters in PubMed, and only date (1970–2014) filter for the remaining three databases. The reference lists of all relevant articles were also screened manually to identify further potentially relevant articles.

The inclusion criteria were as follows: (1) case reports, case series, review articles and retrospective studies; (2) studies reporting the accidental aspiration and ingestion of foreign objects during the dental procedure, dental treatment, and dental practice. (3) studies reporting at least the following information: dental procedure and foreign objects, site of involvement and symptoms, treatment modality and follow-up. (4) studies published in English.

The exclusion criteria were as follows: (1) studies contained limited data including conference abstracts and letters to journal editors, and opinion articles; (2) studies reporting the accidents happening in time other than dental treatment; (3) studies only reporting the prevention and treatment measure of aspiration or ingestion without cases.

Two reviewers independently judged the study eligibility, and any disagreement was resolved by consensus.

The descriptive variables were extracted and collected thoroughly, including journals and reported year, patients' age, gender, general conditions, dental procedure, location for procedure, clinical experience of the involving dentists, tooth position of procedure, possible causes, foreign objects, site of involvement, symptoms, treatment time and treatment modality, anesthesia during procedure and treatment for the accident, and follow-up.

Statistical analysis
SPSS version 13.0 for Windows was used for statistical analysis. The descriptive statistics were made on all the descriptive variables from the selected articles.

Results
A total of 617 cases reported were included and analyzed in this review. Most cases were recorded in detail, while some important variables were incomplete. The statistical analysis results were listed below based on the different descriptive variables.

Variables recorded in detail
Journals and reported year
There were altogether 45 articles published by 37 kinds of journals on aspiration and ingestion during dental procedure. Table 1 showed the analysis on cases number from the articles. Figure 1 showed cases number and their reported year (except four reviews).

More than 80 % of the articles (37/45) were from dental journals. Among them, 19 articles were from comprehensive dentistry [8, 9, 11, 13–28], 6 from oral sugery [10, 29–33], 6 from endodontics [7, 34–37], 3 from prosthodontics [1, 38, 39], 2 from implantation [4, 40] and 2 from orthodontics [41, 42]. The others 8 were from the fields of gastroenterology [43], respiration [44], laryngology [45], pediatrics [46] and comprehensive medicine [4, 47–49].

Age and gender
Figure 2 showed aspiration and ingestion were more seen in patients at 60–79 years old and 10–19 years old, respectively. Of all the 49 cases in case reports, the

Table 1 Analysis on cases number from the articles (case number)

	Year	Aspiration	Ingestion	Total
Review from France [7]	1994–2004	44	464	508
Review from Japan [8]	2008–2009	0	11	11
Review from Japan [9]	2006–2010	0	23	23
Review from USA [13]	1992–2002	1	25	26
Case reports	1971–2014	20	29	49
Total number		65	552	617

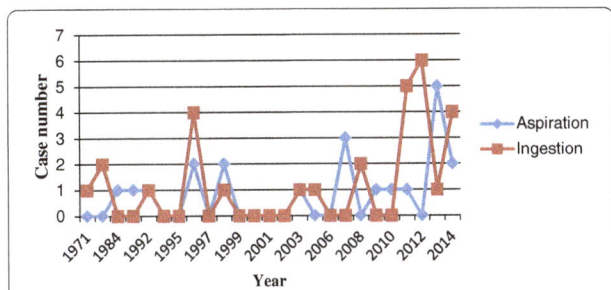

Fig. 1 Analysis on cases number and its happened year. Showed cases number and their reported year (except four reviews)

aspiration and ingestion case number were 18 and 15 in male, 2 and 12 in female. There were even 2 cases did not specify gender [27].

Dental procedure and foreign objects

Aspiration happened more during implantation [10, 19, 30, 33, 40, 46], prosthodontics [13, 14, 20, 28], and restorative dentistry [11, 14, 22, 28, 45]. Ingestion happened more during prosthodontics [9, 13, 29, 39] and RCT [9, 11, 13, 16–19, 24, 27, 34, 35, 37, 43, 49] (Fig. 3). Table 2 listed the top five kinds of foreign objects that were aspirated and ingested in the case reports and reviews.

Site of involvement and symptoms

For the aspirated cases, 7 cases were found foreign objects at right bronchus [10, 11, 14, 22, 30, 31, 33], 6 at left bronchus [15, 19, 36, 44, 45, 48], 5 at right lung [13, 14, 20, 28, 40], 1 at lung without description on left or right [28], and the other one at the piriform fossa [10]. For the ingested cases, 24 cases were found at stomach [4, 9, 11, 16, 18, 21, 27, 29, 32, 35, 37, 42, 47, 49], 10 at intestine [9, 27, 46], 11 at stomach and intestine [8], and esophagus (5 cases) [9, 23, 25].

Of all the 49 cases, 9 aspirated cases had symptom, including 7 cough [10, 15, 19, 22, 31, 36, 40], 1 pain [20], 1 gag [28]. Four ingested cases had symptoms, including 3 pain [11, 43, 46] and 1 cough [34]. All the reviews had no description on the symptoms.

Treatment time, modality and follow-up

Table 3 showed two thirds of the aspirated cases (13/20) got immediate treatment [10, 11, 14, 15, 19, 22, 30, 31, 33, 40, 44, 45, 48], while nearly 40 % of ingested cases (12/29) got observation with foreign objects excreted 2 days to 2 weeks later [18, 21, 24, 27, 29, 34, 35, 37, 39, 41, 49]. Among the 34 ingested cases in reviews from Japan [8, 9], only 3 cases retrieved by endoscopic procedure immediately, the others passed through the gastrointestinal tract in a 10-day period.

Of all the 20 aspirated cases, 15 cases had the foreign objects successfully retrieved by bronchoscopy (7 flexible [10, 14, 28, 40, 44, 45], 5 rigid [22, 30, 31, 33, 48] and 3 without description [15, 19, 36]) and 1 case by laryngoscopy [10]. Three cases failed to retrieve the object after bronchoscopy, including 1 observed with excretion until 6 months later [14], 1 had lung wedge resection 3 days later [14], and 1 got recall every month but without final result reported [36]. The last one case got the lobectomy of right lobe when the dental impressions were found aspirated 1 year later [20].

Of all the 29 ingested cases, 12 got foreign bodies excretion, including 10 with observation before [21, 24, 27, 29, 34, 35, 39, 41, 49] and 2 with immediate endoscopy failed before [18, 37], 15 had the objects retrieved by endoscopy (7 immediate [11, 17, 23, 25, 32, 34, 42], 8 several-day later [1, 4, 11, 16, 29, 43, 47]), and the other 2 had laparatomy [38] and colostomy [46], respectively.

For follow-up, only one case reported happening acute airway obstruction after bronchoscopy [33]. The symptom finally disappeared after suitable treatment. There were no adverse events or description to the other cases.

Variables recorded incompletely
General conditions

There were only 12 cases (12/617) reporting patients with general disease, including 6 cases of cerebrovascular disease [9, 19], 2 cases of tumor excision [33, 38], 1 case of attention deficit hyperactivity disorder [15], 1 case of low intelligence quotient [17], 1 case of dental retardation [21] and 1 case of cleft palate [41].

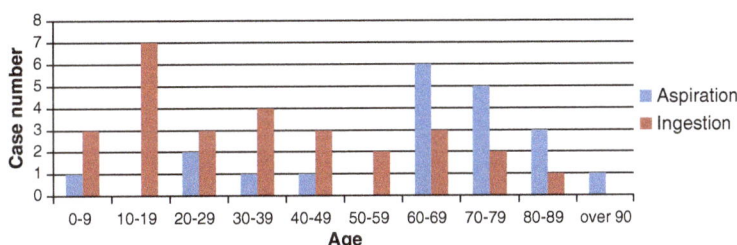

Fig. 2 Analysis on the patient's age of the cases. Showed that aspiration and ingestion were more seen in patients at 60–79 years old and 10–19 years old, respectively

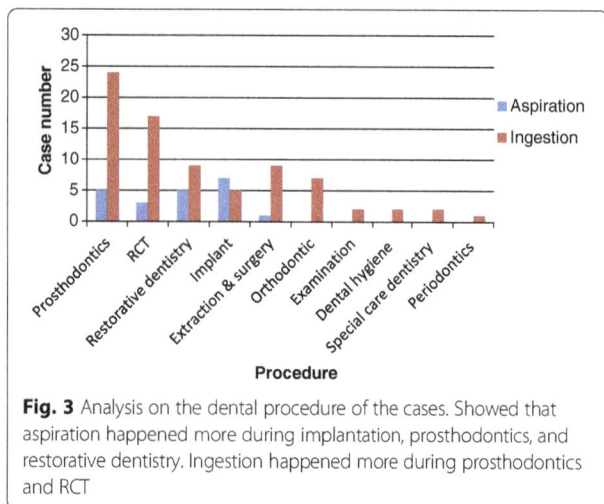

Fig. 3 Analysis on the dental procedure of the cases. Showed that aspiration happened more during implantation, prosthodontics, and restorative dentistry. Ingestion happened more during prosthodontics and RCT

Location for procedure and clinical experience of the involving dentists

In the case reports, there were 14 cases happened at private clinic/hospital [10, 15, 16, 19, 22, 25, 30, 34, 36, 37, 40, 41], 17 cases happened at dental clinic or department in hospital or college hospital [1, 4, 14, 17, 18, 21, 23, 24, 27, 32, 33, 35, 38, 39, 42, 49]; the other 18 cases had no description. In four reviews, there were 60 cases from dental clinics of university hospital [8, 9, 13], the other 508 cases were from general dental clinic [7].

Only two reviews from Japan made detailed analysis on clinical experience of the involving dentists [8, 9]. Both of them thought the accidental ingestion occurred more frequently when procedures were being conducted by practitioners with less experience (5 to 10 years [8], less than 5 years [9]).

Tooth position of procedure and causes

In the case reports, only 16 cases [10, 15–17, 23, 24, 27, 28, 31, 34, 35, 49] were recorded detailed tooth position of procedure. Two reviews reported the ingestion occurred more frequently during treatment of lower molars [8, 9]. The other two reviews had no description [7, 13].

In the case reports, only 14 cases mentioned the causes, including 6 cases of closing mouth and moving

head [15, 17, 25, 34, 41, 46], 3 of discomfort and uncooperative [18, 23, 33], 2 of gagging reflex [24, 31], 2 of instrument fatigue [21, 27], and 1 of no floss tie [11]. All the reviews had no description on the causes.

Anesthesia during procedure and treatment for the accident

During the procedure, only 5 cases received local anesthesia (3 aspirated [1, 23, 43], 2 ingested [31, 33]), 2 cases received sedation (1 aspirated [10], 1 ingested [32]). The other 43 cases and 4 reviews did not receive any anesthesia nor had the record.

During the treatment for aspiration, there were 10 cases received general anesthesia [14, 15, 19, 20, 30, 31, 33, 36, 48], 3 cases received sedation [10, 40], 2 cases received local anesthesia [22, 44], and the other 5 cases had no record [11, 14, 28, 45]. During the treatment for ingestion, there were 7 cases received general anesthesia [17, 23, 25, 29, 39, 46, 47], 2 cases received sedation [32, 42], the other 20 cases did not receive any anesthesia nor had the record.

Discussion

Aspiration or ingestion of foreign objects including instruments, materials or even tooth is a relatively uncommon risk during dental procedures [14]. Yet, it is reported to be the second most common reason for foreign body aspiration in the lung [13]. Actually, the accidents could happen during various dental procedures due to some factors and associated with certain incidence, suggesting the importance of patient's safety and instituting precautions and countermeasures at all times.

However, most literature only reported one or several cases with limited information on the description of the accidents. There were hardly any review on making comprehensive record and discussion of accidental cases.

Therefore, thorough documentation of the accident is stressed in this study so as to arouse the dental personnel's attention, and further to facilitate analysis of the literature, and summarize the prevention and treatment measures on accidental aspiration and ingestion.

In this article, a total of 617 cases reported by 45 articles were reviewed. The statistical analysis was based on

Table 2 The top five kinds of foreign objects aspirated and ingested (case number)

Foreign objects	Case reports		Foreign objects	Reviews	
	Aspiration	Ingestion		Aspiration	Ingestion
Endodontic file (& reamer)	3	11	Prosthesis & crown	32	171
Screwdriver (& screw)	6	6	Bur	0	126
Crown & bridge	3	1	Endodontic file	1	57
Bur & drill	3	0	Inlay core	7	49
Rubber dam clamp	0	2	Broach	0	27

Table 3 Treatment time of the aspirated and ingested cases (number)

	Immediate	2d	3d	4d	5d	7d	2w	5w	2 m	1y	3y	7y	Total
Aspiration	13	2	1	1				1		1	1		20
Ingestion (treatment)	7	1	1		1	3	2		1			1	17
Ingestion (observation and excretion)		2	5	1	2	1	1						12

the different descriptive variables. Most reports made detailed records on patients' age, gender, dental procedure and foreign objects, site of involvement and symptoms, treatment time and modality, and follow-up.

Figures and tables showed there were more accidental cases happened in recent years. Aspirated and ingested cases were more seen in older patients and younger patients, respectively. Male patients suffered more cases than female patients. And the cases were more seen in the fine, cumbersome, and time-consuming procedure. In addition, any kinds of foreign objects could be aspirated or ingested regardless of the shape, size, and even length.

In aspirated cases, foreign objects were found more at right bronchus or lung because the connection from the trachea to the right bronchus is a less marked angle; moreover, the right bronchus has a greater diameter than the left [4, 5, 50]. In ingestion cases, the site of involvement was probably related with the time after the accident. If the checking time is short after the ingestion, the object may be in the stomach; otherwise it will be in the intestine. Since half of the aspirated patients and more than 90 % of the ingested patients had no symptom, it suggested to us that once the instruments, material and even tooth could not be found during procedure, possible aspiration and ingestion might be detected.

From the results, it suggests that once aspiration is confirmed, immediate treatment should be done, since the majority of the cases need endoscopy or even surgery. However, once ingestion is confirmed, observation could be performed until the foreign object excreted. If there is no possible of excretion [18], endoscopy should be chosen. The follow-up also suggested that the treatment was suitable and the complications were under control. The prognosis was pretty good.

However, there were still some important variables recorded incompletely. It showed that only 12 cases reported patient's general conditions. The finding contradicts the widely held belief that patients with a neuromuscular disease or a physical handicap are at high risk of aspirating or ingesting dental foreign objects.

The results also showed that even 18 cases did not report the location of the accident, that only a small number of cases recorded detailed tooth position, and that only a few cases recorded the clinical experience and occupations of the involving dentists though it

was found even lecturer and assistant professor with more than 20 years' experience can make mistakes in this respect [9].

As for the causes, it has been reported [4, 5, 14, 51] that psychotic individuals, alcoholics, mentally disabled individuals, patients who are nervous or restless, and patients who wear dentures ascribed to reduced tactile sensitivity of the palatal mucosa are at high risk of inhaling and swallowing foreign objects, but there were only few records in the dental procedure literature we studied [15, 21]. On the contrary, other possible factors were not recorded in detail, including supine positioning, excessive gag reflex or unexpected patient movement, inadequate lighting, ineffective assistants, instrument fatigue, difficulty of access (posterior areas), and compromised direct view.

In addition, local anesthesia and intravenous sedation had been suggested as the possible reason, since sedation decreases the protective swallowing and coughing reflexes [14, 15]. However, the reason was in controversy since most cases during the procedure in the study did not receive any anesthesia nor had the record. The anesthesia during the treatment for the accidents was recorded incompletely, too.

From above, it could be seen that the missing information have had an effect on the comprehensive analysis of the results. Therefore, it is necessary to emphasize the importance of the thorough documentation and make each dental personnel to do a comprehensive understanding, learning and mastering the treatment and prevention on the accidental aspiration and ingestion.

On the one hand, the proposed treatment algorithm is critical for the management of the complications which could be summarized from the literatures.

Firstly, when accidental event occurs, it is essential that clinicians and their staff remain calm and composed. The patient must be reassured and carefully evaluated [15, 16, 52].

Secondly, thorough clinical and radiological evaluations are required [16]. Early location of an aspirated or ingested foreign body facilitates appropriate and timely treatment management and referral [37]. In cases of aspiration, both posterior-anterior and lateral X-ray films should be taken to confirm the location of foreign objects in the respiratory tract [19]. If the objects (e.g. impression materials or resins) are made of substances that lack of radiopacity, diagnostic bronchoscopy or computed tomography is necessary for their localization.

Thirdly, a prompt decision must be made whether to actively remove the object or to let it pass naturally. The subsequently appropriate actions must be taken to prevent potentially serious complications, and may ultimately save the patient's live [15, 16].

When the object is located in the oral cavity, finger sweeps is the simplest way. When the object is impacted in the airway, noninvasive procedures for managing airway obstruction include back blows in infants, the Heimlich maneuver, abdominal or chest thrusts in pregnant or obese patients [53].

Once aspirated object is confirmed, urgent management with a flexible or hard fiber optic bronchoscope should be performed [54, 55], otherwise it can obstruct the airway [41] or cause pneumonia or a pulmonary abscess [11]. This technique has a success rate of 99 %, with a failure rate of 2.4 to 5 % [10]. And the failed cases require surgical intervention of lobectomy.

If an object is swallowed and impacted in the esophagus, prompt removal is required because the esophagus lies in close proximity with the thoracic great vessels, the pericardium, the pleura and the tracheo-bronchial passages [56–58]. If the object goes into the stomach, there is a greater than 90 % chance, especially for some small (less than 2 cm), blunt objects, that it will pass through the gastrointestinal tract as a result of peristaltic movement without complications [30, 57–59]. Conservative management should include radiographic surveillance and periodic stool inspection [52]. However, sharp, pointed objects are associated with a higher risk of perforation. The perforation is most likely to take place in the esophagus, the pylorus, the duodenum, the duodenojejunal flexure and the ileocaecal region [60]. Thus, early endoscopic removal should be undertaken [55]. If patients develop symptoms of pain, nausea, vomiting, tenderness or abdominal guarding, perforation should be suspected, and if objects remain lodged longer than 2 weeks, surgical intervention is required [17, 59].

Fourthly, the patient should be observed until the object is removed or expelled [21]. A post-operative radiograph should be taken to confirm that the aspirated or ingested instrument has been excreted or removed [52].

Fifthly, thorough documentation of the accident is required as discussed above. Further documentation may include notation of initial and follow-up medical care, clinical experience of the involving assistant or nurse, copies of radiographic reports confirming the diagnosis and notation of removal/expulsion of the objects [21].

On the other hand, prevention through precautionary methods is the most appropriate method to minimize the occurrences of aspiration of dental instruments.

Firstly, every dental personnel should consider the possibility of such emergencies in its standard operating procedures and be well prepared for them [42]. One must be educated and trained regularly to recognize emergencies and how to prevent and minimize adverse events in the work environment [61, 62]. Individual responsibilities must be delegated to offset any confusion in the event of an emergency so as to organize smooth support and cooperative procedures that can be implemented promptly if accidental ingestion or aspiration occurs [9]. To have available the name, address, and telephone number of an endoscopist and a hospital where full service is available is also necessary.

Secondly, patient's thorough medical and dental history should be reviewed [50]. Special considerations should be associated with those patient populations at high risk, and schedule short appointments to them during the morning are most effective [19].

Thirdly, patients should have enough pre-operation educattion. The dental stuff must ensure complete cooperation and active involvement of patients and their accompany [61].

Fourthly, all the instruments should be periodically check and carefully examined before use for signs of wear or work fatigue and replace those that warrant replacement [10, 11, 21, 42]. For example, burs should be fully seated into the handpiece and locked into position [36]. Dental mirrors should be screwed in tightly before being inserted in the mouth [1]. Broken burs and instruments should be retrieved and matched up with retained fragments to ensure that all pieces have been recovered [10].

Finally, standard operating procedures with precautions must be taken during any practices. These precautions include appropriate anesthesia and treatment selection, proper body and head positioning, adequate lighting and four-handed dentistry with an attentive assistant and high-speed evacuation, routinely use of a rubber dam and a properly fitting clamp [10, 21], using a 4 × 4 inch gauze as a protective barrier in the oral cavity distal to the working area [1, 13, 15, 16], tethering small instrument, cast post, core and crown with a ligature to improve the gripping and reduce the possibility of falling from the hands [13, 63–67].

Of course, there were some limitations in the study. For example, articles in languages other than English were not included in the study. Articles published with only abstract or few details were also not included. These limitations may result in a slight bias in statistical analysis. In addition, some meaningful features were not analyzed. For example, the qualification of the dentists or doctors undergoing the procedure was not analyzed since they were recorded only in a few articles.

Conclusions

Although aspiration and ingestion of foreign objects are rare and risky complication during dental procedure, thorough documentation of the accidental aspiration and ingestion of foreign objects during dental procedure is necessary so as to provide enough information for the treatment and prevention.

Acknowledgements
Not applicable

Funding
No funding.

Authors' contributions
RH and HZ carried out the studies and drafted the manuscript. YD, XY and GX made the literature search and helped to draft the manuscript. PX, CS, SJ and YM participated in the design of the study and performed the statistical analysis. RH and KH conceived of the study and make the critical revision. All authors read and approved the final manuscript.

Competing interests
The authors declare that they have no competing interests.

Author details
[1]State Key Laboratory of Military Stomatology & National Clinical Research Center for Oral Diseases & Shaanxi Clinical Research Center for Oral Diseases, Department of Oral Surgery, School of Stomatology, the Fourth Military Medical University, Xi'an City, Shaanxi Province 710032, China. [2]Department of Stomatology, Research Institute of Surgery & Daping Hospital, The Third Military Medical University, Chongqing City 400042, China.

References
1. Pull Ter Gunne L, Wismeijer D. Accidental ingestion of an untethered instrument during implant surgery. Int J Prosthodont. 2014;27(3):277–8.
2. Bernal-Sprekelsen M, Hildmann H. Ingestion and aspiration of foreign bodies. Anesth Pain Control Dent. 1992;1(1):42–5.
3. Parolia A, Kamath M, Kundubala M, Manuel TS, Mohan M. Management of foreign body aspiration or ingestion in dentistry. Kathmandu Univ Med J (KUMJ). 2009;7:165–71.
4. Worthington P. Ingested foreign body associated with oral implant treatment: report of a case. Int J Oral Maxillofac Implants. 1996;11(5):679–81.
5. Ireland AJ. Management of inhaled and swallowed foreign bodies. Dent Update. 2005;32:83–6. 89.
6. Grossman LI. Prevention in endodontic practice. J Am Dent Assoc. 1971;82(2):395–6.
7. Susini G, Pommel L, Camps J. Accidental ingestion and aspiration of root canal instruments and other dental foreign bodies in a French population. Int Endod J. 2007;40(8):585–9.
8. Hisanaga R, Hagita K, Nojima K, Katakura A, Morinaga K, Ichinohe T, Konomi R, Takahashi T, Takano N, Inoue T. Survey of accidental ingestion and aspiration at Tokyo Dental College Chiba Hospital. Bull Tokyo Dent Coll. 2010;51:95–101.
9. Obinata K, Satoh T, Towfik AM, Nakamura M. An investigation of accidental ingestion during dental procedures. J Oral Sci. 2011;53(4):495–500.
10. Fields Jr RT, Schow SR. Aspiration and ingestion of foreign bodies in oral and maxillofacial surgery: a review of literature and report of five cases. Int J Oral Maxillofac Surg. 1998;56:1091–8.
11. Abusamaan M, Giannobile WV, Jhawar P, Gunaratnam NT. Swallowed and aspirated dental prostheses and instruments in clinical dental practice: a report of five cases and a proposed management algorithm. J Am Dent Assoc. 2014;145(5):459–63.
12. Black RE, Johnson DG, Matlak ME. Bronchoscopic removal of aspirated foreign bodies in children. J Pediatr Surg. 1994;29:682e684.
13. Tiwana KK, Morton T, Tiwana PS. Aspiration and ingestion in dental practice: A 10-year institutional review. J Am Dent Assoc. 2004;135:1287–91.
14. Cossellu G, Farronato G, Carrassi A, Angiero F. Accidental aspiration of foreign bodies in dental practice: clinical management and prevention. Gerodontology. 2013. doi:10.1111/ger.12068.
15. Mahesh R, Prasad V, Menon PA. A case of accidental aspiration of an endodontic instrument by a child treated under conscious sedation. Eur J Dent. 2013;7(2):225–8. doi:10.4103/1305-7456.110191.
16. Mohan R, Rao S, Benjamin M, Bhagavan RK. Accidental ingestion of a barbed wire broach and its endoscopic retrieval:prevention better than cure. Indian J Dent Res. 2011;22(6):839–42. doi:10.4103/0970-9290.94681.
17. Bhatnagar S, Das UM, Chandan GD, Prashanth ST, Gowda L, Shiggaon N. Foreign body ingestion in dental practice. J Indian Soc Pedod Prev Dent. 2011;29(4):336–8. doi:10.4103/0970-4388.86387.
18. Venkataraghavan K, Anantharaj A, Praveen P, Rani SP, Krishnan BM. Accidental ingestion of foreign object: Systematic review, recommendations and report of a case. Saudi Dent J. 2011;23(4):177–81. doi:10.1016/j.sdentj.2010.10.007. Epub 2010 Nov 9.
19. Deliberador TM, Marengo G, Scaratti R, Giovanini AF, Zielak JC, Baratto FF. Accidental aspiration in a patient with Parkinson's disease during implant-supported prosthesis construction: a case report. Spec Care Dentist. 2011; 31(5):156–61. doi:10.1111/j.1754-4505.2011.00202.x.
20. Sopeña B, García-Caballero L, Diz P, De la Fuente J, Fernández A, Díaz JA. Unsuspected foreign body aspiration. Quintessence Int. 2003;34(10):779–81.
21. Hodges ED, Durham TM, Stanley RT. Management of aspiration and swallowing incidents: a review of the literature and report of case. ASDC J Dent Child. 1992;59(6):413–9.
22. Goldberg NB, Goldbert AF, Rubenstein L. Instrument aspiration. Quintessence Int. 1989;20(8):603–5.
23. Alexander RE, Delhom JJ. Rubber dam clamp ingestion, an operative risk: report of case. J Am Dent Assoc. 1971;82(6):1387–9.
24. Saraf HP, Nikhade PP, Chandak MG. Accidental ingestion of endodontic file: a case report. Case Rep Dent. 2012;2012:278134. doi:10.1155/2012/278134. Epub 2012 Apr 17.
25. Oncel M, Apiliogullari B, Cobankara FK, Apiliogullari s. Accidental swallowing of the head of a dental mirror: Report of a rare case. J Dent Sci. 2012;7(2):199 202.
26. Zitzmann NU, Elsasser S, Fried R, Marinello CP. Foreign body ingestion and aspiration. Oral Surg Oral Med Oral Pathol Oral Radiol Endod. 1999;88(6):657–60.
27. Govila CP. Accidental swallowing of an endodontic instrument. A report of two cases. Oral Surg Oral Med Oral Pathol. 1979;48(3):269–71.
28. Cameron SM, Whitlock WL, Tabor MS. Foreign body aspiration in dentistry: a review. J Am Dent Assoc. 1996;127(8):1224–9.
29. Santos Tde S, Antunes AA, Vajgel A, Cavalcanti TB, Nogueira LR, Laureano F. Foreign body ingestion during dental implant procedures. J Craniofac Surg. 2012;23(2):e119–23. doi:10.1097/SCS.0b013e31824cda32.
30. Pingarrón Martín L, Morán Soto MJ, Sánchez Burgos R, Burgueño GM. Bronchial impaction of an implant screwdriver after accidental aspiration: report of a case and revision of the literature. Oral Maxillofac Surg. 2010;14(1):43–7. doi:10.1007/s10006-009-0178-0.
31. Elgazzar RF, Abdelhady AI, Sadakah AA. Aspiration of an impacted lower third molar during its surgical removal under local anaesthesia. Int J Oral Maxillofac Surg. 2007;36(4):362–4. Epub 2006 Nov 15.
32. Dhanrajan P. Swallowing of tonsillar pack in recovery following general anaesthesia. Br J Oral Maxillofac Surg. 2013;51(6):e132–4.
33. Bergermann M, Donald PJ, aWengen DF. Screwdriver aspiration: A complication of dental implant placement. Int J Oral Maxillofac Surg. 1992;21(6):339–41.
34. Lambrianidis T, Beltes P. Accidental swallowing of endodontic instruments. Endod Dent Traumatol. 1996;12(6):301–4.
35. Mejia JL, Donado JE, Posada A. Accidental swallowing of a dental clamp. J Endod. 1996;22(11):619–20.
36. Israel HA, Leban SG. Aspiration of an endodontic instrument. J Endod. 1984;10(9):452–4.

37. Kuo SC, Chen YL. Accidental swallowing of an endodontic file. Int Endod J. 2008;41:617–22.

38. de Souza JG, Schuldt Filho G, Pereira Neto AR, Lyra Jr HF, Bianchini MA, Cardoso AC. Accident in implant dentistry:involuntary screwdriver ingestion during surgical procedure. A clinical report. J Prosthodont. 2012;21(3):191–3. doi:10.1111/j.1532-849X.2011.00826.x.

39. Ulusoy M, Toksavul S. Preventing aspiration or ingestion of fixed restorations. J Prosthet Dent. 2003;89(2):223–4.

40. Kim A, Ahn KM. Endoscopic removal of an aspirated healing abutment and screwdriver under conscious sedation. Implant Dent. 2014;23(3):250–2. doi:10.1097/ID.0000000000000100.

41. Tripathi T, Rai P, Singh H. Foreign body ingestion of orthodontic origin. Am J Orthod Dentofacial Orthop. 2011;139(2):279–83. doi:10.1016/j. ajodo.2009.04.026.

42. Umesan UK, Ahmad W, Balakrishnan P. Laryngeal impaction of an archwire segment after accidental ingestion during orthodontic adjustment. Am J Orthod Dentofacial Orthop. 2012;142(2):264–8. doi:10.1016/j.ajodo.2011.05.025.

43. Lankisch TO, Manns MP, Wedemeyer J. Why men should not iron: unperceived swallowed dental root instrument causes seven years of abdominal pain. Clin Gastroenterol Hepatol. 2008;6(9):xxxii. doi:10.1016/j. cgh.2008.01.018. Epub 2008 Jun 2.

44. Bettschart RW, Bolliger CT. Symptomless aspiration of a dental drill. Respiratio. 2009;78(3):329. Epub 2007 Aug 29.

45. Tu CY, Chen HJ, Chen W, Liu YH, Chen CH. A feasible approach for extraction of dental prostheses from the airway by flexible bronchoscopy in concert with wire loop Snares. Laryngoscope. 2007;117(7):1280–2.

46. Li Voti G, Di Pace MR, Castagnetti M, De Grazia E, Cataliotti F. Needle perforation of the bowel in childhood. J Pediatr Surg. 2004;39(2):231–2.

47. Sankar NS. Accidental ingestion of a dental instrument. J R Soc Med. 1998;91(10):538–9.

48. Ankur Thakral, Subrato Sen, V.P. Singh, N. Ramakrishna, V.B. Mandlik. Aspiration of an endodontic file. Medical J Armed Forces India.2013, In Press, Corrected Proof, Available online 20 November 2013

49. Baghele ON, Baghele MO. Accidental ingestion of BiTine ring and a note on inefficient ring separation forceps. Ther Clin Risk Manag. 2011;7:173–9.

50. Zitzmann NU, Fried R, Elsasser S, Marinello CP. The aspiration and swallowing of foreign bodies. The management of the aspiration or swallowing of foreign bodies during dental treatment. [In French, German.] Schweiz Monatsschr Zahnmed 2000;110:619–32.

51. Whitten BH, Gardiner DL, Jeansonne BG, Lemon RR. Current trends in endodontic treatment: report of a national survey. J Am Dent Assoc. 1996;127:1333–41.

52. Uyemura MC. Foreign body ingestion in children. Am Fam Physician. 2006;73(8):1332.

53. Hoekelman RA, Friedman SB, Nelson NM, Seidel HM. Primary Pediatric Care, 2nd ed. CV Mosb Year Book, St. Louis, 1992. 263-263, 1249-1251.

54. Dikensoy O, Usalan C, Filiz A. Foreign body aspiration: clinical utility of flexible bronchoscopy. Postgrad Med J. 2002;78:399–403.

55. Soergel KH, Hogan WJ. Therapeutic endoscopy. Hosp Pract. 1983;18:81–92.

56. Milton TM, Hearing SD, Ireland AJ. Ingested foreign bodies associated with orthodontic treatment: Report of three cases and review of ingestion/ aspiration incident management. Br Dent J. 2001;190:592–6.

57. Samdani T, Singhal T, Balakrishnan S, Hussain A, Grandy-Smith S, El- Hasani S. An apricot story: View through a keyhole. World J Emerg Surg. 2007;2:20.

58. Chung YS, Chung YW, Moon SY, Yoon SM, Kim MJ, Kim KO, et al. Toothpick impaction with sigmoid colon pseudodiverticulum formation successfully treated with colonoscopy. World J Gastroenterol. 2008;14:948–50.

59. Webb WA. Management of foreign bodies of the upper gastrointestinal tract. Gastroenterology. 1988;94:204–16.

60. Allwork JJ, Edwards IR, Welch IM. Ingestion of a quadhelix appliance requiring surgical removal: a case report. J Orthod. 2007;34(3):154–7.

61. Umesan UK, Chua KL, Balakrishnan P. Prevention and management of accidental foreign body ingestion and aspiration in orthodontic practice. Ther Clin Risk Manag. 2012;8:245–52. doi:10.2147/TCRM.S30639.

62. Rohida NS, Bhad WA. Accidental ingestion of a fractured Twin-block appliance. Am J Orthod Dentofacial Orthop. 2011;139(1):123–5.

63. Wilcox CW, Wilwerding TM. Aid for preventing aspiration/ingestion of single crowns. J Prosthet Dent. 1999;81:370–1.

64. American Academy on Pediatrics; American Academy on Pediatric Dentistry. Guideline for monitoring and management of pediatric patients during and after sedation for diagnostic and therapeutic procedures. Pediatr Dent 2008-2009;30:143-

65. Al-Rashed MA. A method to prevent aspiration or ingestion of cast post and core restorations. J Prosthet Dent. 2004;91(5):501–2.

66. Nakajima M, Sato Y. A method for preventing aspiration or ingestion of fixed restorations. J Prosthet Dent. 2004;92(3):303.

67. Wilwerding TM. Preventing aspiration or ingestion of single fixed restorations. J Prosthet Dent. 1990;63(4):489.

20

Assessing degradation of composite resin cements during artificial aging by Martens hardness

Stefan Bürgin, Nadja Rohr[*] ⓘ and Jens Fischer

Abstract

Background: Aim of the study was to verify the efficiency of Martens hardness measurements in detecting the degradation of composite resin cements during artificial aging.

Methods: Four cements were used: Variolink II (VL2), RelyX Unicem 2 Automix (RUN), PermaFlo DC (PDC), and DuoCem (DCM). Specimens for Martens hardness measurements were light-cured and stored in water at 37 °C for 1 day to allow complete polymerization (baseline). Subsequently the specimens were artificially aged by water storage at 37 °C or thermal cycling (n = 6). Hardness was measured at baseline as well as after 1, 4, 9 and 16 days of aging. Specimens for indirect tensile strength measurements were produced in a similar manner. Indirect tensile strength was measured at baseline and after 16 days of aging (n = 10). The results were statistically analyzed using one-way ANOVA (α = 0.05).

Results: After water storage for 16 days hardness was significantly reduced for VL2, RUN and DCM while hardness of PDC as well as indirect tensile strength of all cements were not significantly affected. Thermal cycling significantly reduced both, hardness and indirect tensile strength for all cements. No general correlation was found between Martens hardness and indirect tensile strength. However, when each material was analyzed separately, relative change of hardness and of indirect tensile strength revealed a strong linear correlation.

Conclusions: Martens hardness is a sensible test method to assess aging of resin composite cements during thermal cycling that is easy to perform.

Keywords: Resin composite cement, Martens hardness, Indirect tensile strength, Aging, Thermal cycling

Background

Advances in CAD/CAM technology have increased the application of all-ceramic restorations in dentistry [1, 2]. In clinical use, ceramic has proven to be a reliable restorative material showing survival rates of up to 93% after 10 years [3–8]. Ceramic materials provide high aesthetic options but they are susceptible to tensile stress, which implies a higher risk of failures during functional loading, such as veneer chipping or fractures [9–11]. To prevent any tensile stress in the ceramic, the restoration should not exhibit mechanical retention on the prepared tooth [12]. Therefore, a stable adhesive cementation is

decisive for the long term success of ceramic restorations [13]. Further, it has been shown that the strength of ceramic restorations is doubled when adhesively cemented, because the intaglio surface of the restoration is shielded from tensile stress [14].

Adhesive cementation is technique-sensitive and requires several steps. The hydrophilic tooth surface must be conditioned in order to remove the smear layer and to create a micro-structured surface. In a second step the tooth surface must be primed in order to make it wettable to a hydrophobic resin composite cement. Priming is accomplished by bifunctional monomers in the primer such as HEMA, which are applied at first and bind to the tooth substance with a hydrophilic end while the hydrophobic end contains a polymerizable group that can bind to the resin composite cement [15].

---

* Correspondence: nadja.rohr@unibas.ch

Division of Dental Materials and Engineering, Department of Reconstructive Dentistry and Temporomandibular Disorders, University Center for Dental Medicine Basel, University of Basel, Hebelstrasse 3, 4056 Basel, Switzerland

Efforts were made to simplify the process of surface conditioning for adhesive cementation [16]. Therefore, besides the traditional "etch and rinse" systems, which require all steps of surface treatment, self-adhesive cements were developed, comprising monomers with phosphate groups, which are able to chemically bond to the tooth substance.

In the oral cavity restorations are subjected to mechanical, chemical and thermal stress and thus undergo a process of aging. To simulate the effect of the humid environment in the oral cavity by laboratory testing, storage in water or artificial saliva at 37 °C may be performed. To simulate the effect of temperature changes in the oral cavity, thermal cycling is usually applied [17–20]. Specimens are in turn immersed in water of 5 °C and 55 °C, simulating extreme situations with exposure to ice cream and hot beverages.

To analyze the effect of aging, specimens for flexural strength test can be used [21]. But the preparation of these specimens is time consuming and complex. An alternative is to use the indirect tensile strength test [22–25]. In contrast to flexural specimens the preparation of indirect tensile specimens is less complex. However, as any chemical stress on restorative materials generated in the oral cavity particularly affects the superficial layers of the respective material, assessment of aging effects might also be achieved by hardness measurement, which is a very easily performed test. The only requirement is an even and smooth surface of the specimen. A further advantage of hardness measurements is that multiple measurements can be performed on one specimen, thus alterations over time can be followed.

Published results investigating correlations between strength and hardness of resin composite materials are not consistent. In various studies it has been demonstrated that hardness of composite filling materials is not affected by thermal cycling, while flexural strength decreases significantly under the same conditions [26–29]. In contrast to these findings Medeiros et al. [24] report on a positive correlation between Vickers hardness and indirect tensile strength when investigating the aging of a composite resin restorative material, while Aguiar et al. [25] observed the opposite. However, they both used micro-hardness, which measures only the most superficial layer of the specimens and all measurements were performed after only 24 h water storage. Further, it is unknown whether these observations also apply for resin composite cements.

In all studies Vickers hardness was used. Compared to other hardness test methods, Martens hardness has the advantage that not only plastic but also elastic deformation is measured, which is closer to flexural or indirect tensile strength measurements. Hence, the aim of this study was to analyze the efficiency of Martens hardness measurements in assessing the effect of artificial aging on resin composite cements. Previous investigations with one cement have shown that 16 days of aging by water storage or thermal cycling are sufficient to detect aging effects [23]. Therefore, hardness measurements were performed after water storage at 37 °C or thermal cycling up to 16 days. Indirect tensile strength tests before aging and after 16 days of aging were conducted for the reason of comparison.

Methods

Cements

Four different resin composite cements were used in this study, three conventional multi-step materials and one self-adhesive cement (Table 1).

Specimen preparation for Martens hardness measurements

To measure Martens hardness, specimens with dimensions of $25.0 \times 2.0 \times 2.0$ mm were produced in sets of 6 as described in ISO 4049. The cements were mixed according to the manufacturer's instructions and filled into cavities of a customized Teflon mold. Glass slabs 1 mm in thickness and covered with a transparent Mylar foil (Hawe Transparent Strips, KerrHawe, Bioggio, Switzerland) were placed on both sides of the mold to keep the cement in place.

Light-curing was performed with a polymerization lamp (Elipar, 3 M ESPE, Seefeld, Germany) providing an intensity of 1200 mW/cm^2. The exit window of the light-curing device had a diameter of 8 mm. It was positioned directly on the glass slab, which means in a well-defined distance of 1 mm to the specimen's surface. Light-curing was started in the center of the specimen. After light exposure the exit window was moved to the section next to the center overlapping the previous section by half the diameter of the exit window (i.e. 4 mm). The procedure was reiterated until the specimen on the one side of the center had been completely exposed to the light. Thereafter the section on the other side of the center was light-cured in the same manner. The whole procedure was repeated from the rear side of the specimen. Duration of each light exposure was 10 s (PDF, RUN, and VL2) or 20 s (DCM) according to the manufacturers' instructions.

Specimen preparation for indirect tensile strength tests

To measure indirect tensile strength, cylindrical test specimens (3 mm in height and 3 mm in diameter) were produced in sets of 10 using a customized Teflon mold. The cements were mixed according to the manufacturer's instructions and filled into the cavities of the Teflon mold. A glass slab covered with a transparent

Table 1 Summary of cements used

Name	Abbreviation	Manufacturer	Composition	Mixing mode
Variolink II	VL2	Ivoclar Vivadent, Schaan, Liechtenstein	Matrix: Bis-GMA, urethane dimethacrylate, triethylene glycol dimethacrylate Fillers: barium glass, ytterbium trifluoride, Ba-Al-fluorosilicate glass, spheroid mixed oxide	hand mixing
RelyX Unicem 2 Automix	RUN	3 M ESPE, Seefeld, Germany	Matrix: methacrylate monomers, methacrylated phosphoric esters, initiator components, stabilizers, rheological additives, pigments, Fillers: alkaline (basic) fillers, silanated fillers	automix tip
PermaFlo DC	PDC	Ultradent Products, Jordan, Utah, USA	Matrix: Bis-GMA, triethylene glycol dimethacrylate Fillers: no indications	automix tip
DuoCem	DCM	Coltène/Whaledent, Altstätten, Switzerland	Matrix: methacrylate monomers Fillers: barium glass, amorphous silic acid, fluoride	automix tip

Mylar foil was pressed on each side of the mold and kept in place with a clamp. Each specimen was light-cured on both sides for 20 s. After demolding excess material was carefully removed.

Measurement of Martens hardness

Martens hardness was measured with a universal testing machine (ZHU 2.5, Zwick/Roell, Ulm, Germany), using a Vickers indenter. A load of 10 N was applied. The crosshead speed was set to 5 N/min. Each hardness value was calculated as mean of three indentations. Furthermore, plastic and elastic indentation work was registered.

Measurement of indirect tensile strength

To measure indirect tensile strength, specimens were loaded in a universal testing machine (Z020, Zwick/Roell, Ulm, Germany) perpendicular to the cylinder axis until fracture. The crosshead speed was set to 1 mm/min. The indirect tensile strength was calculated according to the following equation:

$$\sigma = 2F/\pi dh$$

F = load at fracture; d = diameter of the specimen; h = height of the specimen

Endpoint of post-polymerization

To identify the endpoint of post-polymerization after light-curing, specimens for hardness measurement were prepared (n = 6). The specimens were removed from the mold immediately after light-curing and Martens hardness was measured. Subsequently the specimens were stored in deionized water at 37 °C. Martens hardness was measured on all specimens after 1, 6, 12, 24, 48 and 96 h storage time.

Artificial aging

From each cement 2 sets of specimens for Martens hardness measurements were prepared. On all specimens hardness was measured immediately after light-curing. Subsequently, the specimens were stored in water for 1 day at 37 °C to allow complete polymerization and hardness was measured again prior to aging (baseline value).

Indirect tensile strength after light-curing was measured with 1 set of specimens. All further sets of specimens were stored in deionized water at 37 °C for 1 day to allow complete polymerization. Indirect tensile strength after 1 day of water storage was measured with 1 set of specimens (baseline value).

For each cement, 1 set of specimens for Martens hardness measurements and 1 set for indirect tensile strength tests were stored in deionized water at 37 °C, 1 set of specimens for Martens hardness measurements and 1 set for indirect tensile strength tests were thermo-cycled. For thermal cycling a customized device was used. The specimens were immersed alternately in water baths of 5 °C and 55 °C, using a sieve for storage and transportation. The cycle duration was 1 min with a dwell time of

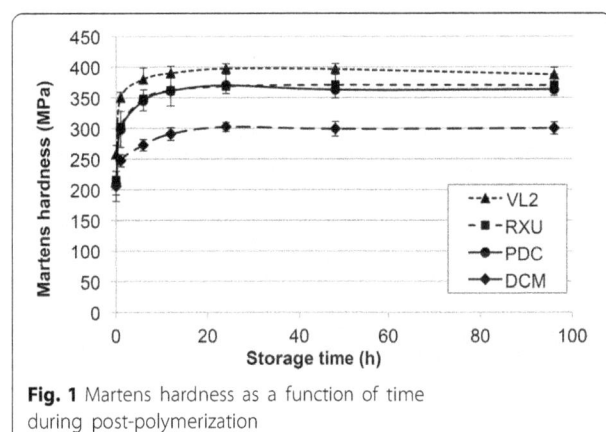

Fig. 1 Martens hardness as a function of time during post-polymerization

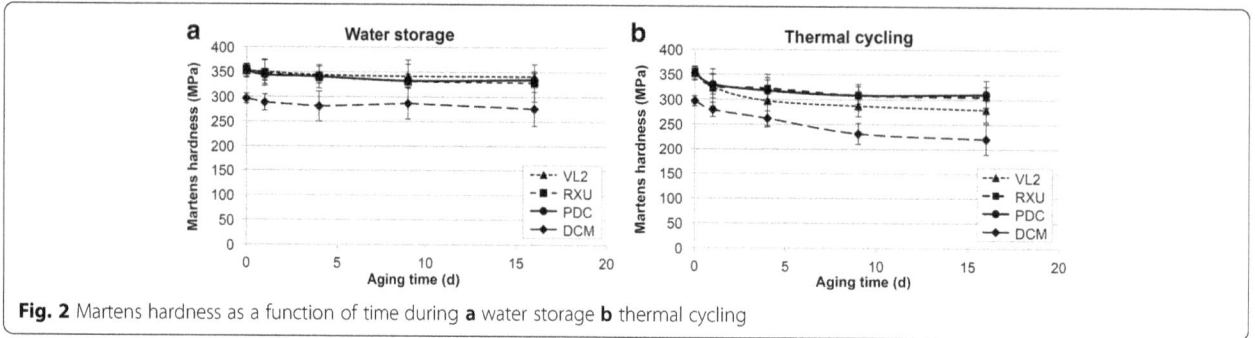

Fig. 2 Martens hardness as a function of time during **a** water storage **b** thermal cycling

28 s in each bath and a transfer time of 2 s between the baths.

Hardness was measured after 1, 4, 9, and 16 days of storage on the same specimens. Indirect tensile strength was measured after 16 days of aging. For PDC an additional value of indirect tensile strength after 4 days of thermal cycling was obtained with one more set of specimens.

Statistics

All groups were tested for normal distribution with Shapiro-Wilk test. The groups were normal distributed and therefore compared using one-way analysis of variance (ANOVA, SPSS, SPSS Inc., Chicago, IL, US). All results with a P-value < 0.05 were considered as statistically significantly different.

Results

Endpoint of post-polymerization

In the first 24 h of water storage an increase in hardness was found in all 4 cements. Then hardness remained constant (Fig. 1).

Effect of aging

Short-term water storage for 16 days slightly affected Martens hardness (Fig. 2a). After thermal cycling the effect was more pronounced and already evident after 1 day of aging (Fig. 2b).

Figure 3a and b are provided to compare the means and standard deviations of Martens hardness and indirect tensile strength, respectively, after light-curing, at baseline (1 day water storage at 37 °C), after 16 days aging by water storage at 37 °C and after 16 days aging by thermal cycling.

In all cases baseline values for hardness and indirect tensile strength were significantly higher than after light-curing ($p < 0.001$). After water storage for 16 days hardness was significantly reduced for VL2 ($p = 0.008$), RUN ($p = 0.006$), DCM ($p = 0.022$) and PDC ($p < 0.001$) while indirect tensile strength of all cements were not significantly affected ($p > 0.05$). Thermal cycling for 16 days in all cases significantly reduced hardness and indirect tensile strength in comparison to the respective baseline values ($p < 0.01$).

The ratio of the plastic and elastic indentation work significantly dropped after complete polymerization, compared to the situation directly after light-curing, but no further change was observed during aging (Fig. 4).

Correlation between Martens hardness and indirect tensile strength

Although the patterns of Martens hardness (Fig. 3a) and indirect tensile strength (Fig. 3b) are similar, no general correlation between both values was found. However, a strong linear correlation was observed for each particular material (Fig. 5). In addition, when plotting the

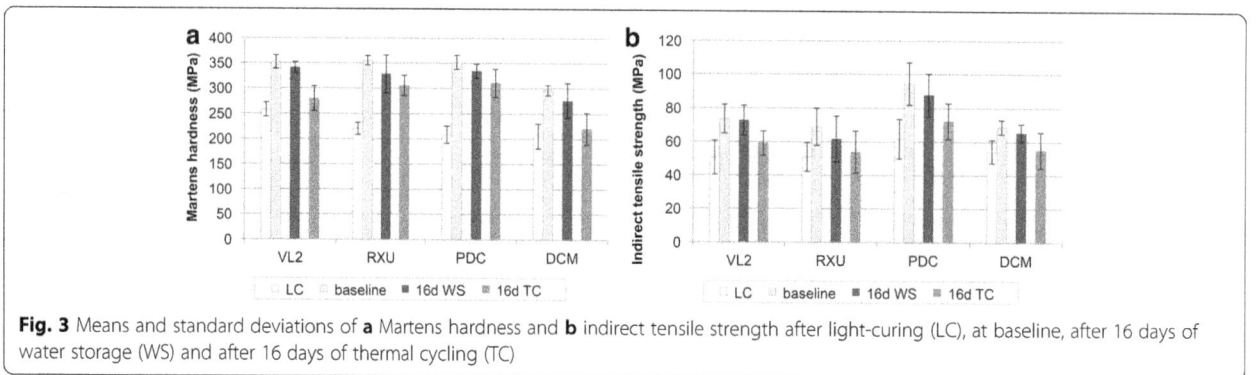

Fig. 3 Means and standard deviations of **a** Martens hardness and **b** indirect tensile strength after light-curing (LC), at baseline, after 16 days of water storage (WS) and after 16 days of thermal cycling (TC)

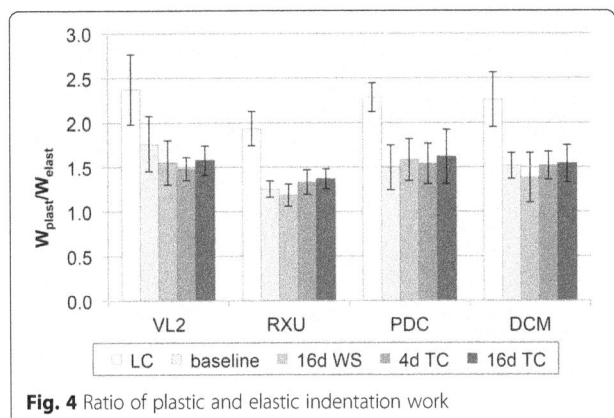

Fig. 4 Ratio of plastic and elastic indentation work

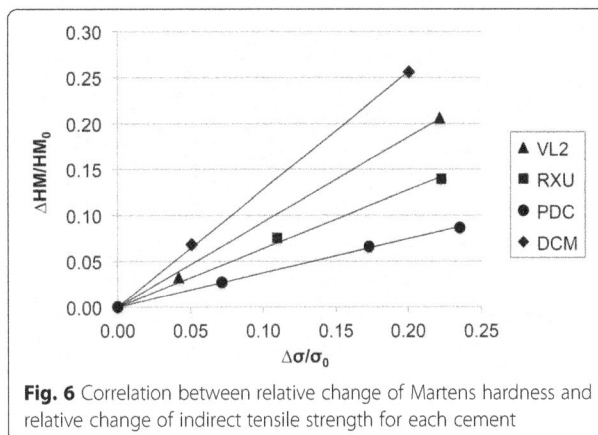

Fig. 6 Correlation between relative change of Martens hardness and relative change of indirect tensile strength for each cement

relative change of Martens hardness (absolute decrease of Martens hardness [ΔHM] divided by the baseline value [HM_0]) against the relative change of indirect tensile strength (absolute decrease of indirect tensile strength [$\Delta\sigma$] divided by the baseline value [σ_0]) a strong linear correlation is obvious with all 4 regression curves running through the origin (Fig. 6).

Discussion

Endpoint of post-polymerization

The obtained results when following the polymerization process after light-curing suggest that hardness measurements correlate with the degree of polymerization of the cements. To the knowledge of the authors the use of Martens hardness measurements in order to characterize the progress of polymerization is not published yet. However, the process of polymerization of resin cements was previously characterized using Knoop-hardness [30, 31]. Vickers [32, 33] and Knoop hardness [34] have been applied to test the degree of polymerization [32, 34] and polymerization shrinkage [33]. All 4 tested cements reached a constant level of hardness after 1 day of storage time, indicating that the polymerization was substantially finished. It was reasoned from the results that in a laboratory test setup a

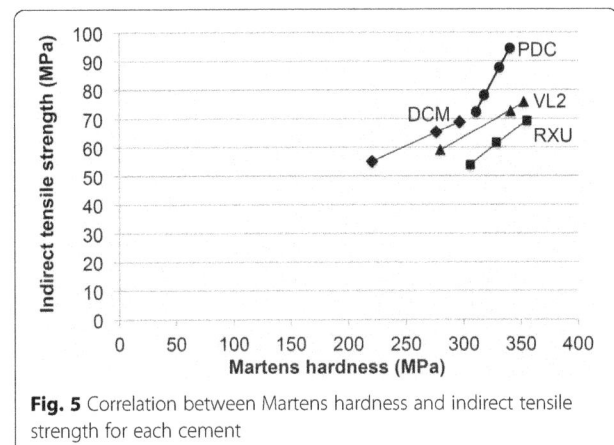

Fig. 5 Correlation between Martens hardness and indirect tensile strength for each cement

1 day water storage at 37 °C is recommended for all 4 cements to allow complete polymerization.

Artificial aging

In the present study the effect of short-term water storage at 37 °C on indirect tensile strength is not as effective as observed in a previous investigation, where 16 days of water storage significantly reduced the indirect tensile strength of a different cement [22]. Therefore, the immersion time in water over 16 days was too short to produce a measurable effect with Martens hardness.

In the present as well as in a previous study [22] thermal cycling revealed to be more effective. However, published results in general are not consistent. That may be explained to some extent by the various methods, which differ in the duration for one cycle and the temperature or the storing medium. Some authors determined a slight decrease [26, 29] while others found a slight increase in strength [27–29].

A specific correlation between Martens hardness and indirect tensile strength for each cement was observed in the present study. A study with a similar test design, which evaluated Vickers hardness and indirect tensile strength was published by Medeiros et al. [23]. Artificial aging of one light-cured composite resin restorative material was carried out by storing the specimens in alcohol, acetic acid, or propionic acid. Regression between mean values of Vickers hardness and indirect tensile strength reveal a linear correlation. Aguiar et al. [25] did not find any correlation between hardness and indirect tensile strength when investigating several different materials. Both results correspond to the present findings. For one single material a correlation between hardness and indirect tensile strength is given, but when comparing multiple materials, no general correlation can be found.

The most important finding in the present study is the fact that the relative variations of Martens hardness and indirect tensile strength following aging reveal a very strong linear correlation specific for each cement, with the regression line running exactly through the point of origin. However, a comparison between different materials must be performed carefully.

Aging in water resulted in significant differences between Martens hardness but not for indirect tensile strength values for all cements when compared to baseline. Therefore measuring Martens hardness can be considered a more sensitive test method for evaluating aging procedures of resin composite cements than indirect tensile strength test.

The invariable ratio between plastic and elastic indentation work during aging indicates that no structural changes in the materials such as an embrittlement occurred which could have changed elasticity or plasticity.

Limitations of the study
It is proposed that 10,000 cycles may represent 1 year of service [18]. In the present study thermal cycling was performed over 16 days indicating more than 2 years of service. For water storage at 37 °C an immersion time of 16 days was too short to induce same degradations as they were found for specimens that were aged by thermal cycling. Martens hardness and indirect tensile strength measurements seem to be suitable methods to detect surface degradations induced by aging. However, further investigations are required to test the change in depth of the specimens over time.

Conclusions
Within the limitations of this study it can be concluded that:

- For artificial aging of resin composite cements thermal cycling (5 °C/55 °C) is more effective than water storage at 37 °C.
- Degradation of resin composite cements after artificial aging may be detected by Martens hardness measurements.
- The relative changes in Martens hardness and indirect tensile strength induced by aging are strongly correlated within one material.

Abbreviations
DCM: DuoCem; HM: Martens hardness; PDC: PermaFlo DC; RUN: RelyX Unicem 2 Automix; VL2: Variolink II

Acknowledgements
The materials were kindly provided by VITA Zahnfabrik, Bad Säckingen, Germany.

Funding
No funding.

Authors' contributions
SB collected the data and wrote the manuscript. NR proofread the manuscript and helped with the interpretation of the data and the statistical analysis. JF designed the concept, interpreted the data and proofread the manuscript. All authors read and approved the final manuscript.

Competing interests
The authors declare that they have no competing interests.

References
1. Fasbinder DJ. Clinical performance of chairside CAD/CAM restorations. J Am Dent Assoc. 2006;137(Suppl):22–31.
2. Kelly JR, Nishimura I, Campbell SD. Ceramics in dentistry: historical roots and current perspectives. J Prosthet Dent. 1996;75:18–32.
3. Reiss B, Walther W. Clinical long-term results and 10-year Kaplan-Meier analysis of Cerec restorations. Int J Comput Dent. 2000;3:9–23.
4. Land MF, Hopp CD. Survival rates of all-ceramic systems differ by clinical indication and fabrication method. J Evid Based Dent Pract. 2010;10:37–8.
5. Mehl A, Hickel R. Current state of development and perspectives of machine-based production methods for dental restorations. Int J Comput Dent. 1999;2:9–35.
6. Wiedhahn K, Kerschbaum T, Fasbinder DF. Clinical long-term results with 617 Cerec veneers: a nine-year report. Int J Comput Dent. 2005;8:233–46.
7. Steeger B. Survival analysis and clinical follow-up examination of all-ceramic single crowns. Int J Comput Dent. 2010;13:101–19.
8. Pjetursson BE, Sailer I, Zwahlen M, Hämmerle CH. systematic review of the survival and complication rates of all-ceramic and metal-ceramic reconstructions after an observation period of at least 3 years. Part I: Single crowns. Clin Oral Implants Res. 2007;18 Suppl 3:73–85.
9. Bindl A, Lüthy H, Mörmann WH. Strength and fracture pattern of monolithic CAD/CAM-generated posterior crowns. Dent Mater. 2006;22:29–36.
10. Kvam K. Fracture toughness determination of ceramic and resin-based dental composites. Biomaterials. 1992;13:101–4.
11. Schmidt KK, Chiayabutr Y, Phillips KM, Kois JC. Influence of preparation design and existing condition of tooth structure on load to failure of ceramic laminate veneers. J Prosthet Dent. 2011;105:374–82.
12. Guess PC, Schultheis S, Wolkewitz M, Zhang Y, Strub JR. Influence of preparation design and ceramic thicknesses on fracture resistance and failure modes of premolar partial coverage restorations. J Prosthet Dent. 2013;110:264–73.
13. Holderegger C, Sailer I, Schuhmacher C, Schläpfer R, Hämmerle CH, Fischer J. Shear bond strength of resin cements to human dentin. Dent Mater. 2008;24:944–50.
14. Addison O, Sodhi A, Fleming GJ. Seating load parameters impact on dental ceramic reinforcement conferred by cementation with resin-cements. Dent Mater. 2010;26:915–21.
15. Abedin F, Ye Q, Parthasarathy R, Misra A, Spencer P. Polymerization behavior of hydrophilic-rich phase of dentin adhesive. J Dent Res. 2015;94:500–7.
16. Hitz T, Stawarczyk B, Fischer J, Hämmerle CH, Sailer I. Are self-adhesive resin cements a valid alternative to conventional resin cements? A laboratory study of the long-term bond strength. Dent Mater. 2012;28:1183–90.
17. Gal M, Darvell B. Thermal cycling procedures for laboratory testing of dental restorations. J Dent. 1999;27:89–99.
18. Morresi AL, D'Amario M, Capogreco M, Gatto R, Marzo G, D'Arcangelo C, Monaco A. Thermal cycling for restorative materials: does a standardized protocol exist in laboratory testing? A literature review. J Mech Behav Biomed Mater. 2014;29:295–308.
19. Chadwick RG. Thermocycling–the effects upon the compressive strength and abrasion resistance of three composite resins. J Oral Rehabil. 1994;21:533–43.
20. Hirabayashi S, Nomoto R, Harashima I, Hirasawa T. The surface degradation of various light-cured composite resins by thermal cycling. Shika Zairyo Kikai. 1990;9:53–64.
21. Drummond JL. Degradation, fatigue, and failure of resin dental composite materials. J Dent Res. 2008;87:710–19.

22. Blumer L, Schmidli F, Weiger R, Fischer J. A systematic approach to standardize artificial aging of resin composite cements. Dent Mater. 2015;31:855–63.

23. Medeiros IS, Gomes MN, Loguercio AD, Filho LE. Diametral tensile strength and Vickers hardness of a composite after storage in different solutions. J Oral Sci. 2007;49:61–6.

24. Aguiar FH, Braceiro AT, Ambrosano GM, Lovadino JR. Hardness and diametral tensile strength of a hybrid composite resin polymerized with different modes and immersed in ethanol or distilled water media. Dent Mater. 2005;21:1098–103.

25. Brosh T, Ganor Y, Belov I, Pilo R. Analysis of strength properties of light-cured resin composites. Dent Mater. 1999;15:174–9.

26. Fischer J, Roeske S, Stawarczyk B, Hämmerle CH. Investigations in the correlation between Martens hardness and flexural strength of composite resin restorative materials. Dent Mater J. 2010;29:188–92.

27. Borba M, Della Bona Á, Cecchetti D. Flexural strength and hardness of direct and indirect composites. Braz Oral Res. 2009;23:5–10.

28. Hahnel S, Henrich A, Bürgers R, Handel G, Rosentritt M. Investigation of mechanical properties of modern dental composites after artificial aging for one year. Oper Dent. 2010;35:412–9.

29. dos Reis AC, de Castro DT, Schiavon MA, da Silva LJ, Agnelli JA. Microstructure and mechanical properties of composite resins subjected to accelerated artificial aging. Braz Dent J. 2013;24:599–604.

30. Rasetto FH, Driscoll CF, von Fraunhofer JA. Effect of light source and time on the polymerization of resin cement through ceramic veneers. J Prosthodont. 2001;10:133–9.

31. Santos Jr GC, El-Mowafy O, Rubo JH, Santos MJ. Hardening of dual-cure resin cements and a resin composite restorative cured with QTH and LED curing units. J Can Dent Assoc. 2004;70:323–8.

32. Gregor L, Bouillaguet S, Onisor I, Ardu S, Krejci I, Rocca GT. Microhardness of light- and dual-polymerizable luting resins polymerized through 7.5-mm-thick endocrowns. J Prosthet Dent. 2014;112:942–8.

33. Frassetto A, Navarra CO, Marchesi G, Turco G, Di Lenarda R, Breschi L, Ferracane JL, Cadenaro M. Kinetics of polymerization and contraction stress development in self-adhesive resin cements. Dent Mater. 2012;28:1032–9.

34. Yoshida K, Meng X. Microhardness of dual-polymerizing resin cements and foundation composite resins for luting fiber-reinforced posts. J Prosthet Dent. 2014;111:505–11.

21

Influence of interradicular and palatal placement of orthodontic mini-implants on the success (survival) rate

Jan Hourfar[1], Dirk Bister[2], Georgios Kanavakis[3], Jörg Alexander Lisson[1] and Björn Ludwig[1,4*]

Abstract

Background: The purpose of this retrospective cohort study was to investigate the success rates of orthodontic mini-implants (OMIs) placed in different insertion sites and to analyse patient and site- related factors that influence mini-implant survival.

Methods: Three hundred eighty-seven OMIs were inserted in 239 patients for orthodontic anchorage and were loaded with a force greater than 2 N. Two different insertion sites were compared: 1. buccal inter-radicular and 2. palatal, at the level of the third palatal ruga. Survival was analysed for location and select patient parameters (age, gender and oral hygiene). The level of statistical significance was set at $p < 0.05$.

Results: The overall success rate was 89.1%. There were statistically significant differences between insertion sites; success rate was 98.4% for OMIs placed in the anterior palate and 71% for OMIs inserted buccal between roots ($p < 0.001$).

Conclusions: Success rate of OMIs was primarily affected by the insertion site. The anterior palate was a more successful location compared to buccal alveolar bone.

Background

The introduction of temporary anchorage devices (TADs) for skeletal anchorage in orthodontics promised to improve biomechanical possibilities for tooth movement [1, 2]; orthodontic mini-implants (OMIs) are the smallest TADs available [3]. Due to their reduced size, OMIs can be inserted at various sites in both jaws [4].

OMIs are generally well accepted by patients [5]; they offer affordable support for anchorage demanding orthodontic biomechanics [4]. Other TADs such as orthodontic mini-plates need soft tissue surgery and are comparatively complex to insert and use; insertion is usually undertaken by oral surgeons. OMIs however can be relatively easily placed and removed, causing little discomfort to the patient [6]; this can be undertaken by the orthodontist during a routine visit [7].

A large body of evidence on success rates [6, 8–40] of OMIs exists, showing an average of approximately 84% [8, 9]. However, considerable variation between different anatomical insertion sites has been reported [41]. A meta-analysis of 52 studies on OMIs reported an overall failure rate of 13.5% [42].

Parasagittal insertion of OMIs in the anterior palate has one of the highest success rates [4]. A prospective study of Straumann® palatal implants revealed success rates of 95.7% [43]. A systematic review [9] showed that palatal implants have a better success rate compared to inter-radicular OMIs. The Straumann® palatal implant has a surface area of about 54 mm^2 whilst two joined OMIs feature a larger combined surface area (2 × 45.34 mm^2) [44]. The success of OMIs may hence be correlated to an increased implant-to-bone contact area rather than the properties of the screws themselves or other proposed factors.

A number of orthodontic appliances, (e.g. for rapid palatal expansion (RPE) [45] or maxillary molar distalization [46]) utilise two OMIs that are usually inserted parasagittal in the anterior palate. Parasagittal insertion is mandatory for OMI-supported RPE, whereas various

* Correspondence: bludwig@kieferorthopaedie-mosel.de
[1]Department of Orthodontics, Saarland University, Homburg, Germany
[4]Private Practice, Am Bahnhof 54, 56841 Traben-Trarbach, Germany
Full list of author information is available at the end of the article

designs have been described for distalization of molars in the upper jaw, some of which use inter-radicular insertion sites [47].

Success rates greater than 80% [8, 9] should encourage orthodontists to use OMIs. Knowledge of insertion sites with high success rates is therefore crucial as it will affect clinical decision making. Success rates of two joined palatal OMIs have not yet been compared to success rates of appliances supported by inter-radicular insertion sites and to our knowledge no conclusive data on this subject is currently available.

The purpose of this retrospective cohort study was to investigate the success rates of orthodontic mini-implants (OMIs) placed either on the buccal side between roots of the teeth or palatally at the level of the third palatal ruga, and also to determine patient related factors that may have an impact on success rates.

Methods

Study sample

All OMIs had identical dimensions (diameter 1.7 mm; length 8 mm), and were manufactured by the same company (OrthoEasy®, Forestadent, Pforzheim, Germany). Other inclusion criteria were: complete patient records including panoramic and cephalometric radiographs, intraoral photographs of applied orthodontic biomechanics and oral hygiene index measurements (Approximal Plaque Index (API) score) at every visit.

After application of the inclusion criteria, the search generated 239 patient records that were eligible for this investigation (137 females and 102 males). The median age of the patients was 13.8 years (interquartile range (IQR) 11.0–16.9 years). A total of 387 OMIs were inserted: 190 in the anterior palate and 197 in buccal inter-radicular sites.

Methodology

All OMIs were inserted in a private orthodontic practice over a three years observation period. This implant system has an anodized surface, features a self-tapping and self-drilling design and is made from titanium-vanadium alloy (Ti-6Al-4 V). Following patient consultation and written consent, 0.2 ml to 0.5 ml of local anaesthetic were used (Ultracain® D-S, Sanofi-Aventis Deutschland GmbH, Frankfurt, Germany), and OMIs were inserted without soft tissue incision or predrilling. The OMIs were inserted at two different sites:

1. Buccal in either upper or lower jaw, using the cortical bone between the roots at the height of the mucogingival line, (Fig. 1a and b) [48].
2. Palatal immediately posterior to the third palatal rugae (Fig. 1c) [49, 50]. Palatal insertion always included the use of two OMIs that were connected by the orthodontic appliance.

All buccal OMIs were loaded on the day of insertion. The typical use was molar protraction with a force >2 N, using standardized Nickel-Titanium (NiTi) coil springs (Fig. 1a and b, Fig. 2c).

Palatal OMIs were loaded within 3 days after placement as the attached appliance had to be manufactured in a dental laboratory. All OMIs were used for direct anchorage. All biomechanics applied to the OMIs produced a force of >2 N and all palatal appliances worked bilaterally therefore exerting equal forces to both implants.

The palatal OMIs used in this study were either for maxillary molar distalization [46] (Fig. 2a), or rapid palatal expansion using a hybrid RPE ("hybrid hyrax", Wilmes et al. [45]) (Fig. 2b). Both of these appliances were directly attached to the OMIs and exerted equal forces of (>2 N) per implant; the exact force values have been previously investigated elsewhere [46, 51].

OMIs remaining in situ over the entire period of treatment that required anchorage were recorded as successful. Premature loss or if removal of the OMI became necessary before achieving the defined treatment aims were charted unsuccessful.

Data collection and statistical analysis

All data were tabulated in a Microsoft Excel® 2007 file (Microsoft Corp., Richmond, Wash., USA). SPSS® for Windows version 22.0 (IBM Corp., Armonk, NY, USA) was used for all statistical analyses. The following parameters were analysed in relation to OMI success rates: 1) insertion site (anatomy); and 2) patient demographic data

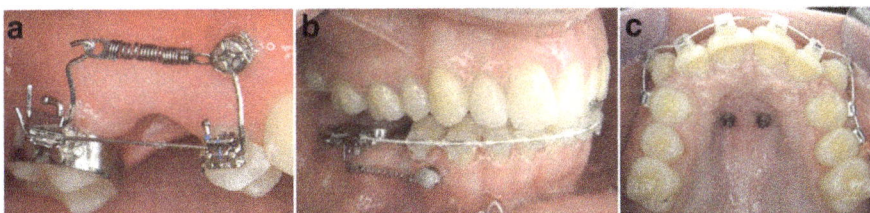

Fig. 1 Vestibular inter - radicular insertion was at the height of the muco-gingival line in the maxilla (**a**) and the mandible (**b**). **c** Palatal orthodontic mini-implants were place only in the anterior palate, directly posterior to the third palatal rugae

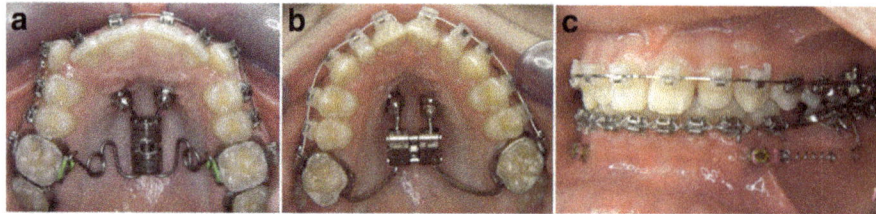

Fig. 2 a Distalization of posterior teeth utilizing palatal orthodontic mini-implants **b** Rapid palatal expansion with hybrid RPE, anchored on two palatal orthodontic mini-implants. **c** Space closure utilising vestibular orthodontic mini-implants

(age, gender and oral hygiene). Normal distribution of metrical parameters was assessed using Kolmogorov-Smirnov (K-S) tests. Comparisons between nominal variables were performed with the Pearson's chi-squared test or Fisher's exact test for non-parametric data. Continuous data not following a normal distribution were analysed using Mann-Whitney U test and descriptive statistics; median and interquartile range (IQR) are displayed accordingly. Survival rates were calculated with the Kaplan-Meier estimator, and their significance was evaluated with log rank tests. Additional Cox regression analysis of multiple variables was performed. Statistical significance was set at $p < 0.05$.

Results

Three hundred twenty-eight out of 387 orthodontic mini-implants were considered successful; the overall success rate was 84.8% over the observation period.

Analysis by anatomical site

Significant differences in success rates were observed between the palatal and the inter-radicular insertion site (Table 1). The success rate of palatal OMIs was 98.9%. Only 2 out of 190 palatal OMIs were lost. Those were inserted in the same patient, providing anchorage for molar distalization; The implants had to be removed before the treatment objectives had been achieved because they were loose.

Interradicular OMIs were successful in 71.1% of the cases. There was no statistically significant difference in success rates between maxillary inter-radicular and mandibular inter-radicular OMIs ($p = 0.628$).

Analysis by patient factors

Patient parameters that were assessed included, age and gender (Table 2) and these parameters had an impact on

success rates. OMIs inserted in patients older than 30 years were found to have a 29.5% failure rate compared to those used in younger patients that showed lower failure rates of 14.8% (20–30 years) and 13.3% (6–20 years). However, this difference was statistically significant only for the youngest group (6–20 years). A significant difference in success rates was also noted between male and female patients.

Survival rate analysis

Survival rates based on Kaplan-Meier estimates were calculated from day of insertion until day of implant loss, early or scheduled removal of mini-implants. 59 OMIs were either lost or removed prematurely. Analysis of survival rates for the anterior palate compared to inter-radicular insertion sites demonstrated a better performance of palatal OMIs (Fig. 3). Those remained in place for 24.4 months on average. Interradicular insertion showed higher loss rates in the first 13 months with an average survival of 17.4 months. The correlation between insertion site and the failure rate of OMIs was statistically significant ($p < 0.001$). The results of the Cox-Regression are displayed in Table 3.

Table 2 Relationship of success rates of OMIs to oral hygiene, age and gender

patient factor		n (total)	success rate		p-value
			%	n	
oral hygiene	good (API < 30%)	352	84.9	299	0.743
	poor (API > 30%)	35	82.9	29	
		387		328	
age	6–20 years old	316	86.7	274	0.002**
	20–30 years old	27	85.2	23	0.287
	> 30 years old	44	70.5	31	0.494
		387		328	
gender	male	160	80.0	128	0.029*
	female	227	88.1	200	
		387		328	

*$p < 0.05$; **$p < 0.01$

Table 1 Success rates by insertion site

Insertion site	n	success rate		p-value
		%	absolute numbers	
anterior palate	190	98.9	188	< 0.001
inter-radicular	197	71.1	140	
total	387	84.8	328	

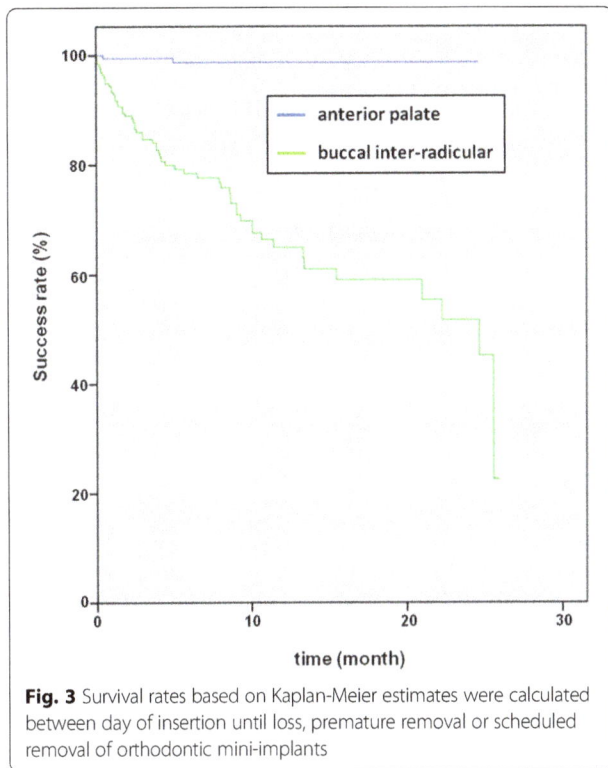

Fig. 3 Survival rates based on Kaplan-Meier estimates were calculated between day of insertion until loss, premature removal or scheduled removal of orthodontic mini-implants

Discussion

During the last decade, numerous studies have assessed the success rates of orthodontic mini-implants [6, 8–11, 14, 16, 17, 19, 20, 22–28, 31, 32, 36, 38, 39] and reported values ranging between 66% and 100% [41]. Results from these investigations reveal a mean success rate of 85.50% (median value 85.46%), which is very close to the results (83.6%) of two systematic reviews [8, 9]. The success rate of our retrospective cohort study (84.8%) is similar.

Approximately half (50.9%) of all OMIs in this study were inserted in the anterior palate, and 98.9% of those were successful. However, palatal OMIs were always inserted and used in pairs. Connecting two OMIs may be the reason for better stability due to the increased surface area of two mini-implants [52]. Two palatal OMIs provide a nearly identical surface area as one standard size palatal implant. The failure rate of the latter has been reported to be between 4.3% and 9% [43, 53–55]. Only in one patient in our cohort both palatal OMIs were lost; these were providing skeletal anchorage for a distalization appliance.

Table 3 Parameters according to Cox regression analysis

variable	hazard ratio	95% CI	p
insertion site	0.036	0.009–0.150	<0.001
age	1.000	0.977–1.023	0.970
gender	1.565	0.928–2.640	0.093
oral hygiene	2.227	0.931–5.329	0.072

CI confidence interval

Orthodontic mini-implants inserted in the buccal alveolus were successful in 71.1% of all cases and similar values have also been reported by other investigators [10, 11, 17, 24, 38, 39].

Success rates were significantly influenced by the combination of load and insertion site. In our investigation palatal OMIs were nearly always successful. Buccal mini-implants were clearly less successful. 59 (15.3%) out of 387 inserted OMIs were lost, and 57 of those had been inserted buccal between roots to support space closure mechanics. It appears that the combination of inter-radicular insertion combined with the type of use resulted in a poorer survival rate.

Existing evidence suggests that moderate loading of OMIs is preferable [56, 57]. Osseointegrated dental implants, featuring treated surfaces, larger diameters and lengths, are probably better suited for the application of heavy loads [58]. Bicortical insertion of OMIs has also been recommended for improved stability when heavy forces are applied [59, 60].

Anchorage design might have an effect on success rates. The findings of Antoszewska et al. [10] indicated that indirect use seemed to have a higher success rate (96.96%) than direct loading (92.60%) but this difference was not statistically significant. In our study, all OMIs were directly loaded, which might have influenced the success rate for buccal inter-radicular insertion (71.1%). In addition all directly loaded OMIs in the palate were joint to one appliance, while the buccal inter-radicular OMIs were used individually and this may have had an impact on success rates.

Other than oral hygiene, gender and age revealed statistically significant differences, but only for younger patients (6–20 years). It is remarkable that OMIs inserted in patients older than 30 years had a failure rate that was twice as high (29.5%) compared to those used in younger patients: 14.8% (20–30 years) and 13.3% (6–20 years), respectively. These differences might be explained by the fact that OMIs in the older patient group (>30 years) were mostly used for molar protraction with forces >2 N, with an associated success rate of 70.5%.

Throughout the entire study period, 59 of 387 OMIs were lost or removed prematurely with an average survival time of 24.4 months. OMIs inserted between roots demonstrated considerably higher loss rates within the first 5 months, with an average survival of 17.4 months. Consequently, the correlation between insertion site and loss of OMIs was highly significant ($p < 0.001$), confirming results from previous research [10, 39].

In summary, our investigation was a large retrospective cohort study and our results concur with previous research [24, 61]. Apart from location and application of OMI we also investigated selected patient related factors. To our knowledge this is the first time that success rates of two joined parasagittal palatal OMIs were compared to inter-radicular insertion sites, adding new data supporting the exiting body of evidence. Maybe not surprisingly the success rate of palatal OMIs of our study was very similar to that of the Straumann® palatal implant [43]. This suggest that two joined palatal OMIs might be used as an alternative for a palatal implant; OMIs can be loaded immediately compared to palatal implants that require 12 weeks' for osseointegration. However once osseointegrated, palatal implants remain absolutely stable when loaded compared to OMIs [62, 63]. A drawback of our investigation is the retrospective design which may have introduced bias and prospective data from a randomized trials may make results more reliable [64].

Extensive research has been undertaken [42, 65] trying to analyse risk factors for OMI failure but many questions remained unanswered [42]. Further research, ideally using prospective randomized designs or a prospective cohort investigation in this field are needed.

Conclusions

This retrospective investigation demonstrated that the success rate of OMIs loaded with forces greater than 2 N was mainly affected by the site of their insertion. Two OMIs inserted in the anterior palate, joined together and used for direct anchorage offered survival rates close to 100%. Individually used OMIs inserted between roots in the buccal alveolus resulted in significantly lower (71.1%) success rates; there was no statistically significant difference for upper and lower buccal insertion sites.

Acknowledgement
The authors express their thanks to Mrs. J. Pasch for participating in the collection of data.

Funding
None.

Authors' contributions
JH conceived the project, gathered and processed the data, created the material presented (tables, electronic images, references, et cetera) and drafted the manuscript. JAL, DB and GK critically revised the manuscript. BL reviewed the process and critically revised the manuscript. All authors read and approved the final manuscript.

Competing interests
The authors declare that they have no competing interests.

Author details
[1]Department of Orthodontics, Saarland University, Homburg, Germany. [2]Department of Orthodontics, Guy's and St Thomas' NHS Foundation Trust and King's College Dental Institute, London, UK. [3]Department of Orthodontics, Tufts University School of Dental Medicine, Boston, USA. [4]Private Practice, Am Bahnhof 54, 56841 Traben-Trarbach, Germany.

References
1. Baumgaertel S, Razavi MR, Hans MG. Mini-implant anchorage for the orthodontic practitioner. Am J Orthod Dentofac Orthop. 2008;133:621–7.
2. Papadopoulos MA, Tarawneh F. The use of miniscrew implants for temporary skeletal anchorage in orthodontics: a comprehensive review. Oral Surg Oral Med Oral Pathol Oral Radiol Endod. 2007;103:6–15.
3. McGuire MK, Scheyer ET, Gallerano RL. Temporary anchorage devices for tooth movement: a review and case reports. J Periodontol. 2006;77:1613–24.
4. Baumgaertel S. Temporary skeletal anchorage devices: the case for miniscrews. Am J Orthod Dentofac Orthop. 2014;145:560.
5. Zawawi KH. Acceptance of orthodontic miniscrews as temporary anchorage devices. Patient Prefer Adherence. 2014;8:933–7.
6. Kuroda S, Sugawara Y, Deguchi T, Kyung HM, Takano-Yamamoto T. Clinical use of miniscrew implants as orthodontic anchorage: success rates and postoperative discomfort. Am J Orthod Dentofac Orthop. 2007;131:9–15.
7. American Association of Orthodontics (AAO). Temporary Anchorage Devices (TADs). For predictable tooth movement. [https://nf.aaoinfo.org/eweb/ DynamicPage.aspx?Action=Add&ObjectKeyFrom=1A83491A-9853-4C87-86A4F7D95601C2E&WebCode=ProdDetailAdd&DoNotSave=yes&ParentObject= CentralizedOrderEntry&ParentDataObject=Invoice%20Detail&ivd_formkey= 69202792-63d7-4ba2-bf4e-a0da41270555&ivd_cst_key=00000000-0000-0000-0000-000000000000&ivd_prc_prd_key=0A27B9E1-2BE3-465F-B3E0-34C218E 99CA1. Accessed: 13–07-2014].
8. Crismani AG, Bertl MH, Celar AG, Bantleon HP, Burstone CJ. Miniscrews in orthodontic treatment: review and analysis of published clinical trials. Am J Orthod Dentofac Orthop. 2010;137:108–13.
9. Schätzle M, Mannchen R, Zwahlen M, Lang NP. Survival and failure rates of orthodontic temporary anchorage devices: a systematic review. Clin Oral Implants Res. 2009;20:1351–9.
10. Antoszewska J, Papadopoulos MA, Park HS, Ludwig B. Five-year experience with orthodontic miniscrew implants: a retrospective investigation of factors influencing success rates. Am J Orthod Dentofac Orthop. 2009;136:158–9.
11. Baek SH, Kim BM, Kyung SH, Lim JK, Kim YH. Success rate and risk factors associated with mini-implants reinstalled in the maxilla. Angle Orthod. 2008; 78:895–901.
12. Basha AG, Shantaraj R, Mogegowda SB. Comparative study between conventional en-masse retraction (sliding mechanics) and en-masse retraction using orthodontic micro implant. Implant Dent. 2010;19:128–36.
13. Berens A, Wiechmann D, Dempf R. Mini- and micro-screws for temporary skeletal anchorage in orthodontic therapy. J Orofac Orthop. 2006;67:450–8.
14. Chaddad K, Ferreira AF, Geurs N, Reddy MS. Influence of surface characteristics on survival rates of mini-implants. Angle Orthod. 2008;78:107–13.
15. Chen CH, Chang CS, Hsieh CH, Tseng YC, Shen YS, Huang IY, et al. The use of microimplants in orthodontic anchorage. J Oral Maxillofac Surg. 2006;64:1209–13.
16. Chen YJ, Chang HH, Huang CY, Hung HC, Lai EH, Yao CC. A retrospective analysis of the failure rate of three different orthodontic skeletal anchorage systems. Clin Oral Implants Res. 2007;18:768–75.
17. Cheng SJ, Tseng IY, Lee JJ, Kok SH. A prospective study of the risk factors associated with failure of mini-implants used for orthodontic anchorage. Int J Oral Maxillofac Implants. 2004;19:100–6.
18. Hedayati Z, Hashemi SM, Zamiri B, Fattahi HR. Anchorage value of surgical titanium screws in orthodontic tooth movement. Int J Oral Maxillofac Surg. 2007;36:588–92.
19. Justens E, De Bruyn H. Clinical outcome of mini-screws used as orthodontic anchorage. Clin Implant Dent Relat Res. 2008;10:174–80.
20. Lee SJ, Ahn SJ, Lee JW, Kim SH, Kim TW. Survival analysis of orthodontic mini-implants. Am J Orthod Dentofac Orthop. 2010;137:194–9.
21. Lim HJ, Eun CS, Cho JH, Lee KH, Hwang HS. Factors associated with initial stability of miniscrews for orthodontic treatment. Am J Orthod Dentofac Orthop. 2009;136:236–42.

Influence of interradicular and palatal placement of orthodontic mini-implants on the success...

149

22. Luzi C, Verna C, Melsen B. A prospective clinical investigation of the failure rate of immediately loaded mini-implants used for orthodontic anchorage. Prog Orthod. 2007;8:192–201.

23. Luzi C, Verna C, Melsen B. Guidelines for success in placement of orthodontic mini-implants. J Clin Orthod. 2009;43:39–44.

24. Manni A, Cozzani M, Tamborrino F, De Rinaldis S, Menini A. Factors influencing the stability of miniscrews. A retrospective study on 300 miniscrews. Eur J Orthod. 2011;33:388–95.

25. Miyawaki S, Koyama I, Inoue M, Mishima K, Sugahara T, Takano-Yamamoto T. Factors associated with the stability of titanium screws placed in the posterior region for orthodontic anchorage. Am J Orthod Dentofac Orthop. 2003;124:373–8.

26. Mommaerts MY, Michiels ML, De Pauw GA. A 2-year outcome audit of a versatile orthodontic bone anchor. J Orthod. 2005;32:175–81.

27. Moon CH, Lee DG, Lee HS, Im JS, Baek SH. Factors associated with the success rate of orthodontic miniscrews placed in the upper and lower posterior buccal region. Angle Orthod. 2008;78:101–6.

28. Moon CH, Park HK, Nam JS, Im JS, Baek SH. Relationship between vertical skeletal pattern and success rate of orthodontic mini-implants. Am J Orthod Dentofac Orthop. 2010;138:51–7.

29. Motoyoshi M, Yoshida T, Ono A, Shimizu N. Effect of cortical bone thickness and implant placement torque on stability of orthodontic mini-implants. Int J Oral Maxillofac Implants. 2007;22:779–84.

30. Oh YH, Park HS, Kwon TG. Treatment effects of microimplant-aided sliding mechanics on distal retraction of posterior teeth. Am J Orthod Dentofac Orthop. 2011;139:470–81.

31. Park HS. Clinical study on success rate of microscrew implants for orthodontic anchorage Korean J Orthod. 2003;33:151–6.

32. Park HS, Jeong SH, Kwon OW. Factors affecting the clinical success of screw implants used as orthodontic anchorage. Am J Orthod Dentofac Orthop. 2006;130:18–25.

33. Park HS, Lee SK, Kwon OW. Group distal movement of teeth using microscrew implant anchorage. Angle Orthod. 2005;75:602–9.

34. Park HS, Yoon DY, Park CS, Jeoung SH. Treatment effects and anchorage potential of sliding mechanics with titanium screws compared with the tweed-Merrifield technique. Am J Orthod Dentofac Orthop. 2008;133:593–600.

35. Santiago RC, de Paula FO, Fraga MR, Picorelli Assis NM, Vitral RW. Correlation between miniscrew stability and bone mineral density in orthodontic patients. Am J Orthod Dentofac Orthop. 2009;136:243–50.

36. Tsaousidis G, Bauss O. Influence of insertion site on the failure rates of orthodontic miniscrews. J Orofac Orthop. 2008;69:349–56.

37. Tseng YC, Hsieh CH, Chen CH, Shen YS, Huang IY, Chen CM. The application of mini-implants for orthodontic anchorage. Int J Oral Maxillofac Surg. 2006;35:704–7.

38. Viwattanatipa N, Thanakitcharu S, Uttravichien A, Pitiphat W. Survival analyses of surgical miniscrews as orthodontic anchorage. Am J Orthod Dentofac Orthop. 2009;136:29–36.

39. Wiechmann D, Meyer U, Buchter A. Success rate of mini- and micro-implants used for orthodontic anchorage: a prospective clinical study. Clin Oral Implants res. 2007;18:263–7.

40. Woo SS, Jeong ST, Huh YS. Hwang: a clinical study of the skeletal anchorage system using miniscrews. J Korean Oral Maxillofacial Surg. 2003;29:102–7.

41. Tsui WK, Chua HD, Cheung LK. Bone anchor systems for orthodontic application: a systematic review. Int J Oral Maxillofac Surg. 2012;41:1427–38.

42. Papageorgiou SN, Zogakis IP, Papadopoulos MA. Failure rates and associated risk factors of orthodontic miniscrew implants: a meta-analysis. Am J Orthod Dentofac Orthop. 2012;142:577–95. e577

43. Männchen R, Schatzle M. Success rate of palatal orthodontic implants: a prospective longitudinal study. Clin Oral Implants res. 2008;19:665–9.

44. Nienkemper M, Wilmes B, Pauls A, Drescher D. Multipurpose use of orthodontic mini-implants to achieve different treatment goals. J Orofac Orthop. 2012;73:467–76.

45. Wilmes B, Nienkemper M, Drescher D. Application and effectiveness of a mini-implant- and tooth-borne rapid palatal expansion device: the hybrid hyrax. World J Orthod. 2010;11:323–30.

46. Ludwig B, Glasl B, Kinzinger GS, Walde KC, Lisson JA. The skeletal frog appliance for maxillary molar distalization. J Clin Orthod. 2011;45:77–84.

47. Ozkalayci N, Yetmez M. A new orthodontic appliance with a mini screw for upper molar Distalization. Appl Bionics Biomech. 2016;5728382:27.

48. Ludwig B, Glasl B, Kinzinger GS, Lietz T, Lisson JA. Anatomical guidelines for Miniscrew insertion: vestibular Interradicular sites. J Clin Orthod. 2011;45:165–73.

49. Ludwig B, Glasl B, Bowman SJ, Wilmes B, Kinzinger GS, Lisson JA. Anatomical guidelines for miniscrew insertion: palatal sites. J Clin Orthod. 2011;45:433–41. quiz 467

50. Hourfar J, Ludwig B, Bister D, Braun A, Kanavakis G. The most distal palatal ruga for placement of orthodontic mini-implants. Eur J Orthod. 2015;37:373–8.

51. Sander C, Huffmeier S, Sander FM, Sander FG. Initial results regarding force exertion during rapid maxillary expansion in children. J Orofac Orthop. 2006;67:19–26.

52. Wilmes B, Drescher D, Nienkemper M. A miniplate system for improved stability of skeletal anchorage. J Clin Orthod. 2009;43:494–501.

53. Asscherickx K, Vannet BV, Bottenberg P, Wehrbein H, Sabzevar MM. Clinical observations and success rates of palatal implants. Am J Orthod Dentofac Orthop. 2010;137:114–22.

54. Jung BA, Kunkel M, Gollner P, Liechti T, Wehrbein H. Success rate of second-generation palatal implants. Angle Orthod. 2009;79:85–90.

55. Jung BA, Kunkel M, Gollner P, Liechti T, Wagner W, Wehrbein H. Prognostic parameters contributing to palatal implant failures: a long-term survival analysis of 239 patients. Clin Oral Implants Res. 2012;23:746–50.

56. Owens SE. Clinical and biological effects of the mini implant for orthodontic anchorage: an experimental study in the beagle dog. Tex Dent J. 2005;122:672.

57. Büchter A, Wiechmann D, Koerdt S, Wiesmann HP, Piffko J, Meyer U. Load-related implant reaction of mini-implants used for orthodontic anchorage. Clin Oral Implants Res. 2005;16:473–9.

58. De Pauw GA, Dermaut L, De Bruyn H, Johansson C. Stability of implants as anchorage for orthopedic traction. Angle Orthod. 1999;69:401–7.

59. Brettin BT, Grosland NM, Qian F, Southard KA, Stuntz TD, Morgan TA, et al. Bicortical vs monocortical orthodontic skeletal anchorage. Am J Orthod Dentofac Orthop. 2008;134:625–35.

60. Morarend C, Qian F, Marshall SD, Southard KA, Grosland NM, Morgan TA, et al. Effect of screw diameter on orthodontic skeletal anchorage. Am J Orthod Dentofac Orthop. 2009;136:224–9.

61. Melo AC, Andrighetto AR, Hirt SD, Bongiolo AL, Silva SU, Silva MA. Risk factors associated with the failure of miniscrews - a ten-year cross sectional study. Braz Oral Res. 2016;30

62. Liou EJ, Pai BC, Lin JC. Do miniscrews remain stationary under orthodontic forces? Am J Orthod Dentofac Orthop. 2004;126:42–7.

63. Nienkemper M, Handschel J, Drescher D. Systematic review of mini-implant displacement under orthodontic loading. Int J Oral Sci. 2014;6:1–6.

64. Vandenbroucke JP. Observational research, randomised trials, and two views of medical science. PLoS med. 2008;5:0050067.

65. Dalessandri D, Salgarello S, Dalessandri M, Lazzaroni E, Piancino M, Paganelli C, et al. Determinants for success rates of temporary anchorage devices in orthodontics: a meta-analysis (n > 50). Eur J Orthod. 2014;36:303-13.

22

Expression of cell adhesion molecule CD44 in mucoepidermoid carcinoma and its association with the tumor behavior

Nada Binmadi[1]* ⓘ, Azza Elsissi[1,2] and Nadia Elsissi[2]

Abstract

Background: The most common malignant salivary gland tumors that affect both adult and children is mucoepidermoid carcinoma. It usually affects both minor and major salivary glands but parotid gland is considering the most common site in which this tumor arises. CD44, a trans-membrane glycoprotein, is an adhesion molecule of cell surface that play a role in the connections between cell-cell and cell-matrix. Many malignant tumors express high levels of CD44, thus, CD44 may be used as an indicator of aggressive behavior of some human malignancy. We evaluate CD44 expression in different grades of mucoepidermoid carcinoma and determine whether expression of CD44 can be used to predict tumor aggressiveness.

Methods: Fifteen cases of mucoepidermoid carcinoma were retrieved from the oral pathology archives and grouped according to the histological grade as well as the clinical behavior regarding metastases and/or recurrence. Tissue sections were immunohistochemically stained for CD44. CD44 staining was scored for intensity and proportion of cells stained.

Results: A higher proportion of high-grade tumor tissues showed moderate or strong CD44 staining compared to low-grade tumors. Additionally, CD44 expression was stronger in tumors from patients with recurrences or metastases, but theses differences were not statistically significant.

Conclusion: Our result showed that mucoepidermoid carcinomas are immunohistochemistry positive to CD44 compare to normal. A trend of CD44 expression associated with different histological grading and aggressive behavior of this tumor.

Keywords: Salivary gland tumor, Mucoepidermoid carcinoma, CD44, Adhesion molecules

Background

The most common type of malignant salivary gland tumor affecting both adults and children is mucoepidermoid carcinoma (MEC). It usually affects both minor and major salivary glands, but the parotid gland is considered the most common site at which this tumor arises and usually has better prognosis than other major salivary glands. Histologically, MECs are composed of epidermoid, mucous, and intermediate cells and are graded low, intermediate, or high according to one of the following grading systems: the modified Healey system, the Armed Forces Institute of Pathology (AFIP) grading system, and the Brandwien system. These grading schemes for MEC are important to determine tumor progression and patient management [1, 2].

CD44, a trans-membrane glycoprotein, is a cell surface adhesion molecule that plays a role in cell-cell and cell-matrix interactions. Many malignant tumors, such as head and neck, breast, and prostate cancer, express high levels of CD44 or its variants [3–5]. Thus, CD44 may be used as an indicator of aggressive behavior of some human malignancies. However, the role of CD44 in MEC remains unclear.

CD44 is encoded by a single gene located on the short arm of chromosome 11 in humans and is required to maintain complex tissue morphology. CD44 exists in a

* Correspondence: nmadi@kau.edu.sa
[1]Department of Oral Diagnostic Sciences, King Abdulaziz University, P.O. Box: 80200, Jeddah 21589, Saudi Arabia
Full list of author information is available at the end of the article

standard form (CD44s) and 10 distinct isoforms (CD44v) that arise from alternative splicing of mRNA and further posttranslational glycosylation [6]. The protein is composed of three domains: extracellular, transmembrane, and intracellular. Its extracellular portion contains the N-terminus, which primarily binds to the ligand hyaluronan (HA), where their interaction promotes signal transduction, regulates matrix assembly and cell migration, and maintains proliferation and differentiation of cancer stem cells (CSCs) [7–9]. CD44 is expressed in many normal cells such as lymphocytes, and epithelial and endothelial cells during hematopoiesis, embryonic development and wound healing [5].

Classical CD44 molecules are intimately involved in the pathogenesis of malignancies such as esophageal cancer, breast cancer, gastric cancer, and prostate cancer [4, 5, 7] CD44 has also been reported as a marker of CSCs in prostate, breast, and head and neck cancer and its expression in these tumors is associated with poor prognosis and aggressive behavior [4, 10, 11]. CSCs are stem-like cells that have the potential to regenerate a tumor mass and maintain their renewal ability. Given the important functions of CD44 in cell-cell and cell-matrix interactions, CSCs are usually postulated to play a vital role in cancer metastasis and aggressiveness.

MEC comprises 12–29 % of malignant tumors [1]. The histogenesis of salivary gland mucoepidermoid carcinoma still remains a controversial topic. Some believe that this tumor originates from myoepithelial cells, the excretory or the intercalated duct cells, or intermediate cells. Histologically, MECs are classified as low, intermediate, or high grade on the basis of the following features: the presence of cellular differentiation, cystic spaces, proportion of mucous cells, growth pattern, type of invasion, and cytological atypia. Many MECs were found to be positive for translocation of cyclic AMP response element-binding protein (CREB)-regulated transcription coactivator (CRTC1-MAML2) t(11;19) [12]. The prognosis of MEC depends mostly on the histological grade, since high-grade MEC is a highly aggressive tumor, while its low-grade variant usually demonstrates a more benign nature.

The treatment of choice in MEC is surgical resection. Whether adjunctive postoperative radiotherapy and/or chemotherapy improve the patient survival rate is not known because of the absence of a systemic analysis of published studies. Metastasis, which can affect patient survival, is a complex process and is not fully understood. We hypothesized that the destruction of adhesions by CD44 provides more free malignant cells that might act to facilitate recurrence and/or metastasis of MECs.

Methods

Tissues from 15 patients with a specific diagnosis of mucoepidermoid carcinoma of the salivary gland from Mansoura University, Egypt, were collected from 2001 to 2006. The Ethics Committee of Mansoura University Hospital authorized the collection of specimens, and follow-up data was obtained from patients' pathology reports. We followed the guidelines of human subjects in the Declaration of Helsinki. The hematoxylin and eosin-stained slides were reviewed and graded in accordance with the Brandwien grading system [13].

Immunohistochemical staining of tissue sections was conducted as follows. After dewaxing and hydration of the tissue sections, antigen retrieval was performed by microwaving in citrate buffer (10 mM citric acid, pH 6.0). Tissue sections were then blocked in 2 % bovine serum and incubated in a moist chamber at 4 °C overnight with anti-CD44 Std-antibody (Thermo Scientific, Clone 156-3C11). The slides were incubated for 10 min at 37 °C with a secondary biotinylated anti-mouse antibody and then incubated with streptavidin-HRP. Specimens were developed with DAB and the nucleus was counterstained with hematoxylin. The sections were photographed under a microscope and analyzed by two pathologists.

Semiquantitative evaluation was performed in tumor tissue using the Allred immunostaining scoring system [14]. The staining intensity was scored as 0 (none), 1 (mild), 2 (moderate), or 3 (strong); and the proportion of stained cells was score as 0 (none), 1 (>0–1 %), 2 (≥1–10 %), 3 (>10–33 %), 4 (>33–66 %) and 5 (>66–100 %). The sum of the proportion score and the intensity score was calculated to obtain a total score that ranged from 0 to 8. The significance of the differences between groups was evaluated using an unpaired Student t test (GraphPad Software, La Jolla, California, United States). P values of <0.05 were considered statistically significant.

Results

The mean age of the 15 patients was 49.7 years (range: 21–70). There were nine (60 %) female and six (40 %) male patients. There were 13 cases from the parotid gland and two from the submandibular gland. Five cases (33.3 %) were classified as low-grade, two cases (13.3 %) as intermediate-grade and eight (53.3 %) as high-grade tumors. Regional lymph node metastasis was noted in eight cases (53.3 %), distant metastases were present in four cases (26.7 %), and local recurrence was found in four patients (26.7 %). Immunohistochemical tissue staining was performed to detect the expression of CD44 in normal salivary glands and in MEC tissue. Representative results are shown in Fig. 1. CD44 expression was found in 13 cases (86.7 %) and considered weak in two (13.3 %), moderate in three (20 %) and strong in eight (53.3 %) cases. Membranous staining was seen in mucous, intermediate, myoepithelial and epidermoid

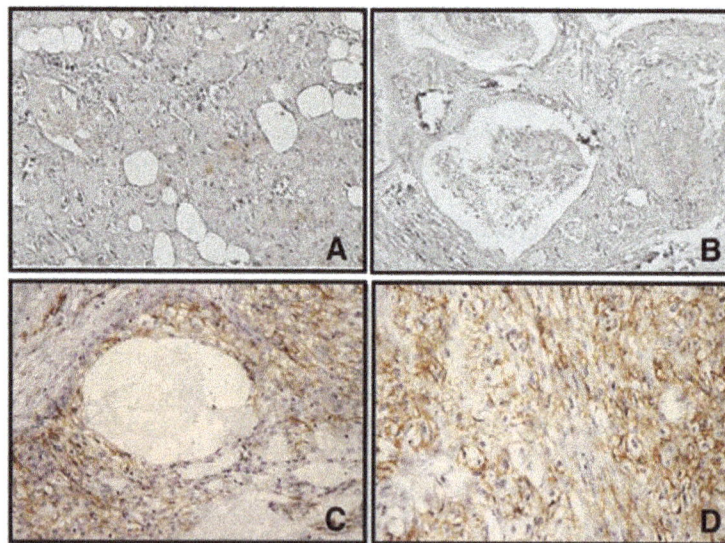

Fig. 1 Immunohistochemistry for CD44 in Mucoepidermoid carcinomas. **a** Normal salivary glands showed weak cytoplasmic stain in ductal epithelium and no immunoreactivity is seen in acinic cells. **b** No or mild CD44 expression was observed in the membrane of mucoepidermoid carcinoma cells (low grade type). **c, d** CD44 expression was strongly expressed in the membrane of the mucoepidermoid carcinoma cells (intermediate and high grade type)

cells in tumor tissues while in normal tissue, staining was positive in lymphocytes, while weak focal cytoplasmic staining was observed in ductal cells. Data on CD44 expression, histological grade, lymph node involvement, recurrence and metastasis are summarized in Table 1. High-grade tumors showed moderate to strong CD44 expression (87.5 %) more frequently than did low-grade tumors (40 %), but this difference was not statistically significant (P =0.2108). CD44 expression was strong in tumors of patients who presented local recurrence and metastasis around 75 % in each group, although this difference in expression compared to tumors of patients who did not have local recurrence or metastasis is failed to meet statistical significant (P = 0.5327, 0.2839). No correlation was found between CD44 expression and

lymph node involvement (P = 0.3599; P < 0.05). Survival data were not available and not included in this study.

Discussion

Mucoepidermoid carcinoma shows widely diverse biological behaviors. High-grade MEC is a highly aggressive tumor, whereas low-grade MEC shows a more benign nature [15]. In our study, MEC was more frequent in the parotid gland of female patients, primarily between the third and sixth decades of life. Molecular alterations associated with histologic and clinical behavior of this tumor are still not clearly understood, and therefore additional studies are necessary. In this study, we examined the expression of CD44 in normal salivary gland and in MEC tissues of different histological grades.

Table 1 CD44 expression according to histological grade of mucoepidermoid carcinoma cases

		Location	CD44 Expression			
		*P/S 13/2	Negative (%)	Weak (%)	Moderate (%)	Strong (%)
Grade						
Low grade		5/0	2/5 (40)	1/5 (20)	1/5 (20)	1/5 (20)
Intermediate grade		1/1	0/2 (0)	0/2 (0)	1/2 (50)	1/2 (50)
High grade		7/1	0/8 (0)	1/8 (12.5)	1/8 (12.5)	6/8 (75)
Lymph node						
Positive	8/15	7/2	0/8 (0)	1/8 (12.5)	2/8 (25)	5/8 (62.5)
Negative	7/15	7/0	2/7 (28.6)	1/7 (14.3)	1/7 (14.3)	3/7 (42.85)
Metastasis	4/15	4/0	0/4 (0)	1/4 (25)	0/4 (0)	3/4 (75)
Recurrence	4/15	3/1	0/4 (0)	0/4 (0)	1/4 (25)	3/4 (75)

*P; Parotid gland. S; Submandibular gland

CD44 is an adhesion molecule and a marker of CSCs that is expressed in several normal and tumor tissues. Metastasis and aggressiveness have been correlated with CD44 expression in breast cancer and renal cell carcinoma [5]. Our immunohistochemistry analysis showed that CD44 expression is substantially upregulated in MEC tissues compared with adjacent normal tissue, indicating that CD44 may contribute to tumorigenicity in MEC, but we failed to observe statistically significant differences in CD44 expression in recurring and metastasized MEC as compared to other MEC. Chang et al. found that the expression of HA but not its receptors CD44 and the hyaluronan receptor for endocytosis (HARE) are associated with MEC metastasis and lymph node involvement [16]. Xing et al. found that HA and CD44 are expressed in most malignant salivary gland tumors including MEC [17].

Analysis of the expression of CD44 and its variant isoforms in salivary gland tumors has yielded different results depending on the type of tumor studied. Fok et al. showed low expression of CD44 in salivary gland tumors (pleomorphic adenoma, polymorphous low grade adenocarcinoma and adenoid cystic carcinoma) compared with normal tissue [18]. This result is consistent with our data showing that low expression of CD44 is associated with less aggressive tumors. Wein et al. reported expression of HA and its associated receptors CD44 and HARE in mucoepidermoid carcinoma [19]. Other studies using qPCR support these findings; CD44 was overexpressed in the tumors from salivary glands compared with normal salivary glands [20]. CD44v3 and v6 variants are widely expressed by the myoepithelial cells of salivary gland tumors and are correlated with the ability to self-renew [21].

We noted a tendency of higher CD44 expression in high-grade tumors compared to low grade, so it can serve as tumor behavior indicator. Since the numbers of cases of each grade of mucoepidermoid carcinoma investigated in this study were relatively small, the relationship between clinicopathological factors and CD44 expression levels in each grade of carcinomas could not be clarified, however, we found that the CD44 staining is varies among different stage of MEC. Another limitation of our study is the incompleteness of patient records, including lack of stage and survival data, which could limit our results.

The mechanism by which a tumor cell invades the surrounding structure is poorly understood in MEC. Several studies suggest that extracellular matrix composition might regulate cell invasion, and that HA and CD44 might facilitate the invasive behavior of tumors [7]. In conclusion, increased expression of CD44 might play an important role in increasing the potential for tumorigenesis; as well as, we found a trend from our results that

the expression of this molecule can be employed as a predictor of tumor behavior and recurrence but further studies with other markers and bigger samples may be more helpful in this regard.

Conclusion

CD44 showed to be expressed by neoplastic cells in MEC like other type of cancer. This expression was not found to correlate with the lymph node involvement of tumor. We observed that CD44 expression was associated with four metastasis cases and four recurrent cases but no significant relation was found and this indicated that CD44 is not a prognostic indicator. In other hand, our study showed a differential staining of CD44 in MEC in different histological grades and this may be an interesting finding that should be explored further in other study with actual correlation with prognosis.

Abbreviations
AFIP: Armed Forces Institute of Pathology; CSCs: cancer stem cells; HA: hyaluronan; HARE: hyaluronan receptor for endocytosis; MEC: Mucoepidermoid carcinoma.

Competing interests
The authors confirm that this article content has no competing interest.

Authors' contributions
AE and NE participated in extracting, collecting the data, staining, and photographing the findings. NB performed the statistical analysis and wrote the manuscript. All authors approved the final manuscript.

Acknowledgement
This study was funded by the Deanship of Scientific Research (DSR), King Abdulaziz University, Jeddah, under grant No. (165-005-D1434). The authors, therefore, acknowledge with thanks technical and financial support from DSR.

Author details
[1]Department of Oral Diagnostic Sciences, King Abdulaziz University, P.O. Box: 80200, Jeddah 21589, Saudi Arabia. [2]Oral Pathology Department, University of Mansoura, Mansoura, Egypt.

References
1. Gnepp DR. Diagnostic Surgical Pathology of the Head and Neck. 2nd ed. Philadilphia: WB Saunders Co; 2009.
2. Speight PM, Barrett AW. Prognostic factors in malignant tumours of the salivary glands. Br J Oral Maxillofac Surg. 2009;47(8):587–93.
3. Naor D, Sionov RV, Ish-Shalom D. CD44: structure, function, and association with the malignant process. Adv Cancer Res. 1997;71:241–319.
4. Naor D, Nedvetzki S, Golan I, Melnik L, Faitelson Y. CD44 in cancer. Crit Rev Clin Lab Sci. 2002;39(6):527–79.
5. Breukelmann D, Bier B, Rempe D, Pschadka G, Bo W. Gains and losses of CD44 expression during breast carcinogenesis and tumour progression. 1998;107–16.
6. Lalit Mohan Negi, Sushama Talegaonkar, Manu Jaggi FJA, Zeenat Iqbal, Khar RK. Role of CD44 in tumour progression and strategies for targeting. J Drug Target. 2012;20(7):561–73.
7. Naor D, Sionov R, Ish-Shalom D. CD44: Structre, Function and Association with the Malignant Process. Adv Cancer Res. 1997;71:241–319.
8. Williams K, Motiani K, Giridhar PV, Kasper S. CD44 integrates signaling in normal stem cell, cancer stem cell and (pre)metastatic niches. Exp Biol Med (Maywood). 2013;238(3):324–38.
9. Page MJ. Chapter 13 The Role of Hyaluronan in Cancer. Chemistry and bioligy of Hyaluronan. 2004. p. 285–305.

10. Simonetti S, Terracciano L, Zlobec I, Kilic E, Stasio L, Quarto M, et al. Immunophenotyping analysis in invasive micropapillary carcinoma of the breast: role of CD24 and CD44 isoforms expression. Breast. 2012;21(2):165–70. Elsevier Ltd.

11. Fitzpatrick SG, Montague LJ, Cohen DM, Bhattacharyya I. CD44 expression in intraoral salivary ductal papillomas and oral papillary squamous cell carcinoma. Head Neck Pathol. 2013;7(2):122–8.

12. Seethala RR. An update on grading of salivary gland carcinomas. Head Neck Pathol. 2009;3(1):69–77.

13. Brandwein MS, Ferlito A, Bradley PJ, Hille JJ, Rinaldo A. Diagnosis and classification of salivary neoplasms: pathologic challenges and relevance to clinical outcomes. Acta Otolaryngol. 2002;122(7):758–64.

14. Allred DC, Allred DC, Harvey JM, Berardo M, Clark GM. Prognostic and predictive factors in breast cancer by immunohistochemical analysis. Mod Pathol. 1998;11(2):155–68.

15. Auclair PL, Goode RK, Ellis GL. Mucoepidermoid carcinoma of intraoral salivary glands. Evaluation and application of grading criteria in 143 cases. Cancer. 1992;69(8):2021–30.

16. Chang SM, Xing RD, Zhang FM, Duan YQ. Serum soluble CD44v6 levels in patients with oral and maxillofacial malignancy. Oral Dis. 2009;15(8):570–2.

17. Xing R, Regezi J a, Stern M, Shuster S, Stern R. Hyaluronan and CD44 expression in minor salivary gland tumors. Oral Dis. 1998;4(4):241–7.

18. Fok TC, Lapointe H, Tuck a B, Chambers a F, Jackson-Boeters L, Daley TD, et al. Expression and localization of osteopontin, homing cell adhesion molecule/CD44, and integrin αvβ3 in pleomorphic adenoma, polymorphous low-grade adenocarcinoma, and adenoid cystic carcinoma. Oral Surg Oral Med Oral Pathol Oral Radiol. 2013;116(6):743–51. Elsevier Inc.

19. Wein RO, McGary CT, Doerr TD, Popat SR, Howard JL, Weigel J a, et al. Hyaluronan and its receptors in mucoepidermoid carcinoma. Head Neck. 2006;28(2):176–81 [Internet].

20. Ianez RCF, Coutinho-Camillo CM, Buim ME, Pinto C a L, Soares F a, Lourenço SV. CD24 and CD44 in salivary gland pleomorphic adenoma and in human salivary gland morphogenesis: differential markers of glandular structure or stem cell indicators? Histopathology. 2013;62(7):1075–82.

21. Fonseca I, Nunes JFM, Soares J. Expression of CD44 isoforms in normal salivary gland tissue : an immunohistochemical and ultrastructural study. 2000;483–8.

23

Granular cell tumors of the tongue: fibroma or schwannoma

Atsushi Musha* ⓘ, Masaru Ogawa and Satoshi Yokoo

Abstract

Background: Granular cell tumors are benign lesions that typically occur in the oral cavity, but can also be found in other sites. However, the characteristics of these tumors are unclear. Thus, the present study aimed to investigate the immunohistological characteristics of these tumors of the tongue.

Methods: Seven patients were treated for granular cell tumors of the tongue at our institution during 2003–2017. Paraffin-embedded specimens were available for all cases; thus, retrospective immunohistochemical analyses were performed.

Results: All cases exhibited cytoplasmic acidophilic granules in the muscle layer of the tumor. Both the normal nerve cells and tumor cells also stained positive for PGP9.5, NSE, calretinin, and GFAP. A nucleus of tumor cells was typically present in the margin. The PAS-positive granules were also positive for CD68 (a lysozyme glycoprotein marker). Various sizes of nerve fibers were observed in each tumor, and granular cells were observed in the nerve fibers of a representative case.

Conclusions: Based on our immunohistological findings, granular cell tumors may be derived from Schwann cells, and the presence of CD68 indicates that Wallerian degeneration after nerve injury may be a contributor to tumor formation. Thus, a safe surgical margin is needed to detect the infiltrative growth of granular cell tumors.

Keywords: Granular cell tumor, Oral cavity, Immunohistochemistry, Wallerian degeneration

Background

Granular cell tumors (GCTs) are rare, benign tumors that were first reported as granular cell myoblastomas in 1926 [1]. The term GCT was first introduced in the 2005 version of the World Health Organization's Classification of Tumors [2]. Contrary to the belief that GCTs have a myogenic origin, an immunohistochemical study [3] has revealed that GCTs are of neural origin, with diffuse expression of S-100 protein present in almost every case. However, there is no clear consensus regarding the mechanism of GCT development. GCTs display cytoplasmic acidophilic granule-like structures, and exhibit many polygonal neoplastic cells that multiply in an alveolar configuration. Because GCTs lack a capsule, they have poorly differentiated margins and frequently exhibit recurrence [4, 5]. Thus, curative treatment for GCTs requires a sufficient clear surgical margin. GCTs are frequently detected in soft tissues throughout the body, especially the skin and oral cavity [5], although the origin of this tumor remains unclear. Therefore, we aimed to evaluate the immunohistological characteristics of oral GCTs of the tongue.

Methods
Case selection

We retrospectively reviewed records from cases of oral GCTs of the tongue, treated in our hospital during a 15-year period (2003–2017), and identified 7 cases that had been treated by resection. The

* Correspondence: musha@gunma-u.ac.jp
Department of Oral and Maxillofacial Surgery, Plastic Surgery, Gunma University Graduate School of Medicine, Gunma, Japan

Table 1 Characterization of the selected antibodies and their expression in granular cell tumors from various sites

Marker	Dilution	Supplier	Character
S-100 protein (rabbit polyclonal antibody)	1:300	DakoCytomation	E-F hand family (granule cells, glia cells, Schwann cells)
Vimentin (mouse monoclonal antibody)	1:300	DakoCytomation	Intermediary filament (granule cells)
PGP 9.5 (mouse monoclonal antibody)	1:300	DakoCytomation	Nerve cells (cell body, axon, granule cells)
NSE (mouse monoclonal antibody)	1:1000	DakoCytomation	Nerve cells (axis-cylinder process)
Calretinin (rabbit polyclonal antibody)	1:10	Spring Biosciences	E-F hand family (Schwann cells, central nerve neurons, mast cells)
GFAP (mouse monoclonal antibody)	1:1000	Novocastra Laboratories	Glia fiber-related acid protein, Schwann cells
CD68 (mouse monoclonal antibody))	1:300	Thermo Fisher Scientific	Highly glycosylated membrane proteins, glycoproteins
Ki-67 (mouse monoclonal antibody)	1:400	DakoCytomation	Proliferation marker

Abbreviations: *NSE* neuron-specific enolase, *GFAP* glial fibrillary acidic protein, *PGP* protein gene product

specimen submission forms were used to extract the data on patient's age and sex, and the location of the lesion. Paraffin-embedded specimens were available for all cases, which allowed us to perform detailed histopathological and immunohistochemical analyses. All patients had provided informed consent for treatment, and this study's retrospective design was approved by our Institutional Review Board (reference number: 150,033).

Morphological assessment

Slides were stained with hematoxylin and eosin to evaluate the following morphological parameters: surgical margin status, presence of pseudocarcinomatous hyperplasia and cytoplasmic acidophilic granules. We also determined the presence of a capsule in these samples.

Immunohistochemical analysis

We stained the slides with antibodies against the following proteins to determine the development mechanism and origin of the GCTs (Table 1):

S-100, a protein from the E-F hand family and a marker widely used in immunostaining of GCTs [5]. The protein was extracted from the brain and is typically found in granule cells, glial cells and Schwann cells.

Vimentin, a protein from the intermediary filament family and associated with the cytoskeleton. It is typically found in granule cells, but has low specificity [5].

The PGP9.5 protein, is seen in nerve cells (cell body and axon) and neuroendocrine cells in the peripheral nervous system. This protein is extracted from the brain, and GCTs exhibit a broad range of staining intensities for PGP9.5 [5, 6].

The NSE protein is a marker of nerve cells (axis cylinder process) and neuroendocrine cells in the peripheral nervous system. This protein is highly specific for nerve cells (axis cylinder process) in all organs, and is produced in large quantities by neuroendocrine cell-derived tumors. Thus, NSE has been used for the diagnosis and monitoring of small-cell lung cancer, neuroblastoma, and neuroendocrine tumors [7].

The calretinin protein, an E-F hand family protein produced in the central nervous system (similar to S-100) [5]. Calretinin is typically found in Schwann

Table 2 Clinical characteristics

Case	Age (years)	Sex	Major complaint	Location	Size (mm)	Mucosal color	Lingual trauma from occlusion	Follow-up (months)
1	45	F	Hard lump	Tongue	8 × 8	Normal	+	202
2	43	F	Hard lump	Tongue	20 × 29	Normal	+	177
3	53	F	Hard lump	Tongue	7 × 7	Normal	−	162
4	39	M	Hard lump	Tongue	5 × 5	Normal	−	147
5	35	F	Hard lump	Tongue	7 × 7	Normal	−	108
6	62	M	Hard lump	Tongue	16 × 17	Normal	+	65
7	70	F	Hard lump	Tongue	13 × 18	Normal	−	40

Abbreviations: *F* female, *M* male

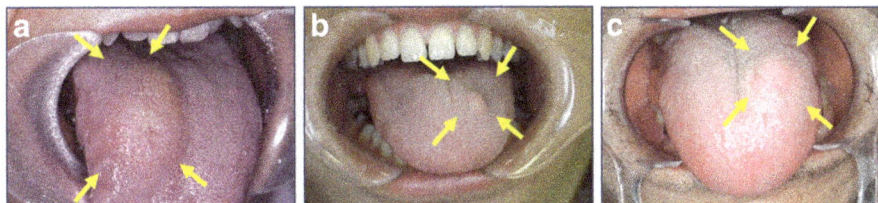

Fig. 1 Granular cell tumors of the tongue (arrows). **a** Case 2, **b** Case 5, and **c** Case 6

cells, neurons of the central nervous system and mast cells.

The GFAP protein is associated with glial fiber-related acid protein and Schwann cells, and is an intermediate filament protein, specific to astroglial cells [8]. The expression of GFAP increases in cases of cerebral damage, dementia, prion disease, and neurologic diseases such as multiple sclerosis.

The CD68 protein is associated with highly glycosylated membrane proteins, glycoproteins, and mucin-like membrane proteins of lysozymes [9]. This protein is typically found in macrophages, fibroblasts, and Schwann cells.

The Ki-67 protein, a cell proliferation marker used to examine the proliferation status of tumor cells [10].

Results

All 7 GCTs occurred in the tongues of middle-aged or elderly patients, all of whom had presented with a hard lump in their tongue (Table 2, Fig. 1). The tumor dimensions ranged from 5 to 29 mm. In all cases, the clinical diagnosis was fibroma. No cases of recurrence were observed over a maximum follow-up period of 15 years.

All cases exhibited cytoplasmic acidophilic granules in the tumor muscle layer. A nucleus of tumor cells was typically present in the marginal regions. In none of the cases the lesion was covered by a capsule and only 3 cases exhibited pseudocarcinomatous hyperplasia. All surgical margins were >10 mm.

Immunohistochemical findings are summarized in Table 3. All cases stained positively for PAS, S-100 protein, vimentin, PGP 9.5, NSE, calretinin, GFAP, and CD68 (Figs. 2 and 3). Co-expression of PGP 9.5, NSE, calretinin, and GFAP in the tumor cells and normal nerve cells was observed in all cases (Fig. 3). The PAS-positive granules were also positive for the lysozyme glycoprotein marker, CD68 (Fig. 4). Nerve fibers of various sizes were observed in each tumor and granular cells were observed in the nerve fibers from a representative case (Case 2; Fig. 5). The tumors exhibited sporadic staining for Ki-67, with a mean Ki-67 index of 1.89% (low cell proliferation index; Table 3).

Discussion

GCTs are relatively rare benign tumors that can occur throughout the body. The tongue is involved in $\geq 60\%$ of oral GCTs, although these tumors can also be found in the head and neck region, buccal mucosa, hard palate, lips and gingiva [3]. A previous study [11] indicated that women are more likely to develop

Table 3 Histopathological and immunohistochemical characteristics in 7 cases of GCT of the tongue

Case	Capsule	PCH	S-100 protein	Vimentin	PGP 9.5	NSE	Calretinin	GFAP	CD68	PAS	Ki-67 index (%)[a]
1	–	–	+	+	+	+	+	+	+	+	2.57
2	–	+	+	+	+	+	+	+	+	+	3.22
3	–	+	+	+	+	+	+	+	+	+	1.21
4	–	–	+	+	+	+	+	+	+	+	0.42
5	–	–	+	+	+	+	+	+	+	+	1.83
6	–	+	+	+	+	+	+	+	+	+	1.63
7	–	–	+	+	+	+	+	+	+	+	2.42

Abbreviations GCT granular cell tumors, GFAP glial fibrillary acidic protein, NSE neuron-specific enolase, PAS periodic acid-Schiff, PCH pseudocarcinomatous hyperplasia, PGP protein gene product
[a]The Ki-67 index was calculated as the percentage of positive cells in a minimum sample of 1000 cells. Mean Ki-67 index, 1.89%

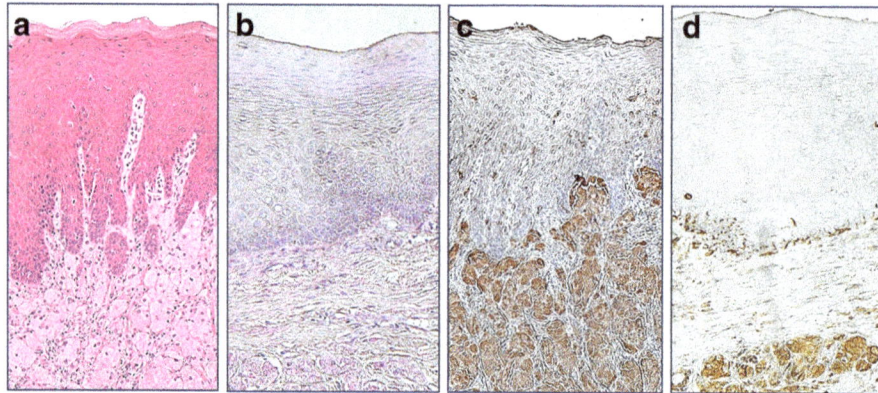

Fig. 2 a Pseudoepitheliomatous hyperplasia associated with granular cell tumors (hematoxylin and eosin staining). All cases stained positive for **b** periodic acid-Schiff, **c** S-100 protein, and **d** vimentin (magnification, 100×)

GCTs than men and we observed similar distribution. It is difficult to confirm a clinical diagnosis of GCT, since these tumors do not have clear clinical characteristics. The first treatment of choice is surgical resection. Since the tumor does not have a capsule and presents with undefined borders, careful resection with clear margins is essential to avoid recurrence [11], an event observed in approximately 20% of cases because of the presence of a resected stump [12]. Although malignant changes (histologic evidence of vesicular nucleus with a prominent nucleolus, high mitotic activity, high nucleus-to-cytoplasm ratio and pleomorphism) are relatively rare, and seen in 1–2% of cases [13, 14], prevention of a malignant transformation may also aid in preventing recurrence. Thus, a broad surgical margin is needed to prevent recurrence. In the present study, the tumors had relatively small volumes, and a 10-mm margin, based on palpation of the tumor mass, was considered sufficient. It is unclear whether a 10-mm margin can be

used for all GCTs, although a 10-mm margin from the palpated mass may be appropriate in cases of GCT with small sizes.

Several theories have been proposed regarding the origin of GCTs. In 1926 Abrikosoff described this tumor as a "granular cell myoblastoma", because of the presence of striated muscle blast cells. However, different reports [15–18] have suggested different origins, such as myogenic, neurogenic, histiocytic and fibroblastic. Nevertheless, based on the presence of the highly specific S-100 protein, it is highly likely that Schwann cells are involved, which was first described in 1982, alongside glial cells [11], resulting in a name change for these tumors to GCT in the 2005 version of the World Health Organization's Classification of Tumors [2].

In the present study, all cases exhibited PAS-positive granules in the tumor cells alongside positive staining for S-100 protein and vimentin (Fig. 2). Furthermore, the tumor cells and normal nerve cells

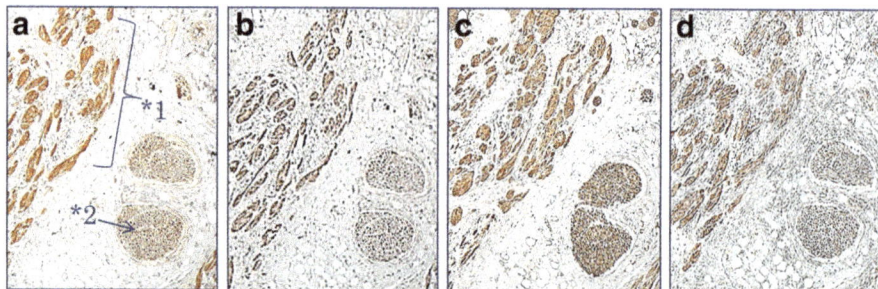

Fig. 3 Immunohistochemistry revealed that the tumor cells (*1) and normal nerve cells (*2) expressed **a** protein gene product 9.5, **b** neuron-specific enolase, **c** calretinin, and **d** glial fibrillary acidic protein (magnification, 40×)

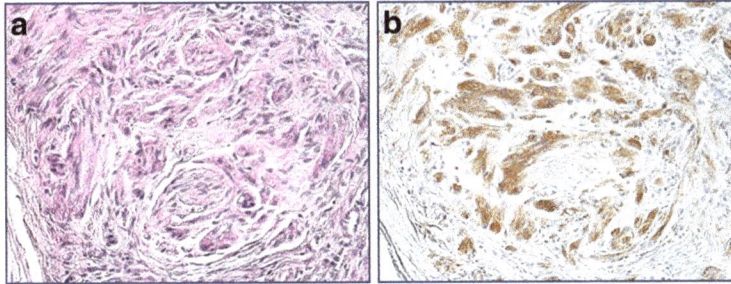

Fig. 4 Granules stained positive for **a** periodic acid-Schiff and **b** the lysozyme glycoprotein marker, CD68 (magnification, 200×)

exhibited co-expression of nerve markers PGP 9.5, NSE, calretinin, and GFAP (Fig. 3), suggesting that the nervous system plays a role in the development of this tumor. Besides, varying thicknesses of funiculi were present in all of the tumors and Schwann cells exhibited findings that were comparable to those of granule cells (Fig. 5). These findings suggest that GCTs may originate from Schwann cells.

The cytoplasmic granular structures of the tumor cells are lysozymes, as they show positive staining for CD68 (Fig. 4), and are reported to contain glycogen, a myelin-like structure, and a phospholipid membrane [19]. As such, neurodegenerative injury has been suggested to be involved in the development and reproduction of GCT cells [20]. In our study, lingual trauma from occlusion was observed in 3 cases, leading to a conclusion that the development of GCT may involve Wallerian degeneration after axonal injury, which generates an axon fragment (i.e., glycogen and the myelin-like structure) with Schwann cells. This fragment may lead to a malignant transformation that can result in cancerous growth and the development of GCT (Fig. 6). An amputation neuroma may also be another cause. Though there are few reports of GCT occurring in such a situation, it is extremely unlikely that both will occur simultaneously. Hence, GCTs can arise in all soft tissues that might experience mechanical stimulation. It should be kept in mind that various other factors, besides Wallerian degeneration, may influence the developmental process in locations not exposed to mechanical injury (e.g., the lungs) [12].

All 7 cases exhibited a low Ki-67 index, which explained the favorable prognoses in our patients, with no signs of recurrence seen after a follow-up period

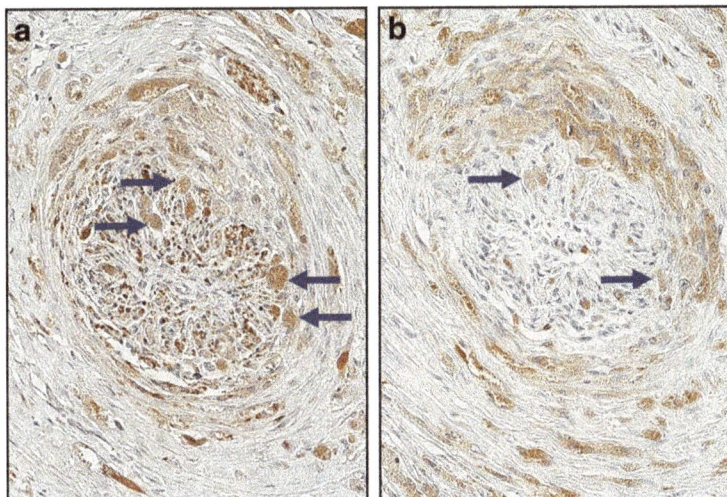

Fig. 5 Granular cells (arrows) were observed in a nerve fiber from a representative case that was stained for **a** protein gene product 9.5 and **b** CD68 (magnification, 200×)

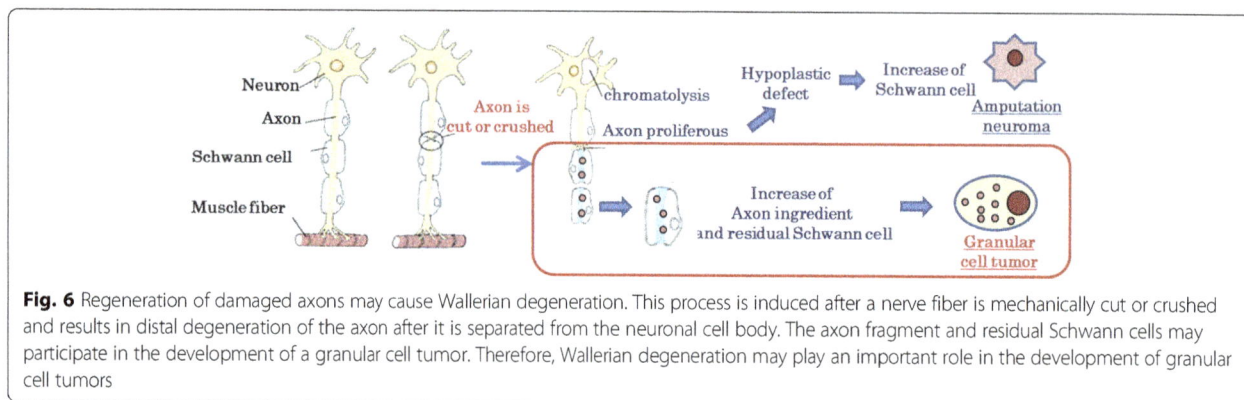

Fig. 6 Regeneration of damaged axons may cause Wallerian degeneration. This process is induced after a nerve fiber is mechanically cut or crushed and results in distal degeneration of the axon after it is separated from the neuronal cell body. The axon fragment and residual Schwann cells may participate in the development of a granular cell tumor. Therefore, Wallerian degeneration may play an important role in the development of granular cell tumors

of 15 years. Previous studies had revealed that a Ki-67 index of >10% was associated with local GCT recurrence [10].

Conclusions

Our immunohistological findings suggest that GCTs are derived from Schwann cells. Furthermore, the CD68-positive findings indicate that Wallerian degeneration may also contribute to nerve injury. A safe surgical margin is needed to identify infiltrative growth of GCTs.

Abbreviations
GCT: Granular cell tumors; GFAP: Glial fibrillary acidic protein; NSE: Nerves-specific enolase; PAS: Periodic acid Schiff; PGP: Protein gene product

Acknowledgements
We would like to thank Editage (www.editage.jp) for English language editing.

Funding
None.

Author's contributions
AM made the initial diagnosis, prepared the first draft of the manuscript and took the required photos. AM, MO and SY planned the treatment. AM and SY analyzed the collected data and contributed to the final drafting of the manuscript. All authors have read and approved the final manuscript.

Competing interest
The authors declare that they have no competing interests.

References
1. Abrikossoff A. Ueber Myome, ausgehend von der quergestreifen willkurlichen. Muskulatur. Virchows Arch Pathol Anat. 1926;260:215–33. [in German]
2. Speight P. Granular cell tumor. In: Barnes L, Eveson JW, Reichart P, Sidransky D, editors. World Health Organization classification of Tumours. Pathology and genetics. Head and neck tumours. Lyon: IARC Press; 2005. p. 185–6.
3. Stewart CM, Watson RE, Eversole LR, Fischlschweiger W, Leider AS. Oral granular cell tumors: a clinicopathologic and immunocytochemical study. Oral Surg Oral Med Oral Pathol. 1988;65:427–35.
4. Meissner M, Wolter M, Schöfer H, Kaufmann R. A solid erythematous tumour. Granular cell tumour (GCT). Clin Exp Dermatol. 2010;35:e44–5.
5. Vered M, Carpenter WM, Buchner A. Granular cell tumor of the oral cavity: updated immunohistochemical profile. J Oral Pathol Med. 2009;38:150–9.
6. Mahalingam M, Lo-Piccolo D, Byers HR. Expression of PGP 9.5 in granular sheath tumors: an immunohistochemical study of six cases. J Cutan Pathol. 2001;28:282–6.
7. Fendler WP, Wenter V, Thornton HI, Ilhan H, von Schweinitz D, Coppenrath E, et al. Combined Scintigraphy and tumor marker analysis predicts unfavorable histopathology of Neuroblastic tumors with high accuracy. PLoS One. 2015;10:e0132809.
8. Nielsen AL, Holm IE, Johansen M, Bonven B, Jørgensen P, Jørgensen AL. A new splice variant of glial fibrillary acidic protein, GFAP epsilon, interacts with the presenilin proteins. J Biol Chem. 2002;277:29983–91.
9. Kunisch E, Fuhrmann R, Roth A, Winter R, Lungerhausen W, Kinne RW. Macrophage specificity of three anti-CD68 monoclonal antibodies (KP1, EBM11, and PGM1) widely used for immunohistochemistry and flow cytometry. Ann Rheum Dis. 2004;63:774–84.
10. Fanburg-Smith JC, Meis-Kindblom JM, Fante R, Kindblom LG. Malignant granular cell tumor of soft tissue: diagnostic criteria and clinicopathologic correlation. Am J Surg Pathol. 1998;22:779–94.
11. Tsuchida T, Okada K, Itoi E, Sato T, Sato K. Intramuscular malignant granular cell tumor. Skelet Radiol. 1997;26:116–21.
12. Lack EE, Worsham GF, Callihan MD, Crawford BE, Klappenbach S, Rowden G, et al. Granular cell tumor: a clinicopathologic study of 110 patients. J Surg Oncol. 1980;13:301–16.
13. Budiño-Carbonero S, Navarro-Vergara P, Rodríguez-Ruiz JA, Modelo-Sánchez A, Torres-Garzón L, Rendón-Infante JI, et al. Granular cell tumors: review of the parameters determining possible malignancy. Med Oral. 2003;8:294–8.
14. Torrijos-Aguilar A, Alegre-de Miquel V, Pitarch-Bort G, Mercader-García P, Fortea-Baixauli JM. Cutaneous granular cell tumor: a clinical and pathologic analysis of 34 cases. Actas Dermosifiliogr. 2009;100:126–32. [in Spanish]
15. Murray MR. Cultural characteristics of three granular-cell myoblastomas. Cancer. 1951;4:857–65.
16. Fisher ER, Wechsler H. Granular cell myoblastoma–a misnomer. Electron microscopic and histochemical evidence concerning its Schwann cell derivation and nature (granular cell schwannoma). Cancer. 1962;15:936–54.
17. Azzopardi JG. Histogenesis of granular-cell myoblastoma. J Pathol Bacteriol. 1956;71:85–94.
18. Pearse AG. The histogenesis of granular-cell myoblastoma (? Granular-cell perineural fibroblastoma). J Pathol Bacteriol. 1950;62:351–62.
19. Sobel HJ, Marquet E, Schwarz R. Is schwannoma related to granular cell myoblastoma? Arch Pathol. 1973;95:396–401.
20. Coleman MP, Freeman MR. Wallerian degeneration, wld(s), and nmnat. Annu Rev Neurosci. 2010;33:245–67.

24

Novel methodologies and technologies to assess mid-palatal suture maturation: a systematic review

Darren Isfeld[1], Manuel Lagravere[2]*, Vladimir Leon-Salazar[3,4] and Carlos Flores-Mir[5]

Abstract

Introduction: A reliable method to assess midpalatal suture maturation to drive clinical decision-making, towards non-surgical or surgical expansion, in adolescent and young adult patients is needed. The objectives were to systematically review and evaluate what is known regarding contemporary methodologies capable of assessing midpalatal suture maturation in humans.

Methods: A computerized database search was conducted using Medline, PubMed, Embase and Scopus to search the literature up until October 5, 2016. A supplemental hand search was completed of references from retrieved articles that met the final inclusion criteria.

Results: Twenty-nine abstracts met the initial inclusion criteria. Following assessment of full articles, only five met the final inclusion criteria. The number of subjects involved and quality of studies varied, ranging from an in-vitro study using autopsy material to prospective studies with in vivo human patients. Three types of evaluations were identified: quantitative, semi-quantitative and qualitative evaluations. Four of the five studies utilized computed tomography (CT), while the remaining study utilized non-invasive ultrasonography (US). No methodology was validated against a histological-based reference standard.

Conclusions: Weak limited evidence exists to support the newest technologies and proposed methodologies to assess midpalatal suture maturation. Due to the lack of reference standard validation, it is advised that clinicians still use a multitude of diagnostic criteria to subjectively assess palatal suture maturation and drive clinical decision-making.

Keywords: Cone-beam computed tomography, Palatal suture, Maxillary expansion

Background

Rapid maxillary expansion (RME) is indicated for a number of clinical situations namely when a posterior crossbite exists (unilateral or bilateral) or limited buccal overjet in patients with constricted maxillary base [1]. Maxillary transverse deficiency may be skeletal, dental or both skeletal and dental in origin [1–3]. Expansion in the transverse dimension has not only been used to improve interdigitation of the occlusion and improved function but also to increase arch perimeter to resolve maxillary crowding [2]. Recently contemporary orthodontics has focused on smile esthetics with emphasis on transverse arch dimensions and minimizing buccal corridor visibility [1, 4]. Those patients with dentofacial deformity or cleft lip and palate with constricted maxillary segments are candidates for RME or possible surgical expansion [2] dependent upon the time of treatment intervention. Additionally, there has been increased interest in the use of RME to increase nasal airway volume and/or function [1, 2].

Treatment options available to clinicians for maxillary expansion include tooth-borne expanders with or without an acrylic support [2, 5], bone-borne maxillary expansion devices supported by temporary (skeletal) anchorage devices [5], as well as surgically assisted rapid palatal expansion [1, 3]. The treatment of choice is dependent on numerous clinical indications including;

* Correspondence: manuel@ualberta.ca
[2]School of Dentistry, University of Alberta, Edmonton, 11405 - 87th avenue, Edmonton, AB T6G 1C9, Canada
Full list of author information is available at the end of the article

the extent of correction required, whether skeletal or dentoalveolar correction is indicated, and perceived efficacy of expansion based on timing of treatment [6].

The amount of skeletal or dentoalveolar effect of the RME is directly correlated with the stage of skeletal maturation of the palatal suture. Treatment timing of transverse deficiencies is recommended relatively early up to peak skeletal growth velocity [6]; however, there is significant variation in the timing of skeletal maturation amongst individuals [2, 6] as the palatal suture fusion is poorly correlated with patient age and sex [3]. Failure to properly identify key clinical signs and provide individual assessment to identify a patient's ideal expansion treatment option can lead to iatrogenic side effects and co-morbidities [3, 6]. Common side effects of poorly timed and failed conventional RME therapy include acute pain [2], gingival recession, dehiscence formation, palatal mucosa necrosis, buccal dentoalveolar tipping and poor long term expansion stability [3, 6]. Conversely prematurely committing a patient to surgically assisted expansion ascribes a patient to a potential significant burden of treatment including increased cost, pain and healing time.

Numerous methodologies have been proposed to discern the architecture and degree of palatal suture fusion including animal and human histologic studies, evaluation of occlusal radiographs, and CT of both autopsy material and animal specimens [3]. Such methodologies presented inherent difficulties in assessing the degree of palatal suture fusion. As defined previously, histological evaluation is the reference standard to evaluate midpalatal suture maturation, unfortunately implementation on active orthodontic patients would require an invasive biopsy, precluding its use [7, 8]. Conversely, serial occlusal radiographic assessment is limited in diagnostic quality due to superimposition of nearby anatomical structures [3]. Cone-beam CT (CBCT) allows for 3D rendering of the maxillofacial complex without superimposition of nearby anatomy and delivers a lower absorbed dose of radiation to the patient than medical CT [3]. To date, however, there has been no validated non-ionizing method to assess palatal suture maturation.

The objectives of this systematic review are to thoroughly describe and evaluate the contemporary technologies and methodologies capable of assessing midpalatal suture maturation.

Methods

The Preferred Reporting Items for Systematic Reviews and Meta-Analysis (PRISMA) statement checklist was followed; however, several points did not apply to this systematic review. This is a review of both in vitro and in vivo studies rather than solely in vivo studies, convoluting the direct comparison of results amongst these types of studies and their possible clinical inferences. No protocol registration was done.

Eligibility criteria

Both in vitro and in vivo studies will be included to identify all diagnostic modalities of palatal suture maturation. The intervention(s) will be any diagnostic method that is designed to evaluate the degree of ossification and/or interdigitation of the midpalatal suture (the outcome). Comparison will be to other diagnostic interventions designed to evaluate the same outcome variable.

The "participants" will be any human subjects or human specimens being investigated for the degree of midpalatal suture maturation. No animal studies were considered as their applicability in humans would be questionable.

Information sources

A computerized database search was conducted using Medline, PubMed, Embase and Scopus to search the literature ranging from 1980 up until October 5, 2016. A supplemental hand search was completed of references from retrieved articles that met the final inclusion criteria.

Search

Terms and their respective truncations used in the literature search (Appendix 1) were specific to each database. Searches were conducted with the help of a senior librarian who specializes in the health sciences. The selection process was carried out together by two researchers (DAI and HE). All references were managed by reference manager software EndNote to eliminate duplicates.

Study selection

The inclusion criterion "*Diagnostic methods to evaluate cranial suture ossification/maturation*" was utilized to initially identify possible articles from the published abstract results of the database search. If an abstract was not available, the full text was reviewed for appropriateness of inclusion. Any disagreement on the inclusion of a study was resolved by discussion amongst the reviewers.

Once these abstracts were selected, full articles were retrieved and inclusion in the systematic review was dependent of fulfilling a final inclusion criterion. The final selection criterion was as follows: "*In vitro and in vivo human subject studies that describe a novel diagnostic method or technology to assess midpalatal suture maturation/ossification over time*". Once more, any disagreement on the inclusion of a study following this final criterion was resolved by discussion amongst the reviewers. The references cited in the finally selected articles were also screened for any applicable references missed in the electronic database search.

Studies describing diagnostic methodologies applied to theoretical models without practical application were excluded. One article was excluded since no German translation was obtained. No other language restrictions were applied.

Data collection process
Data extraction was performed and collected by a researcher (DAI).

Data items
The variables collected included a description of the type of study, type and number of subjects, study objectives, inclusion criteria, imaging modality used, region(s) investigated, and methodology to evaluate degree of ossification/maturation of midpalatal suture (Tables 1 and 2).

Summary measures
The outcome measures included quantitative and/or qualitative results attained with applicable units to describe bone density, ossification or maturation of the palatal suture.

Synthesis of results
As the data was not considered homogeneous enough a meta-analysis was not conducted.

Results
Study selection
Twenty-nine abstracts met the initial inclusion criteria. Following retrieving of the full articles, only five met the final inclusion criteria. Reasons for exclusion due to final inclusion criteria are stated in Additional file 1. A hand-search of the reference lists from the articles that met the final inclusion criteria identified no new articles. Therefore, a total of five articles were finally considered (Fig. 1).

Study characteristics
The methodology of each selected article was summarized in Table 1 and results in Table 2. Study parameters, including the type of study, imaging modality used, methodology to determine the ossification/maturation of the palatal suture and the number of subjects amongst other variables were vastly different amongst the studies meeting the final inclusion criteria.

The studies varied significantly in the number of subjects evaluated and quality of evidence. The studies ranged from having three human subjects in a prospective study [9] to 140 human subjects in a cross-sectional study [3]. The types of studies ranged across the hierarchy of evidence from an in-vitro study [10] to prospective in vivo studies [9, 11].

The only study characteristic common to all studies was the region of interest (ROI) investigated, generally speaking, the maxilla. Four of the five studies [3, 9, 10, 12] had a single common ROI which was the palatal suture. One study [11] evaluated four ROIs in the palatal suture and surrounding hard tissue.

All studies but one utilized CT in some form. The types of CT scanners utilized in the four studies included multi-slice low-dose computed tomography (brand information not given) [11], dental CBCT [3] and the extremely high resolution Micro-CT [10]. One study [9] utilized a less invasive modality of US, specifically using color-coded US duplex scanner (Aplio 80, Toshiba, Tokyo, Japan).

To measure the degree of maturation/ossification at the palatal suture, one of three types of evaluations were utilized amongst the five studies: quantitative, semi-quantitative and qualitative.

Franchi et al [11] performed a quantitative evaluation of the palate using one blinded operator to calculate the radiodensity (Hounsfield units [HU]) of the ossification at the palatal suture from T0 (pre-expansion) and T2 (at 6 months retention).

Korbmacher et al. [10] also performed a quantitative evaluation of sutural maturation by measuring the maturation of the palate cadaver specimens at one time point. In the coronal plane, an obliteration index (%) and mean obliteration index (%) was calculated by comparison of the total length of the suture to the length that has ossified (evaluated every 370 μm). The degree of interdigitation of the palatal suture in the axial plane was assessed by calculating the interdigitation index, a comparison of the sutural distance (μm) to linear sutural distance (μm).

Angelieri et al [3] developed a novel qualitative methodology for individual evaluation of midpalatal suture maturation. Two evaluators defined the maturational stages (A-E) via comparison of the morphological description of the palatal suture found in previous histologic studies [13–15] to the appearance of the suture in the axial plane generated from a standardized CBCT protocol of 140 subjects during initial records [3] To assess the reliability of defining the maturational stages (A-E) a validation study utilizing 30 random axial CBCT cross-sections of the midpalatal suture was performed by three evaluators and weighted kappa coefficients calculated [3].

Kwak et al [12] utilized an objective and quantitative method of fractal analysis, a methodology established previously for the evaluation of mammalian cranial sutures, [16] to be used for the first time in conjunction with CBCT imaging to evaluate the maturity of the midpalatal suture [12]. The cross-sectional study involved 131 subjects (69 men and 62 women) with a mean age

Table 1 Summary of articles that met final inclusion criteria

Author(s)	Franchi et al. [11]	Sumer et al. [9]	Korbmacher et al. [10]	Angelieri et al. [3]	Kwak et al. [12]
Type of Study	Prospective study	Prospective study	In-vitro study	Cross-sectional	Cross-sectional
Human Subjects or Material	Human subjects	Human subjects	Human autopsy material	Human Subjects	Human subject
Study Objective(s)	Assess the midpalatal suture density via lowdose computed tomography (CT) prior to RME (T0), at the end of active RME (T1), and following a 6 month retention period (T2).	Evaluate the efficacy of ultrasonography (US) to generate a qualitative assessment of ossification post-SARME.	Quantification of sutural morphology via micro-CT and its association with age.	To validate and present a novel classification system for the individual assessment of midpalatal suture morphology using CBCT.	Evaluate the correlation of fractal patterning to ossification of the palatal suture via CBCT evaluation and determine whether fractal analysis of the midpalatal suture can be used to assess the maturation of the suture.
# of Subjects and Inclusion Criteria (if applicable)	17 patients, 7 male, 10 female, mean age of 11.2 years old, range of 8–14 years old. Inclusion criteria: patients with constricted maxillary arches with or without unilateral or bilateral posterior crossbite, and within cervical vertebral maturation (CS1–CS3)	3 patients; bilateral transverse maxillary deficiencies requiring SARME. Age, sex and developmental characteristics of subjects not given.	28 human-palate specimens, (11 female, 17 male) aged 14–71. The palatal specimens were categorized by the donor's age into age groups (< 25 years, 25 years to <30 years, ≥ 30 years).	140 subjects (86 female, 56 male), age range from 5.6 to 58.3 years old, Inclusion criteria: patients who are undergoing initial records for orthodontic treatment and who have received no previous orthodontic treatment.	131 subjects, (69 men and 62 women), mean age mean age of 24.1 ± 5.9 years (male subjects 23.1 ± 5.8 years, female subjects 25.2 ± 5.9 years) Age range of18.1–53.4 years old. No specific inclusion criteria noted
Study's Expansion Modality, Expansion protocol, Average amount of Expansion (mm)	Modality: butterfly palatal expander Protocol: standard protocol – activated twice per day (0.25 mm per turn) for 14 days. Retention period of 6 months than appliance removed. Amount of expansion: 7 mm in all subjects	Modality: SARME (tooth borne Hyrax). Protocol: 0.8–0.9 mm expansion/day in two daily activation steps until desired expansion achieved, ~14 days. Retention period of 6 months, then hyrax removed. Amount of expansion: not specified but based on clinical needs of patient.	Not applicable, no expansion performed.	Not applicable, no expansion performed.	Not applicable, no expansion performed
Imaging Modality	Multi-slice low-dose Computed tomography (brand information not given). Standardized axial CT images parallel to the palatal plane and passing through the furcation of maxillary right first molar, scans acquired and magnified (3×) with Light-Speed 16 software (General Electric Medical System, Milwaukee, WI).	Color-coded Ultrasonography duplex scanner (Aplio 80, Toshiba Tokyo, Japan) with 7.5-MHz linear-array transducer	Scanco Micro-CT 40 (Scanco Medical, Bassersdorf, Switzerland) 70 kV, 114 µA. Isotropic voxel size 37 µm. Maximum scanning time of 200 min/specimen. Data analyzed using V4.4A software (Scanco Medical, Bassersdorf, Switzerland). 3D reconstruction via AMIRA 3.00 software m(TGS, Mercury Computer Systems, San Diego, CA). Bone volume and quantification via Image Tool 3.00 software (UTHSCSA, San Antonio, TX),	iCAT cone-beam 3-dimensional imaging system (Imaging Sciences International, Hatfield, PA). 11 cm Minimum FOV. Scantime from 8.9 to 20 s resolution of 0.25 to 0.30 mm. Image analysis using InvivoS (Anatomage, San Jose, CA). A standardized protocol to isolate axial maxillary cross-sections of the palate was presented.	Cone Beam Computed Tomography (CBCT) (Zenith 3D; Vatech Co., Gveonggi-do, Korea) Field of view 20 × 19 cm; current 4.0 mA; scan time 24 s). Images were assessed using CT software (Ez3D 2009; Vatech Co.),

Table 1 Summary of articles that met final inclusion criteria *(Continued,*

Region(s) Investigated	Midpalatal suture and maxilla. 4 regions of interest (ROIs); 1. Anterior sutural ROI (AS ROI): located on the suture 5 mm anterior to nasopalatine 2. Posterior sutural ROI (PS ROI): on suture 5 mm posterior to the nasopalatine duct 3. Anterior bony ROI (AB ROI): control ROI on maxillary bone 3 mm to the right of laterally AS ROI 4. Posterior bony ROI (PB ROI): control ROI on maxillary bone 3 mm right of PS ROI	Midpalatal suture	Midpalatal suture	axial central cross-sectional slices generated and used for assessment of the mid-palatal suture	axial central cross-sectional slices generated and used for assessment of the midpalatal suture. A long and narrow region of interest within the final axial slice highlighting only the suture was considered for fractal analysis, such that the incisive canal was not incorporated, but rather the ROI extended from posterior to the incisive canal to just anterior to the posterior nasal spine.
Method of Measurements (units)	1 trained and blinded operator (R.L.) calculated bone density values in Hounsfield units (HU). RL performed all measurements and repeated all measurements 1 month later. Bone density changes from T0 through T2 at AS ROI and PS ROI contrasted with the Friedman repeated measures ANOVA on ranks and Tukey post-hoc test (SigmaStat 3.5, Systat Software, Point Richmond, CA).	Ultrasonography findings rated via a semi-quantitative bone fill score (0–3). 0 = complete through-transmission of the ultrasound waves, clear gap margins, and no echogenic material; 1 = partial through-transmission of the ultrasound waves, identifiable gap margins, and less than 50% echogenic material; 2 = partial through-transmission of the ultrasound waves, partially obscured gap margins, and greater than 50% echogenic material; 3 = no through transmission of the ultrasound waves, invisible gap margins, and 100% echogenic material. Scores were not supported by histology or CT.	Quantification of 3D Suture Morphology in frontal plane measured: calculated Obliteration index [%], and mean obliteration index [%]. Quantification of 3D Suture Morphology in Axial plane: measured sutural length [μm]: linear sutural distance [μm]: interdigitation index;	Definition of the proposed palatal suture maturational stages (A-E) determined by two operators. The definition of each palatal suture maturational stage derived from the histological appearance of suture described in previous histologic studies.	1 principal investigator trained in the Angelieri et al. [3] method categorized the midpalatal sutures of the patients, and the findings were considered the "ground truth" not "gold standard". Images were reclassified 2 days later two other operators classified 30 images to determine interexaminer reliability. For Fractal analysis, image software (Photoshop CS6 Extended; Adobe Systems, San Jose, CA) was utilized to perform Gaussian blurring and subtract this blurred image from the original, followed by skeletonizing of the binary image, and utilizing the box counting method to determine the fractal dimension. Weighted kappa coefficient was calculated to determine inter- and intra-examiner reliability using MedCalc version 12.3.0 (MedCalc Software, Oostende, Belgium). Fractal dimension at each maturation stage determined by Scheffe's ANOVA test. Spearman's correlation coefficient was calculated to determine the correlation between the fractal analysis and maturation stage. Utilized IBM SPSS Statistics version 21.0 software (IBM Co., Armonk, NY) $P < 0.05$ was considered statistically significant.

Table 1 Summary of articles that met final inclusion criteria *(Continued)*

| Measurement time points | Three time points; Before RME (T0), at the end of RME (T1), and after the 6 month retention period | 5 time points; after RME, at 2and 4 months during the expansion period, 6 months later where appliance removed and 2 months post appliance removal. Note opening of midpalatal suture confirmed by plain radiograph after active expansion. | One time point evaluated | Single time point evaluated prior to RME. Palatal maturational stage reclassified 2 days later for each patient. | Single time point Palatal maturational stage reclassified 2 days later for each patient.) . |

Table 2 Results and conclusions of articles meeting final inclusion criteria

Author(s)	Franchi et al. [11]	Sumer et al. [9]	Korbmacher et al. [10]	Angelieri et al. [3]	Kwak et al. [12]
Result(s)	Bone density in the AS ROI and the PS ROI at T0 (563.3 6183.2 HU and 741.7 6167.1 HU, respectively) were significantly smaller than values in the AB ROI and the PB ROI at T0 (1057.5 6129.4 HU and 1102.8 6160.9 HU, respectively). At T0 there was a significant difference in bone density at AS and PS ROIs, but no difference at T1 and T2. AS and PS ROIs showed significant decreases in density from T0 to T1, significant increases from T1 to T2, and no statistically significant differences from T0 to T2.	No statistics reported. Immediately post expansion all 3 patients had a bone fill score = 0. At 2 and 4 months of expansion there was low echogenicity in the suture (US bone fill score = 1) for 2 of 3 subjects. The remaining patient had a bone fill score = 2 at 2 and 4 months respectively. At 6 months post expansion and 2 months after expander removal, 2 of the 3 patients showed a qualitative increase in echogenic material in the suture was seen but less than 100% therefore had a bone fill score = 2, and the remaining patient demonstrated 100% echogenic material, bone fill score = 3. All trends in scores over time were qualitatively confirmed with plain radiographic images.	Frontal plane: No age dependent significance was found for the mean obliteration index ($P = 0.244$). The mean obliteration index was low, varying in all groups (minimum 0%; maximum 7.3%). Middle-aged group's mean obliteration index tended to be higher than that of either the younger or older age groups but no significant difference was calculated. The highest mean obliteration index (of 7.3%) was found in a 44-year-old male. The oldest individual with a mean obliteration index of 0% was a 71-year-old female. At least one frontal slice per palate – even in the oldest age group – exhibited a suture completely open cranio-caudally. Axial plane: No significant differences detected in all age groups regarding means and standard deviations for suture length, linear sutural distance, and interdigitation index. Interdigitation index computed revealed no significant age-dependent differences ($P = 0.633$). High standard deviation values for suture length, linear sutural distance and interdigitation index were seen in the <25 yo group and >30 yo group, while the 25–30 yo group had far less variation Mean error of measurement amounted to 0.12% for the obliteration index, 2.4% for the suture length, and 0.41% for the linear sutural distance.	The intraexaminer and interexaminer reproducibility values demonstrated agreement, with weighted kappa coefficients from 0.75 (95% CI, 0.57–0.93) to 0.79 (95%CI, 0.60–0.97), and the reproducibility of examiners with the ground truth demonstrated agreement with weighted kappa coefficients from 0.82 (95% CI, 0.64–0.99) to 0.93 (95% CI, 0.86–1.00). From the 140 subject sample, stage A was observed in children from 5 to approximately 11 years of age, a 13 year old boy was the sole exception. Should be noted there was no fusion of the palatal suture in subjects aged 5 to almost 11 years old. Stage B was observed primarily up to 13 years of age but also 6 of 32 subjects (23% of boys, 15.7% of girls) aged 14 to 18 years old. Stage C primarily depicted from 11 to 18 years of age, with exception being two 10-year-old girls (8.3% of girls) and 4 of 32 adults (15.7% of girls, 7.7% of boys). Stage D was observed in 1 of 24 girls aged 11– <14 years old, and 3 of 19 girls aged 14–18 years old, as well as in 3 of 13 males aged 14–18 years old and >18 years old respectively. Stage E was observed in 5 of 24 females aged 11– < 14 years old and 8 of 19 females aged 14–18 years old and 8 of 19 females aged >18 years old. Stage E was observed in far less males, approximately 9 of 13 males aged >18 years old only.	The intra- and inter-examiner reliability analysis demonstrated agreement for fractal dimension, with a weighted kappa coefficient of 0.84 (95% [CI] 0.74–0.93) and 0.67 (95% CI 0.38–0.95) to 0.72 (95% CI 0.48–0.97) respectively. No subjects had a CVM of 1–IV nor maturational stage A present. 13 of 21 subjects with CVM V were found to have maturational stage B or C (61.9%; males 77.8%, females 50.0%). 42 of 110 subjects with CVM VI were found to have maturational stage B or C (38.2%; males 41.6%, females 34.0%). Post-hoc analysis demonstrated that maturational stages B, C, D and E were related to differences in mean fractal dimension ($P < 0.05$). A negative correlation existed between fractal dimension and maturation stage (−0.623, $P < 0.001$). Male and Female correlation coefficients determined to be −0.649 ($P < 0.001$) and −0.569 ($P < 0.001$) respectively. A receiver operating characteristic (ROC) curve determined the boundary between maturation stages A–C and D or E. Fusion of palatal suture was determinable as a fractal dimension. Fractal dimension is a statistically significant indicator capable of predicting dichotomous maturation stages ((A, B, & C) vs. (D or E) (area under ROC curve [AUC] = 0.794, $P < 0.001$). At optimal fractal dimension cut-off value of 1.0235, statistical analysis to evaluate the predictive ability of fractal analysis to determine maturation stage ((A, B, & C) vs. (D or E)), noted the following values; specificity 86.6%, Sensitivity 64.9%, false positive rate 35.1%, false negative rate 13.4%, positive predictability

Table 2 Results and conclusions of articles meeting final inclusion criteria *(Continued)*

Conclusion(s)				
Prepubertal subjects demonstrated a lower bone density at the mid palatal suture as compared to the lateral control ROIs on ossified maxillary bone. The post-expansion low bone density at the sutural ROIs supported findings that prepubertal RME effectively opens the suture. Six months of retention following RME allows reorganization and ossification of the midpalatal suture with sutural bone density values similar to pre-RME values.	Ultrasound bone fill scores increased directly with the duration of time post active expansion (authors referred to this as part of the expansion period) Non-invasive US can yield accurate information regarding bone formation at the midpalatal suture in patients undergoing SARME.	Authors note Micro CT analysis disproves the hypothesis of progressive closure of the suture directly related to patient age. Skeletal age and/or calculation of an obliteration index is not useful in terms of diagnostic criteria to drive clinical decision making regarding the perceived efficacy of non-surgical RME. Micro-CT Quantification of the midpalatal suture yields very low obliteration and age- independent interdigitation in the coronal plane. All calculated parameters demonstrated substantial inter-individual and intra-sutural variation.	Utilizing CBCT to assess the midpalatal suture avoids any overlapping of soft and hard tissues. Authors note that their proposed methodology may be useful in reliably driving clinical decision making as it relates to pursing a non-surgical (RME) or surgical expansion intervention (SARME).	80.3%, and negative predictability 74.6%. Adult patients possess a greater proportion of non-fused palatal sutures than what is assumed. Therefore age of the patient should not drive SARME initiation. Authors report a significant correlation between fractal dimension and degree of maturation of the midpalatal suture Determination of the fractal dimension cut-off value could be used as a reference to pursue RME vs. SARME Fractal analysis can be utilized to evaluate the degree of maturation at the palatal suture.

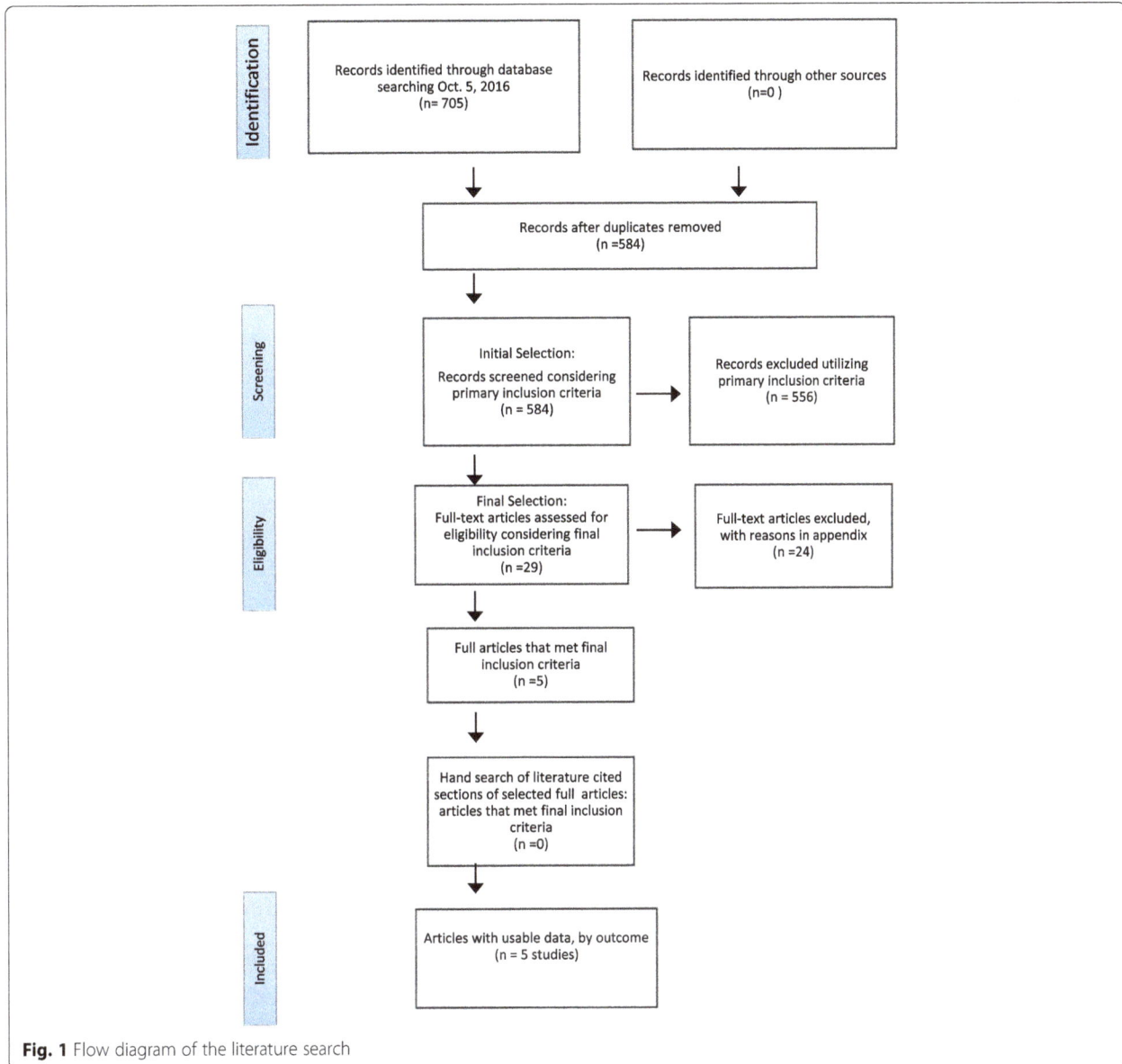

Fig. 1 Flow diagram of the literature search

of 24.1 ± 5.9 years. Each subject underwent CBCT imaging, followed by significant image processing to evaluate Cervical Vertebrae Maturation (CVM) stage, palatal stage of maturation (A-E, as defined by Angelieri et al. [3]) and isolation of a ROI for the calculation of the fractal dimension of the palatal suture. To assess the intra- and inter-reliability of defining the maturational stages (A-E), 30 random axial CBCT cross-sections of the mid-palatal suture were staged by two other evaluators under controlled conditions and weighted kappa coefficients calculated, analogous to the study by Angelieri et al. [3] Statistical analysis included utilizing Scheffe's ANOVA to compare the fractal dimension for each individual maturation stage (A-E) and subsequent Spearman's coefficient calculation to ascertain the correlation between fractal dimension and maturation stage. The generation

of a receiver operating characteristic (ROC) curve was used to develop an optimal fractal dimension cut-off value and sensitivity, specificity, false positive rate, false negative rate, positive predictability, and negative predictability calculated. For all statistical analysis, results were considered statistically significant at $P < 0.05$ [12].

Sumer et al. [9] utilized US to evaluate palatal sutural mineralization in three patients at five different time points; once after the 14 day surgically-assisted RME (SARME) expansion protocol, 2 months post-expansion, 4 months post-expansion, at time of removal of the tooth-borne expander (6 months post-expansion) and 2 months after appliance removal. The authors report that the ultrasound probe was used intra-orally on the skin that overlies the palatal suture, obtaining axial scans with the probe directed perpendicular to the length of the suture [9]. The authors assigned semi-quantitative bone fill scores (0–3). A bone fill score = 0 was characterized by open suture with clean gap margins and 0% echogenic material. A bone fill score = 1 was characterized by partial ultrasound transmission, localization of gap margins, and reduced echogenic material of ≤50%. A bone fill score = 2 was characterized by partial ultrasound transmission, marginally visible gap margins, and increased echogenic material of >50%. A bone fill score = 3 was characterized by no ultrasound transmission, 100% echogenic readings, and unidentifiable gap margins. The bone filling trends were qualitatively supported by comparison to conventional occlusal radiography [9].

Synthesis of results
Due to high methodological heterogeneity among the included studies a meta-analysis was not supported.

Risk of bias across studies
Each proposed technology or methodology to assess the maturation of the palatal suture lacked validation with a reference standard, namely histological evaluation. There was a lack of homogeneity in the quality of evidence amongst all five studies, ranging from an in-vitro study on human autopsy material [10] to human subject prospective studies [9, 11]. Sample sizes across all studies varied greatly, from 3 subjects [9] to a high of 140 subjects in a human subject cross-sectional study [3].

Additional analysis
Not applicable due to lack of meta-analysis.

Discussion
Summary of evidence
Modality #1 – Multi-slice low-dose CT and quantitative bone density measurements (HU).
A technique to assess palatal suture maturation includes the use of multi-slice low-dose CT to capture axial slices of the maxilla and quantitatively measure the bone density at a particular ROI in HU [11]. It is known that CT is an excellent modality to evaluate the localized architecture of cancellous and cortical bone of the jaws; [17] however, less is known regarding the quantitative measurement of bone density, the HU scale. Hus were first utilized in dentistry to evaluate the pre-surgical bone density of implant sites [17–19]. The HU scale is a linear transformation of tissue attenuation coefficients where air is defined as −1000 HU, distilled water at standardized conditions equal to 0 HU and very dense bone defined as ≥1000 HU [17]. Consequently the authors considered and utilized the calculated Hus as an applicable unit of measurement to quantitatively assess mineralization at the palatal suture [11].

Franchi et al. [11] utilized the Houndsfield quantitative scale to evaluate the radiodensity of four previously mentioned ROI in the maxilla, 2 sutural and 2 bony areas. Pre-expansion (T0) statistical analysis noted a significant difference between the anterior and postural sutural regions (563.3 ± 183.29 HU and 741.7 ± 167.1 HU) and anterior and posterior bony areas (1057.5± 129.4 HU and 1102.8 ± 160.9 HU) ($P < 0.05$) (Table 2). Further statistical analysis yielded a significant difference between the anterior sutural and posterior sutural landmarks at T0 ($P < 0.05$), but no significant differences of these sutural areas at T1 or T2 ($P > 0.05$, Mann-Whitney). A significant difference between the radiodensity of the anterior and postural sutural ROIs between T0 and immediately post-expansion (T1), but no difference between their radiodensities when comparing pretreatment (T0) and the post-expansion retention phase (T2) readings ($P < 0.05$) (Table 2).

Throughout the course of the study, trends in bone density measurements at the suture and its comparison to lateral bony sites followed conventional expectations of successful RME. Pre-expansion the measured HU at the anterior sutural region was significantly smaller than that of the posterior sutural site, and the applied expansion protocol introduced differential sutural opening with greatest opening at the anterior sutural region consistent with the pre-expansion HU scores. Additionally, the results measured at T2 at the end of the 6 month RME retention protocol, were congruent with previous histologic findings, namely post-expansion evidence of reorganization and sutural interdigitation [20].

An inherent advantage of using a low-dose CT protocol, where the voltage was decreased to 80 kV (KV), is subjecting the patient to a lower absorbed dose required for children undergoing radiologic evaluation [21]. Additionally, when the kilovoltage is reduced, image contrast of anatomical structures increases while still acceptable for assessing bone quality via this protocol [21]. Future areas of interest relating to the findings and protocol of this study would include further studies to define an anterior sutural HU: postural sutural HU ratio that best predicts the success of RME treatment. Conversely, further studies could elucidate specific ratios comparing sutural radiodensity to maxillary bony radiodensity that may predict an improved expansion prognosis.

It has to be noted that the reliability of using HU between subjects and within the same subjects the same day has not been demonstrated. Therefore some variation could be due to such factors. Also, not all studies specified patient orientation when taking the images thus effect of patient positioning on the image and HU or grey values is another aspect that should be tested.

Modality #2 – Micro-CT quantification of 3D palatal suture in the frontal and axial planes.

Korbmacher et al. [10] proposed assessing palatal suture maturation via micro-CT scanning and calculation of a number of developed indices, namely the obliteration index (%) and mean obliteration index (%) in the frontal plane, as well as, suture length [μm], linear sutural distance [μm] and interdigitation index in the axial plane.

Korbmacher et al. [10] evaluated 28 human palate specimens in the frontal and axial planes. In the frontal plane there was no demonstrated age dependent difference in the mean obliteration index between specimens (P = 0.244). The specimens were classified into one of three age groups (<25 years of age (yo), ≥25 to <30 yo and ≥30 yo) and results demonstrate that the frontal plane obliteration index varied across age groups between a minimum index of 0% to a maximum interdigitation of 7.3% (44 yo patient) (Table 2). Although the ≥25 to <30 yo age group consistently had a higher obliteration index in the frontal plane compared to other age groups, the results were not significant. Across all age groups, each subject had at least one frontal sutural cross-section that was devoid of interdigitation (mean obliteration index of 0%), with the oldest patient exhibiting a frontal plane mean obliteration index of 0% being a 71yo female. Investigation into the degree of interdigitation in the axial plane demonstrated no significant age-dependent differences in the calculated interdigitation index (P = 0.633). The authors did report a large standard deviation in the interdigitation index in the axial plane in the youngest and oldest age groups, and considerably less variation in the calculated index in the middle (<25 yo group and >30 yo) group [10] (Table 2).

Results indicated a generally low obliteration index amongst all subjects as well as an age-independent degree of interdigitation in the axial plane; however, across all measured indices there was significant intra-sutural and inter-subject variation [10]. This was the first time micro-CT was used on human samples and although this methodology was not implemented as part of an active expansion study, its principles can still be important to evaluate the pre-expansion maturity of the palatal suture. Additionally, it could be applied during mid-expansion protocol to evaluate the efficacy of treatment via calculation of the above noted indices and evaluation of the sutural architecture.

A limiting feature of the Korbmacher et al. [10] modality is the fact cadaver specimens were used, making direct translation of this study's findings poorly applicable to clinical practice [15]. Considering the limitations of the gantry size of the micro-CT unit, and maximum scanning time used (200 min), micro-CT is best used on ex-vivo samples, and very small in-vivo samples to avoid an excessive absorbed dose emitted to patients [22].

Consequently, the use of micro-CT for in-vivo radiologic evaluation of the palate is impractical at this time. Therefore continued improvements to micro-CT technology including decreasing the emitted radiation while maintaining superior resolution, is necessary prior to implementation of such a technique on active RME patients.

An area of interest is the development of a CT-based strain assessment of peri-sutural and maxillary tissues; the development of which the authors believe will help facilitate predicting the success of RME treatment [10].

Modality #3 - US and assignment of semi-quantitative bone fill scores (0–3).

Sumer et al. [9] utilized US to evaluate sutural mineralization at five time points during the SARME and retention protocol for three patients, scoring each patient's palatal suture calcification via assignment of semi-quantitative bone fill scores (0–3).

US findings in the Sumer et al. [9] study demonstrated that immediately post-expansion all subjects had a bone fill score = 0. (Table 2) Two of the three subjects at 2 and 4 months post-expansion were identified as having a bone score = 1, while the remaining subject was determined to have a bone fill score = 2 for these same time periods. Following the removal of the tooth-borne appliance at 6 months and 2 months subsequent to that during continued fixed appliance therapy, the bone scores for two of the subjects demonstrated increased mineralization and identification of echogenic material, having bone fill scores =2. The remaining patient received a bone fill score = 3 due to incomplete transmission of the waves and 100% echogenicity measured at these respective time points [9]. (Table 2) It should be noted that no statistics were reported by the authors.

The results of this study follow those of a similar animal study, [23] such that there was a statistically significant increase in bone fill scores that were directly related to the length of time the patient has been in retention post expansion. A major advantage to US is its low cost and non-invasiveness, [9, 23, 24] as well as improved usability compared to other methodologies, with the ability to perform real-time chair side evaluations with smaller hand held units. Additionally, US is a reliable method to image early bone formation as demonstrated by previous studies involving distraction osteogenesis [9, 23, 24]. A study comparing US to normal panoramic radiography, demonstrated that the efficacy of US to measure an osteotomy gap during distraction osteogenesis is equal to that of conventional radiography [9, 25]. US also demonstrated increased reliability compared to panoramic radiography to evaluate the maturation of early bone formation [9, 25] in the distraction gap. A disadvantage to US is its inability to penetrate cortical bone [9] However, following SARME or successful RME the osteotomy gap and its margins are easily visualized [9]. An area of significant future interest is to ascertain whether this technology can penetrate an immature midpalatal suture prior to the start of RME treatment, and allow the clinician to perform a chair side subjective evaluation of the bone maturity and interdigitation along the whole length of the suture. Limitations to this study included a very small sample size of three patients and lack of a gold standard (histology) or CT to validate the findings. Consequently, an area of future research is the use of this technology and bone fills scores in a similar larger sample size study in conjunction with a gold standard methodology to support the findings [9].

Modality #4 - CBCT and proposed maturation stages.

Angelieri et al. [3] utilized a standardized methodology to capture axial CBCT cross-sections of the palatal suture to provide individual staging of midpalatal suture maturation from the authors' proposed maturation stages (A-E).

As it relates to Angelieri et al. [3] a validation study performed reported a weighted Kappa statistic for intra- and interexaminer reliability to be κ =0.75 (95% Confidence Interval (CI), 0.64–0.99) and be κ =0.79 (95% CI, 0.60–0.97) (no P-value reported), respectively. Due to a lack of an histologic or microCT gold standard, the authors also reported examiner reliability compared to the "ground truth", a descriptor used to represent consensus among examiners with the principal investigator' radiographic evaluations or other interpretations. Examiner reliability with ground truth ranged from κ = 0.82 (95% CI, 0.64–0.99) to κ =0.93 (95% CI, 0.86–1.00) (no P-value reported) [3].

Results of the validation study demonstrated "almost perfect" inter-examiner reliability with the "ground truth", however, the authors did not report appropriate P-values with their statistics. As was mentioned before, there was no reference standard utilized during the validation study, but rather utilized what the authors termed the "ground truth", [3] the professional opinion of the principal investigator when utilizing their own proposed maturation stages to classify each patient's sutural maturation. Due to the lack of a gold standard, nor listed P-values, the results of the validation should be interpreted with caution. An additional limitation of this methodology is the proposed novel palatal suture maturation classification system itself. The authors developed the stages (A-E) based on comparison of CBCT axial cross-sections of the palatal suture to the perceived likeness of this radiographic morphology to the histological morphology of the suture as determined by

previous studies [13–15]. Theoretically direct comparison of the histological morphology to the CBCT morphology of the suture is incompatible due to the histological assessment being on the microscopic scale as compared to the macro or eye level scale of sutures depicted in the CBCT axial slices. Consequently, any inference or direct translation of the sutural histological appearance and subsequent development of CBCT based sutural maturation stages is not possible. Therefore, the findings and developed maturational stages should be used with caution, and should not drive clinical decision making. Rather, at best, this maturational staging may be used as part of an extended protocol to subjectively assess palatal suture maturity during the treatment planning process. Future studies to thoroughly validate the proposed maturation stages to an available gold standard are advised.

Modality #5 – CBCT and fractal analysis to quantitatively ascertain degree of sutural maturation per proposed maturation stages of Anglieri et al. [3]

Kwak et al. [12] utilized CBCT imaging in conjunction with quantitative fractal analysis to ascertain if this analysis can be correlated to the maturational stage of each subjects palatal suture. Conceptually fractal analysis is based on the observation that cranial sutures can be visualized as a fractal pattern, [16] the dimensions of which are directly related to localized stresses experienced [12]. Additionally, the closer the approximation of two articulating bones, the more complex sutural morphology [12] suggestive of a more mature suture. Conceptually sound, fractal analysis has demonstrated its applicability in various areas dental research [26].

Fractal dimension intra- and inter-reliability results from the Kwak et al. [12] study demonstrated agreement with calculated weighted kappa coefficients of 0.84 (95% CI 0.74–0.93) and 0.67 (95% CI 0.38–0.95) to 0.72 (95% CI 0.48–0.97), respectively (Table 2). The CVM index inter- and intra-examiner reliability demonstrated agreement with weighted kappa coefficients from 0.69 (95% CI 0.53–0.86) and 0.71 (95% CI 0.56–0.86), respectively. The authors reported that none of the patients investigated possessed a CVM 1-IV nor was any subject classified as having palatal suture maturational stage A. It was found that 13 of 21 subjects with CVM V were classified as having maturational stage B or C (61.9%; males 77.8%, females 50.0%). Additionally, 42 of 110 subjects with CVM VI were classified as having maturational stage B or C (38.2%; males 41.6%, females 34.0%). Post-hoc analysis demonstrated that maturational stages B, C, D and E were related to differences in mean fractal dimension (P < 0.05). A negative correlation existed between fractal dimension and maturation stage (−0.623, $P < 0.001$). Male and female correlation coefficients were determined to be −0.649 ($P < 0.001$) and −0.569 ($P < 0.001$) respectively. A ROC curve was generated and determined the boundary between dichotomous maturation stages A–C and D or E, allowing for fractal dimension to be used to identify midpalatal suture fusion. Predictive statistical analysis noted that fractal dimension is a statistically significant indicator capable of predicting dichotomous maturation stages ((A, B, & C) vs. (D or E) (area under ROC curve [AUC] = 0.794, $P < 0.001$) [12] (Table 2).

The study notes a significant correlation between fractal patterning and degree of maturation of the midpalatal suture, and consequently the authors feel that fractal analysis can provide an objective and quantitative methodology to assess palatal suture maturity [12].

Disadvantages of this methodology include requiring significant training and proficiency in classifying the maturation stage of palatal sutures as proposed by Angelieri et al. [3]. Another disadvantage is requiring the clinician to have significant familiarity with image processing and possessing necessary software. Consequently, the time, cost and resources to do so may be prohibitive to clinicians. Additionally, this modality relies on complex statistical analyses to determine the variable (optimal cut-off value) to predict the dichotomous maturation stage of the patient's palatal suture. Kwak et al. [12] argue that if an individual's fractal dimensions can be compared, it may provide a straightforward and clinically viable method to assess the maturation of the palatal suture and aid in clinical decision making as it relates to the modality of expansion at the diagnostic record visit [12]. Conversely, the authors do note a variety of methods to calculate fractal dimensions and the fact these varying techniques produce different fractal dimension values. Consequently, Kwak et al. [12] argue for a more agreed upon method for its calculation to be utilized clinically.

Performing and interpreting these analyses requires significant advanced knowledge of statistics. Ultimately it is the view of the authors that this methodology is impractical in terms of time, cost, resources and knowledge required to complete this methodology for each patient as part of their diagnostic work up in day-to-day clinical practice.

Furthermore, as was stated previously in the discussion, utilization of the crudely proposed maturational staging as defined by Angelieri et al. [3] should be used with caution and lacks validation to a reference standard as does this study as mentioned by Kwak et al. [12]. Further areas of interest include

the development of a ratio comparing the fractal dimensions of a mature coronal suture to that of the midpalatal suture [12]. Additionally, improvement in the accuracy of the methodology may be gained by refinement and minimization of the number of actions needed to determine fractal dimensions [12].

Limitations

As mentioned before significant methodological differences were identified (sample size, in vitro vs. in vivo, imaging technique used, lack of adequate reference standard). The results were non-homogenous consequently a meta-analysis could not be performed, nor direct comparison of the studies possible, limiting any major conclusions regarding these newer contemporary methodologies to assess midpalatal sutural maturation. Overall, these studies did not present solid evidence of their validity for the accurate determination of the maturation of the palatal suture. As a consequence of this weak body of evidence, it is of utmost importance that clinicians use a multitude of diagnostic criteria to properly direct clinical decision making as it pertains to the maturity of the mid palatal suture and appropriate modality of expansion, namely RME or SARME. It is worth noting that expansion does not solely involve the palatal suture but also the circummaxillary sutures, this would also be a limitation present.

Conclusions

- Only a weak limited body of evidence exists to support the newest technologies and proposed methodologies that evaluate the extent of mid palatal suture maturation.
- All discussed novel methodologies lack validation with histological reference/gold standard. Consequently, it is still advised that clinicians use a multitude of diagnostic criteria to subjectively assess palatal suture maturation and drive clinical decision-making as it relates to the appropriate treatment of maxillary skeletal transverse deficiency in late adolescents and young adults (RME vs. SARME).
- Future considerations in the imaging and assessment of the midpalatal sutural maturation will likely include some form of invasive CT technology, and proposed methodologies should follow appropriate ALARA radiation safety protocols.
- Non-invasive imaging technologies such as ultrasound present a promising and biologically safer alternative to assess midpalatal sutural ossification.

Appendix

Table 3 Database search and results

Database	Keywords	New
Medline	(1) Palate.mp or exp. palate/ or ex palate, Hard/ (2) Cranial suture. mp or exp. cranial sutures (3) Maturation.mp (4) Interdigitation.mp or exp. cranial sutures (5) Ossification.mp 1 and 2 and (3 or 4 or 5)	221
Pubmed	(("palate") AND "cranial sutures") AND (("maturation" OR "interdigitation" OR "ossification"))	31
Embase	(1) Palate.mp or exp. palate/ or ex primary palate/ or exp. secondary palate or exp., hard palate/ (2) Cranial suture. mp or exp. cranial suture; (3) Exp maturation/ or exp. bone maturation/ or maturation.mp (4) Interdigitation.mp (5) Ossification.mp or exp. ossification/ 1 and 2 and (3 or 4 or 5)	31
Scopus	Palate AND cranial sutures AND (maturation OR interdigitation OR ossification) Subjects limited to Medicine, biochemistry, genetics and molecular biology, dentistry Documents limited to articles only	422

Abbreviations
CBCT: Cone-beam computed tomography; CT: Computed tomography; 2D: Two-dimensional; 3D: Three-dimensional; RME: Rapid maxillary expansion; SARME: Surgically assisted rapid maxillary expansion; US: Ultrasonography; PRISMA: Preferred Reporting Items for Systematic Reviews and Meta-Analysis; ROI: Region of Interest; HU: Hounsfield Units; CVM: Cervical Vertebrae Maturation; ROC: Receiver Operating Characteristic; T0: Pre-expansion; T1: Post-expansion; T2: Retention phase; KV: Kilovolts; CI: Confidence interval

Acknowledgements
Not applicable.

Funding
There is no source of funding for the research reported.

Authors' contributions
DI collected the data, analyzed and interpreted the results and wrote the manuscript. CF, VLS and ML mentored DI and participated in planning the study, analyzing the data, and writing the manuscript. All authors read and approved the final manuscript.

Competing interests
The authors declare they have no competing interests in this work.

Author details
[1]Orthodontic Graduate Program, School of Dentistry University of Alberta, Edmonton, AB, Canada. [2]School of Dentistry, University of Alberta, Edmonton, 11405 - 87th avenue, Edmonton, AB T6G 1C9, Canada. [3]Division of Pediatric Dentistry, School of Dentistry, University of Minnesota, Minneapolis, MN, USA. [4]Orthodontic Graduate Program, School of Dentistry, University of Alberta, Edmonton, AB, Canada. [5]School of Dentistry, University of Alberta, Edmonton, AB, Canada.

References
1. McNamara JA. Maxillary transverse deficiency. Am J Orthod Dentofac Orthop. 2000;117:567–70.
2. Bishara SE, Staley RN. Maxillary expansion: clinical implications. Am J Orthod Dentofac Orthop. 1987;91:3–14.
3. Angelieri F, Cevidanes LH, Franchi L, Gonçalves JR, Benavides E, McNamara JA Jr. Midpalatal suture maturation: classification method for individual assessment before rapid maxillary expansion. Am J Orthod Dentofac Orthop. 2013;144:759–69.
4. Isiksal E, Hazar S, Akyalcin S. Smile esthetics: perception and comparison of treated and untreated smiles. Am J Orthod Dentofac Orthop. 2006;129:8–16.
5. Lin L, Ahn HW, Kim SJ, Moon SC, Kim SH, Nelson G. Tooth-borne vs bone-borne rapid maxillary expanders in late adolescence. Angle Orthod. 2015;85:253–62.
6. Baccetti T, Franchi L, Cameron CG, McNamara JA Jr. Treatment timing for rapid maxillary expansion. Angle Orthod. 2001;71:343–50.
7. Melsen B. Palatal growth studied on human autopsy material. A histologic microradiographic study. Am J Orthod. 1975;68:42–54.
8. Persson M, Thilander B. Palatal suture closure in man from 15 to 35 years of age. Am J Orthod. 1977;72:42–52.
9. Sumer AP, Ozer M, Sumer M, Danaci M, Tokalak F, Telcioglu NT. Ultrasonography in the evaluation of midpalatal suture in surgically assisted rapid maxillary expansion. J Craniofac Surg. 2012;23:1375–7.
10. Korbmacher H, Schilling A, Püschel K, Amling M, Kahl-Nieke B. Age-dependent three-dimensional microcomputed tomography analysis of the human midpalatal suture. J Orofac Orthop. 2007;68:364–76.
11. Franchi L, Baccetti T, Lione R, Fanucci E, Cozza P. Modifications of midpalatal sutural density induced by rapid maxillary expansion: a low-dose computed-tomography evaluation. Am J Orthod Dentofac Orthop. 2010;137:486–8. discussion 12A-13A
12. Kwak KH, Kim SS, Kim YI, Kim YD. Quantitative evaluation of midpalatal suture maturation via fractal analysis. Korean J Orthod. 2016;46:323–30.
13. Persson M, Magnusson BC, Thilander B. Sutural closure in rabbit and man: a morphological and histochemical study. J Anat. 1978;125:313–21.
14. Cohen MM Jr. Sutural biology and the correlates of craniosynostosis. Am J Med Genet. 1993;47:581–616.
15. Sun Z, Lee E, Herring SW. Cranial sutures and bones: growth and fusion in relation to masticatory strain. Anat Rec A Discov Mol Cell Evol Biol. 2004;276:150–61.
16. Yu JC, Wright RL, Williamson MA, Braselton JP 3rd, Abell ML. A fractal analysis of human cranial sutures. Cleft Palate Craniofac J. 2003;40:409–15.
17. Shapurian T, Damoulis PD, Reiser GM, Griffin TJ, Ran WM. Quantitative evaluation of bone density using the Hounsfield index. Int J Oral Maxillofac Implants. 2006;21:290–7.
18. Duckmanton NA, Austin BW, Lechner SK, Klineberg IJ. Imaging for predictable maxillary implants. Int J Prosthodont. 1994;7:77–80.
19. Norton MR, Gamble C. Bone classification: an objective scale of bone density using the computerized tomography scan. Clin Oral Implants Res. 2001;12:79–84.
20. Cleall JF, Bayne DI, Posen JHM, Subtelny JD. Expansion of the midpalatal suture in the monkey. Angle Orthod. 1965;35:23–35.

21. Ballanti F, Lione R, Fanucci E, Franchi L, Baccetti T, Cozza P. Immediate and post-retention effects of rapid maxillary expansion investigated by computed tomography in growing patients. Angle Orthod. 2009;79:24–9.

22. Perilli E, Parkinson IH, Reynolds KJ. Micro-CT examination of human bone: from biopsies towards the entire organ. Ann Ist Super Sanita. 2012;48:75–82.

23. Thurmüller P, Troulis M, O'Neill MJ, Kaban LB. Use of ultrasound to assess healing of a mandibular distraction wound. J Oral Maxillofac Surg. 2002;60:1038–44.

24. Hughes CW, Williams RW, Bradley M, Irvine GH. Ultrasound monitoring of distraction osteogenesis. Br J Oral Maxillofac Surg. 2003;41:256–8.

25. Bruno C, Minniti S, Buttura-da-Prato E, Albanese M, Nocini PF, Pozzi-Mucelli R. Gray-scale ultrasonography in the evaluation of bone callus in distraction osteogenesis of the mandible: initial findings. Eur Radiol. 2008;18:1012–7.

26. Sánchez I, Uzcátegui G. Fractals in dentistry. J Dent. 2011;39:273–92.

25

Head circumference - a useful single parameter for skull volume development in cranial growth analysis?

Markus Martini[1,4]* , Anne Klausing[1], Guido Lüchters[2], Nils Heim[1] and Martina Messing-Jünger[3]

Abstract

Background: The measurement of maximal head circumference is a standard procedure in the examination of childrens' cranial growth and brain development. The objective of the study was to evaluate the validity of maximal head circumference to cranial volume in the first year of life using a new method which includes ear-to-ear over the head distance and maximal cranial length measurement.

Methods: 3D surface scans for cranial volume assessment were conducted in this method comparison study of 44 healthy Caucasian children (29 male, 15 female) at the ages of 4 and 12 months.

Results: Cranial volume increased from measurements made at 4 months to 12 months of age by an average of 1174 ± 106 to 1579 ± 79 ml. Maximal cranial circumference increased from 43.4 ± 9 cm to 46.9 ± 7 cm and the ear-to ear measurement increased from 26.3 ± 21 cm to 31.6 ± 18 cm at the same time points. There was a monotone association between maximal head circumference (HC) and increase in volume, yet a backwards inference from maximal circumference to the volume had a predictive value of only 78% (adjusted R^2). Including the additional measurement of distance from ear to ear strengthened the ability of the model to predict the true value attained to 90%. The addition of the parameter skull length appeared to be negligible.

Conclusion: The results demonstrate that for a distinct improvement in the evaluation of a physiological cranial volume development, the additional measurement of the ear-to ear distance using a measuring tape is expedient, and, especially for cases with pathological skull changes, such as craniosynostosis, ought to be conducted.

Keywords: Head circumference, Validity, Ear-to-ear measurement, Skull volume, 3d scan, Cranial growth

Background

The measurement of maximal head circumference ([HC] or occipito-frontal circumference [OFC]) has been a standard procedure in the examination of childrens' cranial growth and brain development for decades [1–4]. It is a quick, simple and economic screening method without the danger of exposure to radiation. Early detection of pathological changes are ascertained with this method. Normative data for pediatric cranial circumference and braincase volume are of multidisciplinary interest. In addition to its primary importance for differential diagnosis and therapy decisions for neurosurgical, maxillofacial- and plastic surgery, [5, 6], as well as for anthropological study of evolution [7, 8], these measurements are of immense importance to pediatric doctors and neurologists [9–13]. The collection of exact cranial volume data and anthropometric parameters is, for this reason, the subject of countless studies [14–19]. Improvements in cranial volume measurement methods rely increasingly on 3D databases. This type of data acquisition can occur in a semi-automatic manner using CT [20–22] or MRT segmentation, or, most recently, via 3D photography in combination with traditional methods of measurement [18, 23–25].

The goal of this study was to examine whether head circumference measurement alone is a good predictor of

---

* Correspondence: markus.martini@ukbonn.de; markus.martini@ukb.uni-bonn.de
[1]Department of Maxillofacial and Plastic Surgery, University of Bonn, Sigmund-Freud Str. 25, 53127 Bonn, Germany
[4]Department of Oral, Maxillofacial and Plastic Surgery, University of Bonn, Welschnonnenstraße 17, D – 53111 Bonn, Germany
Full list of author information is available at the end of the article

cranial volume, and whether the addition of head length and head height measurements increase the predictability of skull volume. Such additional measures included the ear-to-ear distance over the vertex to be measured for the skull height calculation as well as the head length over the top of the head point. Since cranial growth in the time between birth and the 12th month of life is the strongest [5], this evaluation focused on this period.

Methods

Approval for the study was obtained from the local Ethic Committee of the Medicine faculty of the University of Bonn. The study was performed at the Department of Maxillofacial and Plastic Surgery at the University of Bonn and 44 healthy 4-month-old Caucasian children (29 male, 15 female) who had an unremarkable general medical history, normal course of pregnancy and unremarkable head form were included. Assessments were conducted between the ages of 4 months and 12 months from 2014 to 2016 and included a single 3D optical image scan of every child's head without follow up.

First, 3D optical image scans of the cranium and facial surface, with the help of an optical 3D sensor (3D–Shape®, Erlangen, Deutschland). These data were triangulated and fused using Software Slim3D (3D–Shape®, Erlangen, Deutschland). After converting to a STL- format, cephalometric analysis of the data followed with the help of Software Onyx Ceph™ (Image Instruments GmbH, Chemnitz, Deutschland). Several reference parameters were identified for each patient's cranium using Onyx Ceph™ including: three medians (Glabella [Gl], Opistocranion [Oc], the point at the top of the head [ToH]), and two bilateral (Preauricular [Pa], Infraorbital [Or]) soft tissue reference points. The Preauricular and Infraorbital points defined the horizontal plane (H), in accordance with the commonly used Frankfort horizontal plane.

After generation of the 3D data set and voxelization, intracranial volume was calculated based on the total sum of all voxels located within the space between the vertex and the angularized cranial base plane (H).

Beside the maximal head circumference (HC) the cranial length (CL) from glabella to opistocranion (Gl-ToH-Oc) and the cranial height (CH), measured from cranial ear base to ear base on the contralateral side (Pa-ToH-Pa = ear-to-ear measurement; EtEm; Fig. 1) were determined using the software Onyx Ceph. Regarding the sample size the suggestion of Babyak and Rothman were followed by taking 10 to 15 observations per predictor variable (HC, CL, CH) to avoid overfitting in a multiple regression i.e. a too heavy influence by random error in the data [26, 27]. Statistical analysis was conducted using STATA 14.2 (College Station, Texas, USA), which included Pearson correlation, multiple linear regression, likelihood

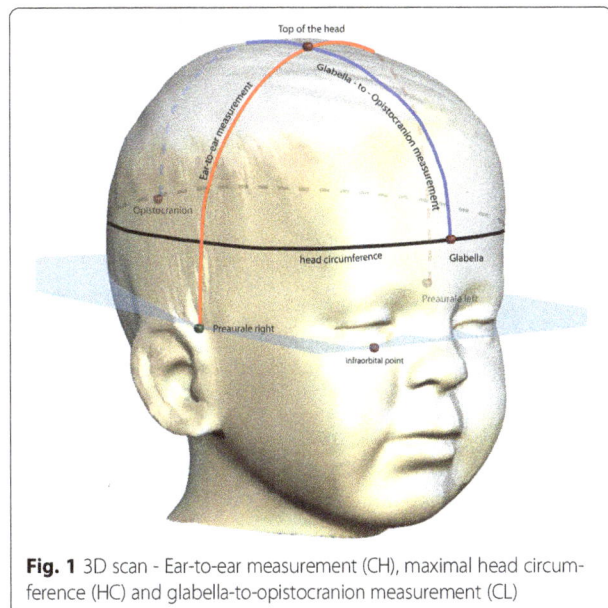

Fig. 1 3D scan - Ear-to-ear measurement (CH), maximal head circumference (HC) and glabella-to-opistocranion measurement (CL)

ratio tests, and Bland-Altman plots. Means and standard deviations are given and effect sizes are reported as partial eta^2.

Results

The average cranial volume for all children during the course of this study expanded from 1174 ± 106 ml (4 months) to 1579 ± 79 ml (12 months). The average intracranial volume growth among the 29 boys (1351 ± 155 ml) was larger than that of the 15 girls (1213 ± 113 ml). In the same period, maximum cranial circumference increased from 43.4 ± 9 cm to 46.9 ± 7 cm, the cranial length increased from 23.6 ± 13 cm to 25.3 ± 13 cm and the ear-to-ear measurement increased from 26.3 ± 21 cm to 31.6 ± 18 cm (Fig. 2). The maximal cranial circumference and measured volumes showed statistically significant linear correlations across all children (Pearson $r = 0.8828$; $p = 0.000$). For any given cranial circumference, 78% (R^2) of the volume variability was explained by the model (Fig. 3).

To examine the question of whether the predictiveness can be improved by the addition of further parameters, various models were compared. It was assumed that cranial volume at the base of the skull approximates the volume of a half ellipsoid. Hence, a spherical volume calculation was made based on the ear-to-ear measurements as well as the length-girth measurement, analogue to earlier studies [28–30]. The mathematically determined cranial volumes using HC, CL and CH were compared with the voxel-based cranial volume calculation made by the software program OnyxCeph using Bland-Altman plots. These showed no clear differences in the degree of agreement of the cranial volumes

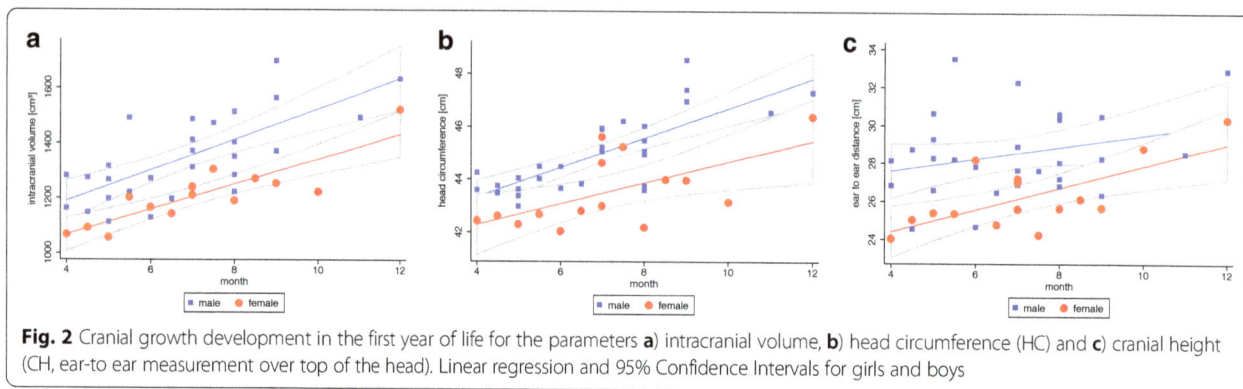

Fig. 2 Cranial growth development in the first year of life for the parameters **a**) intracranial volume, **b**) head circumference (HC) and **c**) cranial height (CH, ear-to ear measurement over top of the head). Linear regression and 95% Confidence Intervals for girls and boys

between the two measurement methods. Variabilities using the two methods were also equivalently large.

Next, the predictiveness of three different multiple linear regression models were compared. First, Model A included head circumference (HC), cranial height (CH) and cranial length (CL). This model achieved highly accurate volume correspondence of 90% (adjusted R^2). The average variance inflation factor (VIF) of 1.5 (range 1.4–1.7) eliminated the issue of collinearity. Statistically significant effects were shown for the predictors maximal circumference ($p = 0.000$) and ear-to-ear distance ($p = 0.000$). Cranial length (Gl-ToH-O), however, showed no statistically significant effect ($p = 0.907$). After a z-transformation, the maximal cranial circumference proved to be the most influential variable (beta = 0.69), followed by cranial height (beta = 0.40) and cranial length (beta = –0.007). This was also reflected by the differences in effect size quantified as partial eta^2 (HC: 74%; CH: 54%; CL: 0.03%;).

Further, a reduced model based on head circumference and cranial height (Model B: HC and CH), was compared to Model A (HC, CH and CL) using a likelihood ratio test. This yielded no significant difference in predictiveness of calculated volume (B vs. A, LR: $p = 0.902$).

Hence, the addition of CL had no effect on predictive value. Sex was then added as a predictor (Model C: HC, CH, Sex), which, in turn, rendered no increase in explanatory power (B vs. C, LR: $p = 0.135$). Figure 4 and Table 1 moreover show that estimated coefficients did not significantly differ in the two models. According to the principle of parsimony (Occam's razor), Model B with the variables head circumference and ear-to-ear measurement should be preferred, since both Model A and B had an adjusted R^2 von 90% (Table 1).

To calculate the expected cranial volume with a given HC and CL, coefficients and absolute terms were derived from linear regression model and transferred to the formula as follows: Vol. (cm3) $\triangleq 68 \cdot HC + 27 \cdot CL - 2472$.

Discussion

In the first 2 years of life the infant skull experiences its greatest structural and geometric change [31]. Intracranial volume doubles during the first 6–9 months of life [5], and increases by another 20% in the subsequent 6 months

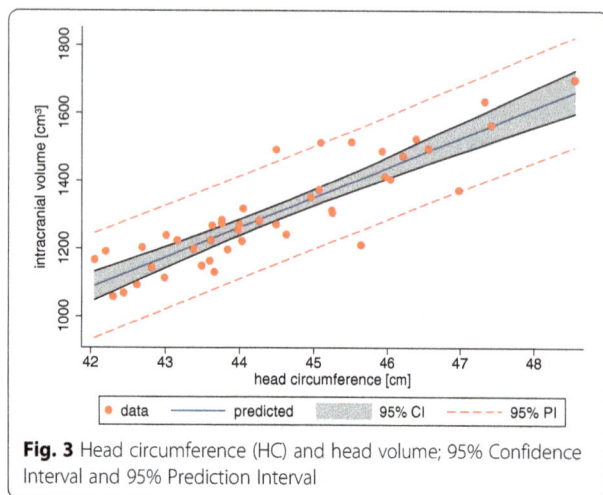

Fig. 3 Head circumference (HC) and head volume; 95% Confidence Interval and 95% Prediction Interval

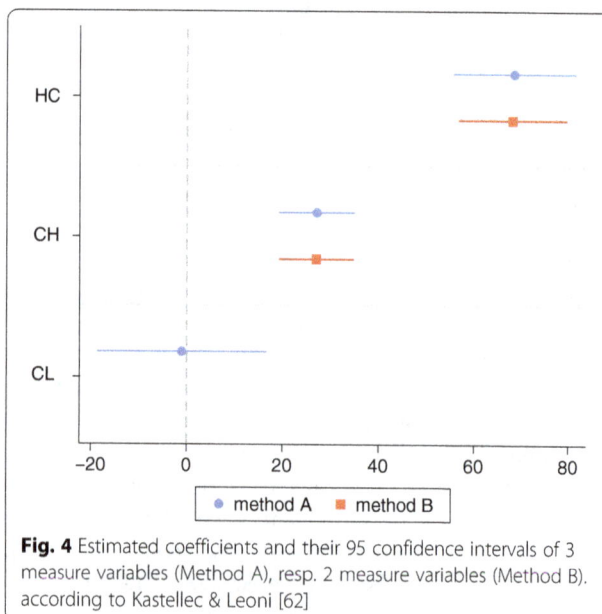

Fig. 4 Estimated coefficients and their 95 confidence intervals of 3 measure variables (Method A), resp. 2 measure variables (Method B). according to Kastellec & Leoni [62]

Table 1 Impact of 3 measure variables (Method A: head circumference [HC], cranial height [CH], cranial length [CL], 2 measure variables (Method B: HC, CH) and with added gender and age (Method C); n.s. not significant; * $p < 0.05$; ** $p < 0.01$; *** $p < 0.001$

Variable	Method A	Method B	Method C
HC	68.40***	68.07***	70.25***
CH	27.03***	26.96 ***	28.86***
CL	−1.03 n.s.		
sex			−26.87 n.s.
Intercept	−2463.02***	−2471.68***	−2603.73***
adj. R^2	0.89	0.90	0.90

[5]. A significant positive correlation between brain volume and cranial circumference has been demonstrated by postmortem studies and CT examinations of deceased newborns [32, 33], in line with MRI studies of older children [4]. For this reason, the head circumference measure (HC) is a recognized, well-established screening parameter for intracranial volume [34–36]. This measure should, however, not be accepted without reservation, since maximal head circumference primarily reflects expansion of the base of the skull [22, 29, 37, 38].

Estimating skull volume is based, on the one hand, on country-specific HC growth reference charts, which are periodically updated [10, 13]. On the other, a wide variety of specific craniometric ratios attempt to estimate the change in skull volume and make allowances for brain configuration [29, 39]. Further, early on Buda et al. [37] pointed out that the HC in children with non-normally shaped skulls is not a valid indicator of cranial volume [37]. Skull morphology appears too complex to be represented via any single parameter, according to Marcus et al. [21], in contrast to Rijken [40]. Our own examinations of healthy children showed invalidity in the relation between HC and cranial volume (Fig. 3). The relationship was monotonously linear, yet it was not completely reliable, and showed small skull volumes for large HCs and vice versa, in line with Treit [11]. This can not be explained merely by sex-specific differences in skull form in which girls have shorter and broader skulls compared to boys [29]. At the end of the exponential skull growth phase at the age of 2 years up to the 6th year of life, the attained HC gained high reliability with $r = 0.93$ according to Rollins [10], a reliability that is reached in this study only after the addition of two further parameters (cranial height and length) for the age range 4–12 months.

Likewise, as mentioned above, the lack of validity of maximal head circumference for estimating skull volume is problematic when referencing norm values, regardless of which pathological group is used for comparison. One problem for intracranial volume determination is the

lack of adequate reference material and normative age- and sex-adapted control groups based on the same evaluation procedures [41]. Even now, the most commonly referenced skull volume estimation method dates from the early 1960s which utilizes a two-dimensional radiological dataset and mathematical calculations based on the assumption of a proximal spherical volumetric relationship to estimate skull volume [42]. This estimation technique has found application by numerous authors [22, 28, 29, 38, 43] and including additional usage of a multiplier for 2D radiographic pictures [37, 42, 44]. However, the reliability 2D skull image evaluation is very limited due to inadequate reproducibility [45–47] and this method is not commensurate with modern standards of analysis. Moreover aside from country-specific living standards [13] cohort analyses show that the average HC is larger now than it was 50 years ago [29, 48]. Hence, a current comparison of HC in the literature with volume data that are even additional 10 years older warrants, at the very least, an age correction. Generally the reference data are based on segmentation of CT or MRI scans [5, 11, 14, 22] or 3D optical surface scans of healthy children [24, 25, 49]. Based on these findings, a critical debate followed regarding older publications [22, 50–52]. Recently Tenhagen [53] and Van Lindert et al. [54] compared these three different techniques and endorsed the optical 3D scan method due to its many advantages.

Intracranial volume calculation based on CT-scans uses the Cavalieri principle: the cranial volume is calculated as the sum of the surface products taking into account the CT layer thickness cranial of the foramen magnum to the vertex [5, 14, 15, 23, 41, 55]. The axial layers in sequential CTs are generally aligned with the osseous frontobase and are, therefore, valid for intracranial volume detection. Modern spiral CTs even allow a multiplanar reconstruction with free H-plane referencing. Analysis software for modern 3D photogrammetry also enables free angulation of the caudal layers for volume calculations from the sum of the individual volume elements between the triangle network of the Vertex – surface data set and the specified cranial base layer (Fig. 5).

Thus, 3D photogrammetry as employed by Meyer-Marcotty et al. (analogous to MRI examinations by Tenhagen, [53]) used a caudal bounded layer through the reference points of both tragi and nasion to calculate normal volume [24]. In contrast, Seeberger [25] set this further caudal under the nose, defined via the subnasal point. Tenhagen's intention in using a steep angle of the layer was to account for the specialness of occipital bossing in patients with scaphocephaly. They rejected the widely recognized Frankfort horizontal plane in favor of the nasion as a reference point, as Acer et al. did as

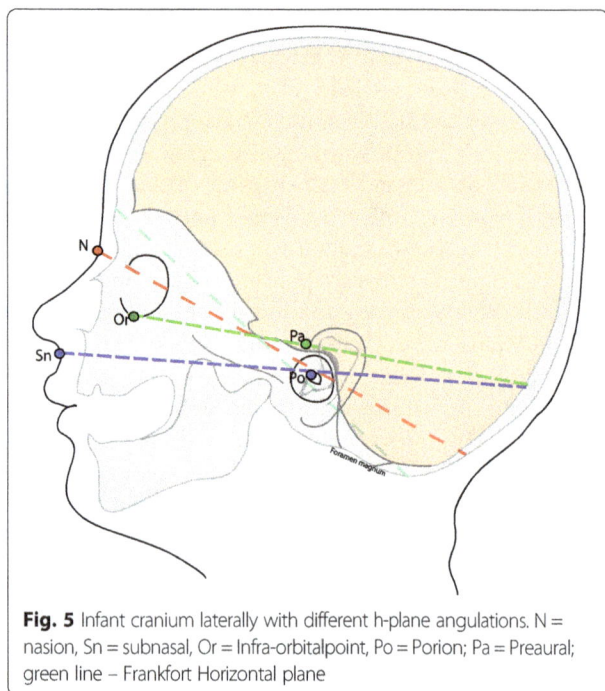

Fig. 5 Infant cranium laterally with different h-plane angulations. N = nasion, Sn = subnasal, Or = Infra-orbitalpoint, Po = Porion; Pa = Preaural; green line – Frankfort Horizontal plane

well [15]. In selecting the subnasal point as a reference instead of the nasion, it should be taken into consideration that the intracranial volume estimates take large parts of the mid-face into account. Hence, Seeberger's values are commensurately larger than those of Meyer-Marcotty et al. (with 100.32 cm^3 at the age of 6 months and 112.05 cm^3 at the age of 12 months). It can be problematic that, depending on the quality of the 3D laser scan image, the tragus point may be difficult to identify. In this study, therefore, the preaural point was chosen instead to define the Frankfort horizontal plane, since it is consistently easy to identify the cranial base of the ear as a reference point, and easily measurable with a tape measure for clinical examinations. Generally, the fact that the precision of the validity of the intracranial volume varies depending on the selected layer and the individual inclination of the skull base should be considered.

3D photography and CT-analysis were combined by Toma et al. [23] in their skull form analysis in children with scaphocephaly. In addition to the Cavalieri principle for volume calculation, a lot-based cranial height measurement (auricular head height: Vertex to Frankfort horizontal plane) was also used, among others parameters, to distinguish pathology from normal. As the authors point out with regret within the text of their article, such a comparison was not possible for cranial height for lack of norm values. This absence of data is due, on the one hand, to the danger of radiation exposure during CT scan for subjects, which also renders this method inappropriate for routine measurement.

On the other hand, there is also limited availability of special cephalometric measurement devices. In the clinical context, quantification of cranial measures is conducted with such instruments such as a craniometer, head spanner or anthropometric calipers. With the help of a craniometer, maximal cranial length (glabella-opistocranion) and maximal cranial width (euryon-euryon) measured through the head-center can be directly measured and the cranial volume can be determined [28, 56]. Indices such as the auricular head height via head spanner or cranial width [57] and cranial height measurements [39, 58] with the help of the spreading caliper of Hrdlička are only available in special centers and norm values with sufficiently large samples are hardly possible to generate.

Further, the possibility of 3D photocephalometry is not available to every investigator. As this study based on 3D surface scanning shows, just using a tape measure to measure to parameters enables calculation of a good approximation to the true intracranial volume. The method introduced here attained the same correlation factor (0.91) as that of 3D Photogrammetry with CT [59]. The volumes measured in this study concurred with those of the 3D surface-scan studies of Meyer-Marcotty and Seeberger regarding the 6 and 12-month evaluations of Caucasian children (see Table 2). These volumes were, however, distinctly above those of the CT based investigations by Toma [23], Abbott [14] and Sgouros [22]. The ear-to-ear measurements as well as the HC-measurements were, on the whole, slightly larger than those reported in Hou et al. for one-year-old Chinese children with 48 cm versus 47 cm and 33 cm versus 27 cm, respectively [60], whereby the HC data in this study corresponded to the percentile curves of German children in the normal range.

The visual imaging-based measurement methods a) cranial height in the form of ear-to-ear distance over the vertex, as well as b) the cranial length, measured as the distance from glabella to external occipital protuberance over the Vertex, which have been described in the literature [60, 61], were examined here for their validity with regard to volume calculation. The use of these measures (CH and CL) in addition to HC assessed with a measuring tape, decisively raise the predictive power of cranial volume of the children in the first year of life from 78% to 90%, whereby the ear-to-ear measurement is of particular relevance. This is independent of age or sex (Table 1). Hence, in daily clinical practice the predictive value of HC and CH are sufficiently high. Dolichocephalic and turicephalic head shapes can also be detected quickly, easily and validly in children with putatively normal skull shapes merely using a measuring tape, and the skull shape can be specified quantitatively as well. As far as we know, this is the first demonstration of the

Head circumference - a useful single parameter for skull volume development in cranial...

181

Table 2 Volume measurement (ml) according to age 1(6 months) and age 2 (12 months), relevant sample size and imaging method. In case that only graphics were presented instead of numerical values, the figures were reconstructed from these graphics using the software Digitizelt 2.2 (Braunschweig, Germany; Table 2)

	Imaging Method	Number	Age 1	Volume	Number	Age 2	Volume
Treit 2016 [11]	MRT	15	6 ± 1	1145 ± 113	22	12 ± 1	1239 ± 112
Lichtenberg 1960 [42]	X-ray		7 ± 1	920 ± 136		10 ± 1	990 ± 118
Toma 2010 [23]	CT		5–6	799		11 ± 2	997
Abbott 2000 [14]	CT	63	6 ± 1	853 ± 134		12 ± 1	1079 ± 72
Sgouros 1999 [22]	CT		6 ± 1	829 ± 104		12 ± 1	1026 ± 52
Meyer-Marcotty 2014 [24]	3D–Scan	52	6 ± 0.5	1229 ± 100	52	12 ± 0.5	1460 ± 112
This study 2017	3D–Scan	8	6 ± 0.5	1228 ± 116	3	12 ± 0.5	1551 ± 74
Seeberger 2016 [25]	3D–Scan	246	0–6	1336 ± 207	301	7–12	1527 ± 168

relationship between volume and measuring tape measurements.

There are several limitations inherent in our study. The database of this study with 44 children ranging in age from 4 to 12 months is too small to derive normative data, and requires a more extensive investigation. In addition, in as much as further studies are based on 3D photography, which reference planes should be used to optimally determine the approximate true intracranial volume needs to be explored. On the whole, the scan-based volume estimates are necessarily larger than those of real intracranial volumes, since they include in the thickness of skin, hair, cranial vault and cerebrospinal fluid space: These estimates, therefore, must lie above estimates any based on CT and autopsy findings.

Conclusion

These results demonstrate that a clear improvement is made to the assessment of a physiological cranial volume development in children up to 12 months by the mere addition of ear-to-ear distance by means of a measuring tape, in addition to the HC. This is particularly useful for detecting pathological cranial changes as in micro- or macrocephaly or for more complex conditions, such as craniosynostoses.

Abbreviations
CH: Cranial height; CL: Cranial length; Gl: Glabella; H: Horizontal plane; HC: Maximal head circumference,; Oc: Opistocranion; OFC: Occipito-frontal circumference; Or: Infraorbital; Pa: Preauricular; ToH: Top of the head; VIF: Variance inflation factor

Acknowledgements
Not applicable.

Funding
Not applicable: Neither the authors nor the institutions received third party funding associated with the study.

Authors' contributions
MM conceived the study, carried out design and coordination and wrote the manuscript, AK and NH collected and evaluated the data, GL performed the statistical analysis, MMJ participated in acquisition of the patients and data collection. All authors read and approved the final manuscript.

Competing interests
The authors declare that they have no competing interests or commercial associations that might post a conflict of interest in connection with the submitted article.

Author details
[1]Department of Maxillofacial and Plastic Surgery, University of Bonn, Sigmund-Freud Str. 25, 53127 Bonn, Germany. [2]Center for Development Research (ZEF), University of Bonn, Walter-Flex-Str. 3, 53113 Bonn, Germany. [3]Department of Neurosurgery, Asklepios Children's Hospital, Arnold-Janssen-Str. 29, 53757 Sankt Augustin, Germany. [4]Department of Oral, Maxillofacial and Plastic Surgery, University of Bonn, Welschnonnenstraße 17, D – 53111 Bonn, Germany.

References
1. Gale CR, Walton S, Martyn CN. Foetal and postnatal head growth and risk of cognitive decline in old age. Brain. 2003;126:2273–8.
2. Bray PF, Shields WD, Wolcott GJ, Madsen JA. Occipitofrontal head circumference-an accurate measure of intracranial volume. J Pediatr. 1969; 75:303–5.
3. Vernon PA, Wickett JC, Bazana PG, Stelmack RM. The neuropsychology and psychophysiology of human intelligenc. In: Sternberg RJ, editor. Handbook of intelligence. Cambridge: Cambridge University Press; 2000. p. 245–64.
4. Bartholomeusz HH, Courchesne E, Karns CM. Relationship between head circumference and brain volume in healthy normal toddlers, children, and adults. Neuropediatrics. 2002;33:239–41.
5. Kamdar MR, Gomez RA, Ascherman JA. Intracranial volumes in a large series of healthy children. Plast Reconstr Surg. 2009;124:2072–5.
6. MacLullich AM, Ferguson KJ, Deary IJ, Seckl JR, Starr JM, Wardlaw JM. Intracranial capacity and brain volumes are associated with cognition in healthy elderly men. Neurology. 2002;59:169–74.
7. Falk D, Hildebolt C, Smith K, Morwood MJ, Sutikna T, Brown P, Jatmiko, Saptomo EW, Brunsden B, Prior F. The brain of LB1, Homo Floresiensis. Science. 2005;308:242–5.
8. Falk D, Hildebolt C, Smith K, Morwood MJ, Sutikna T, Jatmiko, Wayhu Saptomo E, Prior F. LB1's virtual endocast, microcephaly, and hominin brain evolution. J Hum Evol. 2009;57:597–607.
9. Ivanovic DM, Leiva BP, Perez HT, Olivares MG, Diaz NS, Urrutia MS, Almagia AF, Toro TD, Miller PT, Bosch EO, Larrain CG. Head size and intelligence, learning, nutritional status and brain development. Head, IQ, learning, nutrition and brain. Neuropsychologia. 2004;42:1118–31.

10. Rollins JD, Collins JS, Holden KR. United States head circumference growth reference charts: birth to 21 years. J Pediatr. 2010;156:907–13. 913 e901-902

11. Treit S, Zhou D, Chudley AE, Andrew G, Rasmussen C, Nikkel SM, Samdup D, Hanlon-Dearman A, Loock C, Beaulieu C. Relationships between head circumference, brain volume and cognition in children with prenatal alcohol exposure. PLoS One. 2016;11:e0150370.

12. van der Linden V, Pessoa A, Dobyns W, Barkovich AJ, Junior HV, Filho EL, Ribeiro EM, Leal MC, Coimbra PP, Aragao MF, et al. Description of 13 infants born during October 2015-January 2016 with congenital Zika virus infection without Microcephaly at birth - Brazil. MMWR Morb Mortal Wkly Rep. 2016; 65:1343–8.

13. von der Hagen M, Pivarcsi M, Liebe J, von Bernuth H, Didonato N, Hennermann JB, Buhrer C, Wieczorek D, Kaindl AM. Diagnostic approach to microcephaly in childhood: a two-center study and review of the literature. Dev Med Child Neurol. 2014;56:732–41.

14. Abbott AH, Netherway DJ, Niemann DB, Clark B, Yamamoto M, Cole J, Hanieh A, Moore MH, David DJ. CT-determined intracranial volume for a normal population. J Craniofac Surg. 2000;11:211–23.

15. Acer N, Sahin B, Bas O, Ertekin T, Usanmaz M. Comparison of three methods for the estimation of total intracranial volume: stereologic, planimetric, and anthropometric approaches. Ann Plast Surg. 2007;58:48–53.

16. Lee MC, Shim KW, Yun IS, Park EK, Kim YO. Correction of Sagittal Craniosynostosis using distraction Osteogenesis based on strategic categorization. Plast Reconstr Surg. 2017;139:157–69.

17. Heller JB, Heller MM, Knoll B, Gabbay JS, Duncan C, Persing JA. Intracranial volume and cephalic index outcomes for total calvarial reconstruction among nonsyndromic sagittal synostosis patients. Plast Reconstr Surg. 2008; 121:187–95.

18. Kyriakopoulou V, Vatansever D, Davidson A, Patkee P, Elkommos S, Chew A, Martinez-Biarge M, Hagberg B, Damodaram M, Allsop J, et al. Normative biometry of the fetal brain using magnetic resonance imaging. Brain Struct Funct. 2016. :https://doi.org/10.1007/s00429-016-1342-6.

19. Delye H, Clijmans T, Mommaerts MY, Sloten JV, Goffin J. Creating a normative database of age-specific 3D geometrical data, bone density, and bone thickness of the developing skull: a pilot study. J Neurosurg Pediatr. 2015;16:687–702.

20. Smith K, Politte D, Reiker G, Nolan TS, Hildebolt C, Mattson C, Tucker D, Prior F, Turovets S, Larson-Prior LJ. Automated measurement of skull circumference, cranial index, and braincase volume from pediatric computed tomography. Conf Proc IEEE Eng Med Biol Soc. 2013;2013:3977–80.

21. Marcus JR, Domeshek LF, Das R, Marshall S, Nightingale R, Stokes TH, Mukundan S Jr. Objective three-dimensional analysis of cranial morphology. Eplasty. 2008;8:e20.

22. Sgouros S, Goldin JH, Hockley AD, Wake MJ, Natarajan K. Intracranial volume change in childhood. J Neurosurg. 1999;91:610–6.

23. Toma R, Greensmith AL, Meara JG, Da Costa AC, Ellis LA, Willams SK, Holmes AD. Quantitative morphometric outcomes following the Melbourne method of total vault remodeling for scaphocephaly. J Craniofac Surg. 2010;21:637–43.

24. Meyer-Marcotty P, Bohm H, Linz C, Kochel J, Stellzig-Eisenhauer A, Schweitzer T. Three-dimensional analysis of cranial growth from 6 to 12 months of age. Eur J Orthod. 2014;36:489–96.

25. Seeberger R, Hoffmann J, Freudlsperger C, Berger M, Bodem J, Horn D, Engel M. Intracranial volume (ICV) in isolated sagittal craniosynostosis measured by 3D photocephalometry: a new perspective on a controversial issue. J Craniomaxillofac Surg. 2016;44:626–31.

26. Babyak MA. What you see may not be what you get: a brief, nontechnical introduction to overfitting in regression-type models. Psychosom Med. 2004;66:411–21.

27. Rothman KJ. Epidemiology - an introduction. Toronto: Oxford University Press; 2012. p. 226.

28. Dekaban AS. Tables of cranial and orbital measurements, cranial volume, and derived indexes in males and females from 7 days to 20 years of age. Ann Neurol. 1977;2:485–91.

29. Vannucci RC, Barron TF, Lerro D, Anton SC, Vannucci SJ. Craniometric measures during development using MRI. NeuroImage. 2011;56:1855–64.

30. Bergerhoff W. Determination of cranial capacity from the roentgenogram. Fortschr Geb Rontgenstr Nuklearmed. 1957;87:176–84.

31. Slovis T. Anatomy of the skull. 11th ed. Amsterdam: Mosby Elsevier; 2007.

32. Cooke R, Lucas A, Yudkin P, Pryse-Davies J. Head circumference as an index of brain weight in the fetus and newborn. Early Hum Dev. 1977;1:145–9.

33. Lindley A, Benson J, Grimes C, Cole T, Herman A. The relationship in neonates between clinically measured head circumference and brain volume estimated from head CT-scans. Early Hum Dev. 1999;56:17–29.

34. Bruner E. Geometric morphometrics and paleoneurology: brain shape evolution in the genus homo. J Hum Evol. 2004;47:279–303.

35. Holloway RL. The evolution of the primate brain: some aspects of quantitative relations. Brain Res. 1968;7:121–72.

36. Howells WW. Howells' craniometric data on the internet. Am J Phys Anthropol. 1996;101:441–2.

37. Buda FB, Reed JC, Rabe EF. Skull volume in infants. Methodology, normal values, and application. Am J Dis Child. 1975;129:1171–4.

38. Scheffler C, Greil H, Hermanussen M. The association between weight, height, and head circumference reconsidered. Pediatr Res. 2017. :https://doi.org/10.1038/pr.2017.3.

39. Kolar JC, Munro IR, Farkas LG. Patterns of dysmorphology in Crouzon syndrome: an anthropometric study. Cleft Palate J. 1988;25:235–44.

40. Rijken BF, den Ottelander BK, van Veelen ML, Lequin MH, Mathijssen IM. The occipitofrontal circumference: reliable prediction of the intracranial volume in children with syndromic and complex craniosynostosis. Neurosurg Focus. 2015;38:E9.

41. Fischer S, Maltese G, Tarnow P, Wikberg E, Bernhardt P, Tovetjarn R, Kolby L. Intracranial volume is normal in infants with sagittal synostosis. J Plast Surg Hand Surg. 2015;49:62–4.

42. Lichtenberg R. Radiographie du crâne de 226 enfants normaux de la naissance à 8 ans: Impressions digtiformes, capacite; angles et indices, Thèse pour le Doctorat en médicine. Paris: University of Paris; 1960.

43. Menichini G, Ruiu A. On the radiological evaluation of the cranial capacity in infants. Minerva Pediatr. 1960;12:1358–63.

44. Mackinnon IL, Kennedy JA, Davis TV. The estimation of skull capacity from roentgenologic measurements. Am J Roentgenol Radium Therapy, Nucl Med. 1956;76:303–10.

45. Lavelle CL. Craniofacial growth in patients with craniosynostosis. Acta Anat (Basel). 1985;123:201–6.

46. Tng TT, Chan TC, Hagg U, Cooke MS. Validity of cephalometric landmarks. An experimental study on human skulls. Eur J Orthod. 1994;16:110–20.

47. Ward RE, Jamison PL. Measurement precision and reliability in craniofacial anthropometry: implications and suggestions for clinical applications. J Craniofac Genet Dev Biol. 1991;11:156–64.

48. Nellhaus G. Head circumference in children with idiopathic hypopituitarism. Pediatrics. 1968;42:210–1.

49. Schweitzer T, Bohm H, Linz C, Jager B, Gerstl L, Kunz F, Stellzig-Eisenhauer A, Ernestus RI, Krauss J, Meyer-Marcotty P. Three-dimensional analysis of positional plagiocephaly before and after molding helmet therapy in comparison to normal head growth. Childs Nerv Syst. 2013;29:1155–61.

50. Posnick JC, Bite U, Nakano P, Davis J, Armstrong D. Indirect intracranial volume measurements using CT scans: clinical applications for craniosynostosis. Plast Reconstr Surg. 1992;89:34–45.

51. Gault DT, Renier D, Marchac D, Ackland FM, Jones BM. Intracranial volume in children with craniosynostosis. J Craniofac Surg. 1990;1:1–3.

52. Netherway DJ, Abbott AH, Anderson PJ, David DJ. Intracranial volume in patients with nonsyndromal craniosynostosis. J Neurosurg. 2005;103: 137–41.

53. Tenhagen M, Bruse JL, Rodriguez-Florez N, Angullia F, Borghi A, Koudstaal MJ, Schievano S, Jeelani O, Dunaway D. Three-dimensional handheld scanning to quantify head-shape changes in spring-assisted surgery for Sagittal Craniosynostosis. J Craniofac Surg. 2016;27:2117–23.

54. van Lindert EJ, Siepel FJ, Delye H, Ettema AM, Berge SJ, Maal TJ, Borstlap WA. Validation of cephalic index measurements in scaphocephaly. Childs Nerv Syst. 2013;29:1007–14.

55. Gosain AK, McCarthy JG, Glatt P, Staffenberg D, Hoffmann RG. A study of intracranial volume in Apert syndrome. Plast Reconstr Surg. 1995;95:284–95.

56. Manjunath KY. Estimation of cranial volume: an overview of methodologies. J Anat Soc India. 2002;51:85–91.

57. Steele DG, Bramblett CA. The anatomy and biology oft he human skeleton. Texas: A&M University Press; 2007.

58. Farkas LG. Anthropometry of the head and face in medicine. New York: Elsevier; 1981.

59. McKay DR, Davidge KM, Williams SK, Ellis LA, Chong DK, Teixeira RP, Greensmith AL, Holmes AD. Measuring cranial vault volume with three-dimensional photography: a method of measurement comparable to the gold standard. J Craniofac Surg. 2010;21:1419–22.

60. Hou HD, Liu M, Gong KR, Shao G, Zhang CY. Growth of the skull in young children in Baotou, China. Childs Nerv Syst. 2014;30:1511–5.

61. Christofides EA, Steinmann ME. A novel anthropometric chart for craniofacial surgery. J Craniofac Surg. 2010;21:352–7.

62. Kastellec JP, Leoni EL. Using graphs instead of tables in political science. Perspectives on Politics. 2007;5:755–71.

26

Oral microbiota carriage in patients with multibracket appliance in relation to the quality of oral hygiene

Katharina Klaus[1]*[iD], Johanna Eichenauer[2], Rhea Sprenger[3] and Sabine Ruf[1]

Abstract

Background: The present study aimed to investigate the prevalence of oral microbiota (*Candida* species (spp.), *Streptococcus mutans*, and *Lactobacilli*) in patients with multibracket (MB) appliances in relation to the quality of oral hygiene.

Saliva and plaque samples were collected from three groups of 25 patients each (good oral hygiene (GOH), poor oral hygiene (POH), and poor oral hygiene with white spot lesions (POH/WSL)). Counts of colony forming units (CFU) of the investigated oral microbiota were compared using Chi-square and Mann–Whitney U tests.

Results: Both saliva and plaque samples showed a high prevalence of *Candida* spp. in all patients (saliva: 73.4 %, plaque: 60.9 %). The main *Candida* species was *C. albicans*. The salivary CFU of *Candida* spp. in the GOH group was significantly lower than that in the POH group ($p = 0.045$) and POH/WSL group ($p = 0.011$). *S. mutans* was found in the saliva and plaque samples of all patients. *Lactobacilli* were found in the saliva samples of all patients and in 90.7 % of the plaque samples. In the saliva samples, the CFU of *Lactobacilli* were more numerous in the POH and POH/WSL groups than in the GOH group ($p = 0.047$).

Conclusions: The investigated sample of patients showed a high carriage of oral *Candida* spp. Patients with WSL formation during MB appliance treatment exhibited higher counts of *Candida* and *Lactobacilli* compared with patients with good oral hygiene. Independent of oral hygiene quality, *S. mutans* was detected in all patients.

Keywords: *Candida*, *Streptococcus mutans*, *Lactobacilli*, Oral hygiene, Fixed appliance, White spot lesions

Background

The insertion of a multibracket (MB) appliance induces a change in the number and composition of oral microflora. Besides the increase in potential cariogenic bacteria such as *Streptococcus mutans*, *Lactobacilli*, and periodontal pathogenic microorganisms, a marked increase in oral yeasts also occurs [1–6]. In particular, colonization with *Candida albicans* is of interest for orthodontists because of the fungus' possible cariogenic effect [7–10], which has been demonstrated in vitro [11–13] and in vivo [14–20].

During orthodontic treatment with MB appliances, the development of white spot lesions (WSL) is an undesirable side effect with an incidence rate of 30 %–70 % [6, 21, 22]. WSL can develop as quickly as within 4 weeks [23]. Although patients with poor oral hygiene (POH) during treatment are reportedly affected [6, 24, 25], WSL are quite unpredictable from a clinical perspective. Some patients develop WSL despite acceptable oral hygiene, while others with consistently POH remain unaffected.

Therefore, the present pilot study aimed to analyze and compare oral microbiota in patients with MB appliances, with special emphasis on *Candida* spp. colonization. The quality of oral hygiene and the development of WSL were considered in this study. The null hypothesis was no difference in the amount of *Candida*, *S. mutans*, and *Lactobacilli* colonization among patients with good oral hygiene (GOH), POH, or POH with WSL.

* Correspondence: Katharina.Klaus@dentist.med.uni-giessen.de
[1]Department of Orthodontics, Justus-Liebig University Giessen, Schlangenzahl 14, 35392 Giessen, Germany
Full list of author information is available at the end of the article

Methods

Ethical approval was granted by the ethical committee of the medical faculty of the Justus-Liebig-University of Giessen, Germany (No. 95/08).

Patients were selected from the Department of Orthodontics at Justus-Liebig-University Giessen, Germany. In general, after placement of a MB appliance, all patients of the department received the same standardized oral care instructions regarding frequency, technique, and duration of daily tooth brushing with fluoridated toothpaste, use of interdental brushes, and additional weekly fluoride gel application.

The inclusion criteria comprised patients aged 11 years or older without craniofacial anomalies, general diseases, or drug intake undergoing active MB appliance treatment in both jaws for at least three months. All selected patients were prospectively monitored for the quality of their oral hygiene at three consecutive regular appointments.

Dental plaque at selected index teeth (13, 21, 24, 33, 41, and 44) was visually inspected, and oral hygiene was categorized as follows:

1. GOH: no visible dental plaque on index teeth and no signs of gingival inflammation.
2. Average oral hygiene (AOH): small amounts of dental plaque on index teeth and mild signs of gingival inflammation.
3. POH: massive dental plaque on index teeth especially between the bracket and gingival margin, as well as marked signs of gingival inflammation.
4. POH with new WSL (POH/WSL): massive dental plaque on index teeth especially between the bracket and gingival margin, as well as marked signs of gingival inflammation and development of WSL during MB treatment. Possible pre-orthodontic WSL were excluded by analyzing the pre-treatment intraoral images.

Patients with consistent scorings of GOH or POH with/without WSL formation for three consecutive appointments were considered for possible inclusion in the present study. Patients with AOH were excluded. Written informed consent was obtained from the patients and their parents. For each group (GOH, POH, and POH/WSL), the first 25 patients fulfilling the abovementioned criteria were included.

The study appointment occurred during the next regular control appointment. Patients were instructed to stop oral hygiene for 24 h before the appointment (tooth brushing/antibacterial oral rinsing) to ensure a sufficient amount of plaque for sampling even in patients with GOH.

The dental status was checked using a slight modification of the DMF-T-index [26]. The index was modified to assess orthodontic patients. Tooth agenesis, extractions

caused by orthodontic treatment plan, and impacted teeth were not scored as missing teeth.

The plaque samples were obtained by sterilized swabs (Nerbe plus, Winsen/Luhe, Germany) from the enamel surfaces along the gingival margin of the index teeth. In all patients of the POH/WSL group, a second plaque sample was obtained from the affected WSL surface regions with a probe tip and then applied on a second swab.

Saliva secretion was stimulated by chewing a paraffin wax pellet over a period of 5 min. The entire amount of saliva produced during that period was collected in a single-use plastic cup. From this sample, 2 ml of saliva was extracted using a sterile syringe (B. Braun, Melsungen, Germany) and used for further analysis.

Candida counts were identified with Sabouraud agar (Merck, Darmstadt, Germany) for the saliva samples. Depending on the number of colony forming units (CFU) per milliliter of saliva, counts were categorized into 0 (none), 1 (isolated, <10 CFU/ml), 2 (moderate, $10–10^2$ CFU/ml), 3 (many, $10^2–10^3$ CFU/ml), and 4 (massive, $>10^3$ CFU/ml). *Candida* species were differentiated by an Auxacolor™ 2-Test (Bio-Rad, Marnes-la-Coquette, France). Furthermore, the amounts of *S. mutans* and *Lactobacilli* were counted using the CRT® bacteria test (Ivoclar Vivadent, Schaan, Liechtenstein). The number of CFU per milliliter of saliva was categorized as 0 (none), 1 (moderate, $<10^5$ CFU/ml), and 2 (many, $\geq10^5$ CFU/ml). For plaque samples, the test manufacturers recommended classifying the occurrence of *S. mutans*, *Lactobacilli*, and *Candida* in terms of a binary (yes/no) decision only, because the plaque samples have no defined volume.

Statistical analysis was performed by IBM SPSS Statistics 22 (IBM Company, Chicago, IL, USA). Descriptive data analysis was conducted by exploring means, standard deviations, minima, and maxima. The data were not normally distributed, and the differences between groups were assessed using the Chi-square and Mann–Whitney U tests.

Results

The general descriptive characteristics of the final patient sample are given in Table 1. The mean age of the total sample was 14.4 ± 1.5 years and did not differ significantly among the three oral hygiene groups. The gender distribution was nearly equal in the total sample and in the POH/WSL group. Female predominance was found in the GOH group, whereas male predominance was noted in the POH group. The DMF-T-index was generally very low (mean range: 0–0.1) and did not differ among the oral hygiene groups.

At the time of saliva and plaque sample collection, the mean wearing time of the MB appliance in the GOH group (14.9 ± 7.9 months) was insignificantly higher than

Table 1 Demographic characteristics of the studied patient sample ($n = 75$) and their fixed appliance treatment duration at the time of the study

Group	Age (years) mean ± SD	Male	Female	MB in situ (months) mean ± SD
Total sample	14.4 ± 1.8	36	39	16 ± 9.2
GOH	14.6 ± 1.8	6	19	14.9 ± 7.9
POH	14.0 ± 1.4	16	9	13.4 ± 6.7
POH/WSL	14.6 ± 1.3	14	11	19.6 ± 11.3

SD standard deviation, *MB* multibracket appliance, *GOH* good oral hygiene, *POH* poor oral hygiene, *POH/WSL* poor oral hygiene with white spot lesions

that in the POH group ($13.4 ± 6.7$ months). The POH/WSL group showed the longest wearing period ($19.6 ± 11.3$ months) with a significant difference from the other groups ($p = 0.017$).

Analysis of the saliva samples revealed that 73.4 % of the patient sample were *Candida* carriers. About half of the carrier samples (49.4 %, $n = 37$) showed isolated to moderate numbers of CFU, whereas 24 % ($n = 18$) presented many to massive CFU. CFU of *Candida* spp. were significantly lower in the GOH group than in the POH group ($p = 0.045$) and POH/WSL group ($p = 0.011$) (Fig. 1). Saliva samples of *Candida* carriers ($n = 54$) showed *C. albicans* in 83.3 % ($n = 45$), *C. dubliniensis* in 14.8 % ($n = 8$), and *C. albicans II* in 1.9 % ($n = 1$). No significant difference in the distribution of species was found among the different oral hygiene groups.

S. mutans and *Lactobacilli* were detected in the saliva samples of all patients. Patients with POH irrespective of WSL formation presented higher counts of *S. mutans*, but the difference was not statistically significant (Fig. 2). High *Lactobacilli* CFU were noted in 52 % of patients in the GOH group. A comparable amount of CFU was

found in 60 % and 84 % of patients in the POH group and POH/WSL group, respectively. This difference was statistically significant ($p = 0.047$; Fig. 3). For the saliva samples, the null hypothesis regarding *S. mutans* was accepted but rejected in *Candida* and *Lactobacilli*.

Analysis of the plaque samples revealed a 60.9 % prevalence of *Candida* carriers in the total sample. In the POH/WSL patients, the plaque samples from the index teeth showed an insignificantly higher *Candida* prevalence (62.4 %). The second plaque samples from the affected white spot enamel regions exhibited only a slightly and insignificantly different prevalence of 64 %.

Among the *Candida* carriers ($n = 46$), 82.6 % ($n = 38$) of the carriers showed *C. albicans*, 15.2 % ($n = 7$) presented *C. dubliniensis*, and *C. albicans II* was found in 2.2 % ($n = 1$). As in the saliva samples, the distribution of *Candida* species revealed no statistically significant difference among the oral hygiene groups. Similar to the saliva samples, *S. mutans* was verified in the plaque samples of all patients, whereas *Lactobacilli* were found in 90.7 % ($n = 68$) of all plaque samples. For the plaque samples, the null hypothesis regarding all types of microbiota was accepted.

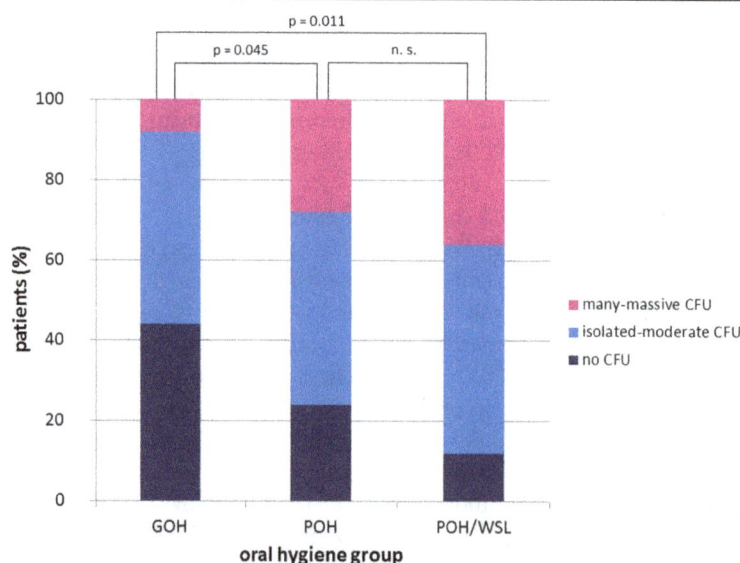

Fig. 1 Relative *Candida* carriage in patients' saliva in relation to the oral hygiene groups. A significant difference was found between the GOH and POH groups ($p = 0.045$), as well as between the GOH and POH/WSL groups ($p = 0.011$)

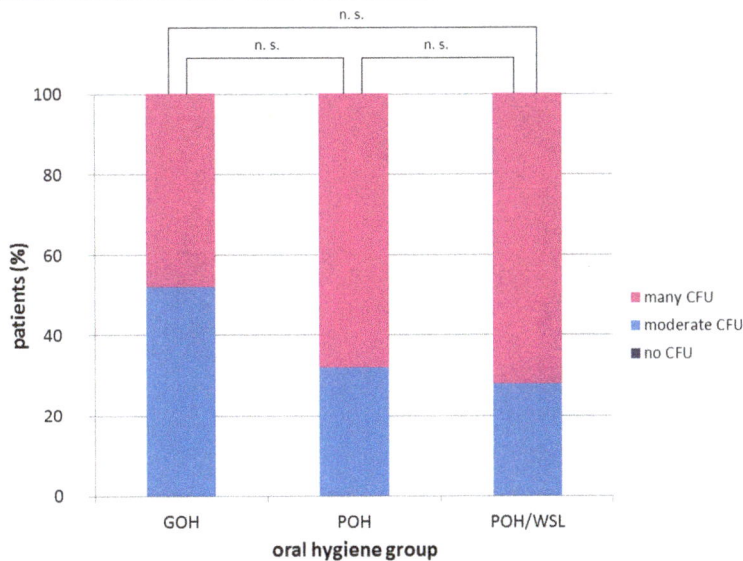

Fig. 2 Relative *S. mutans* carriage in patients' saliva in relation to the oral hygiene groups. No significant difference was found among the groups

Discussion

Counts of oral microbiota peak at about three months after insertion of a fixed appliance [3, 27–30]. Although most studies [3, 28–30] reported a slight decrease thereafter, Arslan et al. [27] found a consistent increase in *Candida*, *S. mutans*, and *Lactobacilli* counts up to 12 months of treatment. Despite the slight decrease reported by the other studies, patients showed consistently higher counts of oral microbiota compared with pretreatment [28–30]. In the present patient sample, the mean treatment duration at the study appointment ranged between 13.4 and 19.6 months with a significantly longer treatment time in the POH/WSL group, which was far longer than that in all other studies in the literature. For the POH/WSL group in the present study, the influence of oral microbiota or longer treatment duration on the development of WSL could not be clarified. However, given the cross-sectional design of the present study, the development of microbial counts in all the investigated groups during the treatment period remains unclear.

In the current literature, oral *Candida* carrier rates vary between 28.6 % and 57.2 %, depending on the age of the examined individuals and the microbiological sampling method [31–36]. During orthodontic treatment, an even greater variation with prevalence rates between 8.3 % and 78.8 % was reported [1, 3, 27, 37]. The results of the present study corresponded to the top end of these data with *Candida* prevalence in dental plaque of 60.9 % and in saliva of 73.4 % of the patients.

Unfortunately, no standard currently exists for oral microbiological sampling. According to the literature, the most popular sampling methods are stimulated and unstimulated saliva samples, centrifuged saliva samples, swabs from oral mucosa, plaque samples, and imprint cultures from different sites in the oral cavity [20]. When comparing results achieved by different sampling methods and different culture media [38], centrifuged saliva samples and imprint cultures showed a significantly higher sensitivity in detecting oral yeasts [39] than cultures from the other sampling methods. In the current literature, studies with patient samples comparable with the present investigation [1, 3, 27, 37] used various sampling methods (Table 2). Hägg et al. [3] used three different sampling methods, and the method closest to the sampling collection in our study (pooled plaque) revealed a clearly lower *Candida* rate (22.2 %), in contrast to our study. Furthermore, 18.5 % of their patients became *Candida* carriers during treatment. In the present work, the incidence rates of *Candida* infection could not be revealed because of the cross-sectional design of the study.

In concordance with the present findings, the current literature on oral yeast carriage indicated *C. albicans* as the dominant species both in orthodontic-treated patients [3, 27, 37] and untreated individuals [31, 33]. In our sample, *C. dubliniensis* was the second most frequent species and one patient presented *C. albicans II*; the literature reported other additional *Candida* strains. Given that *C. albicans* and *C. dubliniensis* present pronounced morphological similarities and some common tests are unable to differentiate them reliably [16], *C. dubliniensis* was possibly undetected in other investigations.

In general, the current literature agreed that *S. mutans* and *Lactobacilli* are characteristic for deep carious lesions [14, 15, 40–42] and therefore not for initial carious lesions such as WSL. Aas et al. [40] verified high concentrations

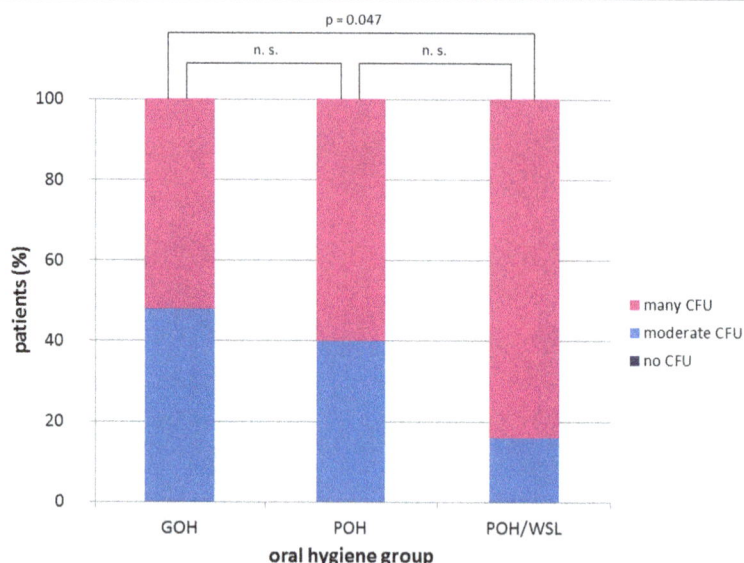

Fig. 3 Relative *Lactobacilli* carriage in patients' saliva in relation to the oral hygiene groups. A significant difference was observed between the GOH and POH/WSL groups (*p* = 0.047)

of *Actinomyces* and non-*S. mutans*–*Streptococci* in initial lesions, but they additionally emphasized that bacterial profiles in initial lesions are more complex than in advanced destruction stages. Badet and Thebaud [41] revealed a strong correlation between the DMF-T-index and amount of *Lactobacilli* counts and furthermore showed that *Lactobacilli* are not isolated from initial carious lesions because of weak adherence potential; retentive niches for adherence are required by *Lactobacilli*. A fixed orthodontic appliance inevitably presents retentive niches, so whether the high *Lactobacilli* counts in the present study are associated with WSL development or simply caused by better possibilities for plaque accumulation remains unclear.

However, an in vivo study by Arneberg et al. [43] revealed higher bacterial counts for *S. mutans* and *Lactobacilli* at initial carious lesion surfaces compared with the unchanged control surfaces of neighboring teeth, suggesting the participation of these microorganisms even in initial enamel lesions.

The association of *C. albicans* with dental caries has been frequently investigated in patients with severe early childhood caries [17–19, 44–46]. Current in vitro and in vivo studies [12, 13] demonstrated a symbiosis between *C. albicans* and *S. mutans* in dental plaque, in which the two microbiota strains stick together because of extracellular polysaccharides. During the maturation of dental plaque, large microcolonies of *S. mutans* and *C. albicans* can be observed after 42 h [13]. Falsetta et al. [13] investigated the effect of *S. mutans* and *C. albicans* in rodents and showed that co-infected animals present significantly more severe carious lesions, whereas rodents infected with either *S. mutans* or *C. albicans* revealed initial carious lesions. In the present study, a statistically significant relationship between the quality of oral hygiene and *Candida* colonization could only be demonstrated for the saliva samples. Furthermore, the present patient sample showed high counts of *S. mutans* and *Lactobacilli* in POH or POH/WSL patients (significant for *Lactobacilli* in saliva only). In other words, all three

Table 2 Oral microbiological sampling methods and investigated time points used in previous studies to analyze *Candida* carriage in orthodontic patients

Study group	Time points of investigation		Type of appliance		Saliva sampling	Plaque sampling	Oral mucosa sampling
	Before insertion	During treatment	Fixed	Removable			
Current study	-	x	x	-	**stimulated saliva**	**pooled plaque**	-
Addy et al. 1982 [1]	-	x	x	x	-	-	imprint culture
Hägg et al. 2004 [3]	x	x	x	-	oral rinse	**pooled plaque**	imprint culture
Arslan et al. 2008 [27]	x	x	x	-	**stimulated saliva**	**pooled plaque**	-
Arendorf, Addy 1985 [37]	x	x	-	x	-	-	imprint culture

Comparable study methods are highlighted in bold text

microorganisms investigated in the present study influenced caries development, but the relative amount of their contribution and possible timing of their contribution remain unknown.

The first possible limiting factor of the present study is the lack of precise knowledge on the age and maturity of the dental plaque analyzed, because one cannot be sure that all patients followed the instructions to stop their oral hygiene for 24 h before the study appointment. Even if the patients followed this instruction, we are uncertain of the events that occurred during the previous days. Additionally, patients received no standardized information regarding eating or drinking between the appointments and before sample collection. Perhaps the comparability could have been improved slightly if all patients had a professional cleaning of their teeth, followed by the sampling appointment after a determined time period.

Furthermore, we cannot exclude the Hawthorne effect, because the knowledge about study participation and the special reminders about the study appointment given by the study team can evoke patient's behavior modification [47]. Moreover, such knowledge and reminders possibly influenced oral hygiene and in turn the oral microbiota in the weeks before study sampling.

One could also question the categorization of the patients into the GOH and POH groups based on the subjective judgement of the treating orthodontists instead of an objective measurement. However, even with objective measurements, cut-off values for the groups have to be defined, which still provide ample space for large variations in the quality of oral hygiene. Nevertheless, a quantitative plaque assessment would have improved the comparability with the results of Hägg et al. [3] and Arslan et al. [27].

Given the present results, oral *Candida* counts and *S. mutans* or *Lactobacilli* counts showed no clear interrelation to the development of WSL. The current literature revealed that the abovementioned organisms participated in initial enamel caries formation. Further prospective longitudinal clinical trials concerning changes in oral microbiota during MB treatment are required to clarify the developmental process of WSL.

Conclusions

The investigated sample of patients showed a high carriage of oral *Candida* spp., *S. mutans*, and *Lactobacilli*. Patients with WSL formation during MB appliance treatment showed higher counts of *Candida* and *Lactobacilli* compared with patients with GOH. Independent of oral hygiene quality, *S. mutans* was detected in all patients.

Abbreviations

AOH: Average oral hygiene; CFU: Colony forming units; GOH: Good oral hygiene; MB: Multibracket; POH: Poor oral hygiene; POH/WSL: Poor oral hygiene with white spot lesions; Spp: Species; WSL: White spot lesions

Acknowledgements

The authors are grateful to Mrs. Ingrid Heidmann (Department of Periodontology and Department of Paediatric Dentistry of Justus-Liebig-University Giessen, Germany) for handling the microbial samples.

Funding

The authors declare that no funding was granted to the study by any company or institution.

Authors' contributions

JE and RS participated in the design and coordination of the study and carried out the collection of samples. KK carried out the collection of samples, analysis and interpretation of data, and drafted the manuscript. SR participated in the design of the study and gave final approval of the version to be published.

Competing interests

The authors declare that they have no competing interests.

Author details

[1]Department of Orthodontics, Justus-Liebig University Giessen, Schlangenzahl 14, 35392 Giessen, Germany. [2]Private orthodontic practice, Rosengasse 2, 35305 Grünberg, Germany. [3]Private orthodontic practice, Marktgasse 2, 72070 Tübingen, Germany.

References

1. Addy M, Shaw C, Hansford P, Hopkins M. The effect of orthodontic appliances on the distribution of Candida and plaque in adolescents. Br J Orthod. 1982;9:158–63.
2. Freitas AO, Marquezan M, Nojima Mda C, Alviano DS, Maia LC. The influence of orthodontic fixed appliances on the oral microbiota: A systematic review. Dental Press J Orthod. 2014;19:46–55.
3. Hägg U. Kaveewatcharanont P; Samaranayake YH, Samaranayake LP: The effect of fixed orthodontic appliances on the oral carriage of Candida species and Enterobacteriaceae. Eur J Orthod. 2004;26:623–9.
4. Hibino K, Wong PW, Hägg U, Samarayanake LP. The effects of orthodontic appliances on Candida in the human mouth. Int J Paed Dent. 2009;19:301–8.
5. Ren Y, Jongsma MA, Mei L, Van der Mei HC, Busscher HJ. Orthodontic treatment with fixed appliances and biofilm formation—a potential public health threat? Clin Oral Investig. 2014;18:1711–8.
6. Topaloglu-Ak A, Ertugrul F, Eden E, Ates M, Bulut H. Effect of orthodontic appliances on oral microbiota—6 month follow-up. J Clin Pediatr Dent. 2011;35:133 6.
7. De Carvalho FG, Silva DS, Hebling J, Spolidorio LC, Spolidorio DM. Presence of mutans streptococci and Candida spp. in dental plaque/dentine of carious teeth and early childhood caries. Arch Oral Biol. 2006;51:1024–8.
8. Hossain H, Ansari F, Schulz-Weidner N, Wetzel WE, Chakraborty T, Domann E. Clonal identity of Candida albicans in the oral cavity and the gastrointestinal tract of pre-school children. Oral Microbiol Immunol. 2003;18:302–8.
9. Klinke T, Guggenheim B, Klimm W, Thurnheer T. Dental caries in rats associated with Candida albicans. Caries Res. 2011;45:100–6.
10. Tufekci E, Dixon JS, Gunsolley JC, Lindauer SJ. Prevalence of white spot lesions during orthodontic treatment with fixed appliances. Angle Orthod. 2011;81:206–10.
11. Wetzel WE, Böhmer C, Sziegoleit A. In vitro Karies durch Candida albicans. Acta Med Dent Helv. 1997;2:308–13.
12. Barbieri DSAV, Vicente VA, Fraiz FC, Lavoranti OJ, Svidzinski TIE, Pinheiro RL. Analysis of the in vitro adherence of Streptococcus mutans and Candida albicans. Braz J Microbiol. 2007;38:624–31.
13. Falsetta ML, Klein MI, Colonne PM, Scott-Anne K, Gregoire K, Pai CH, Gonzalez-Begne M, Watson G, Krysan DJ, Bowen WH, Koo H. Symbiotic relationship between Streptococcus mutans and Candida albicans synergizes virulence of plaque biofilms in vivo. Infect Immun. 2014;82:1968–81.
14. Van Houte J. Role of micro-oganisms in caries etiology. J Dent Res. 1994;73:672–81.
15. Van Houte J, Lopman J, Kent R. The final pH of bacteria comprising the predominant flora on sound and carious human root and enamel surfaces. J Dent Res. 1996;75:1008–14.

16. Wandelt S. Hefen in der menschlichen Mundhöhle und ihre Bedeutung für die Ätiologie der Karies. Dtsch Zahnärztl Z. 1969;24:486–528.

17. Wetzel WE, Sziegoleit A, Weckler C. Karies-Candidose im Milchgebiss. Notabene Medici. 1984;10:845–9.

18. Wetzel WE, Sziegoleit A. Karies-Candidose in Milch-, Wechsel- und bleibenden Gebissen. Hautnah Dermatol. 1990;4:40–5.

19. Wetzel WE, Hanisch S, Sziegoleit A. Keimbesiedlung in der Mundhöhle bei Kleinkindern mit nursing-bottle-syndrom. Schweiz Monatsschr Zahnmed. 1993;103:1107–12.

20. Williams DW, Lewis MAO. Isolation and identification of candida from the oral cavity. Oral Dis. 2000;6:3–11.

21. Enaia M, Bock NC, Ruf S. White-spot lesions during MB appliance treatment: a challenge for clinical excellence. Am J Orthod Dentofacial Orthop. 2011; 140:e17–24.

22. Richter AE, Arruda AO, Peters MC, Sohn W. Incidence of caries lesions among patients treated with comprehensive orthodontics. Am J Orthod Dentofacial Orthop. 2011;139:657–64.

23. Ögaard B, Rölla G, Arends J, Ten Cate JM. Orthodontic appliances and enamel demineralization. Part 2. Prevention and treatment of lesions. Am J Orthod Dentofacial Orthop. 1988;94:123–8.

24. Heymann GC, Grauer D. A contemporary review of white spot lesions in orthodontics. J Esthet Restor Dent. 2013;25:85–95.

25. Lucchese A, Gherlone E. Prevalence of white-spot lesions before and during orthodontic treatment with fixed appliances. Eur J Orthod. 2013;35:664–8.

26. Klein H, Palmer C. Studies on dental caries. Pub Hlth Rep. 1939;53:1353–64.

27. Arslan SG, Akpolat N, Kama JD, Özer T, Hamamci O. One-year follow-up of the effect of fixed orthodontic treatment on colonization by oral candida. J Oral Pathol Med. 2008;37:26–9.

28. Peros K, Mestrovic S, Anic-Milosevic S, Slaj M. Salivary microbial and nonmicrobial parameters in children with fixed orthodontic appliances. Angle Orthod. 2011;81:901–6.

29. Petti S, Barbato E, Simonetti D'Arca A. Effect of orthodontic therapy with fixed and removable appliances on oral microbiota: a six-month longitudinal study. New Microbiol. 1997;20:55–62.

30. Ristic M, Vlohovic Svabic M, Sasic M, Zelic O. Clinical and microbiological effects of fixed orthodontic appliances on periodontal tissues in adolescents. Orthod Craniofacial Res. 2007;10:187–95.

31. Arendorf T, Walker D. The prevalence and intra-oral distribution of Candida albicans in man. Arch Oral Biol. 1980;25:1–10.

32. Darwazeh AMG, Hammad MM, Al-Jamaei AA. The relationship between oral hygiene and oral colonization with Candida species in healthy adult subjects. Int J Dent Hygiene. 2010;8:128–33.

33. Moalic E, Gestalin A, Quinio D, Gest PE, Zerilli A, Le Flohic AM. The extent of oral fungal flora in 353 students and possible relationships with dental caries. Caries Res. 2001;35:149–55.

34. Muzurovic S, Babajic E, Masic T, Smajic R, Selmanagic A. The relationship between oral hygiene and oral colonisation with Candida species. Med Arh. 2012;66:415–7.

35. Roskiewicz D, Daniluk T, Zaremba ML, Cylwik-Rokicka D, Stokowska W, Pawinska M, Dabrowska E, Marcuk-Kolada G, Waszkiel D. Oral Candida albicans carriage in healthy preschool and school children. Adv Med Sci. 2006;51 Suppl 1:187–90.

36. Russell JI, Mac Farlane TW, Aitchison TC, Stephen KW, Burchell CK. Salivary levels of mutans streptococci, Lactobacillus, Candida, and Veilonella species in a group of Scottish Adolescents. Community Dent Oral Epidemiol. 1990;18:17–21.

37. Arendorf T, Addy M. Candida carriage and plaque distribution before, during and after removable orthodontic appliance therapy. J Clin Periodontol. 1985;12:360–8.

38. Hildebrandt GH, Bretz WA. Comparison of culture media and chairside assays for enumerating mutans streptococci. J Appl Microbiol. 2006;100:1339–47.

39. Samaranayake LP, Mac Farlane TW, Lamey PJ, Ferguson MM. A comparison of oral rinse and imprint sampling techniques for the detection of yeast, coliform and Staphylococcus aureus carriage in the oral cavity. J Oral Pathol. 1986;15:386–8.

40. Aas JA, Griffen AL, Dardis SR, Lee AM, Olsen I, Dewhirst FE, Leys EJ, Paster BJ. Bacteria of dental caries in primary and permanent teeth in children and young adults. J Clin Microbiol. 2008;46:1407–17.

41. Badet C, Thebaud N. Ecology of lactobacilli in the oral cavity: a review of literature. Open Microbiol J. 2008;2:38–48.

42. Sansone C, Van Houte J, Joshipura K, Kent R, Margolis HC. The Association of mutans streptococci and non-mutans streptococci capable of acidogenesis at a low pH with dental caries on enamel and root surfaces. J Dent Res. 1993; 72:508–16.

43. Arneberg P, Ögaard B, Scheie AA, Rölla G. Selection of streptococcus mutans and lactobacilli in an intra-oral human caries model. J Dent Res. 1984;63:1197–200.

44. Raja M, Hannan A, Ali K. Association of oral candida carriage with dental caries in children. Caries Res. 2010;44:272–6.

45. Yang XQ, Zang Q, Lu LY, Yang R, Liu Y, Zou J. Genotypic distribution of Candida albicans in dental biofilm of Chinese children associated with severe early childhood caries. Arch Oral Biol. 2012;57:1048–53.

46. Srivastava B, Bhatia HP, Chaudhary V, Aggarwal A, Kumar Singh A, Gupta N. Comparative evaluation of oral Candida albicans carriage in children with and without dental caries: a microbiological in vivo study. Int J Clin Pediatr Dent. 2012;5:108–12.

47. Lied TR, Kazandjian VA. A Hawthorne strategy: implications for performance measurement and improvement. Clin Perform Qual Health Care. 1998;6:201–4.

27

First-in-human study and clinical case reports of the alveolar bone regeneration with the secretome from human mesenchymal stem cells

Wataru Katagiri[*], Masashi Osugi, Takamasa Kawai and Hideharu Hibi

Abstract

Background: Secreted growth factors and cytokines in the conditioned medium from bone marrow-derived mesenchymal stem cells (MSC-CM) have several effects on cell behavior. Our previous studies revealed that MSC-CM enhances bone regeneration by increasing cell mobilization, angiogenesis, and osteogenesis in vitro and in vivo. This clinical study was undertaken to evaluate the safety and use of MSC-CM for alveolar bone regeneration in eight patients who were diagnosed as needing bone augmentation prior to dental implant placement.

Methods: The protocol of this clinical study was approved by the ethics committee of Nagoya University Hospital. MSC-CM was prepared from conditioned medium from commercially available human bone marrow-derived MSCs. Patients were treated with beta-tricalcuim phosphate (β-TCP) or an atelocollagen sponge soaked with MSC-CM. Clinical and radiographic assessments were performed during the follow-up period. Histological assessments were also performed in some cases. Clinical and histological data from patients who underwent the SFE procedure without MSC-CM were also used retrospectively as reference controls.

Results: MSC-CM contained several cytokines such as insulin-like growth factor-1, vascular endothelial growth factor, transforming growth factor-β1, and hepatocyte growth factor in relatively low amounts. No systemic or local complications were reported throughout the study. Radiographic evaluation revealed early bone formation in all cases. Histological evaluation also supported the radiographic findings. Furthermore, infiltration of inflammatory cells was scarce throughout the specimens.

Conclusions: MSC-CM was used safely and with less inflammatory signs and appears to have great osteogenic potential for regenerative medicine of bone. This is the first in-human clinical study of alveolar bone regeneration using MSC-CM.

Keywords: Secretome, Mesenchymal stem cells (MSC), Tissue engineering, Regenerative medicine, Bone

Background

Alveolar bone regeneration with grafting is often carried out prior to placement of dental implants. Several graft materials have been used including autogenous bone, xenogeneic bone, and synthetic bone substitutes. Autogenous bone grafts have been used for a long time with good predictability and are considered the "gold standard" because of their osteoinductive and osteoconductive properties and immunogenic compatibility. However, autogenous

bone must be harvested from a donor site of the patient and is associated with higher morbidity [1, 2]. Xenogeneic bone and synthetic bone substitutes such as deproteinized bovine bone, hydroxyapatite, and calcium triphosphate are often used clinically as osteoconductive scaffolds, but they provide limited osteoinductivity and a potential risk of infection and extrusion [3]. Osteoinductive growth factors such as bone morphogenic protein (BMP)-2 have been used with these osteoconductive materials to promote bone regeneration [4]. However, recent studies have indicated unexpected effects on bone regeneration [5] including induction of a severe inflammatory response,

* Correspondence: w-kat@med.nagoya-u.ac.jp
Department of Oral and Maxillofacial Surgery, Nagoya University Graduate School of Medicine, 65 Tsuruma-cho, Showa-ku, Nagoya 466-8550, Japan

because of the higher dose with clinical application of BMP-2 [6–8].

Recently, the concept of tissue engineering and regenerative medicine has been widely accepted [9], and many clinical studies have been performed including studies of bone and periodontal regenerative medicine.

We previously developed a technique whereby autogenous human mesenchymal stem cells (hMSCs) from the patient's bone marrow are combined with platelet-rich plasma for use as an alternative to such materials with predictable good prognosis [10, 11]. However, clinical use of stem cells requires highly qualified safety investigation and quality management of cell handling, and is very expensive. These limitations currently impede the widespread use of stem cells for alveolar bone regeneration therapy. Moreover, recent studies have revealed that the implanted cells do not survive long [12–14]. As an alternative, the effects of the secretomes, the various factors secreted into the medium, from stem cells on tissue repair and regeneration have attracted much attention [15–17].

We have reported the effects of the secretomes in the conditioned medium from bone marrow-derived mesenchymal stem cells (MSC-CM) on bone and periodontal tissue regeneration in vitro and in vivo. MSC-CM contains several cytokines such as insulin-like growth factor (IGF)-1, vascular endothelial growth factor (VEGF), and transforming growth factor (TGF)-β1. MSC-CM enhances cell proliferation, mobilization, angiogenesis, and expression of osteogenic markers such as *alkaline phosphatase, collagen type I,* and *Runx2* genes [18]. MSC-CM also recruits endogenous stem cells to the grafted site and shows early bone and periodontal regeneration in rat calvarial bone defects and dog periodontal bone defects [19–21]. Furthermore, the concentrations of cytokines contained in MSC-CM are relatively low such that use of MSC-CM does not induce the severe histological inflammatory responses that are observed with the clinical use of recombinant human BMP-2 [18].

Based on these experimental and preclinical studies, we performed a clinical study using MSC-CM for alveolar bone regeneration. Until now, no human study has been reported, and thus, this is the first in-human study using MSC-CM for bone regenerative therapy.

Methods
Cell culture and preparation of MSC-CM
Human MSCs were purchased from Lonza Inc. (Walkersville, MD, USA) and cultured in mesenchymal stem cell basal medium (MSCBM; Lonza Inc.) with MSCGM SingleQuots (Lonza Inc.). Cells of the third passage were used in this study. Cells were maintained at 37 °C in 5 % CO_2/95 % air.

When hMSCs reached 70 % confluency, the medium was refreshed with 10 ml serum-free Dulbecco's modified

Eagle's Medium (DMEM; GIBCO, Rockville, MD, USA) containing antibiotics (100 units/ml penicillin G, 100 μg/ml streptomycin, and 0.25 μg/ml amphotericin B; GIBCO). The cell culture-conditioned media were collected after incubation for 48 h. This medium was defined as MSC-CM.

For clinical use, MSC-CM was then concentrated and stored as described below. Briefly, MSC-CM was centrifuged for 5 min at 1500 rpm and then for another 1 min at 15,000 rpm to remove any cells. Five milliliters MSC-CM was mixed with 45 ml 100 % ethanol and incubated at –20 °C for 1 h. The mixture was centrifuged for 15 min at 15,000 rpm at 4 °C, and the supernatant was discarded. The precipitate was suspended again in cold 90 % ethanol and centrifuged for 15 min at 15,000 rpm at 4 °C. The final precipitate was frozen at –80 °C, lyophilized, and stored at –80 °C until use.

To verify the safety, MSC-CM was examined for not only contamination with bacteria, fungi, or mycoplasmas but also virus infection including hepatitis B and C virus, human immunodeficiency virus, and human T-cell leukemia virus before the following procedures.

Enzyme-linked immunosorbent assay (ELISA)
The levels of IGF-1, VEGF, TGF-β1, hepatocyte growth factor (HGF), fibroblast growth factor (FGF)-2, platelet-derived growth factor (PDGF)-BB, BMP-2, and stromal cell-derived factor (SDF)-1α in MSC-CM were investigated using ELISA. The concentration of these factors was measured using a Human Quantikine ELISA kit (R&D Systems, Minneapolis, MN, USA) according to the manufacturer's instructions. Briefly, 200 μl MSC-CM, DMEM-0 % FBS, or DMEM-30 % FBS were added to 96-well microplates that were coated with a monoclonal antibody recognizing the factor of interest and incubated for 2 h. After washing with phosphate-buffered saline (PBS), a horseradish peroxidase-conjugated antibody against the cytokine or growth factor was added to each well, incubated for 2 h, and washed. Substrate solution was added and incubated for 30 min, and the reaction was terminated by addition of the stop solution. Cytokine levels were determined by measuring the optical density at 450 nm using a microplate spectrophotometer (Benchmark Plus; Bio-Rad, Hercules, CA, USA).

Patient selection
Eight partially edentulous patients who were diagnosed as needing bone augmentation, including maxillary sinus floor elevation (SFE), guided bone regeneration (GBR) and socket preservation (SP), were enrolled in this study. Because of severe alveolar bone atrophy, all the patients had problems with retention of conventional removable dentures, and these procedures and application of dental implants were expected to solve this problem. The

criteria for application of these procedures are <5 mm residual bone from the sinus floor to the alveolar ridge in SFE cases and <10 mm of residual bone height in GBR cases.

After routine oral and physical examinations, patients who did not desire to undergo surgery for autogenous bone harvesting were selected for this study. All patients were healthy and free from any disease that may have influenced the outcome of this study (e.g., diabetes, malignant tumor, autoimmune disease, bone disease, endocrine disease). Each patient provided informed consent after receiving detailed information about the surgical procedures, graft materials, alternative treatments, and uncertainties of using a new method. The ethics committee of Nagoya University Hospital approved this research protocol (No.3437). Clinical, radiographic and histological data from two patients who underwent the SFE procedure without MSC-CM were also used retrospectively as reference controls.

Preparation and application of MSC-CM

During the surgery, MSC-CM was dissolved in 5 ml saline. As a scaffold, porous pure beta-tricalcuim phosphate (β-TCP; Osferion®, Olympus Terumo Biomaterials, Tokyo, Japan) was used in SFE and GBR cases. In some cases with small and four-wall defects in SP cases, a shell-shaped atelocollagen sponge (ACS) (Terudermis®; Olympus Terumo Biomaterials) was also used as a scaffold. β-TCP (1 g) or ACS (8 mm in diameter × 25 mm in length) was soaked with 3 ml of MSC-CM solution for at least 5 min and then used for grafting (Fig. 1).

Surgical procedures

All surgical procedures were conducted under local anesthesia. The SFE procedure was performed using the lateral window approach [22]. Briefly, a window was created with a round diamond burr at the lateral maxillary sinus wall. After removing the bone, the sinus membrane was elevated. The space created by this procedure was filled with the mixture of MSC-CM and β-TCP (MSC-CM/β-TCP). In cases of simultaneous implant placement, Brånemark MkIII Groovy or NobelActive implants (Nobel Biocare, Zürich, Switwerland) were placed into the alveolar bone at a depth of at least 5 mm according to pre-surgical computer simulation. The lateral window was then covered with a bioabsorbable polylactic acid-glycol acid (PLGA) membrane (GC Membrane®, GC, Tokyo, Japan). The mucoperiosteal flap was repositioned and sutured in the usual manner. The GBR procedure was performed after the mucoperiosteal flap was elevated. In cases of simultaneous implant placement, implants were placed in the same manner as described above. Because of the atrophic alveolar bone, exposed threads of the implants were covered with

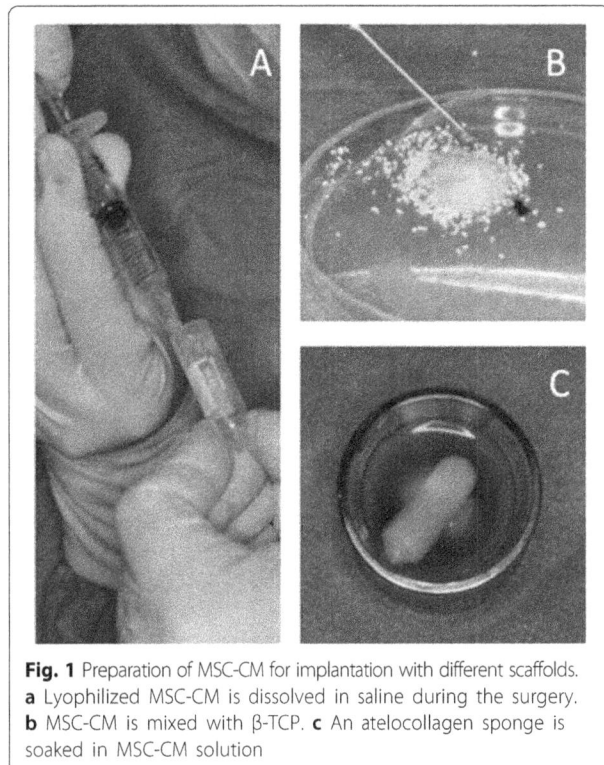

Fig. 1 Preparation of MSC-CM for implantation with different scaffolds. **a** Lyophilized MSC-CM is dissolved in saline during the surgery. **b** MSC-CM is mixed with β-TCP. **c** An atelocollagen sponge is soaked in MSC-CM solution

MSC-CM/β-TCP. In SP cases such as tooth extraction sockets, the bone defects were filled with MSC-CM/ACS. After grafting MSC-CM/β-TCP, the grafted areas were covered with PLGA membranes. Lesions grafted with MSC-CM/ACS were not covered with any membranes, and all lesions were closed with a tension-free mucoperiosteal flap. In all cases, the second-stage surgeries were performed about 6 months after implant placement (first-stage surgery). All surgeries were performed by the same surgeon (W.K.).

Clinical and radiographic observations

After registration, safety evaluations were performed before surgery. Briefly, the drug lymphocyte stimulation test (DLST) and the patch test were performed to evaluate the allergic reaction to MSC-CM. Blood tests were also performed to check for any organ dysfunction and inflammatory and allergic reactions before and after surgery. Computed tomography (CT) scans and panoramic X-ray examinations were performed before and after surgery. Bone biopsies were obtained for histology with a 2-mm-diameter trephine bar at the regenerated bone areas during the second-stage surgery and immersed in 10 % formaldehyde. Paraffin sections were prepared according to standard protocols, and hematoxylin-eosin staining was performed. The protocol for clinical and radiographic observations in this study is shown in Table 1.

Table 1 The schedule of this clinical study

Item		Before registration	After registration	Administration	After administration			
					<1W	1M	3M	6M
Informed consent		●						
Patient background		●	●					
Administration of MSC-CM				●				
Safety evaluation	Observation of medical findings of the oral cavity and whole body	●	●		●	●	●	●
	Blood test		●		●		●	
	DLST and Patch test		●					
Clinical evaluation	X-ray		●		●	●	●	●
	Clinical inspections		●		●	●	●	●
	Bone biopsy (if possible)							●

Results

Cytokines present in MSC-CM

The concentrations of the cytokines IGF-1, VEGF, TGF-β1, HGF, FGF-2, PDGF-BB, BMP-2, and SDF-1α in MSC-CM were quantified with ELISA. Cytokines were not detected in DMEM-0 % and DMEM-30 %. However, MSC-CM contained IGF-1, VEGF, TGF-β1, and HGF at concentrations of 1386 ± 465, 468.5 ± 109, 339.8 ± 14.4, and 20.3 ± 7.8 pg/ml, respectively. The other factors assayed were not detected in MSC-CM (Table 2).

Clinical observations

The eight patients in this study included three men and five women, ranging from 45 to 67 (mean, 57.8 years) years old. SFE was performed in three patients, and GBR was performed in five patients. β-TCP was used in all SFE cases and two GBR cases, whereas ACS was used in two SP cases (Table 3). No systemic or local complications were noted throughout the study. The results of DLST and blood tests showed no abnormal findings except minor inflammatory signs after surgery. Implant placement was performed simultaneously with the bone

Table 2 Cytokines detected in MSC-CM

Cytokines	Concentration (pg/ml)
IGF-1	1386±465
VEGF	465.8±109
TGF-β	339.8±14.4
HGF	20.3±7.8
FGF-2	ND
PDGF-BB	ND
BMP-2	ND
SDF-1	ND

ND Not detected

Table 3 Patient data

Patient	Age(y)	Sex	Location	Surgery	Scaffold
1	46	F	25,26	SFE	TCP
2	67	F	45	SP	ACS
3	45	F	35,36	GBR	TCP
4	51	F	47	SP	ACS
5	63	M	11,21	GBR	TCP
6	67	F	45	SP	ACS
7	59	M	27	SFE	TCP
8	64	M	25,26,27	SFE	TCP

SFE sinus floor elevation, *GBR* guided bone regeneration, *SP* socket preservation, *TCP* β-TCP, *ACS* atelocollagen sponge

augmentation procedure in five cases and was performed within 8 to 9 months after the first surgeries in two cases. All the implants were placed without any problems and showed good initial stabilities.

Radiographic observations

Panorama X-ray and CT images showed early mineralization in the augmented bone. Furthermore, CT images showed that the β-TCP structures gradually become indistinct around 6 months after the first surgery. No bone resorption was observed in any cases, and notable edematous swelling of the maxillary sinus membrane was not obvious throughout the study after the surgery in SFE cases.

Histological observations

Bone biopsies were taken from five cases. Newly formed bone was observed in each specimen. Resorption of β-TCP was found, and replacement with new bone had occurred only 6 months after the first surgery. Furthermore, infiltration of inflammatory cells (e.g., neutrophils, macrophages) was observed less often in these specimens.

Case reports

Case 1

A 46-year-old woman came to the hospital because she had lost her left maxillary teeth because of periodontitis about 3 months before. CT images showed alveolar bone loss at 25 and 26; the thickness of the residual bone was about 3 to 5 mm. SFE and simultaneous implant placement were planned under local anesthesia. Once the lateral maxillary window was opened and the maxillary sinus membrane was elevated, two Brånemark MkIII Groovy 11.5-mm long implants were placed into the prepared cavity (Fig. 2a). Then MSC-CM/β-TCP was implanted into the cavity, especially around the exposed implants. About 0.5 g β-TCP was used to fill the cavity (Fig. 2b). The window was covered with a PLGA membrane, and the wound was closed with a tension-free mucoperiosteal flap. After 6 months, the second-stage surgery was performed. The lateral window was almost covered with newly formed bone and some remnants of β-TCP. Osseointegration of the implants was good, and a bone biopsy was taken from the augmented area (Fig. 2c).

In CT images, the particles of implanted β-TCP were clear 1 month after the first surgery, but became gradually indistinct after 6 months (Fig. 2d-f). Histologic findings also supported this phenomenon. The remnants of β-TCP were resolved from the edge, and replacement with new bone was observed. Interestingly, infiltration of inflammatory cells was not severe, and newly formed bone was seen throughout the specimen (Fig. 2g, h). As a reference control, histology from a patient who had

undergone SFE with β-TCP only (i.e., without MSC-CM) 6 months before is shown in Fig. 3. Replacements of β-TCP with regenerated bone were scarce, and infiltration of inflammatory cells was observed around the particles of β-TCP.

Case 2

A 67-year-old woman presented with severe bone resorption due to periodontitis at 45, and this tooth was extracted 3 weeks prior to the SP procedure. X-ray diagnosis revealed that the residual bone height was appropriate. However, the extraction socket remained, and socket preservation was considered to be ideal for future implant placement. A crestal incision and mucoperiosteal flap were made at the buccal aspect of the right mandibular molar area. Granulation tissue was removed from the flap and bony defect with curettes, and perforation of the surrounding cortical bone was done with a bar to improve the blood supply. MSC-CM/ACS was implanted into the bony defect, and the flap was closed (Fig. 4a, b). Healing was uneventful. CT images showed gradual bone formation in the implanted area (Fig. 4d-f). Six months after MSC-CM/ACS implantation, CT images showed that the extraction socket had almost completely filled with newly formed bone, and placement of the implant was planned 8 months after the first surgery. Prior to implant placement, a bone biopsy was done from where the NobelActive 11.5-mm-long implant would be placed (Fig. 4c). The bone quality was so good that the implant acquired initial stability. H-E staining of the specimen showed dense trabecular bone with little infiltration of inflammatory cells (Fig. 4g, h).

Discussion and conclusions

This study evaluated the safety and efficacy of MSC-CM in a human clinical trial for alveolar bone regeneration. Tissue engineering and regenerative medicine of the bone and periodontal tissue using stem cells has begun to be used clinically [10, 23]. We have developed regenerative medicine for bone and periodontal tissue using autogenous bone marrow-derived MSCs, and this approach is considered an alternative to conventional autogenous bone grafting [11]. However, the use of adult stem cells for tissue regeneration has several problems such as safety and quality management in stem cell handling, and the high cost and strict regulation by authorities currently prevent the popularization of this approach. Moreover, permanent engraftment and transdifferentiation of transplanted adult stem cells have not been confirmed [24]. Recent studies have indicated that the therapeutic effects of transplanted stem cells are considered effective for tissue regeneration and for their interesting role as cellular modulators, not just for their multipotent differentiation ability [25, 26].

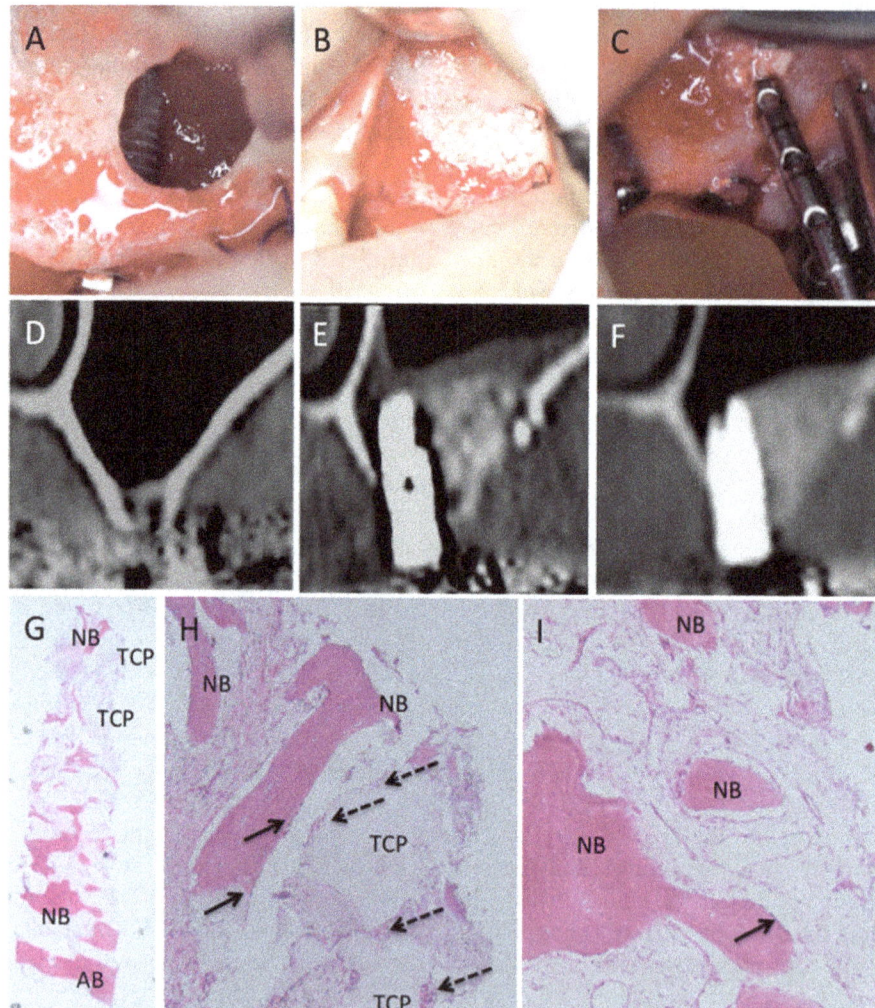

Fig. 2 Clinical, radiographic, and histological observations in Case 1. **a** The implant is placed into the cavity created by the SFE procedure. **b** The cavity is filled with MSC-CM/β-TCP. **c** The second surgery. A bone biopsy was taken from the newly formed bone 6 months after the SFE procedure. **d-f** CT images before and after the SFE procedure. **d** Before the SFE procedure. **e** Three months after the SFE procedure. **f** Six months after the SFE procedure. **g, h, i** Histologic findings of the specimen from the augmented area (H-E stain). **g** Out line of the specimen (×12.5). **h** Nasal side of the specimen (H; ×100). **i** Oral side of the specimen (×100). Newly formed bone was seen throughout the specimen. Arrow indicates the arrangement of osteoblasts along with the newly formed bone. The residual β-TCP granules were seen at the nasal side of specimen. The dotted arrow indicates β-TCP resorption by osteoclasts. (TCP: β-TCP, NB: Newly formed bone)

Transplanted stem cells release several paracrine factors such as cytokines, growth factors, and extracellular matrix molecules that modulate endogenous cellular mobilization, angiogenesis, and cellular differentiation, and induce endogenous stem cells to promote tissue repair and regeneration [15]. Our previous studies revealed that MSC-CM contains several cytokines, such as IGF-1, VEGF, TGF-β1, and HGF, and enhances early bone and periodontal tissue regeneration [18–21]. IGF-1 induces osteoblast proliferation and migration [27, 28] and enhances periodontal regeneration by stimulating periodontal ligament (PDL) cells through the PI3K pathway [29]. VEGF is believed to be the main regulator of angiogenesis, and bone marrow stromal cells secrete sufficient quantities of VEGF to enhance the survival and differentiation of endothelial cells. VEGF also contributes to osteogenesis [30]. TGF-β1 enhances the migration of osteoprogenitor cells, and regulates cell proliferation, differentiation, and extracellular matrix production [31]. TGF-β1 also stimulates PDL regeneration and repair [32] and is expressed during the development of the alveolar bone, PDL, and cementum [33]. HGF has a direct effect on angiogenesis [34]. A previous study demonstrated that a combination of several factors has an additive effect on cellular migration and osteogenic differentiation [35]. Some studies have investigated a combination of two or more factors to promote bone regeneration [35, 36].

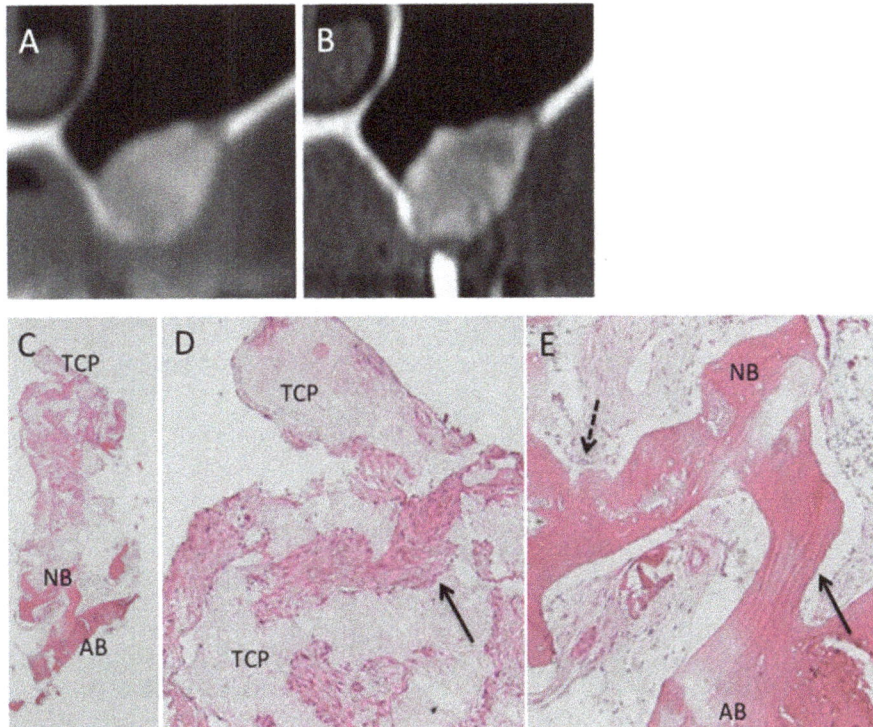

Fig. 3 Histological observation in the reference case. CT images and histology of an SFE case with β-TCP alone are shown. **a**, **b** CT images after the SFE procedure. **a** Three months after the SFE procedure. **b** Six months after the SFE procedure. **c** Outline of the specimen. Newly formed bone is scarce, and β-TCP remains much from nasal part to the middle area of the specimen (H-E, ×12.5). **d** Nasal side of the specimen (×100). **e** Oral side of the specimen (×100). Replacement of new bone is insufficient. The arrow indicates infiltration of inflammatory cells. Arrow indicates the arrangement of osteoblasts along with the newly formed bone. The dotted arrow indicates that osteoclasts, but the number of osteoclasts was less. Infiltration of the inflammatory cells was seen in the oral part of the specimen. (TCP: β-TCP, NB: Newly formed bone, AB: Alveolar bone)

In our study, the advantage of a combination of several factors seems to be versatile effects on bone regeneration. Furthermore, the concentration of each cytokine in MSC-CM may be relatively low and at physiological levels because they were secreted from cells and are not an industrial product such as recombinant BMP-2. BMP-2 has a strong osteoinductive ability, but a high concentration of BMP-2 is required to obtain therapeutic effects on bone regeneration. Cowan et al. suggested that BMP has dose-dependent bone regeneration effects in the rat calvaria model, and the concentration of BMP-2 that induced effective bone regeneration was 240 ng/mm^3 [37]. In MSC-CM, the concentration of each cytokine was around hundreds to thousands of picograms per milliliter.

MSC-CM has other effects as well. Ionescu et al. suggested that conditioned medium from MSCs promotes alternative macrophage activation, producing a wound healing/anti-inflammatory M2 phenotype that is due in part to IGF-1 [38]. We found that only a few inflammatory cells were seen where MSC-CM was implanted in our allogeneic animal study [18–21]. In this clinical study, no patient showed abnormal swelling or delayed healing after surgery. β-TCP has been widely used

clinically both in orthopedic and maxillofacial lesions and produces excellent osteoconductivity; however, β-TCP is resorbed over a long period [39]. In this study, β-TCP mixed with MSC-CM promoted early resorption and replacement of new bone compared with β-TCP without MSC-CM. This phenomenon may have been due not only to the effects of several cytokines that induced several types of cell behavior and angiogenesis as described above, but also alternative macrophage phenotypes that quickly degraded the scaffold. Badylak et al. investigated the two different types of scaffolds. One was a chemically cross-linked scaffold that did not show any significant degradation during the study period following implantation and that resulted in a predominantly M1-type macrophage response. The other was a non-cross-linked scaffold that was rapidly degraded following implantation and that elicited an M2-type response and showed more constructive regeneration of tissue [40]. From this point of view, the cytokines in MSC-CM are considered to induce the resorption of β-TCP and the switching of the phenotype of macrophages from M1 to M2 at an earlier phase of bone regeneration. Interestingly, implantation of MSC-CM/ACS resulted in denser

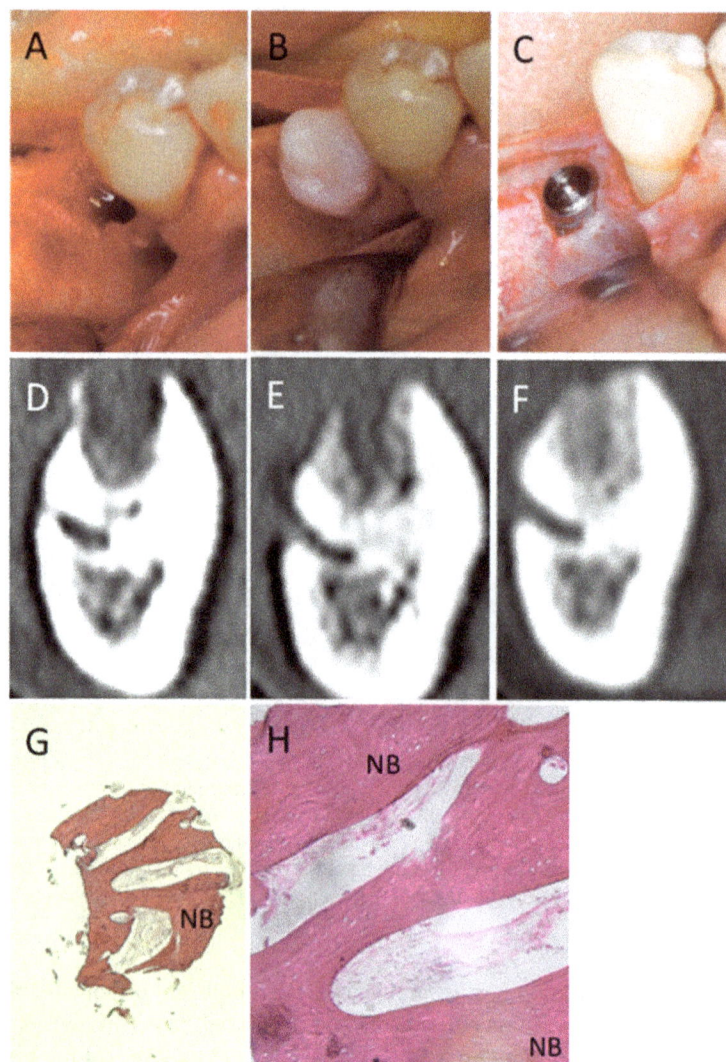

Fig. 4 Clinical, radiographic, and histological observations in Case 2. **a** The extraction socket remains at the distal part of the right mandibular first premolar. **b** The socket was filled with MSC-CM/ACS. **c** The implant placement 8 months after MSC/ACS implantation. The socket is completely regenerated with newly formed bone. A bone biopsy was done where the implant was placed. **d-f** CT images before and after the SP procedure. **d** Before the SP procedure. **e** Three months after the SP procedure. **f** Six months after the SP procedure. **g, h** Histologic findings of the specimen from the augmented area (H-E stain) (G; ×12.5 and H; ×40). Newly formed and mature bone was seen throughout the specimen. No inflammatory cells were seen in this specimen. (NB: Newly formed bone)

new bone formation shown as in case 2. ACS is resorbed more easily than β-TCP, and this finding is also consistent with the relationship between the mechanical characteristics of the scaffolds and the phenotype of macrophages.

MSC-CM leads to prominent osteoinductivity according to our series of studies. MSC-CM is required at a relatively low physiological dose to produce therapeutic effects, and it may also have an immunomodulatory effect as described above. Further studies will be required to confirm which individual factors are important and indispensable. This implies the possibility of making new agents using these novel concepts for not only bone and

periodontal regeneration but also other systemic diseases that had previously been expected to be treated with transplantation of stem cells.

This is the first-in-human study for alveolar bone regeneration using MSC-CM. Because this study was aimed to assess the safety and response to MSC-CM clinically with a small patients group, we could not deeply show and discuss about the radiographic and histological effects. We have already started the next phase clinical trial to assess the efficacy of MSC-CM on alveolar bone regeneration with more lager patients group. We are planning to report these results will in the future.

Abbreviations

MSC-CM: conditioned medium from bone marrow-derived mesenchymal stem cells; β-TCP: beta-tricalcium phosphate; ACS: atelocollagen sponge; IGF: insulin like growth factor; VEGF: vascular endothelial growth factor; TGF: transforming growth factor; BMP: bone morphogenetic protein; HGF: hepatocyte growth factor; FGF: fibroblast growth factor; PDGF: platelet-derived growth factor; SDF: stromal cell-derived factor; DMEM: Dulbecco's modified eagle's medium; SFE: sinus floor elevation; GBR: guided bone regeneration; SP: socket preservation.

Competing interests

The authors declare that they have no competing interests.

Authors' contributions

WK did main contribution on carrying this clinical study and manuscript preparation. OM did surgical assist in this study. TK mainly prepared MSC-CM with the help of WK and OM. HH participated in designing and coordination of this study. All authors read and approved the final manuscript.

Acknowledgements

The authors wish to thank Tatsuo Hirai, Hideo Tateishi, Yukako Fukada and Erika Sasaki in Fujieda Heisei Memorial Hospital for their help, encouragement and contributions to the completion of this study. The authors also thank Minoru Ueda, Ryoko Yoshimi and the members of the Department of Oral and Maxillofacial Surgery, Nagoya University Graduate School of Medicine for their assistance. This work was supported in part by Grants-in-Aid for Scientific Research (B) (23592883) from the Ministry of Education, Culture, Sports, and Technology of Japan. None of the authors have any conflicts of interest associated with this study.

References

1. Arrington ED, Smith WJ, Chambers HG, Bucknell AL, Davino NA. Complications of iliac crest bone graft harvesting. Clin Orthop Relat Res. 1996;329:300–9.
2. Joshi A, Kostakis GC. An investigation of post-operative morbidity following iliac crest graft harvesting. Br Dent J. 2004;196:167–71.
3. Damien CJ, Parsons JR. Bone graft and bone graft substitutes: a review of current technology and applications. J Appl Biomater. 1991;2:187–208.
4. Herford AS, Boyne PJ. Reconstruction of mandibular continuity defects with bone morphogenic protein-2 (rhBMP-2). J Oral Maxillofac Surg. 2008;66:616–24.
5. Woo EJ. Adverse events reported after the use of recominnant human bone morphogenetic protein 2. J Oral Maxillofac Surg. 2012;70:765–7.
6. Perri B, Cooper M, Lauryssen C, Anand N. Adverse swelling associated with use of rh-BMP-2 in anterior cervical discectomy and fusion: a case study. Spine J. 2007;7:235–9.
7. Vaidya R, Carp J, Sethi A, Bartol S, Craig J, Les CM. Complications of anterior cervical discectomy and fusion using recombinant human bone morphogenetic protein-2. Eur Spine J. 2007;16:1257–65.
8. Kawasaki K, Aihara M, Honmo J, Sakurai S, Fujimaki Y, Sakamoto K, et al. Effects of reconbinant human bone morphogenetic protein-2 on differentiation of cells isolated from human bone, muscle, and skin. Bone. 1998;23:223–31.
9. Langer R, Vacanti JP. Tissue engineering. Science. 1993;260:920–6.
10. Yamada Y, Ueda M, Naiki T, Takahashi M, Hata K, Nagasaka T. Autogenous injectable bone for regeneration with mesenchymal stem cells (MSCs) and platelet-rich plasma (PRP) – Tissue-engineered bone regeneration. Tissue Eng. 2004;10:955–64.
11. Yamada Y, Nakamura S, Ito K, Umemura E, Hara K, Nagasaka T, et al. Injectable bonetissue engineeringusingexpanded mesenchymal stem cells. Stem Cells. 2013;31:572–80.
12. Muller-Ehmsen J, Whittaker P, Kloner RA, Dow JS, Sakoda T, Long TI, et al. Survival and development of neonatal rat cardiomyocytes transplanted into adult myocardium. J Mol Cell Cardiol. 2002;34:107–16.
13. Toma C, Wagner WR, Bowry S, Schwartz A, Villanueva F. Fate of culture-expanded mesenchymal stem cells in the microvasculature: in vivo observations of cell kinetics. Circ Res. 2009;104:398–402.
14. Ide C, Nakai Y, Nakano N, Seo T, Yamada Y, Endo K, et al. Bone marrow stromal cell transplantation for treatment of sub-acute spinal cord injury in rat. Brain Res. 2010;1332:32–47.
15. Chen L, Tredget EE, Wu PYG, Wu Y. Paracrine factors of mesenchymal stem cells recruit macrophages and endothelial lineage cells and enhance wound healing. PLoS One. 2008;3:e1886.
16. Ciapetti G, Granchi D, Baldini N. The combined use of mesenchymal stromal cells and scaf- folds for bone repair. Curr Pharm Des. 2012;18:1796–820.
17. Baglio SL, Pegtel DM, Baldini N. Mesenchymal stem cell secreted vesicles provide novel opportunities in (stem) cell-free therapy. Front Physiol. 2012;3:1–11.
18. Katagiri W, Osugi M, Kawai T, Ueda M. Novel cell-free regenerative medicine of bone using stem cell derived factors. Int J Oral Maxillofac Implants. 2013;28:1009–16.
19. Osugi M, Katagiri W, Yoshimi R, Inukai T, Hibi H, Ueda M. Conditioned media from mesenchymal stem cells enhancedbone regeneration in rat calvarial bone defects. Tissue Eng Part A. 2012;18:14779–1489.
20. Inukai T, Katagiri W, Yoshimi R, Osugi M, Kawai T, Hibi H, et al. Novel application of stem cell-derived factors for periodontal regeneration. Biochem Biophys Res Commun. 2013;430:763–8.
21. Kawai T, Katagiri W, Osugi M, Sugimura Y, Hibi H, Ueda M. Secretomes from bone marrow-derived mesenchymal stromal cells enhance periodontal tissue regeneration. Cytotherapy. 2015;17:369–81.
22. Tatum H. Maxillary and sinus implant reconstructions. Dent Clin North Am. 1986;30:207–29.
23. Okuda K, Yamamiya K, Kawase T, Mizuno H, Ueda M, Yoshie H. Treatment of human infrabony periodontal defects by grafting human cultured periosteum sheets combined with platelet-rich plasma and porus hydroxyapatite granules: case series. J Int Acad Periodontol. 2009;11:206–13.
24. Freyman T, Polin G, Osman H, Crary J, Lu M, Cheng L, et al. A quantitative, randomized study evaluating three methods of mes- enchymal stem cell delivery fol- lowing myocardial infarction. Eur Heart J. 2006;27:1114–22.
25. Parekkadan B, van Poll D, Suganuma K, Carter EA, Berthiaume F, Tilles AW, et al. Mesenchymal stem cell-derived molecules reverse fulminant hepatic failure. PLoS One. 2007;2:e941.
26. Lee JK, Jin HK, Endo S, Schuchman EH, Carter JE, Bae JS. Intracerebral trans- plantation of bone marrow-derived mesenchymal stem cells reduces amyloid-beta deposition and res- cues memory deficits in Alzheimer's disease mice by modulation of immune responses. Stem Cells. 2010;28:329–43.
27. Cornish J, Grey A, Callon KE, Naot D, Hill BL, Lin CQ, et al. Shared pathways of osteoblast mitogenesis induced by amylin, adrenomedullin, and IGF-1. Biochem Biophys Res Commun. 2004;318:240–6.
28. Li Y, Yu X, Lin S, Li X, Zhang S, Song YH. Insulin-like growth factor 1 enhances the migratory capacity of mesenchymal stem cells. Biochem Biophys Res Commun. 2007;356:780–4.
29. Han X, Amar S. Role of insulin-like growth factor-1 signaling in dental fibroblast apoptosis. J Periodontol. 2003;74:1176–82.
30. Kaiglar D, Krebsbach PH, West ER, Horger K, Huang YC, Mooney DJ. Endothelial cell modulation of bone marrow stromal cell osteogenic potential. FASEB J. 2005;19:665–7.
31. Bostrom MP, Asnis P. Transforming growth factor beta in fracture repair. Clin Orthop Relat Res. 1998;355:S124–131.
32. Fujita T, Shiba H, van Dyke TE, Kurihara H. Differential effects of growth factors and cytokines on the synthesis of SPARC, DNA, fibronectin and alkaline phosphatase activity in human periodontal ligament cells. Cell Biol Int. 2004;28:281–6.
33. Gao J, Symons AL, Bartold PM. Expression of transforming growth factor-beta 1 (TGF-beta1) in the developing periodontium of rats. J Dent Res. 1998;77:1708–16.
34. Morishita R, Nakamura S, Hayashi S, Taniyama Y, Moriguchi A, Nagono T, et al. Therapeutic angiogenesis induced by human recombinant hepatocyte growth factor in rabbit hind limb ischemia model as cytokine supplement therapy. Hypertension. 1999;33:1379–84.
35. Ozaki Y, Nishimura M, Sekiya K, Suehiro F, Kanawa M, Nikawa H, et al. Comprehensive analysis of chemotactic factors for bone marrow mesenchymal stem cells. Stem Cells Dev. 2007;16:119–29.
36. Chen L, Jiang W, Huang J, He B, Zuo G, Zhang W, et al. Insulin-like growth factor 2 (IGF-2) potentiates BMP-9-induced osteogenic differentiation and bone formation. J Bone Miner Res. 2010;25:2447–59.
37. Cowan CM, Aghaloo T, Chou YF, Walder B, Zhang X, Soo C, et al. MicroCT evaluation of three-dimensional mineralization in response to BMP-2 doses in vitro and in critical sized rat calvarial defects. Tissue Eng. 2007;13:501–12.

38. Ionescu L, Byrne RN, van Haaften T, Vadivel A, Alphonse RS, Rey-Parra GJ, et al. Stem cell conditioned medium improves acute lung injury in mice: in vivo evidence for stem cell paracrine action. Am J Physiol Lung Cell Mol Physiol. 2012;303:L967–977.

39. Zerbo IR, Zijderveld SA, De Boer A, Bronckers ALJJ, De Lange G, Bruggenkate CMT, et al. Histomorphometry of human sinus floor augmentation using a porous β-tricalcium phosphate: a prospective study. Clin Oral Implants Res. 2004;15:724–32.

40. Badylak SF, Valentin JE, Ravindra AK, McCabe GP, Stewart-Akers AM. Macrophage phenotype as a determinant of biologic scaffold remodeling. Tissue Eng Part A. 2008;14:1835–42.

28

Facial soft tissue changes after nonsurgical rapid maxillary expansion: a systematic review and meta-analysis

Jing Huang[1], Cui-Ying Li[2*] and Jiu-Hui Jiang[1*] (iD)

Abstract

Background: The present systematic review and meta-analysis aimed to test the hypothesis that no facial soft tissue changes occur after nonsurgical rapid maxillary expansion (RME), in order to provide a reference for orthodontists.

Methods: PubMed, EMBASE, Cochrane Library, OVID, MEDLINE, CINAHL, Scopus, and ScienceDirect databases were electronically and manually searched up to December 2017, and randomized controlled, clinical controlled trials, cohort studies and retrospective studies where soft tissue changes were measured before and after nonsurgical RME were identified. Study appraisal and synthesis were performed by two reviewers who completed the study selection and quality assessment procedures independently and in duplicate. Data from the involved studies were pooled using Revman 5.3.

Results: A total of 1762 articles were identified after the removal of duplicates. After selection and quality assessment, 15 studies met the inclusion criteria for the systematic review, and 13 articles were ultimately included in the meta-analysis. The quality of the involved studies was relatively moderate. Pre-expansion, postexpansion, and postretention data were pooled. The nasal width, alar base width, and distances from the lower lips to the E line showed significant changes after expansion. Moreover, after retention, the nasal width, mouth width, upper philtrum width, and distance from the lower lip to the E line showed significant increases relative to the baseline values. Limitations of the present study included the moderate quality of the included studies and the fact that the results were based on short-term observations of patients in the growth phase.

Conclusion: Our findings suggest that RME results in a significantly increased nasal width, mouth width, upper philtrum width, and distance from the lower lip to the E line after the retention phase. However, the clinical importance of these findings is questionable.

Keywords: Maxillary expansion, Nasal changes, Soft tissue changes

Background

Rapid maxillary expansion (RME) is routinely adopted by orthodontists to eliminate skeletal maxillary transverse deficiency; it is especially preferred for patients with posterior crossbite, moderate crowding, and sleep-disordered breathing [1–4]. This treatment approach involves the mechanical separation of the midpalatal suture via disruption of the sutural connective tissue by orthopedic forces in a short period of time. This increases the width of the maxillary segments and achieves harmony between the maxillary and mandibular arches [3, 4].

However, Proffit et al. claimed that RME should be cautiously used in preschool-aged children, who are at high risk for developing undesirable nasal morphological changes [5]. Bailey et al. also reported a case involving a 5-year-old girl who underwent RME and developed an unpleasant nasal shape and dorsal hump after 10 days of treatment [6]. Moreover, Haas et al. and Berger et al. suggested that an increase in the soft nasal width is a potential side effect of orthopedic maxillary expansion [2, 7].

---

* Correspondence: licuiying_67@163.com; drjiangw@163.com
[2]Central Laboratory, Peking University School and Hospital of Stomatology, 22 South Zhongguancun Avenue, Haidian District, Beijing 100081, China
[1]Department of Orthodontics, Peking University School and Hospital of Stomatology, 22 South Zhongguancun Avenue, Haidian District, Beijing 100081, China

One of the primary aims of orthodontists is to improve facial harmony and esthetics while achieving ideal occlusion. Well-balanced facial soft tissue proportions, rather than hard tissue proportions, should be the ultimate aim of orthodontic treatment [8]. Berger et al. initially associated soft tissue alterations with skeletal changes after RME through an analysis of soft tissue changes in patients who underwent orthopedically or surgically assisted RME. They analyzed posteroanterior cephalograms and confirmed that the soft tissue changes/skeletal changes ratio was 1:1 [7]. These findings were supported by those in a recent study by Pangrazio-Kulbersh et al., who used cone beam computed tomography (CBCT) [9].

Although several studies have reported the skeletal and dental effects of RME, only a few studies and scarce data have addressed alterations in the overlying soft tissue. To our knowledge, there is no meta-analysis concerning the effects of RME on facial soft tissues.

The objective of this meta-analysis was to investigate the hypothesis that no facial soft tissue changes occur after nonsurgical RME, in order to provide a reference for orthodontists.

Methods

This systematic review and meta-analysis followed the Preferred Reporting Items for Systematic Reviews and Meta-Analyses (PRISMA) guidelines. The study was conducted under the ethical guidelines of the 1975 Declaration of Helsinki and was approved by the review committee of the Peking University School and Hospital of Stomatology.

The meta-analysis was designed and conducted according to instructions from the Cochrane Handbook; its study design, participant, intervention, comparison, and outcome definitions were followed.

Study search

PubMed, EMBASE, Cochrane Library, OVID, MEDLINE, CINAHL, Scopus and ScienceDirect databases were electronically and manually searched up to December 2017. A search strategy was formulated for each database; details are shown in Table 1. Only articles published in English were selected, and those in other languages with no English version available were not considered.

Inclusion criteria

The inclusion criteria for the selected articles were as follows: randomized controlled trials (RCTs), clinical controlled trials (CCTs), cohort studies and retrospective studies including human subjects who underwent nonsurgical RME, and the availability of facial tissue

Table 1 Search strategies for different databases

Database	Search strategy	Results
Pubmed	((orthodontics[MeSH Terms]) AND ((maxillary expansion) OR palatal expansion technique[MeSH Terms])) AND (face[Title/Abstract] OR mouth[Title/Abstract] OR lip[Title/Abstract] OR nose[Title/Abstract] OR nasal[Title/Abstract] OR naso*[Title/Abstract] OR alar[Title/Abstract] OR soft tissue*[Title/Abstract])	668
Embase	#1 'orthodontics'/exp. #2 'palatal expansion technique'/exp. #3 'maxillary expansion' #4 'soft tissue':ab,ti #5 face:ab,ti OR mouth:ab,ti OR lip:ab,ti OR nose:ab,ti OR nasal:ab,ti OR naso*:ab,ti OR alar:ab,ti #6 #2 OR #3 #7 #4 OR #5 #8 #1 AND #6 AND #7	282
Crochrane	#1 MeSH descriptor: [Orthodontics] explode all trees #2 MeSH descriptor: [Palatal Expansion Technique] explode all trees #3 face or mouth or lip or nose or nasal or naso* or alar or 'soft tissue*':ti,ab,kw (Word variations have been searched) #4 'maxillary expansion' (Word variations have been searched) #5 #2 OR #4 #6 #1 AND #3 AND #5	66
Ovid	1. exp. orthodontics/ 2. exp. palatal expansion technique/ 3. maxillary expansion.af. 4. 2 or 3 5. (face or mouth or lip or nose or nasal or naso* or alar or soft tissue*).af. 6. 1 and 4 and 5	603
MEDLINE Complete (EBSCOhost)	AB (face or mouth or lip or nose or nasal or naso* or alar or 'soft tissue*') AND AB orthodontic AND AB ((maxillary expansion) OR (palatal expansion))	154
CINAHL (EBSCOhost)	same as MEDLINE Complete	19
SCOPUS	(TITLE-ABS-KEY(face OR mouth OR lip OR nose OR nasal OR naso* OR alar OR "soft tissue*") AND TITLE-ABS-KEY("maxillary expansion" OR "palatal expansion") AND TITLE-ABS-KEY(orthodontic))	702
Sciencedirect	TITLE-ABSTR-KEY(face OR mouth OR lip OR nose OR nasal OR naso* OR alar OR "soft tissue*") and TITLE-ABSTR-KEY((orthodontic AND ("maxillary expansion" OR "palatal expansion")))	73
In total		2567

measurements obtained before and after RME by direct measurement, two-dimensional (2D) methods, or three-dimensional (3D) methods.

Studies where orthopedic surgery or a surgically assisted technique was used, those where other interventions such as protraction and fixed-bracket therapy were performed during the observational period after RME; those including patients with cleft lip or palate and orthodontic or orthopedic treatment histories; and those categorized as reviews, abstracts, conference papers, case reports, and letters were excluded.

Selection of studies

Two reviewers (JH and JHJ) completed the study search and selection procedures by screening the titles and abstracts of articles identified via the electronic and manual searches. When the titles and abstracts were insufficient for decision making, we obtained the full text to make a judgment. The full texts of all potential studies were collected for further consideration; the two reviewers independently decided whether to include each article according to the selection criteria. Studies that presented only changes between time periods, with no available data for each time point, were excluded from the meta-analysis. Disagreements were resolved through a discussion among all reviewers.

Primary and secondary outcomes

The following transversal measurements were collected as the primary outcomes: nasal width (distance between the most lateral points of the left and right soft alar), alar base width (distance between the most lateral points of insertion of the nose into the face), mouth width, and upper philtrum width.

The secondary outcomes included seven sagittal measurements, including the nasal tip prominence, nasolabial angle, upper lip thickness, basic upper lip thickness (superior sulcus to the skeletal A point), soft pogonion thickness, distance from the upper lip to the E line, and distance from the lower lip to the E line. Moreover, four vertical measurements were recorded, including the upper lip height, lower lip height, lower facial height, and height of nose.

Risk of bias assessment

We compiled and modified a bias assessment scale for this study on the basis of the CONSORT statement. It involved the study design, measurement methods, statistics, and reports to evaluate the value and quality of each included article. As Johnson et al. reported, a sample with 17 per group would have a statistical power of over 80% [10]. For this study, if there was more than one study group, we pooled patients who underwent RME in each article into a total sample. In total, the maximum sum was 17 points; scores of ≥15, scores of < 15 and ≥12 and scores of< 12 were considered to represent high,

moderate, and low quality, respectively. Two reviewers (JH and JHJ) independently evaluated the quality of each article; any disagreement was resolved by discussion with the third reviewer (CYL).

Data extraction and synthesis

Two reviewers (JH and JHJ) separately extracted the relevant data and information. When there were insufficient data in the articles, we contacted the authors by e-mail for additional information.

We pooled the linear and angular changes in certain landmarks, while volumetric analyses and changes in regions were not pooled. Data for more than one RME group were previously synthesized as the sum of the data representing each study.

Statistical analyses were performed using Review Manager 5.3 (The Nordic Cochrane Centre, The Cochrane Collaboration, 2014; Copenhagen, Denmark). Heterogeneity was assessed using the I^2 statistic with a significance level of $\alpha = 0.05$. We adopted the mean difference (MD) with the 95% confidence interval (CI). Continuous data were recorded as MDs, while dichotomous data were expressed as relative risks (RRs). Subgroup analyses were conducted on the basis of measurement intervals. Quantitative synthesis would not be conducted if there was high heterogeneity (> 75%). We applied a random-effects model (REM) when there was moderate heterogeneity (50% to 75%); otherwise, when heterogeneity was lower than 50%, a fixed-effects model (FEM) was used.

Results

Study selection

The study selection flowchart is depicted in Fig. 1. In total, 2571 articles were identified via electronic and manual searches. After the removal of duplicates, we screened the titles and abstracts of 1762 studies. We obtained the full texts of 27 studies for further consideration. Finally, 15 studies met the inclusion criteria for this systematic review, and 13 were included in the meta-analysis. Articles excluded after reading the full texts had been listed in Additional file 1: Table S1 with reasons explained. We compared the results between reviewers; the interexaminer κ-value was 0.95.

Bias assessment

We assessed the eligibility and quality of 15 studies and found that five were of high quality and 9 were of moderate quality; one low-quality study was not included in the meta-analysis. The findings of bias assessment are shown in Table 2.

Characteristics of the involved studies

The detailed characteristics of the included studies are summarized in Table 3. The methodological features

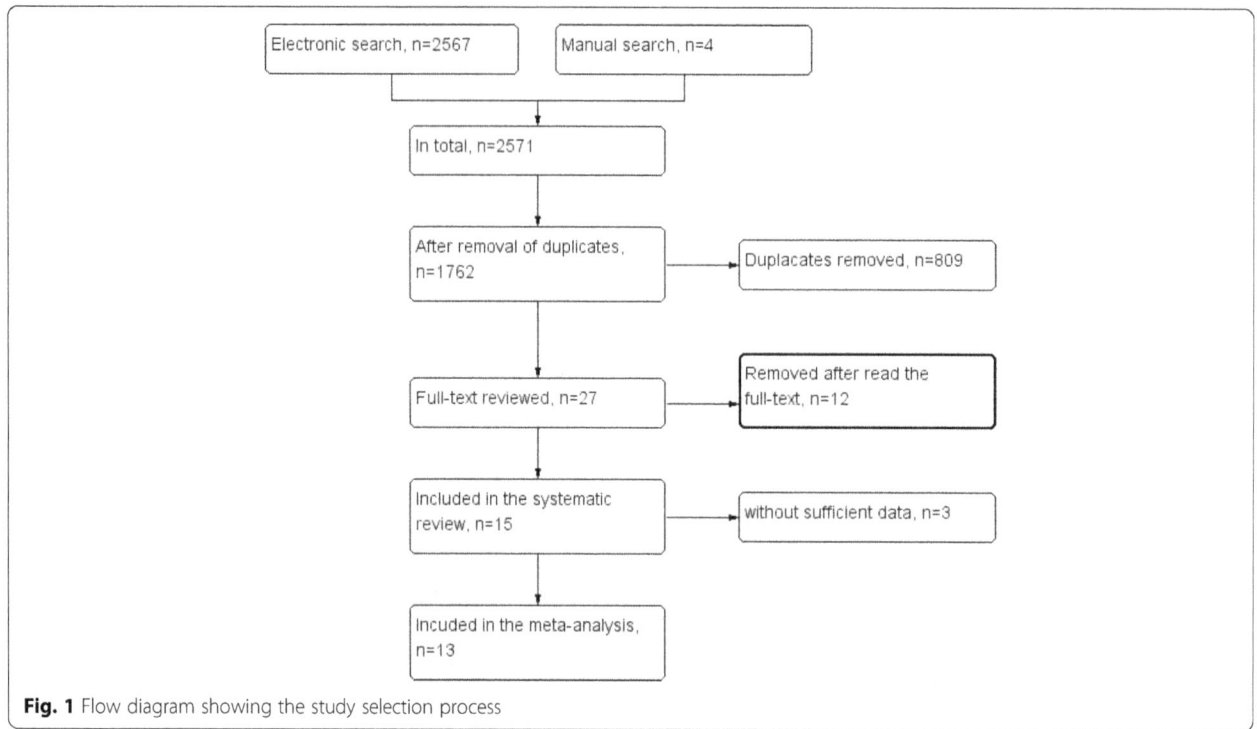

Fig. 1 Flow diagram showing the study selection process

included size, sex, age, appliance, duration of activation, and retention.

Data extraction and synthesis

Two reviewers (JH and JHJ) separately extracted and pooled data based on the primary and secondary outcomes.

We compared measurements obtained before and after expansion, before expansion and after retention, and after expansion and after retention.

Except distance from upper lip to E line, the I^2 values for all the other comparisons were $< 50\%$, indicating high homogeneity among groups for most pooled measurements.

Table 2 Quality assessment of the 15 articles included in the systematic review on changes in soft tissues after rapid maxillary expansion

Quality Assessment Criteria(Point)	1	2	3	4	5	6	7	8	9	10	11	12	13	14[a]	15[a]
Age and gender distribution described(1)	1	1	1	1	1	1	1	1	1	1	1	1	1	1	1
Clinical features fully defined(1)	1	1	1	1	1	1	1	1	1	1	0	1	1	1	1
Sample size: adequate(1)	1	1	1	1	1	1	1	1	1	1	1	1	1	0	1
Presence of a blank control(1)	1	0	1	0	0	1	0	1	0	0	1	0	0	0	0
Prospective(1)	0	1	1	0	1	1	1	1	1	1	1	1	1	1	1
Randomization(1)	0	1	1	0	1	0	0	0	1	0	0	0	0	0	0
Appliances described(1)	1	1	1	1	1	1	1	1	1	1	1	1	1	1	1
Interventions fully described(1)	1	1	1	1	1	1	1	0	0	1	1	1	1	1	1
Follow-up defined(1)	0	1	1	1	1	1	0	1	1	1	1	1	0	0	0
Measurement method: appropriate(1)	1	1	1	1	1	1	1	1	1	1	1	1	1	1	1
Assessor blinding(1)	1	0	1	0	0	0	1	0	1	0	1	0	0	0	0
Reliability testing(1)	1	1	1	1	1	1	1	1	1	1	1	1	1	1	1
No dropouts or explained(1)	1	1	1	1	1	1	1	1	1	1	1	1	1	1	1
Statistical analysis: appropriate(1)	1	1	1	1	1	1	1	1	1	1	1	1	1	1	1
Confounders analysed(1)	1	0	1	0	1	1	1	1	1	1	1	1	1	1	1
Results reported: adequate(1)	1	1	1	1	1	1	1	1	1	1	1	1	1	0	0
Reasonable conclusion(1)	1	1	1	1	1	1	1	1	1	1	1	1	1	1	1
Total	14	14	17	12	15	15	14	14	15	14	15	14	13	11	12

[a]articles included in the systematic review but not in the meta-analysis. The number of articles is the same as that in Table 3

Table 3 Details of included articles

No.	Author& Year	Design	Groups	Size	Males/Females	Average Age(year)	Appliance	Expansion duration	Retention duration	Measurement methods	Measurement time
1	Badreddine 2017 [30]	retrospective	study	20	10/10	8.9±2.16	hyrax expander	3 months	–	CT images	T0,T1
			control	10	5/5	9.2±2.17	–	–	–		
2	Altındıs, 2016 [23]	RCT	banded RME	14	6/8	12.7±0.6	Hyrax screw	–	3 months	3-D image	T0,T2
			bonded RME	14	7/7	12.4±0.8					
			Modified bonded RME	14	5/9	12.5±0.8					
3	Baysal 2016 [14]	RCT	treated	17	9/8	13.4±1.2	bonded acrylic splint expander	–	6 months	poteroanterior cephalogram and 3-D image	T0,T2
			untreated	17	9/8	12.8±1.3	–	–	–		
4	Torun 2016 [35]	retrospective	prepubertal	14	10/18	13.91±1.8	Hyrax screw	3–4 weeks	6 months	CBCT and 3-D image	T0,T2
			postpubertal	14							
5	Halıcıoğlu 2016 [31]	RCT	memory-screw	17	9/8	13±1.29	memory- screw	7.76±1.04 days	6.42±0.59 months	lateral cephalograms	T0,T1,T2
			Hyrax-screw	15	8/7	12.58±1.5	Hyrax- screw	35.46±9.39 days	6.17±0.32 months		
6	Uysal 2015 [36]	CCT	study	20	8/12	13.4±0.99	acrylic bonded RME appliance	average 1.1 months	6 months	lateral and anteroposterior radiographs	T0,T1,T2
			control	16	6/10	13.25±1.19					
7	Longo 2014 [34]	cohort	study	28	14/14	12 years 2 months ±3.1 years	banded Hyrax (24 subjects), banded Haas(3), bonded Hyrax(1)	–	–	direct measurement with caliper	T0,T1
8	Santariello 2014 [37]	CCT	study	61	35/26	10.5±1.8	Hyrax type expander	3–4 weeks	nearly 6 months	direct measurement with caliper	T0,T1,T2
			control	41	15/26	10.7±2.2	–	–	–		
9	Pangrazio-Kulbersh 2012 [9]	RCT	banded maxillary expanders	13	7/6	12.6±1.8	banded maxillary expanders	4–6 weeks	6 months	CBCT and 3-D image	T0,T2
			bonded maxillary expanders	10	5/5	13.5±2.1	bonded maxillary expanders				
10	Santos 2012 [22]	cohort	study	20	10/10	9.3 years ± 10 months	modified acrylic Hyrax device	3–4 weeks	6 months	lateral cephalograms	T0,T1,T2
11	Johnson 2010 [10]	CCT	prepubertal	31	12/19	13.1	Hyrax- type expander	average 35 days	average 5.7 months	direct measurement with caliper	T0,T1,T2
			postpubertal	48	17/31						

Table 3 Details of included articles (Continued)

No.	Author& Year	Design	Groups	Size	Males/Females	Average Age(year)	Appliance	Expansion duration	Retention duration	Measurement methods	Measurement time
12	Kilic 2008 [15]	cohort	study	18	3/15	13.5 ± 1.07	rigid acrylic bonded appliance	–	5.95 ± 0.35 months	lateral cephalograms	T0,T1,T2
13	Karaman 2002 [38]	cohort	study	20	10/10	12.8	modified acrylic bonded appliance	5.2 weeks	–	lateral cephalograms	T0,T1
14[a]	Altorkat 2016 [20]	cohort	study	14	7/7	12.6 ± 1.8	Hyrax screw	–	–	3D stereophoto-grammetry	T0,T1
15[a]	Kim 2012 [24]	cohort	study	23	10/13	12.3 ± 2.6	fixed rapid maxillary expander	average 22.8 days	–	CBCT	T0,T1

[a]Articles included in the systematic review but not in the meta-analysis. T0 = pre-expansion, T1 = postexpansion, T2 = postretention

FEM was used for those comparisons. For upper lip to E line between pre-expansion and postexpansion and between postexpansion and postretention, RME was used.

Comparisons

Ten baseline and postexpansion measurements (compared in at least two of the included studies), 11 baseline and postretention measurements, and five postexpansion and postretention measurements (to determine the extent of relapse) were compared in forest plots as Additional file 2: Figure S1 and the results are summarized in Table 4A, B, and C, respectively.

Table 4 Results of the meta-analysis on changes in soft tissues after rapid maxillary expansion

Outcome	Studies	Subjects	Effect EstimateMD (Fixed, CI 95%)
A.Pre-expansion VS. postexpansion			
Nasal width	5	208	0.84 [0.33, 1.34] [a]
Alar base width	4	188	0.71 [0.19, 1.23] [a]
Nasal tip prominence	3	56	0.59 [−0.26, 1.44]
Nasolabial angle	2	52	−0.06 [−4.36, 4.24]
Upper lip thickness	2	38	−0.01 [− 0.82, 0.79]
Basic upper lip thickness	2	38	0.28 [− 0.65, 1.22]
Soft pogonion thickness	2	38	0.01 [−0.79, 0.81]
upper lip to E line	3	72	0.11 [−0.65, 0.88]
Lower lip to E line	3	72	0.75 [0.51, 0.99] [a]
Height of nose	3	68	1.30 [−0.08, 2.67]
B.Pre-expansion VS. postretention			
Nasal width	6	232	0.87 [0.34, 1.41] [a]
Alar base width	3	158	0.51 [−0.04, 1.06]
Mouth width	2	59	1.84 [0.66, 3.02] [a]
Upper philtrum width	2	45	0.74 [0.12, 1.36] [a]
Nasal tip prominence	4	78	0.26 [−0.99, 1.51]
Nasolabial angle	5	142	−0.88 [−2.96, 1.20]
upper lip to E line	2	52	−0.11 [− 0.33, 0.11]
Lower lip to E line	2	52	0.42 [0.17, 0.66] [a]
Upper lip height	3	87	−0.38 [−1.17, 0.41]
Lower lip height	2	59	0.48 [−0.47, 1.43]
Lower face height	2	59	0.42 [−1.17, 2.01]
C.Postexpansion VS. postretention			
Nasal width	3	160	−0.13 [−0.70, 0.44]
Alar base width	2	140	−0.20 [− 0.80, 0.39]
Nasal tip prominence	2	38	0.19 [−1.25, 1.63]
upper lip to E line	2	52	−0.25 [−1.27, 0.77]
Lower lip to E line	2	52	−0.34 [− 0.57, − 0.11] [a]

A. Pre-expansion versus post-expansion; B. Pre-expansion versus postretention; C. Postexpansion versus postretention. [a]significant

Discussion

In the present study, we included studies that assessed 3D and 2D images and direct measurements. Scholars have believed that images of the craniofacial complex are more accurate with 3D radiography techniques, which avoid the superimposition and image distortion observed with 2D radiography techniques [11, 12]. However, Weinberg et al. suggested that there was high intraobserver precision among 2D, 3D, and direct measurements, which was supported by the findings in a study by Baysal et al. [13, 14].

A flattened nasal shape and development of a dorsal hump are two of the potential negative effects of RME [15]. According to the present study, the nasal width(MD:0.84 mm, 95% CI:0.33, 1.34) and alar base width(MD: 0.71 mm, 95% CI:0.19, 1.23) significantly increased after active expansion, and nasal width(MD: 0.87 mm, 95% CI:0.34, 1.41) continued to show significant increase during retention. According to previous studies evaluating hard tissues, the skeletal nasal cavity width increased by approximately 2.1–4.5 mm via separation of the lateral walls of nasal cavity after RME [4, 10, 16, 17]. Cameron et al. reported that this change effectively enlarged the nasal volume to facilitate respiration, and it was maintained after 8 years of follow-up [18]. Guyuron suggested that the nasal form was mainly controlled by the nasal frame, and that the shape of the nose was probably changed by alterations in the skeleton [19]. Despite the widening effect, Altorkat et al. found a significant increase in the horizontal nasal tip angle (the left alar-pronasal-right alar angle) [20].

RME is performed to relieve transverse constriction of the maxilla via buccal tipping of the posterior teeth and lateral rotation of the two maxillary halves, which increases the transverse dental and skeletal dimensions [3, 21]. Scholars found that the soft tissue changes after RME were consistent with changes in the underlying hard tissues [7] [9]. In our study, the mouth width(MD: 1.84 mm, 95% CI:0.66, 3.02) significantly increased to a mean of 1.84 mm, with an upper 95% confidence limit of 3.02 mm, which indicated possible clinical importance, particularly in larger populations. Soft tissue stretching is probably the reason for the significant increases in the mouth width and upper philtrum width(MD: 0.74 mm, 95% CI:0.12, 1.36) observed after retention in the present study.

With regard to sagittal measurements, the hard tissue responses after RME are still controversial [4, 16, 22]. Lagravère proved that the maxilla moved downward and forward after RME in a meta-analysis, although the findings were not clinically important [21]. The present study showed no significant sagittal changes in the nasomaxillary region. This was supported by the findings in a report by Altorkat et al. [20]. Moreover, Altındiş et al. claimed that there were no significant changes in the soft facial convexity after RME [23]. This was probably because nose flattening was compensated for by forward movement and growth of the maxilla [15]. In the present study, the distance from the lower lips to the E line(MD: 0.75 mm, 95% CI:0.51, 0.99) showed statistically significant changes after expansion, although the changes did not exceed 1 mm, and significantly relapsed after retention(MD: – 0.34 mm, 95% CI:-0.57, – 0.11), which may be related to movement and rotation of the maxilla and mandible. Transversal stretching of the lips was considered the reason for the significant decrease in the lip thickness reported by Kim et al. [24]; however, our findings revealed no significant changes.

Previous studies have supported the conclusion that RME leads to downward and backward rotation of the mandible [3, 4, 22, 25, 26]. Kiliç et al. found that the H angle was significantly increased, with long-term stability, after RME [15]. This probably represents a favorable effect in patients with Class III malocclusion and an undesirable effect in patients with Class II malocclusion. Scholars have indicated that a bonded expander prevents clockwise rotation of the mandible, thus inhibiting an undesirable increase in the facial height [3, 4, 27–29]. In the present study, we found no significant changes in the height of the lower face, nose, or lips.

However, Badreddine found a significant change in the length of the soft tissue of the nose when they compared the treatment group with the control group [30]. This discrepancy may have occurred because of individual differences between groups, and not as an effect of RME. Thus, we evaluated data obtained before expansion and before retention, rather than spontaneous data for the control group, as control data for quantitative analysis; this was done even when a blank control existed, as observed in a study by Halıcıoğlu et al. [31]. On the basis of our findings, the increase in the height of the nose (MD: 1.30 mm, 95% CI: – 0.08, 2.67) after expansion and elongation of the lower face (MD: 0.42 mm, 95% CI: – 1.17, 2.01) could indicate possible esthetic relevance, particularly in larger populations where an increase of > 2 mm is observed.

The effects of various types or designs of expanders and the sex and age of patients were not evaluated because of the small sample size. Torun et al. claimed that there was no significant difference between prepubertal and postpubertal subjects [32]. This was consistent with the findings of Johnson et al., who stated that the maturation status and sex had no significant effects on the soft tissue changes after RME [10].

All studies included in this systematic review enrolled subjects with an average age of 8 to 14 years who were in the active growth phase. As reported by Quintão et al. and Longo et al., the effects of growth on soft tissues could be eliminated as a variable over a 6-month duration [33, 34]. We presumed that growth would not cause substantial interference with the parameters evaluated during the observational period of up to 6–7 months in all studies included in this meta-analysis. None of the involved studies had a follow-up duration beyond the retention period, because RME was usually followed by fixed-bracket therapy or functional orthodontics. Thus, the results of this study were based on short-term studies and observation, leaving long-term stability open to question. Moreover, these factors are obstacles to future research on changes induced by RME [15].

Because RME is more broadly utilized for adult patients in the current clinical setting, it is crucial to clarify that our findings were based on subjects in the facial skull growth phase, and that the conclusions cannot be extrapolated to the general population. Further studies evaluating soft tissue changes after RME in adults are necessary.

The quality of the articles included in this systematic review was relatively moderate. Only five studies included a blank control group for elimination of the effects of normal growth and development as variables. Randomization was relatively difficult because of ethical problems, and blinding of the assessors was not ensured in over half of the involved studies, which decreased the overall quality. Three of the studies included in the meta-analysis and the two studies included only in the systematic review did not document follow-up data after active expansion; thus, the stability during the retention period remains unknown. Further RCTs with larger samples are necessary to obtain more trustworthy results.

Our findings revealed that most of the evaluated measurements showed a mean change of < 1 mm, which indicated limited clinical or esthetic relevance. In order to provide pertinent and convincing evidence regarding this research question, further investigations with larger samples and appropriate controls are necessary for more accurate evaluation of soft tissue responses after RME and the long-term stability of these changes.

Limitations

This study is limited by the fact that the results and conclusions were based on patients in the growth phase, and that the observational period was only up to 6 months. Therefore, the findings should be cautiously interpreted with regard to patients outside the growth phase and long-term outcomes.

Conclusions

Our findings suggest that RME results in a significantly increased nasal width, mouth width, upper philtrum width, and distance from the lower lip to the E line after the retention phase. However, the clinical importance of these findings is questionable.

Abbreviations

2D: two-dimensional; 3D: three-dimensional; CBCT: cone beam computed tomography; CCT: clinical controlled trial; CI: confidence interval; CINAHL: Cumulative Index to Nursing and Allied Health Literature; FEM: fixed-effects model; MD: mean difference; PRISMA: Preferred Reporting Items for Systematic Reviews Meta-Analyses; RCT: randomized controlled trial; REM: random-effects model; RME: rapid maxillary expansion; RR: relative risk

Acknowledgments

The authors would like to thank the Center Laboratory of the Peking University, School of Stomatology.

Funding

This study was supported by the National Natural Science Foundation of China (Nos. 81171006 and 81571002), the Beijing Natural Science Foundation (No. 7162203), and the Beijing Science and Technology Committee (No. Z121107001012024). The funders played no role in the study design, data collection and analysis, decision to publish, or manuscript preparation.

Authors' contributions

J H, J-H J, and C-Y L conducted the searches, collected data, and performed statistical analyses. JH designed the studies and drafted the manuscript. All authors read and approved the final manuscript.

Competing interests

The authors declare that they have no competing interests.

References

1. Zeng J, Gao X. A prospective CBCT study of upper airway changes after rapid maxillary expansion. Int J Pediatr Otorhinolaryngol. 2013;77:1805–10.
2. Haas AJ. Rapid expansion of the maxillary dental arch and nasal cavity by opening the midpalatal suture. Angle Orthod. 1961;31:73–90.
3. Haas AJ. The treatment of maxillary deficiency by opening the midpalatal suture. Angle Orthod. 1965;35:200–17.
4. Wertz RA. Skeletal and dental changes accompanying rapid midpalatal suture opening. Am J Orthod. 1970;58:41–66.
5. Proffit WR, White RP, Sarver DM. Contemporary treatment of dentofacial deformity. 1st ed. St. Louis: Mosby; 2003.
6. Bailey L, Sarver D, Turvey T, Proffit W III. Class III problems. In: Proffit WR, White RP, Sarver DM, editors. Contemporary treatment of dentofacial deformity. 1st ed. St. Louis: Mosby; 2003. p. 507.
7. Berger JL, Pangrazio-Kulbersh V, Thomas BW, Kaczynski R. Photographic analysis of facial changes associated with maxillary expansion. Am J Orthod Dentofac Orthop. 1999;116:563–71.
8. Sarver DM. Interactions of hard tissues, soft tissues, and growth over time, and their impact on orthodontic diagnosis and treatment planning. Am J Orthod Dentofac Orthop. 2015;148:380–6.
9. Pangrazio-Kulbersh V, Wine P, Haughey M, Pajtas B, Kaczynski R. Cone beam computed tomography evaluation of changes in the naso-maxillary complex associated with two types of maxillary expanders. Angle Orthod. 2012;82:448–57.
10. Johnson BM, McNamara JA, Bandeen RL, Baccetti T. Changes in soft tissue nasal widths associated with rapid maxillary expansion in prepubertal and postpubertal subjects. Angle Orthod. 2010;80:995–1001.
11. Lübbers HT, Medinger L, Kruse A, Grätz KW, Matthews F. Precision and accuracy of the 3dMD photogrammetric system in craniomaxillofacial application. J Craniofac Surg. 2010;21:763–7.
12. Lane C, Harrell W Jr. Completing the 3-dimensional picture. Am J Orthod Dentofac Orthop. 2008;133:612–20.
13. Weinberg SM, Naidoo S, Govier DP, Martin RA, Kane AA, Marazita ML. Anthropometric precision and accuracy of digital three-dimensional photogrammetry: comparing the Genex and 3dMD imaging systems with one another and with direct anthropometry. J Craniofac Surg. 2006;17:477–83.
14. Baysal A, Ozturk MA, Sahan AO, Uysal T. Facial soft-tissue changes after rapid maxillary expansion analyzed with 3-dimensional stereophotogrammetry: a randomized, controlled clinical trial. Angle Orthod. 2016;86:934–42.
15. Kiliç N, Kiki A, Oktay H, Erdem A. Effects of rapid maxillary expansion on Holdaway soft tissue measurements. Eur J Orthod. 2008;30:239–43.
16. da Silva Filho OG, Montes LA, Torelly LF. Rapid maxillary expansion in the deciduous and mixed dentition evaluated through posteroanterior cephalometric analysis. Am J Orthod Dentofac Orthop. 1995;107:268–75.
17. Doruk C, Bicakci AA, Basciftci FA, Agar U, Babacan H. A comparison of the effects of rapid maxillary expansion and fan-type rapid maxillary expansion on dentofacial structures. Angle Orthod. 2004;74:184–94.
18. Cameron CG, Franchi L, Baccetti T, McNamara JA Jr. Long-term effects of rapid maxillary expansion: a posteroanterior cephalometric evaluation. Am J Orthod Dentofac Orthop. 2002;121:129–35. quiz 193
19. Guyuron B. Precision rhinoplasty. Part II: Prediction Plast Reconstr Surg. 1988;81:500–5.
20. Altorkat Y, Khambay BS, McDonald JP, Cross DL, Brocklebank LM, Ju X. Immediate effects of rapid maxillary expansion on the naso-maxillary facial soft tissue using 3D stereophotogrammetry. Surgeon. 2016;14:63–8.
21. Lagravere MO, Major PW, Flores-Mir C. Long-term skeletal changes with rapid maxillary expansion: a systematic review. Angle Orthod. 2005;75:1046–52.
22. dos Santos BM, Stuani AS, Stuani AS, Faria G, Quintão CC, Stuani MB. Soft tissue profile changes after rapid maxillary expansion with a bonded expander. Eur J Orthod. 2012;34:367–73.
23. Altındiş S, Toy E, Başçiftçi FA. Effects of different rapid maxillary expansion appliances on facial soft tissues using three-dimensional imaging. Angle Orthod. 2016;86:590–8.
24. Kim KB, et al. Evaluation of immediate soft tissue changes after rapid maxillary expansion. Dent Press J of Orthod. 2012;17:157–64.

25. da Silva Filho OG, Boas MC, Capelozza FL. Rapid maxillary expansion in the primary and mixed dentitions: a cephalometric evaluation. Am J Orthod Dentofac Orthop. 1991;100:171–9.

26. Sandikçioğlu M, Hazar S. Skeletal and dental changes after maxillary expansion in the mixed dentition. Am J Orthod Dentofac Orthop. 1997;111:321–7.

27. Sarver DM, Johnston MW. Skeletal changes in vertical and anterior displacement of the maxilla with bonded rapid palatal expansion appliances. Am J Orthod Dentofac Orthop. 1989;95:462–6.

28. Cozza P, Giancotti A, Petrosino A. Rapid palatal expansion in mixed dentition using a modified expander: a cephalometric investigation. J Orthod. 2001;28:129–34.

29. Handelman CS, Wang L, BeGole EA, Haas AJ. Nonsurgical rapid maxillary expansion in adults: report on 47 cases using the Haas expander. Angle Orthod. 2000;70:129–44.

30. Badreddine FR, Fujita RR, Cappellette M Jr. Short-term evaluation of tegumentary changes of the nose in oral breathers undergoing rapid maxillary expansion. Braz J Otorhinolaryngol. 2017. https://doi.org/10.1016/j.bjorl.2017.05.010. [Epub ahead of print].

31. Halicioglu K, Yavuz I. A comparison of the sagittal and vertical dentofacial effects of maxillary expansion produced by a memory screw and a hyrax screw. Aust Orthod. 2016;32:31–40.

32. Torun GS. Soft tissue changes in the orofacial region after rapid maxillary expansion: a cone beam computed tomography study. J Orofac Orthop. 2017;78:193–200.

33. Quintão C, Helena I, Brunharo VP, Menezes RC, Almeida MA. Soft tissue facial profile changes following functional appliance therapy. Eur J Orthod. 2006;28:35–41.

34. Longo PC. Dimensional changes of facial soft tissue associated with rapid palatal expansion. Ann Arbor: Marquette University; 2014. p. 82.

35. Torun GS. Soft tissue changes in the orofacial region after rapid maxillary expansion : A cone beam computed tomography study. J Orofac Orthop 2017:78(3):193–200.

36. Uysal İÖ, Zorkun B, Yüce S, Birlik M, Polat K, Babacan H. Morphological Nasal Changes Associated with Rapid Maxillary Expansion. Hızlı Üste Çene Genişletilmesinde Morfolojik Burun Değişiklikleri. 2015:136–43.

37. Santariello C, Nota A, Baldini A, Ballanti F, Cozza P. Analysis of Rapid Maxillary Expansion Effects on Nasal Soft Tissues Widths. Minerva Stomatol 2014:63:307–14.

38. Karaman AI, Basciftci FA, Gelgo¨r I, Demir A. Examination of soft tissue changes after rapid maxillary expansion. World J Orthod 2002:3(3):217–22

29

Incidence of pulp sensibility loss of anterior teeth after paramedian insertion of orthodontic mini-implants in the anterior maxilla

Jan Hourfar[1], Dirk Bister[2], Jörg A. Lisson[3] and Björn Ludwig[3,4*]

Abstract

Background: The aim of this retrospective investigation was to evaluate the incidence of loss to pulp sensibility testing (PST) of maxillary front teeth after paramedian (3 to 5 mm away from the suture) orthodontic mini-implant (OMI) insertion in the anterior palate.

Methods: A total of 284 patients (102 males, 182 females; mean age was 14.4 years (±8.8) years at time of OMI-Insertion) with a total of 568 OMIs (1.7 mm diameter, length 8 mm) were retrospectively investigated. A binomial regression analysis was performed to explore covariates, such as age, gender, inclination of upper central incisors, dentition status and insertion position of OMIs that could have contributed to loss of sensibility. Statistical significance was set at $p < 0.05$.

Results: Loss of response to PST was encountered during retention in 3 out of 284 patients and the respective OMIs had been placed at height of the second rugae (R-2). Affected teeth were a right canine, a left lateral and a left central incisor. Subsequent root canal treatment was successful. Results of the binomial regression analysis revealed that the covariate insertion position (R-2) of OMIs ($p = 0.008$) had statistically significant influence on loss of response to PST.

Conclusions: (1) Although there was no radiographic evidence for direct root injury, the proximity of the implants to the anterior teeth was nevertheless statistically related to loss of PST. (2) In all cases of PST loss OMIs were inserted at the second rugae. Therefore OMIs should be placed either more posteriorly, at the third rugae or in the median plane. (3). Loss of PST was not increased for patients with palatal OMI (0.18%) compared to samples without OMI (0.25%).

Keywords: Orthodontic mini-implant, Paramedian insertion, Maxilla, Pulp sensibility loss, Anterior teeth

Background

Sensibility is defined as the ability to respond to a stimulus and testing of the dental pulp, which can be performed using different techniques. In clinical practice commercially available refrigerant sprays (cold - tests) are often used for pulp sensibility testing (PST) [1] and the response is recorded as positive or negative. Various

---

* Correspondence: bludwig@kieferorthopaedie-mosel.de
[3]Department of Orthodontics, University of Saarland, Homburg/Saar, Germany
[4]Private Practice, Am Bahnhof 54, 56841 Traben-Trarbach, Germany
Full list of author information is available at the end of the article

factors such as previous trauma [2], patient age [3], periodontal attachment loss [4] or medications (sedatives, tranquilizers, analgesics) [5] are known to have an influence on the response. It is known that orthodontic tooth movement can affect PST response temporarily [6], but sensibility is thought to return to normal after completion of treatment. The authors state that there is no agreement in the literature regarding potential long-term sequelae: reported pulpal responses after orthodontics included circulatory vascular stasis and necrosis [7]. Cases of pulpal necrosis following orthodontic therapy have been occasionally reported [8, 9], but this is unusual.

Adjunctive procedures such as extensive enamel stripping [10] and subtractive Odontoplasty [11, 12] may lead to a critical rise in intrapulpal temperature [10] with subsequent pulp necrosis [13]. Clinicians performing PSTs use the qualitative sensory manifestations to extrapolate the state of the pulp to assess the "vitality" of the tooth [1, 14]. "Sensibility" and "vitality" are hence often used interchangeably [1, 5], although it is well known that PST can produce false positive and false negative results for vitality.

Orthodontic mini-implants (OMIs) have changed orthodontic paradigms by broadening the spectrum of dental movements [15]. Numerous risks and complications associated with the use of OMIs have been described before and specific complications such as unintentional root damage [16, 17], if severe enough can lead to loss of sensibility and vitality.

The anterior palate is most suitable [18] as insertion site for OMIs because of high success rates [19] and ideal anatomical conditions. Palatal bone quality and quantity for safe insertion of OMIs has been well documented [20–22]. Despite these findings, unintentional root damage of a lateral incisor after paramedian OMI-Insertion in the anterior palatal vault has been reported [23].

The aim of this retrospective investigation was to evaluate incidence of response loss to PST of maxillary front teeth after paramedian OMI insertion in the anterior palate.

Methods
Patients and treatment protocol
Patients
Patients with no history of previous orthodontic treatment and need for OMI supported orthodontic biomechanics were included. All patients received treatment by a single orthodontist (B. L.) in a specialist orthodontic practice (Traben-Trarbach, Germany), including fixed orthodontic appliances with OMI placement. As previously described [24–26], two OMIs were inserted symmetrically parasagittal (3 to 5 mm away from the suture) [27] into the anterior palate for appliance attachment. OMIs were loaded two weeks after insertion, because of manufacture of the appliances attached to them.

Inclusion criteria:

Unrestored maxillary permanent front teeth without history of trauma and previous dental treatment

Exclusion criteria:

- systemic diseases/disorders
- craniofacial malformations
- chemo and/or radiotherapy during tooth development
- accidents/craniofacial trauma

- history of previous surgery requiring endotracheal intubation
- dental malformations
- severe crowding of the upper front teeth
- periodontal disease
- history of previous orthodontic treatment
- tooth agenesis (except for third molars) or tooth loss
- enamel stripping or occlusal adjustments to the upper front teeth
- medications such as sedatives, tranquilizer, analgesics

Skeletal anchorage
Only one type of mini-implant (1.7 mm diameter, length 8 mm) was used (OrthoEasy®, Forestadent, Pforzheim, Germany). This implant system has an anodized surface and features a self-tapping and cutting design and is made from Titanium-alloy (Ti-6Al-4 V). Following patient consultation and consent, 0.2 ml to 0.5 ml of local infiltration anaesthesia (Ultracain® D-S, Sanofi-Aventis Deutschland GmbH, Frankfurt, Germany) was used. The OMIs were inserted without soft tissue incision or pre-drilling, perpendicular to the bone surface, using a motorised dental handpiece at an insertion speed of 60 RPM. Torque limitation was 30 Ncm. All OMIs were removed at debond.

Bonding and debonding of the fixed appliance
Bonding and removal of the fixed appliances followed a standardized protocol. Self- ligating steel Brackets (Quick®, Forestadent, Pforzheim, Germany) were indirectly bonded applying a light cure bonding material (Transbond® Supreme LV, 3 M Unitek, Monrovia, Calif., USA). A halogen light was used for curing composite material according to manufacturer instructions.

Bracket removing pliers were used for debonding. The residual adhesive on each tooth was removed with fluted tungsten carbide burs and the surface finished using silicone carbide polishers. All clean-up procedures included water-cooling.

Pulp sensibility testing
Thermal PST (cold test) of the maxillary front teeth was performed just prior to OMI-insertion, at debond of the fixed appliance/OMI-removal and 24 month post debond. Endo-Ice® (Coltène/Whaledent Inc., Cuyahoga Falls, Ohio, USA), producing a temperature of −50 °C was used. The product was applied to the teeth using a cotton wool pad. Response was recorded as either positive or negative.

Records included full documentation for the entire treatment including appropriate radiographs.

Diagnosis of radiographic material
All radiographs were taken with an Orthophos® XG 3 (Sirona, Bensheim, Germany).

Panoramic x-rays (OPGs)

OPGs were available pre-treatment (initial diagnostics) and were used for the diagnosis of bony and dental anomalies/pathologies prior to OMI-insertion.

Cephalometric analysis

Using the pre-treatment cephalograms (initial diagnostics) the inclination of upper central incisors (U1/ANS-PNS) prior to OMI-insertion was measured (Fig. 1), and 108° ± 5° [28] was regarded as a standard mean value.

Assessment of OMIs' insertion positions

Position of the OMIs were assessed using the plaster working models for the appliances.

Because palatal rugae have been previously described as stable, clinically visible structures [29], the insertion positions of the OMIs were classified in relation to the medial ends of palatal rugae:

1. at second rugae (R-2)
2. between second and third rugae (R-2/3)
3. at third rugae (R-3)

Data collection and statistical analysis

Data was collated using Microsoft Excel® 2007, (Microsoft Corp., Redmond, Wash., USA). All cephalometric angular measurements and the assessment of the implant position were re-measured after three months by the same operator. Average intra-examiner reliability calculated by the coefficient of variation (COV) was 0.01 for the former and using the intraclass correlation coefficient (ICC) was 1.0 for the latter.

A binomial logistic regression analysis was performed to explore covariates, such as age, gender, Inclination of upper centrals, dentition status and insertion position of OMIs that could possibly have contributed to loss of sensibility. Statistical analysis was performed using SPSS® for Windows®, version 22.0 (IBM Corp., Armonk, New York, USA). Statistical significance was set at $p < 0.05$.

Results

A total of 284 patients (102 males, 182 females) with a total of 568 OMIs met the inclusion criteria. All patients were of Caucasian origin. At the time of OMI-insertion the mean age was 14.4 years ± 8.8 years. 169 patients were in mixed dentition, and 109 patients were in permanent dentition. Average inclination of upper incisors (U1/ANS-PNS) was 109.81° ± 8.37°; they were hence slightly proclined. Most OMIs were inserted at the third rugae (Table 1). In none of the patients root injuries were diagnosed on the available radiographs.

Loss of response to pulp sensibility testing (PST)

Loss of response to PST was encountered in 3 (1.06%) out of 284 patients or 0.53% per OMI. The percentage was 0.18% ($n = 3$) for the 1704 maxillary incisors and canines and 0.18% ($n = 2$) for the 1136 maxillary incisors respectively. PST was found negative in the three affected patients in the second half of two year retention phase following debond of the fixed appliances. Affected maxillary teeth were: A right canine, a left lateral and a left central incisor. Details are in Table 2.

The three affected patients initially presented with painful teeth and were hence referred to an endodontic specialist for further clinical and radiographic diagnosis. All affected teeth received root canal treatment. After successful treatment the symptoms resolved. Interestingly, no root injury was diagnosed on the intraoral films during endodontic treatment.

Results of the binomial logistic regression analysis revealed that covariates gender ($p = 0.996$), age at OMI-Insertion ($p = 0.456$), Inclination of upper incisors (U1/ANS-PNS) ($p = 0.289$) and dentition status ($p = 0.587$) had no statistically significant influence on loss of response to

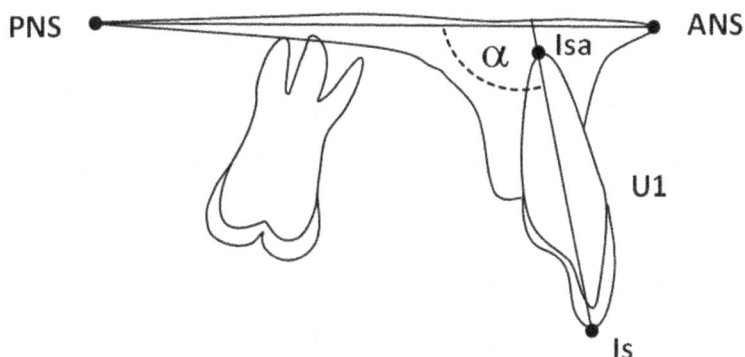

Fig. 1 Inclination of upper central incisors. Measurement of the Inclination of upper central incisor (U1/ANS-PNS) between the palatal plane (ANS-PNS) and the long axis of U1 (Is-Isa)

Table 1 Distribution of OMIs insertion positions' in relation to palatal rugae

Insertion position	Number	Percent
second rugae (R-2)	76	13.4
between second and third rugae (R-2/3)	24	4.2
third rugae (R-3)	468	82.4

PST, whereas the insertion position of OMIs (p = 0.008) had.

Discussion

Loss of response to PST and vitality respectively was encountered in 3 out of 284 patients of our sample. The percentage was 0.18% for the 1704 maxillary incisors and canines and 0.18% for the 1136 maxillary incisors respectively. Interestingly, these results are very similar to those of an investigation by Bauss et al. [30]. They also found a small percentage of 0.25% (n = 2) for 800 healthy non-traumatized permanent incisors in 200 randomly selected patients who underwent fixed treatment without OMI placement.

In all affected patients of our sample, symptoms that led to referral to an endodontic specialist were encountered during retention. Occurrence of symptoms was late, considering loss of vitality was only detected long after OMI removal and debond. However, considerable variation has been described in the literature [23, 31–33] and loss of vitality can occur up to 2 years after OMI placement [32] because root injury can remain symptomless over a long period of time. Er et al. [23] reported a periradicular lesion caused by unintentional root damage after paramedian placement of two OMIs (1.5 mm diameter, length 10 mm) in the anterior palate for a distalizing appliance in a 22-year-old female, thus requiring endodontic treatment. Two months after OMI-insertion, the patient complained of pain and the right maxillary lateral incisor was endodontically treated.

Root perforations after buccal interradicular insertion of OMIs have also been reported: two cases of maxillary first molars [32, 33] and a mandibular right lateral incisor [31]. In the latter additional periapical surgery was performed for retrograde root canal treatment.

Table 2 Details of affected patients

Gender	Patient 1	Patient 2	Patient 3
	female	female	female
Age (years)	37	11	12
Inclination U1 (degrees)	99.20	98.50	110.50
OMIs insertion positions	R-2	R-2	R-2
Affected tooth (FDI-Notation)	13	22	21

R-2, OMI's insertion position at second rugae

After loss of response to PST, patients were referred to an endodontic specialist who diagnosed pulp necrosis and undertook endodontic treatment. Because no root injury could be diagnosed on the available plain film radiographs and all patients were free of symptoms after treatment, no additional cone beam computed tomography (CBCT) was performed, although this would have been the modality of choice to diagnose the exact location of the possible root injury site [34]. Therefore, we cannot completely exclude root perforations due to OMI insertion and this has to be kept in mind when considering the results of this investigation.

It was well known that OMIs did not remain stationary during orthodontics [35] and primary (direct) and secondary (migration) displacement has been observed. Primary displacement is due to the elastic characteristics of the bone whereas the latter occurs under orthodontic loading over time, caused by remodeling processes of the bone. In a systematic review by Nienkemper et al. [36] secondary displacement of OMIs was found 0.23 to 1.08 mm for the head, 0.1 to 0.5 mm for the body and 0.1 to 0.83 mm for the tip. Maximum values ranged from 1.0 to 4.1 mm for the head, 1.0 to 1.5 mm for the body and 1.0 to 1.92 mm for the tip. Tipping angles ranging from 1.0 to 2.65° were noted. The mean extrusion of OMIs ranged from 0.1 to 0.8 mm and intrusion of up to 0.5 mm was also observed. In our study OMIs were removed at the time of debond and the tip of displaced OMIs might have interfered with the tissues supplying surrounding teeth with innervation and vascularity.

Besides possible complications with the use of OMIs [16, 17] affecting PST response and pulp vitality, numerous relationships between orthodontics and adjunctive procedures respectively and the state of the dental pulp were also described [37–39]. Patients requiring adjunctive procedures to orthodontics on maxillary front teeth such as approximal enamel reduction [10] and occlusal adjustments [11, 12] were not included, because pulpal temperature may have risen critically during the procedure [10].

It has been reported that orthodontic tooth movements like intrusion might also influence PST response [7, 40]. Radiographic examination, albeit limited to two-dimensional plain film radiographs, did not reveal any close proximity between the OMIs and the roots of the teeth. It is therefore unlikely that direct Injury led to loss of vitality.

However loss of response to PST and vitality might have been caused by orthodontics itself. This may be relevant for the canine that required root canal treatment, as direct injury of this tooth during OMI-Insertion in the anterior palate was unlikely to have caused this issue and has never before been reported in literature. Moreover the patient was an adult (37 years) and older than the other patients affected (11 and 12 years). Hamersky et al. suggested [41] that orthodontic forces cause biochemical and biologic pulpal tissue changes and that orthodontic forces may be less safe as the age of the patient increases. Open apices allow vessels to enter the pulp and the increased amount of loose connective tissue in this apical area may help to maintaining pulpal blood flow during orthodontic force application; this argument has also been made by other authors [42, 43]. Remarkably Ingle et al. [44] found that the maxillary canine, which is generally not affected by dental trauma, appears to be the tooth most susceptible to pulp hemorrhage and necrosis when exposed to orthodontic force application, suggesting ischemic infarction as most likely cause.

The possibility of dental trauma before, during and subsequent to orthodontic treatment plays an important role when interpreting the results of our study. Incidence of dental trauma is subject to continuous investigation [45–47] and data from the United States revealed that 25% of the population from 6 to 50 years of age may have suffered dental trauma to the anterior teeth [45]. Surprisingly, some patients are unaware of this and many choose not to seek dental treatment [45, 48] and taking a past dental history is likely to be unreliable. Most dental injuries occur during the first two decades of life; the most accident-prone time was found from the age 8 to 12 years [46, 48]. Dental trauma is more frequent in boys than girls however there is considerable variation [47]. Maxillary central incisors, followed by the lateral incisors are most frequently involved [49]. One investigation evaluated pulp vitality in teeth suffering trauma during orthodontic therapy; prevalence of pulp necrosis was 18.6% [30] and this was much higher than our findings.

We excluded patients who had a past history of general anaesthesia; dental trauma during endotracheal intubation anaesthesia is one of the most common encountered adverse events of general anaesthesia [50]. Maxillary central incisors are affected most frequently [51]. Incidence of dental trauma reporting was found to be smaller than 0.2% [52] when assessed by anaesthesiologists compared to 12.1% [53] when assessed by dentists. It was suggested that examinations should hence be conducted by dental surgeons [54].

Alomari et al. [6] examined PST response using electric pulp testing (EPT) during and after orthodontic treatment. The threshold of response to PST using EPT was found to vary during but returned to pre-treatment values towards the end of the retention phase. The authors suggested that responses to electrical pulp testing, should be interpreted with caution during orthodontics and that a negative PST response does not always indicate pulpal necrosis.

In daily clinical practice a refrigerant spray (RS) is often used for practical reasons [55] and in our study we also used a RS producing a local temperature of -50 °C. There is little evidence which cold delivery method is most accurate in determining pulp responsiveness. Jones et al. [56] compared carbon dioxide dry ice sticks (CO_2) with RS and concluded that RS and CO2 were equivalent in determining pulpal responsiveness, but the response elicited from the refrigerant spray (RS) was faster.

To distinguish between "sensibility" and "vitality" advanced techniques such as Laser-Doppler techniques (Laser Doppler Flowmetry - LDF) to measure intrapulpal blood flow can be used [1, 5]. LDF was found to be a reliable method. However, it is technique-sensitive [57] and extra-pulpal blood flow, mainly from the periodontal ligament, may contaminate the signal [58]. Moreover LDF is time-consuming [57, 59] and hence not always practical for routine clinical use.

Regression analysis showed that only the insertion position of the OMIs was a statistically significant covariate ($p = 0.008$) for loss of vitality. In the three patients affected by a negative response to cold testing the OMIs were inserted at the second rugae (R-2), and we must assume that a more posterior insertion directed to the third rugae (R-3) is more likely to preserve vitality. This is in agreement with a recent investigation by Hourfar et al. [21] which examined bone availability for OMI insertion in relation to the palatal rugae. Most bone was found in the vertical dimension at the first and second rugae for 8 mm long OMIs. Yet they stated that it was challenging to access the area of the second rugae clinically: OMIs would have to be inserted vertically to avoid damage to the incisor roots and perpendicular insertion to the bone surface might not be suitable for this area.

The inclination of upper incisors (U1/ANS-PNS) was not a statistically significant covariate ($p = 0.289$) although a slight tendency towards proclination was noted within in the sample.

To our knowledge, this study is the first retrospective study that investigates the relationship between OMI positioning and loss of PST response and pulp vitality.

Time delay of endodontic complications was accounted for in our study design by investigating the patients 24 months after debond. We propose further research using prospective designs to verify the outcome of our investigation.

Conclusions

- Although there was no radiographic evidence of OMI induced trauma to the teeth that lost vitality, the proximity of the implants to the anterior teeth was positively and related to loss of PST ($p = 0.008$).
- In all cases of PST loss OMIs were inserted at the second rugae (R-2) and we therefore we recommend

that OMIs should be placed either more posteriorly, at the third rugae (R-3), or in the median plane. This will decrease risk of trauma to the roots of the anterior teeth.

- PST/vitality loss post OMI-insertion in the anterior palate was only 0.18%. We conclude that the risk of palatal OMIs leading to loss of PST/vitality of the upper front teeth is small.

Acknowledgement
The authors express their thanks to Mr. J. Hammer for participating in the collection of data.

Funding
None.

Authors' contributions
JH conceived the project, gathered and processed the data, created the material presented (tables, electronic images, references, et cetera) and drafted the manuscript. DB translated and critically revised the manuscript. JAL critically revised the manuscript. BL reviewed the process and critically revised the manuscript. All authors read and approved the final manuscript.

Competing interests
The authors declare that they have no competing interests.

Author details
[1]Department of Orthodontics, University of Heidelberg, Heidelberg, Germany. [2]Department of Orthodontics, Guy's and St Thomas' NHS Foundation Trust and King's College Dental Institute, London, UK. [3]Department of Orthodontics, University of Saarland, Homburg/Saar, Germany. [4]Private Practice, Am Bahnhof 54, 56841 Traben-Trarbach, Germany.

References
1. Chen E, Abbott PV. Dental pulp testing: a review. Int J Dent. 2009;365785:12.
2. Bastos JV, Goulart EM, de Souza Cortes MI. Pulpal response to sensibility tests after traumatic dental injuries in permanent teeth. Dent Traumatol. 2014;30:188–92.
3. Farac RV, Morgental RD, Lima RK, Tiberio D, dos Santos MT. Pulp sensibility test in elderly patients. Gerodontology. 2012;29:135–9.
4. Rutsatz C, Baumhardt SG, Feldens CA, Rosing CK, Grazziotin-Soares R, Barletta FB. Response of pulp sensibility test is strongly influenced by periodontal attachment loss and gingival recession. J Endod. 2012;38:580–3.
5. Gopikrishna V, Pradeep G, Venkateshbabu N. Assessment of pulp vitality: a review. Int J Paediatr Dent. 2009;19:3–15.
6. Alomari FA, Al-Habahbeh R, Alsakarna BK. Responses of pulp sensibility tests during orthodontic treatment and retention. Int Endod J. 2011;44:635–43.
7. Veberiene R, Smailiene D, Danielyte J, Toleikis A, Dagys A, Machiulskiene V. Effects of intrusive force on selected determinants of pulp vitality. Angle Orthod. 2009;79:1114–8.
8. Spector JK, Rothenhaus B, Herman RI. Pulpal necrosis following orthodontic therapy. Report of two cases. N Y State Dent J. 1974;40:30–2.
9. Fonseca GM, Guzmán AE. Orthodontic Forces Causing Damage the Pulpal Condition. Report of Two Cases. Int J Odontostomat. 2010;4:271–6.
10. Baysal A, Uysal T, Usumez S. Temperature Rise in the Pulp Chamber during Different Stripping Procedures. Angle Orthod. 2007;77:478–82.
11. Zachrisson BU, Mjor IA. Remodeling of teeth by grinding. Am J Orthod. 1975;68:545–53.
12. Tuverson DL. Orthodontic treatment using canines in place of missing maxillary lateral incisors. Am J Orthod. 1970;58:109–27.
13. Zach L, Cohen G. Pulp Response to Externally Applied Heat. Oral Surg Oral Med Oral Pathol. 1965;19:515–30.
14. Rowe AH, Pitt Ford TR. The assessment of pulpal vitality. Int Endod J. 1990; 23:77–83.
15. Carrillo R, Buschang PH. Palatal and mandibular miniscrew implant placement techniques. J Clin Orthod. 2013;47:737–43.
16. Kravitz ND, Kusnoto B. Risks and complications of orthodontic miniscrews. Am J Orthod Dentofacial Orthop. 2007;131:S43–51.
17. Kuroda S, Tanaka E. Risks and complications of miniscrew anchorage in clinical orthodontics. Jpn Dent Sci Rev. 2014;50:79–85.
18. Ludwig B, Glasl B, Bowman SJ, Wilmes B, Kinzinger GS, Lisson JA. Anatomical guidelines for miniscrew insertion: palatal sites. J Clin Orthod. 2011;45:433–41.
19. Baumgaertel S. Temporary skeletal anchorage devices: The case for miniscrews. Am J Orthod Dentofacial Orthop. 2014;145:560.
20. Winsauer H, Vlachojannis C, Bumann A, Vlachojannis J, Chrubasik S. Paramedian vertical palatal bone height for mini-implant insertion: a systematic review. Eur J Orthod. 2014;36:541–9.
21. Hourfar J, Ludwig B, Bister D, Braun A, Kanavakis G. The most distal palatal ruga for placement of orthodontic mini-implants. Eur J Orthod. 2015;37: 373–8.
22. Hourfar J, Kanavakis G, Bister D, Schatzle M, Awad L, Nienkemper M, Goldbecher C, Ludwig B. Three dimensional anatomical exploration of the anterior hard palate at the level of the third ruga for the placement of mini-implants - a cone-beam CT study. Eur J Orthod. 2015;37:589–95.
23. Er K, Bayram M, Tasdemir T. Root canal treatment of a periradicular lesion caused by unintentional root damage after orthodontic miniscrew placement: a case report. Int Endod J. 2011;44:1170–5.
24. Ludwig B, Glasl B, Kinzinger GS, Walde KC, Lisson JA. The skeletal frog appliance for maxillary molar distalization. J Clin Orthod. 2011;45:77–84.
25. Wilmes B, Nienkemper M, Drescher D. Application and effectiveness of a mini-implant- and tooth-borne rapid palatal expansion device: the hybrid hyrax. World J Orthod. 2010;11:323–30.
26. Ludwig B, Zachrisson BU, Rosa M. Non-compliance space closure in patients with missing lateral incisors. J Clin Orthod. 2013;47:180–7.
27. Bernhart T, Vollgruber A, Gahleitner A, Dörtbudak O, Haas R. Alternative to the median region of the palate for placement of an orthodontic implant. Clin Oral Implants Res. 2000;11:595–601.
28. Houston WJB, Stephens CD, Tulley WJ. A textbook of orthodontics. Wright, Oxford. Oxford: Wright; 1992.
29. Christou P, Kiliaridis S. Vertical growth-related changes in the positions of palatal rugae and maxillary incisors. Am J Orthod Dentofacial Orthop. 2008; 133:81–6.
30. Bauss O, Rohling J, Meyer K, Kiliaridis S. Pulp vitality in teeth suffering trauma during orthodontic therapy. Angle Orthod. 2009;79:166–71.
31. Hwang YC, Hwang HS. Surgical repair of root perforation caused by an orthodontic miniscrew implant. Am J Orthod Dentofacial Orthop. 2011;139: 407–11.
32. Lim G, Kim KD, Park W, Jung BY, Pang NS. Endodontic and surgical treatment of root damage caused by orthodontic miniscrew placement. J Endod. 2013;39:1073–7.
33. McCabe P, Kavanagh C. Root perforation associated with the use of a miniscrew implant used for orthodontic anchorage: a case report. Int Endod J. 2012;45:678–88.
34. Shokri A, Eskandarloo A, Noruzi-Gangachin M, Khajeh S. Detection of root perforations using conventional and digital intraoral radiography, multidetector computed tomography and cone beam computed tomography. Restor Dent Endod. 2015;40:58–67.
35. Liou EJ, Pai BC, Lin JC. Do miniscrews remain stationary under orthodontic forces? Am J Orthod Dentofacial Orthop. 2004;126:42–7.
36. Nienkemper M, Handschel J, Drescher D. Systematic review of mini-implant displacement under orthodontic loading. Int J Oral Sci. 2014;6:1–6.
37. von Bohl M, Ren Y, Fudalej PS, Kuijpers-Jagtman AM. Pulpal reactions to orthodontic force application in humans: a systematic review. J Endod. 2012;38:1463–9.
38. Javed F, Al-Kheraif AA, Romanos EB, Romanos GE. Influence of orthodontic forces on human dental pulp: a systematic review. Arch Oral Biol. 2015;60:347–56.
39. Meeran N. Iatrogenic possibilities of orthodontic treatment and modalities of prevention. J Orthod Sci. 2013;2:73–86.
40. Veberiene R, Smailiene D, Baseviciene N, Toleikis A, Machiulskiene V. Change in dental pulp parameters in response to different modes of orthodontic force application. Angle Orthod. 2010;80:1018–22.
41. Hamersky PA, Weimer AD, Taintor JF. The effect of orthodontic force application on the pulpal tissue respiration rate in the human premolar. Am J Orthod. 1980;77:368–78.

42. Unsterseher RE, Nieberg LG, Weimer AD, Dyer JK. The response of human pulpal tissue after orthodontic force application. Am J Orthod Dentofacial Orthop. 1987;92:220–4.

43. Stenvik A, Mjor IA. Pulp and dentine reactions to experimental tooth intrusion. A histologic study of the initial changes. Am J Orthod. 1970;57:370–85.

44. Ingle JI, Simon JHS, Walton RE, Pashley DH, Bakland LK, Heithersay GS, Stanley HR. Pulpal pathology: Its etiology and prevention. In: Ingle JI, Bakland LK, editors. Endodontics. fifth ed. Hamilton - London: BC Decker Inc; 2002. p. 95–174.

45. Kaste LM, Gift HC, Bhat M, Swango PA. Prevalence of incisor trauma in persons 6-50 years of age: United States, 1988-1991. J Dent Res. 1996:696-705

46. Glendor U. Epidemiology of traumatic dental injuries–a 12 year review of the literature. Dent Traumatol. 2008;24:603–11.

47. Bastone EB, Freer TJ, McNamara JR. Epidemiology of dental trauma: a review of the literature. Aust Dent J. 2000;45:2–9.

48. Bakland LK. Endodontic considerations in dental trauma. In: Ingle JI, Bakland LK, editors. Endodontics. fifth ed. Hamilton - London: BC Decker Inc; 2002. p. 795–844.

49. Francisco SS, Filho FJ, Pinheiro ET, Murrer RD, de Jesus SA. Prevalence of traumatic dental injuries and associated factors among Brazilian schoolchildren. Oral Health Prev Dent. 2013;11:31–8.

50. Idrees SR, Fujimura K, Bessho K. Dental trauma related to general anesthesia: should the anesthesiologist perform a preanesthetic dental evaluation? Oral Health Dent Manag. 2014;13:271–4.

51. Newland MC, Ellis SJ, Peters KR, Simonson JA, Durham TM, Ullrich FA, Tinker JH. Dental injury associated with anesthesia: a report of 161,687 anesthetics given over 14 years. J Clin Anesth. 2007;19:339–45.

52. Manka-Malara K, Gawlak D, Hovhannisyan A, Klikowska M, Kostrzewa-Janicka J. Dental trauma prevention during endotracheal intubation–review of literature. Anaesthesiol Intensive Ther. 2015;47:425–9.

53. Chen JJ, Susetio L, Chao CC. Oral complications associated with endotracheal general anesthesia. Ma Zui Xue Za Zhi. 1990;28:163–9.

54. Chadwick RG, Lindsay SM. Dental injuries during general anaesthesia. Br Dent J. 1996;180:255–8.

55. Jafarzadeh H, Abbott PV. Review of pulp sensibility tests. Part I: general information and thermal tests. Int Endod J. 2010;43:738–62.

56. Jones VR, Rivera EM, Walton RE. Comparison of carbon dioxide versus refrigerant spray to determine pulpal responsiveness. J Endod. 2002;28:531–3.

57. Evans D, Reid J, Strang R, Stirrups D. A comparison of laser Doppler flowmetry with other methods of assessing the vitality of traumatised anterior teeth. Endod Dent Traumatol. 1999;15:284–90.

58. Jafarzadeh H. Laser Doppler flowmetry in endodontics: a review. Int Endod J. 2009;42:476–90.

59. Abd-Elmeguid A, Yu DC. Dental pulp neurophysiology: part 2. Current diagnostic tests to assess pulp vitality. J Can Dent Assoc. 2009;75:139–43.

30

Morphology of the distal thoracic duct and the right lymphatic duct in different head and neck pathologies: an imaging based study

Ferdinand J. Kammerer*, Benedikt Schlude, Michael A. Kuefner, Philipp Schlechtweg, Matthias Hammon, Michael Uder and Siegfried A. Schwab

Abstract

Background: The purpose of this study was to assess the influence of head and neck pathologies on the detection rate, configuration and diameter of the thoracic duct (TD) and right lymphatic duct (RLD) in computed tomography (CT) of the head and neck.

Methods: One hundred ninety-seven patients were divided into the subgroups "healthy", "benign disease" and "malignant disease". The interpretation of the images was performed at a slice thickness of 3 mm in the axial and coronal plane. In each case we looked for the distal part of the TD and RLD respectively and subsequently evaluated their configuration (tubular, sacciform, dendritic) as well as their maximum diameter and correlated the results with age, gender and diagnosis group.

Results: The detection rate in the study population was 81.2 % for the TD and 64.2 % for the RLD and did not differ significantly in any of the subgroups. The predominant configuration was tubular. The configuration distribution did not differ significantly between the diagnosis groups. The mean diameter of the TD was 4.79 ± 2.41 mm and that of the RLD was 3.98 ± 1.96 mm. No significant influence of a diagnosis on the diameter could be determined.

Conclusions: There is no significant influence of head/neck pathologies on the CT detection rate, morphology or size of the TD and RLD. However our study emphasizes that both the RLD and the TD are detectable in the majority of routine head and neck CTs and therefore reading physicians and radiologists should be familiar with their various imaging appearances.

Keywords: Head and neck pathologies, Distal thoracic duct, Right lymphatic duct, Computed tomography

Background

Computed tomography (CT) is a frequently used imaging method for pathologies of the head and neck, which represents a quite complex anatomic region. Various anatomic structures such as arteries or veins have to be differentiated and assessed by the reading physician, for both pure diagnostic purposes and/or therapy planning. As a CT of the head and neck region usually encloses parts of the upper mediastinum, both the distal thoracic duct (TD) and the right lymphatic duct (RLD) are included in the

examinations as well and are detectable by CT [1]. The function of these main lymphatic vessels is to drain the whole body's lymphatic fluid into the venous system: the right side of the thorax, the right arm and the right side of the head and neck are drained by the RLD into the junction of the right internal jugular and the right subclavian vein. The TD drains the rest of the body into the junction of the left internal jugular and the left subclavian vein.

While there are various reports in the literature about the influence of pathologies of the body trunk (e.g. malignancies, portal venous hypertension, congestive heart failure) on the imaging morphology and function of the main lymphatic vessels [2–9] to the best of our knowledge

---
* Correspondence: ferdinand.kammerer@uk-erlangen.de
Institute of Radiology, University Erlangen-Nuremberg, Maximiliansplatz 1, D-91054 Erlangen, Germany

there exist no data regarding diseases of the head and neck. Therefore the aim of this study was to assess the influence of head and neck pathologies on the morphology of the distal thoracic duct and right lymphatic duct in CT.

Methods

Patients and diagnoses

The study was conducted in accordance with the guidelines of the Declaration of Helsinki and with approval of the ethics committee of the University of Erlangen-Nuremberg (23-06-2015). Written informed consent had been obtained from all patients. Our RIS (radiology information system) was searched for patients who underwent routine CT of the head and neck with intravenous contrast media (CM) application in a retrospective period of 30 months. In order to keep the possibility of any iatrogenic influence on the ducts' morphology as low as possible patients with a history of cervical surgery or radiation and any history of systemic chemotherapy were excluded from evaluation. To asses a potential influence of patient's age on the CT morphology of the RLD and TD two age groups were defined: Age group A consisted of patients ≤ 50 years, age group B of patients > 50 years. Regarding the head and neck diagnoses the patients were divided into three particular diagnosis groups: Diagnosis group 1 included healthy patients without any visible disease on the CT scans. Diagnosis group 2 consisted of patients with benign and diagnosis group 3 of patients with malignant disease. If a pathology was present, its side of the neck was noted, pathologies crossing or reaching the midline were considered as both sided. All malignant lesions were pathologically proven (either before or after the CT scan). Benign lesions were either proven clinically, pathologically or by follow up examinations.

Imaging and reading technique

To avoid any technical bias resulting from different CT technologies only patients examined on one particular scanner at our institution (Somatom Sensation 64, Siemens Healthcare, Erlangen, Germany) were included. Scanning parameters (120 kV, 200 eff. mAs, anatomy based tube current modulation) were identical in all examinations. The collimation was 64 x 0.6 mm. Patients were examined in the supine position with their arms lowered. Intravenous contrast media (Imeron 350, Bracco Imaging, Konstanz, Germany) was applied via an antecubital vein at a flow rate of 2.5 ml/s and the scan was started after a delay of 80 seconds.

All examinations were evaluated on a dedicated PACS (Picture Archiving and Communication System) workstation (syngo.plaza, Siemens, Germany). All examinations were anonymized and randomized. A board-certified radiologist (Siegfried A. Schwab) and a Ph.D. student (Benedikt Schlude) evaluated the distal TD and RLD in consensus on

axial and coronal 3 mm reconstructions in soft tissue windowing (window 400, center 50).

Evaluation

If both sides of the lower neck were not readable because of artifacts (e.g. due to pacemaker material or retained, highly concentrated intravenous CM), the examination was excluded from our evaluation. On the other hand if only one side of the lower neck was unreadable due to artifacts, the other side was included into the evaluation anyway.

Concerning the main lymphatic vessels the readers at first assessed if the RLD and TD could be identified at all. Criterion of identifiability was the visualization of a continuous non venous, non arterial vessel draining into the venous system on either side. In case of the TD there had to be a visible continuity into the upper mediastinum. The RLD or TD were considered as not detectable if their side of the neck was readable but no vessel meeting the criteria of identification was detected.

If the main lymphatic vessels could be identified, their configuration was classified as either tubular, dendritic or sacciform: A tubular classification was chosen, when the vessel was mainly cylindrical in its morphology (Fig. 1). In case of a circumferential convex border of the distal lymphatic vessel, its configuration was considered as sacciform (Fig. 2). A dendritic configuration was considered at the presence of multiple smaller lymphatic vessels conjoining just before the drainage into the veins (Figs. 2 and 3). Moreover the largest transverse diameter of each identifiable main lymphatic vessel was measured and noted. In the dendritic configuration group the overall diameter of the area of confluence of the particular smaller vessels just before draining into the venous system was measured.

During the evaluation in some RLDs and TDs the readers observed very high Hounsfield Units (Fig. 4), which was considered a reflux of CM from the venous into the lymphatic vessel [1, 10]. The presence of this phenomenon was noted for both sides.

Statistical analysis

All statistical evaluations were performed using dedicated software (SAS-Analyst Version 9.2, SAS Institute, USA). Data concerning the detectability of the lymphatic vessels, their diameters and configurations in various subsets of the study population were compared and checked for differences between the diagnosis groups (no pathology, benign pathology, malignant pathology). As both main ducts predominantly drain the lymph of either the right (RLD) or the left (TD) side of the neck, a differentiation between the sides of the pathology regarding the evaluated duct was made. The pathology was considered as ipsilateral if the pathology was on the particular duct's drainage side and as contralateral if it was on the opposite side of the

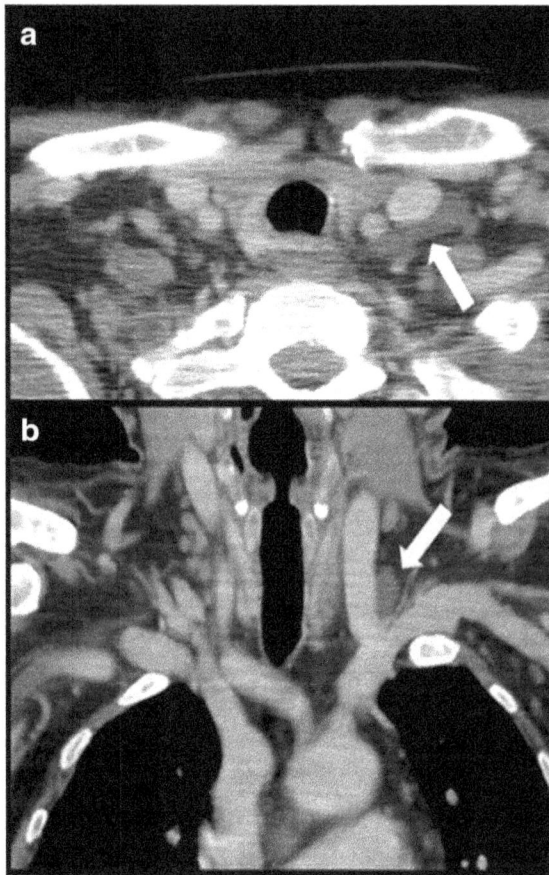

Fig. 1 A 66 year old male with pharyngeal lymphoma. Contrast enhanced computed tomography in the axial (**a**) and coronal (**b**) plane. Tubular (axial plane) configuration of the thoracic duct (arrows)

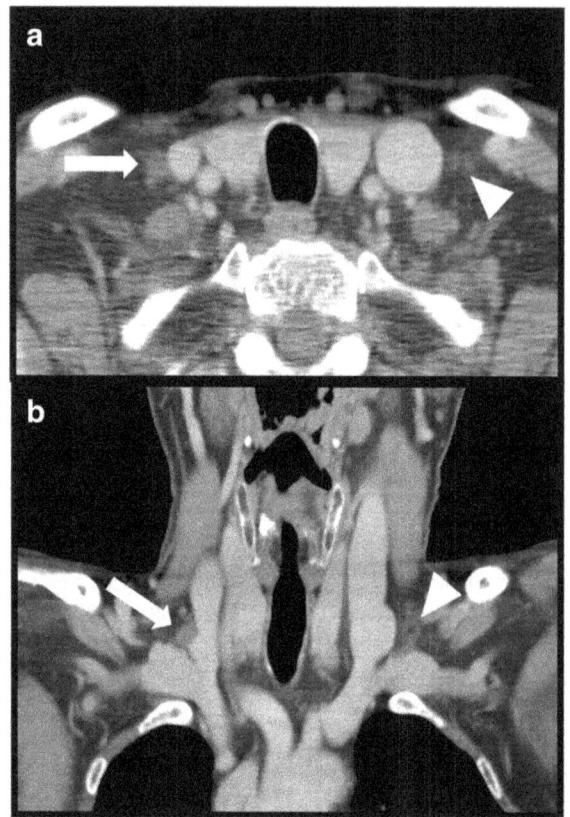

Fig. 2 A 55 year old male with laryngeal carcinoma. Contrast enhanced computed tomography in the axial (**a**) and coronal (**b**) plane. Sacciform configuration of the right lymphatic duct in both planes (arrows). The thoracic duct shows a dendritic morphology (arrowheads)

neck. Furthermore for the analysis of the vessels' diameters the independent variables age (>50 years, $\leq$ 50 years) and gender (female, male) were included in the analysis. As statistical tests were chosen: T-Test, Kruskal-Wallis-Test, Wilcoxon-Test and Chi-Quadrat-Test. P-values < 0.05 were considered significant. Due to the lack of knowledge about the laterality of the injection site of the CM, the frequency of CM reflux into a lymph vessel could not be analyzed statistically.

Results

Within time period of retrospective analysis 457 CTs of the neck were identified. Due to a history of surgery, radiotherapy or chemotherapy or the situation of both sided artifacts 260 examinations had to be excluded from the analysis. Therefore 197 examinations were included into the evaluation. 131 patients (66.5 %) were male (m), 66 (33.5 %) were female (f). Age was between 12 and 89 years (mean 59.0 years). Number of patients $\leq$ 50 years (age group A) was 49, whereas it was 148 for patients > 50 years (age group B). Diagnosis group 1 (no pathology) consisted of 32 patients (16.2 %; 14 m, 18 f).

Diagnosis group 2 (benign pathology) consisted of 47 patients (23.9 %; 20 m, 27 f) and the pathologies noted in this group were: inflammatory/infectious ($n = 25$), benign tumor ($n = 10$), osteonecrosis ($n = 5$), developmental/other ($n = 7$). Diagnosis group 3 (malignant pathology) consisted of 118 individuals (59.9 %; 97 m, 21 f) and the pathologies in this group were: carcinoma ($n = 111$), lymphoma ($n = 4$), sarcoma ($n = 2$) and melanoma ($n = 1$). The benign pathology was right sided in 21, left sided in 15 and on both sides in 11 cases, the numbers for malignant disease were 45, 37 and 36 respectively. While the examinations could be evaluated on the left side of the neck for all 197 patients, this was the case in only 187 patients on the right side due to artifacts.

Detectability of the TD and RLD

The TD could be identified in 160/197 (81.2 %) of the patients; the detectability rate was 87.5 % in diagnosis group 1, 78.8 % in group 2 and 80.5 % in group 3. This difference was not significant ($p = 0.59$). No significant difference between the diagnosis groups for ipsilateral pathologies could be observed (group 2 84.6 %; group 3 76.7 %; $p = 0.37$). Regarding the patients' age the

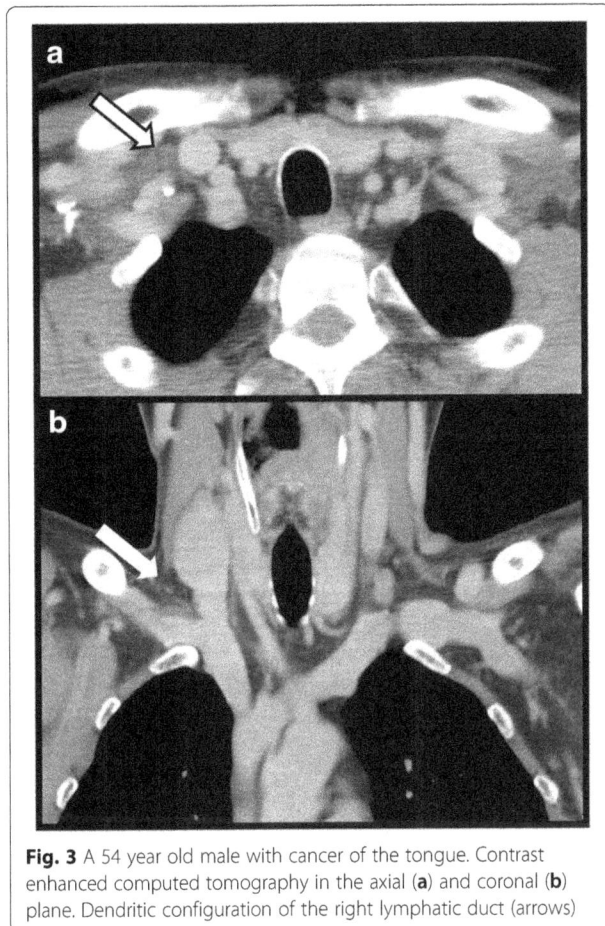

Fig. 3 A 54 year old male with cancer of the tongue. Contrast enhanced computed tomography in the axial (**a**) and coronal (**b**) plane. Dendritic configuration of the right lymphatic duct (arrows)

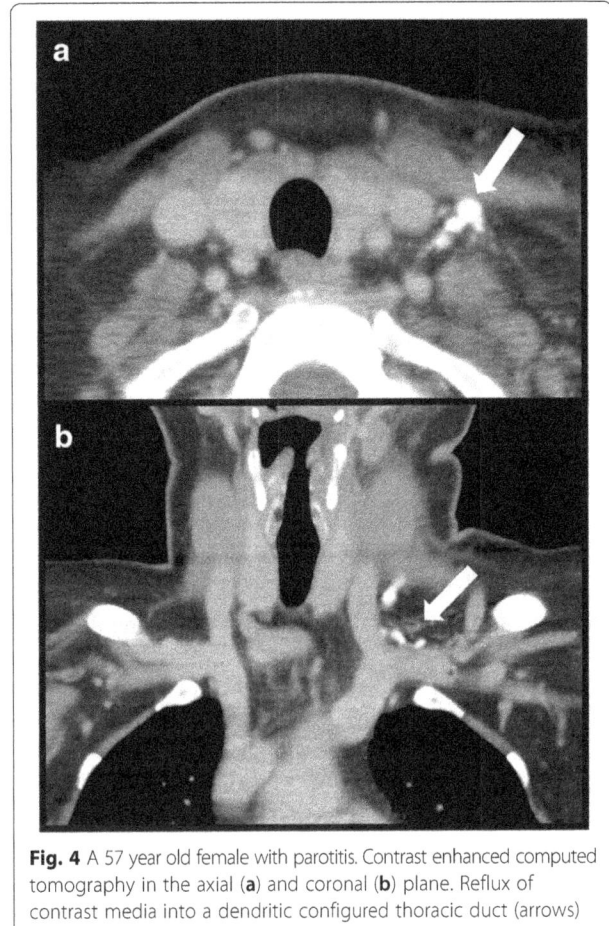

Fig. 4 A 57 year old female with parotitis. Contrast enhanced computed tomography in the axial (**a**) and coronal (**b**) plane. Reflux of contrast media into a dendritic configured thoracic duct (arrows)

detectability rate was 75.5 % in age group A and 83.1 % in group B ($p = 0.24$). In men the TD could be identified in 84.7 % and in women in 83.3 % ($p = 0.16$).

The RLD could be identified in 120/187 (64.2 %) of the patients; the detectability rate was 61.3 % in diagnosis group 1, 65.1 % in group 2 and 64.6 % in group 3. This difference was not significant ($p = 0.93$). Also no significant difference between the diagnosis groups for ipsilateral pathologies could be observed (group 2 67.9 %; group 3 64.9 %; $p = 0.87$). Regarding the patients' age the detectability rate was 63.6 % in age group A and 64.3 % in group B ($p = 0.93$). In men the RLD could be identified in 66.4 % and in women in 59.3 % ($p = 0.35$).

Configuration of the TD and RLD

The configuration of the TD was tubular in 108 (67.5 %), sacciform in 34 (21.3 %) and dendritic in 18 (11.3 %) of all examinations. The distribution was 64.3 %, 21.4 % and 14.3 % for diagnosis group 1, 67.6 %, 27.0 % and 5.4 % in diagnosis group 2 and 68.4 %, 18.9 % and 12.6 % in diagnosis group 3. The distribution of configurations did not differ significantly between the diagnosis groups, no matter if the side of pathology was taken into account ($p = 0.54$) or not ($p = 0.67$). There was no significant

influence of the gender concerning the configuration ($p = 0.65$). However a significant difference in configurations between age groups was found: patients > 50 years showed tubular or dendritic TDs more often than individuals $\leq$ 50 years who had more sacciform TDs ($p = 0.02$).

The configuration of the RLD was tubular in 53 (44.2 %), sacciform in 23 (19.2 %) and dendritic in 44 (36.7 %) of all evaluable examinations. The distribution was 47.4 %, 10.5 % and 42.1 % for diagnosis group 1, 42.9 %, 17.9 % and 39.3 % in diagnosis group 2 and 43.8 %, 21.9 % and 34.2 % in diagnosis group 3. The distribution of configurations did not differ significantly between the diagnosis groups, no matter if the side of pathology was taken into account ($p = 0.82$) or not ($p = 0.84$). Also there was no significant influence of the gender ($p = 0.83$) or age group ($p = 0.10$).

Diameter of the TD and RLD

In all TDs the mean diameter was 4.79 ± 2.41 mm. Males had a mean diameter of 4.96 ± 2.49 mm while the TD in women measured 4.4 ± 2.19 mm. The difference was not significant ($p = 0.15$). Healthy patients (group 1) had a mean diameter of 4.54 ± 2.78 mm, whereas it was $5.08 \pm$

2.37 mm in group 2 and 4.75 ± 2.32 mm in group 3 (Fig. 5). Taking into account only ipsilateral pathologies the mean diameter in group 2 was 4.55 ± 2.02 mm and 4.54 ± 2.24 mm in group 3. Neither of these differences were significant ($p = 0.4$ and $p = 0.88$).

The mean diameter of the RLDs was 3.98 ± 1.96 mm. Males had a mean diameter of 4.08 ± 2.05 mm while the TD in women measured 3.71 ± 1.69 mm. The difference was not significant ($p = 0.31$). Healthy patients (group 1) had a mean diameter of 3.68 ± 1.7 mm, whereas it was 4.04 ± 1.64 mm in group 2 and 4.03 ± 2.13 mm in group 3 (Fig. 6). Taking into account only ipsilateral pathologies the mean diameter in group 2 was 4.16 ± 1.64 mm and 4.04 ± 2.11 mm in group 3. Neither of these differences were significant ($p = 0.74$ and $p = 0.60$).

The mean diameter of the TD was 5.41 ± 2.55 mm in age group A whereas it was 4.6 ± 2.34 mm in age group B ($p = 0.09$). The values for the RLD were 4.07 ± 1.68 mm and 3.95 ± 2.04 mm respectively ($p = 0.74$). On the other hand a significant influence of age regarding the diameter of the TD could be determined in both the univariate ($p = 0.0463$) and multivariate ($p = 0.0481$) regression. This was not the case for the RLD. Figure 7 shows the relation of age and diameter for both the TD and the RLD. Contrary to this regarding healthy individuals (diagnosis group 1) a tendency for smaller diameters in younger individuals could be observed for the TD (4.44 ± 2.07 mm in age group A vs. 4.58 ± 3.11 mm in age group B) exlusively which was not the case for the RLD (4.13 ± 1.46 mm in age group A vs. 3.36 ± 1.86 mm in age group B). However both differences were not significant.

Reflux of CM into the great lymphatic vessels
In 160 identified TDs a CM reflux could be observed in 40 cases (25 %). On the other hand in 120 identified RLDs a CM reflux was found in 21 patients (17.5 %). As

the side of CM injection was not known, statistical analyses seemed not to be reasonable.

Discussion
Altough the main lymphatic vessels (thoracic duct (TD) and right lymphatic duct (RLD)) in the cervical-thoracic junction are rather delicate anatomic structures we were able to identify them in the majority of cases even in routine computed tomography (CT) examinations of the head and neck region. The TDs' identification rate of 81.2 % in our study is quite higher than in previous reports about rates of 55 % and 63 % [1, 11]. This difference is even bigger concerning the identification of the RLD which was 64.2 % in our study and thus much higher than the 4 % in the report of Liu et al. [1]. As the diagnostic benefit of including coronal reformations into the reading of CT scans is well documented for other body regions [12–14], we conjecture that our higher detection rate can be explained by the fact that in our analysis also both the axial and coronal planes were included.

Moreover a difference in the slice thickness between 3 mm in our study and 1.5 mm from Gossner [11] could contribute to the different detection rates due to increased image noise in thinner sections. A detection frequency of 14 % for the distal TD in another study which used 1 mm slices may support this theory [15].

We categorized the morphology of th main lymphatic vessels into three groups (tubular, sacciform, dendritic). For the TD the distribution was tubular > sacciform > dendritic, even in most of the subgroups of patients. Our rate of 11.3 % of the dendritic type is comparable to Kinnaert's analysis [16]. On the other hand the dendritic configuration was not described in other analyses: Liu et al. differentiated tubular (43 %), flared (45 %) and fusiform (12 %) subgroups [1]. Our higher (67.5 %) rate of tubular TDs may be

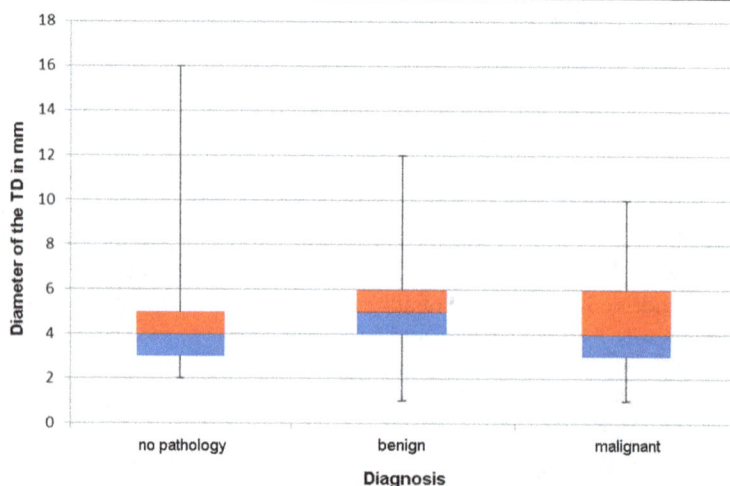

Fig. 5 Box-Whisker-Plot for the diameter of the thoracic duct (TD) depending on diagnosis

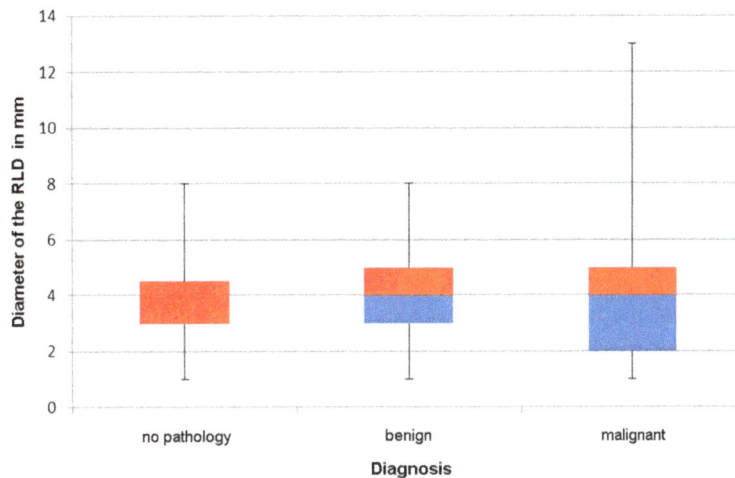

Fig. 6 Box-Whisker-Plot for the diameter of confluence of the right lymphatic duct (RLD) depending on diagnosis

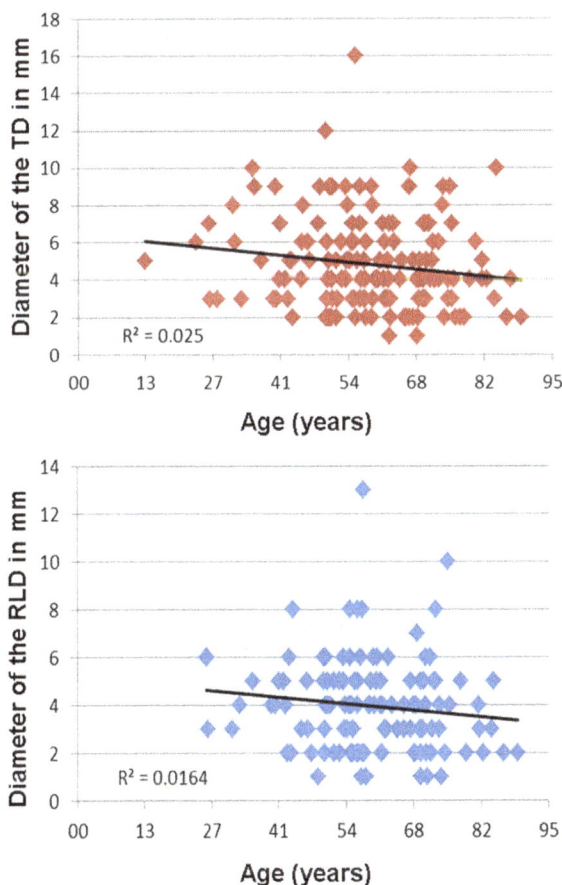

Fig. 7 Diameters of the thoracic duct (TD) and right lymphatic duct (RLD) in millimeters (mm) in relation to patient's age in years

explained by the fact, that in our analysis both healthy and sick patients were included whereas Liu et al. excluded patients with a history of cancer, presence of lymphadenopathy or neck abscesses. This could give rise to the assumption that unhealthy individuals tend to have tubular shaped TDs. However even in our "healthy" subgroup the tubular configuration could be observed in more than 6 out of 10 patients (64.3 %).

There seems to be an influence of patients' age on the distribution of configuration subgroups as the TD was described significantly more often as tubular or dendritic in the elderly (age group B) and as sacciform in the younger (age group A). However to find out if the morphology of the TD is subject to change during lifetime, patients would have to be observed in an additional study for a very long period.

The mean diameter of the TD varies between the reports in literature. While the mean diameter of healthy individuals in our study (4.54 mm) correlates quite well with the CT-based results of Liu et al. (4.8 mm [1]), lower mean diameters from 1.9 to 3.74 mm were reported for MRI [7, 9] and ultrasound [5, 17] (Table 1). This could be explained in some part by the different image resolution

Table 1 Overview of mean imaging based diameters of the thoracic duct in literature

Authors	Imaging Modality	Mean Diameter	Range
Liu et al. [1]	CT	4.8 mm	–
Kiyonaga et al. [15]	CT	2.3 mm	1.1–2.8 mm
Yu et al. [9]	MRI	3.6 ± 0.1 mm	–
Takahashi et al. [7]	MRI	3.75 ± 0.81 mm	2.62–5.57 mm
Seeger et al. [5]	US	2.5 mm	–
Zironi et al. [17]	US	1.9 ± 0.5 mm	–
Parasher et al. [20]	US	2.43 mm	1.5–4 mm

CT computed tomography, *MRI* magnetic resonance imaging, *US* Ultrasound

in different modalities and the possible influence of inspiration and expiration on the TD's calibre [7]. On the other hand not all authors described in detail in what exact anatomic region the diameter of the TD was obtained. However according to Kiyonga et al. this seems to be of minor importance [15].

As it is well documented in literature that pathologies of the body trunk may have an influence on the morphology of the TD (mostly diseases leading to increased hydrostatic pressure as portal hypertension or cardiac congestion) [2–9, 17] the central aim of the study was to investigate this phenomenon for the head and neck region for the first time. Theoretically there are two main causes for a dilatation of the main lymphatic vessels: overproduction or impeded drainage of lymph. Pathologies as inflammations or tumours often cause edema due to increased vessel permeability leading to a higher lymph volume. Moreover pathologies may induce both neohemangiogenesis and neolymphangiogenesis [18]. On the other hand besides compression or direct invasion tumours can also metastasize into the main lymphatic vessels [19] possibly leading to an obstruction of the duct. However in our study we did not find a significant influence of the presence of head and neck pathologies (including benign and malign tumours) on the morphology of the main lymphatic vessels, which correlates well with the results Takahashi et al. presented for malignancies of the body trunk [7].

While there exists quite a lot of literature about imaging of the TD, data about the RLD is very limited and makes comparison of our results almost impossible at the time of writing. We were able to detect the RLD less often than the TD (64.2 % vs. 81.2 %) but with a much higher frequency than Liu et al. reported (4 %, [1]). Analogical with the TD the discrepancy to the results of Liu et al. could be explained by us evaluating multiplanar images leading to a higher detection rate of this rather short anatomic structure. Similar to the findings on the left side we could not observe any significant correlation between the RLD's detection rate or diameter and the presence of head and neck pathologies.

In our entire study population with increasing age a tendency of the diameter of the TD and RLD to decrease could be observed (diagrams 5, 6). Contrary to this regarding healthy individuals exclusively the diameter of the TD seems to increase with age, which correlates with the results of the healthy populations of other studies [1, 17]. The patients' gender in our observation had no significant influence on detection rate or diameter of the main lymphatic vessels as reported before in CT or MRI studies [1, 9]. However Seeger et al. found a significant larger TD in males than in females using ultrasound [5].

As reported before reflux of highly concentrated contrast media from the veins into the RLD and TD can be observed in CT [1, 10]. We found that phenomenon quite more often than Liu et al. reported (21.8 % vs. 9 %), which again may be caused by including the coronal plane into our image evaluation. However as the identification of the injection side (right vs. left arm) was not possible in our retrospective study there seems to be no way of any reasonable statistical evaluation of this interesting finding.

Another limitation of the study lies within the lack of knowledge of individual factors (e.g. cardiac function, renal function, body height and weight) which could influence the detection rate, diameter and morphology of the main lymphatic vessels, too. Therefore our results should be correlated with further prospective evaluations including these informations.

Conclusions

According to our results there is no influence of head and neck pathologies or age on the CT detection rate and morphology of the TD and RLD. On the other hand we could find a tendency of the ducts' diameters to decrease with age. Among the various configurations of the distal TD and the RLD the tubular type predominates. In CT contrast media reflux into the main lymphatic ducts may be seen in more than one fifth of patients. Our study shows that both the RLD and the TD can be detected regularly in routine head and neck CT. Therefore reading physicians and radiologists should be familiar with its various imaging appearances to avoid mistaking these structures for a lesion and to be able to describe its precise location e.g. prior to surgery in order to prevent potential injury. Our higher detection rate of the main lymphatic vessels compared to previous work emphasizes the importance of the inclusion of multiplanar images in the evaluation of the quite complex anatomy of the head and neck region.

Competing interests
The authors declare that they have no competing interests and received no funding for the study.

Authors' contributions
All authors contributed extensively to the work presented in this paper. FJK, BS and SAS made substantial contributions to conception, design, acquisition, analysis and interpretation of data and drafting of the manuscript. MAK, PS, MH and MU made substantial contributions to analysis and interpretation of data, contributed to the writing and reviewed the paper. All authors approved the manuscript prior to submission.

References
1. Liu ME, Branstetter BF, Whetstone J, Escott EJ. Normal CT appearance of the distal thoracic duct. AJR Am J Roentgenol. 2006;187(6):1615–20.
2. Dumont AE. The flow capacity of the thoracic duct-venous junction. Am J Med Sci. 1975;269(3):292–301.
3. Dumont AE, Mulholland JH. Alterations in Thoracic Duct Lymph Flow in Hepatic Cirrhosis: Significance in Portal Hypertension. Ann Surg. 1962;156(4):668–75.

4. Feuerlein S, Kreuzer G, Schmidt SA, Muche R, Juchems MS, Aschoff AJ, et al. The cisterna chyli: prevalence, characteristics and predisposing factors. Eur Radiol. 2009;19(1):73–8.

5. Seeger M, Bewig B, Gunther R, Schafmayer C, Vollnberg B, Rubin D, et al. Terminal part of thoracic duct: high-resolution US imaging. Radiology. 2009;252(3):897–904.

6. Shimada K, Sato I. Morphological and histological analysis of the thoracic duct at the jugulo-subclavian junction in Japanese cadavers. Clin Anat. 1997;10(3):163–72.

7. Takahashi H, Kuboyama S, Abe H, Aoki T, Miyazaki M, Nakata H. Clinical feasibility of noncontrast-enhanced magnetic resonance lymphography of the thoracic duct. Chest. 2003;124(6):2136–42.

8. Witte MH, Dumont AE, Clauss RH, Rader B, Levine N, Breed ES. Lymph circulation in congestive heart failure: effect of external thoracic duct drainage. Circulation. 1969;39(6):723–33.

9. Yu DX, Ma XX, Zhang XM, Wang Q, Li CF. Morphological features and clinical feasibility of thoracic duct: detection with nonenhanced magnetic resonance imaging at 3.0 T. J Magn Reson Imaging. 2010;32(1):94–100.

10. Han DH. Opacification of the distal thoracic duct on CT: not by lymphatic resorption of contrast material. AJR Am J Roentgenol. 2013;200(6):W694.

11. Gossner J. Appearance And Visibility Of The Thoracic Duct On Computed Tomography Of The Chest. Internet J Radiol. 2009;12:2.

12. Hwang SH, Yu JS, Chung JJ, Kim JH, Kim KW. Diagnosing small hepatic cysts on multidetector CT: an additional merit of thinner coronal reformations. Korean J Radiol. 2011;12(3):341–50.

13. Jung SI, Park HS, Yim Y, Jeon HJ, Yu MH, Kim YJ, et al. Added Value of Using a CT Coronal Reformation to Diagnose Adnexal Torsion. Korean J Radiol. 2015;16(4):835–45.

14. Kim HC, Yang DM, Jin W. Identification of the normal appendix in healthy adults by 64-slice MDCT: the value of adding coronal reformation images. Br J Radiol. 2008;81(971):859–64.

15. Kiyonaga M, Mori H, Matsumoto S, Yamada Y, Sai M, Okada F. Thoracic duct and cisterna chyli: evaluation with multidetector row CT. Br J Radiol. 2012;85(1016):1052–8.

16. Kinnaert P. Anatomical variations of the cervical portion of the thoracic duct in man. J Anat. 1973;115(Pt 1):45–52.

17. Zironi G, Cavalli G, Casali A, Piscaglia F, Gaiani S, Siringo S, et al. Sonographic assessment of the distal end of the thoracic duct in healthy volunteers and in patients with portal hypertension. AJR Am J Roentgenol. 1995;165(4):863–6.

18. Nagy JA, Benjamin L, Zeng H, Dvorak AM, Dvorak HF. Vascular permeability, vascular hyperpermeability and angiogenesis. Angiogenesis. 2008;11(2):109–19.

19. Onuigbo WI. The carriage of cancer cells by the thoracic duct. Br J Cancer. 1967;21(3):496–500.

20. Parasher VK, Meroni E, Spinelli P. Anatomy of the thoracic duct: an endosonographic study. Gastrointest Endosc. 1995;42(2):188–9.

31

The influence of dexamethasone on postoperative swelling and neurosensory disturbances after orthognathic surgery: a randomized controlled clinical trial

W. Semper-Hogg[1][*], M. A. Fuessinger[1], T. W. Dirlewanger[1], C. P. Cornelius[2] and M. C. Metzger[1]

Abstract

Background: Orthognathic surgery is associated with considerable swelling and neurosensory disturbances. Serious swelling can lead to great physical and psychological strain. A randomized, prospective, controlled clinical trial was realized in order to evaluate the effect of a preoperative intravenous dexamethasone injection of 40 mg on postoperative swelling and neurosensory disturbances after orthognathic surgery.

Methods: Thirty-eight patients (27 male and 11 female) patients, all with the indication for an orthognathic surgery, were enrolled in this study (mean age: 27.63 years, range: 16–61 years) and randomly divided into two groups (study group/ control group). Both groups underwent either maxillary and/or mandibular osteotomies, resulting in three subgroups according to surgical technique (A: LeFort I osteotomy, B: bilateral sagittal split osteotomy (BSSO), C: bimaxillary osteotomy). The study group received a single preoperative intravenous injection of 40 mg dexamethasone. Facial edema was measured by 3D surface scans on the 1st, 2nd, 5th, 14th and 90th postoperative day. Furthermore, neurosensory disturbances on the 2nd, 5th, 14th and 90th postoperative day were investigated by thermal stimulation.

Results: Facial edema after LeFort I osteotomy, BSSO and bimaxillary osteotomy showed a significant decrease in the study group compared to the control group ($P = 0.048$, $P = 0.045$, $P < 0.001$). The influence of dexamethasone on neurosensory disturbances was not significant for the inferior alveolar nerve ($P = 0.746$) or the infraorbital nerve ($P = 0.465$).

Conclusions: Patients undergoing orthognathic surgery should receive a preoperative injection of dexamethasone in order to control and reduce edema. However, there was no influence of dexamethasone on reduction of neurosensory disturbances.

Keywords: Dexamethasone, Swelling, Orthognathic surgery, Neurosensory disturbance, Edema, Glucocorticoids

Background

Several methods exist to reduce considerable swelling after orthognathic surgery. The most common method to reduce swelling is cooling [1, 2]. Glucocorticoids are also recommended to reduce postoperative edema [3]. They decrease the permeability of the capillaries [4].

Consequently there are less fluid and inflammation mediators entering the concerned tissue [5–7]. Therefore, several trials in oral and maxillofacial surgery have evaluated the use of glucocorticoids to reduce and control the postoperative side effects [5, 8–14]. All these clinical trials were not able to measure the swelling three-dimensionally due to a lack of technical capabilities, such as 3D scanning facilities. Two-dimensional measurements cannot reflect the extension of facial swelling adequately. The three-dimensional volume of swelling in its complete extension should be quantified in the present study. 3D surface

---
* Correspondence: wiebke.semper.hogg@uniklinik-freiburg.de
[1]Department of Oral and Craniomaxillofacial Surgery, Center for Dental Medicine, University Medical Center Freiburg, Hugstetter Straße 55 D, 79106 Freiburg, Germany
Full list of author information is available at the end of the article

The influence of dexamethasone on postoperative swelling and neurosensory disturbances...

227

scans are used more and more frequently in orthognathic and plastic surgery. Few studies in orthognathic surgery have evaluated the postoperative swelling applying this procedure by comparing cooling devices with conventional cooling. Additionally, they evaluated how body mass index, age and sex influence the swelling [2, 15].

Concerning neurosensory disturbances, one of the most frequently described complications after bilateral sagittal split osteotomy (BSSO) is an impairment of the inferior alveolar nerve (IAN) [16]. Many trials have described a large number of different testing methods to quantify these neurosensory disturbances, but comparatively few trials have evaluated a possible effect on the reduction of neurosensory disturbances of glucocorticoids [3, 17–19]. Therefore, further studies are needed [3, 20].

The aim of the present study was to investigate the swelling three-dimensionally at defined time points and to evaluate the effect of a preoperative injection of 40 mg of dexamethasone. The possible effect of glucocorticoids on reduction of neurosensory disturbances was examined.

Methods

The study had been approved by the local ethics committee of the Albert-Ludwigs-Universität Freiburg, Germany (Protocol number: EK 4 / 14).

Study design

A randomized, prospective, controlled trial was carried out at the University of Freiburg in the Department of Oral and Maxillofacial Surgery. Thirty-eight patients (27 male and 11 female, mean age: 27.63 years, range: 16 61 years) with an indication for orthognathic surgery were enrolled in this study. Exclusion criteria were regular drug therapy, psychiatric illness, coagulopathy, diabetes mellitus, and chronical infections. The patients involved were divided into three subgroups, depending on the executed surgery (A: LeFort I osteotomy, B: BSSO, C: bimaxillary osteotomy). The patients of each group were randomly assigned to a study-group and a control-group. Baseline characteristics of the patient collective are shown in Table 1 and the Consort Statement Flow Diagram is presented in Fig. 1. The study-group received a single preoperative injection of 40 mg dexamethasone (Fortecortin Inject, Merck Serono GmbH). Surgery duration was documented in all cases. To homogenize the groups, all participants got a thorough instruction in cooling. This standardized postoperative cooling procedure was important to allow a direct comparison of the swellings. Therefore cooling was realized immediately after the operation for the time of hospitalization (for subgroups A and B 3–4 days, subgroup C 5–7 days). All participants used the same type of cooling device (Hilotherm GmbH,

Argenbühl-Eisenharz, Germany) at a temperature between 17 and 19 °C for 14–16 h/day.

The facial swelling was determined by the three-dimensional scanning device 3dMD (Atlanta, USA) consisting of six vision cameras and a flash light. The scanning system is linked to a personal computer with the relating software 3dMD Patients (3dMD, Atlanta, USA). The result is a polygonal mesh (45.000–60.000 polygons) ready for evaluation. The amount of swelling was measured by the volume (milliliters). 3D surface scans were generated at five different points of time: D1 (first postoperative day, only for subgroups A and B, in subgroup C not possible due to physical impairment after intervention), D2 (second postoperative day), D5 (fifth postoperative day), D14 = (fourteenth postoperative day) and D90 (ninetieth postoperative day) (Figs. 2 and 3). After cutting and customizing the scans by anatomical structures, scans D1-D14 were matched to the reference scan D90. The forehead and the ridge of the nose were used for surface matching because they are barely influenced by the swelling. After surface matching, the volume difference between the masks was calculated.

Neurosensory disturbances were determined by thermal stimulating using the MSA Thermal Stimulator (Somedic AB, Hörby, Sweden). It consists of a thermode and a push-button and is linked to a personal computer with the accompanying software SENSELab MSA v.6.25 (Somedic AB, Hörby, Sweden). Depending on the

Table 1 Baseline charcteristics of the patient collective

	n (%)	
Ethnic group		
Caucasian	38 (100%)	
Gender		
Male	27 (71%)	
Female	11 (29%)	
Age		
< 20 years	6 (15,8%)	
20–30 years	26 (68,4%)	
30–50 years	3 (7.9%)	
> 50 years	3 (7.9%)	
Surgery	12 (31.6%)	7 study group
LeFort I		5 control group
BSSO		(2 lost to follow-up)
Bimaxillary osteotomy	16 (42.1%)	8 study group
		8 control group
	10 (26.3%)	6 study group
		4 control group
		(2 lost to follow-up)

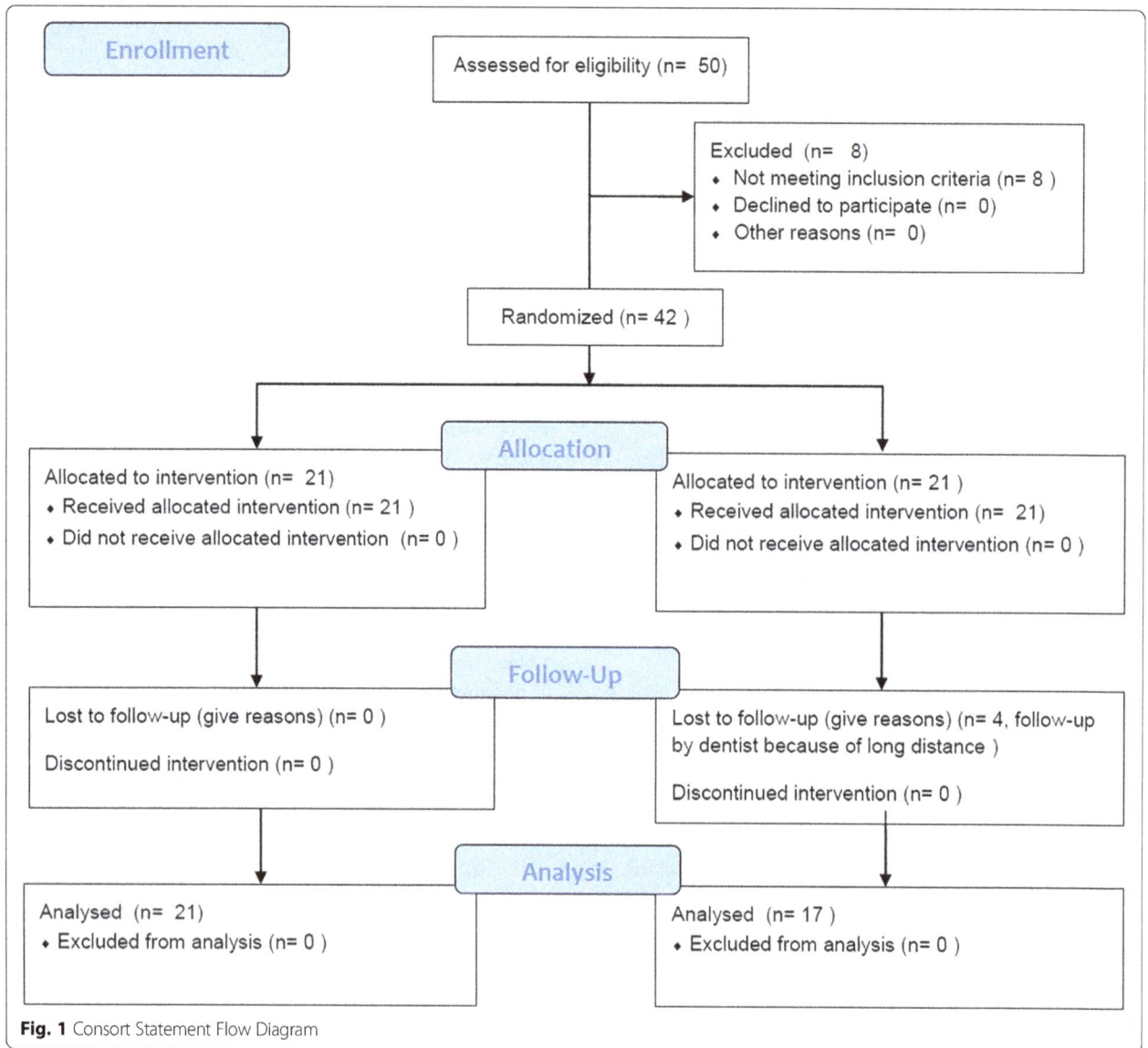

Fig. 1 Consort Statement Flow Diagram

executed surgery, the thermode is placed on the skin above the infraorbital foramen (infraorbitale nerve / LeFort 1 osteotomy) or above the mental foramen (inferior alveolar nerve / BSSO) to evaluate heat and cold thresholds for the inferior alveolar nerve (IAN) or the infraorbital nerve (ION). Each sequence consists of ten single stimulations (five heat- / five cold stim.). The starting temperature is defined at 32 °C (max. 50 °C / min 15 °C). The heat and cold thresholds are calculated as the average of the five single stimulations. These tests were performed on the second, the fifth, the fourteenth and the ninetieth postoperative day.

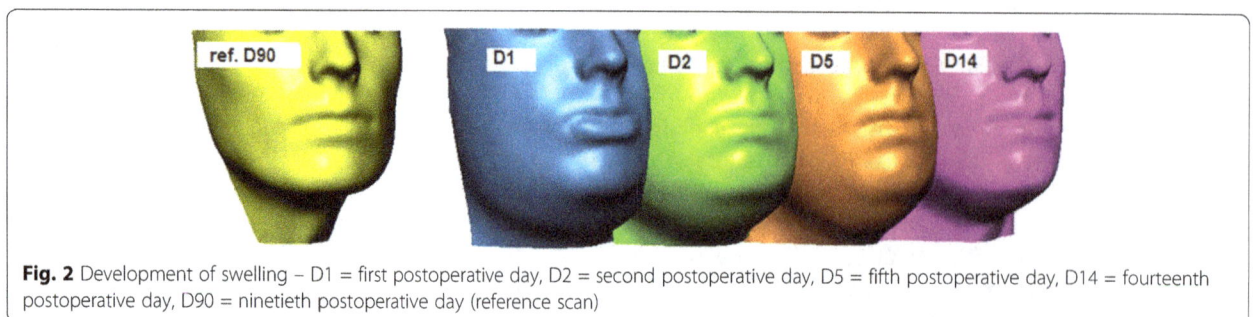

Fig. 2 Development of swelling – D1 = first postoperative day, D2 = second postoperative day, D5 = fifth postoperative day, D14 = fourteenth postoperative day, D90 = ninetieth postoperative day (reference scan)

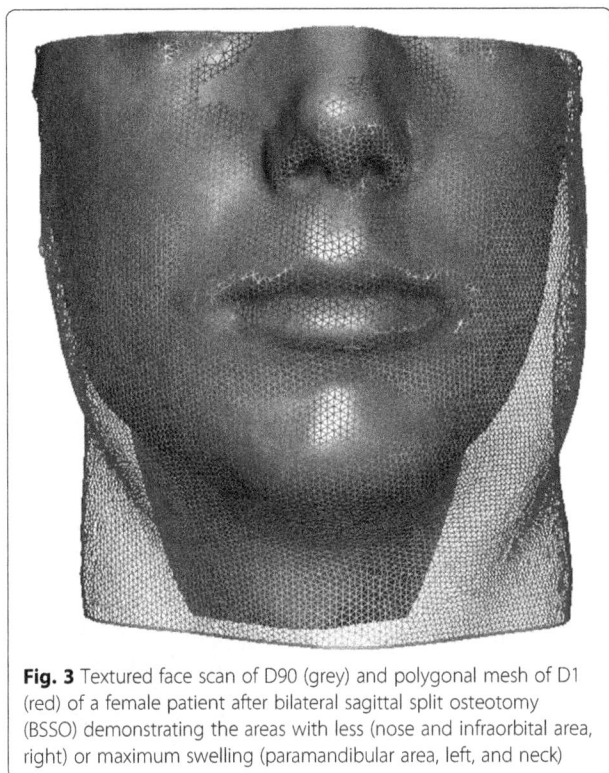

Fig. 3 Textured face scan of D90 (grey) and polygonal mesh of D1 (red) of a female patient after bilateral sagittal split osteotomy (BSSO) demonstrating the areas with less (nose and infraorbital area, right) or maximum swelling (paramandibular area, left, and neck)

Surgical procedure

Each patient received orthodontic treatment preoperatively. The same surgeon performed all operations. Twelve patients underwent LeFort I osteotomies (7 with preoperative dexamethasone injection) and 16 a bilateral sagittal split osteotomy (8 with preoperative dexamethasone injection) as described by Obwegeser/Dal Pont [21]. Bimaxillary surgery was necessary in 10 cases (6 with preoperative dexamethasone injection).

Statistical analysis

For a descriptive analysis mean, median and standard deviation were computed. Statistical analyses were performed by the t-test and the method of Scheffe (adjustment of p-values). Significance level was set on $P < 0.05$. The data were analyzed using the statistical software package STATA 13.1. (StataCorp LP, Texas, USA).

Results

Thirty-eight patients (27 male, 11 female) were included in the study. There were no statistically significant differences between our study and control group concerning age and sex. Mean surgery duration was 97,16 (±41,29) minutes in subgroup A, 142,56 (±29,24) minutes in subgroup B, and 285 (±63,56) minutes in subgroup C.

Postoperative swelling

The degree of swelling was measured by matching a three-dimensional mask in swollen condition (D1-D14) to a reference mask in unswollen condition (D90) and calculating its volume difference. Figs. 2 and 3 illustrates the development of swelling.

The maximum swelling in the LeFort I subgroup was observed on postoperative day one with a significant difference in swelling between the study group and control group with less swelling in the study group (−11%: 53.05 ml (± 30.06) vs. 59.49 ml (±28.28), $p = 0.048$). Fourteen days postoperatively, the remaining swelling differed between the two groups (study group: 16%, 8.84 ml (±5.16) vs. control group: 36%, 21, 45 ml (±18.95) (Fig. 4).

In contrast to LeFort I osteotomies, the maximum of swelling in the BSSO patients was observed on postoperative day two. Less swelling was also observed in the study group (−18%: 127.84 ml (±21.97) vs. 153.95 ml (±53.85), $p = 0.046$). The remaining swelling 14 days postoperatively was about 25% in comparison to its initial value in both groups (study group: 21%, 27.13 ml (±18.40) vs. control group: 24%, 37.13 ml (±21.69) (Fig. 5).

After bimaxillary osteotomies, there was 39% less swelling on postoperative day two in the study group compared to the control group (107.46 ml (±32.78) vs. 175.39 ml (±45.09), $p < 0.001$). Despite the much higher initial swelling in the control group, there were no differences in swelling 14 days postoperatively between the two groups (study group: 32%, 31.9 ml (±10, 25) vs. control group: 22%, 37.8 ml (±22.31)) (Fig. 6).

Postoperative neurosensory disturbances

Neurosensory disturbances were quantified by thermal stimulating in 30 of the 38 patients (20 male, 10 female) of a mean age of 28.11 years.

Statistical analysis showed, that the influence of dexamethasone on the reduction of neurosensory disturbances of the IAN was not significant different between the study and control group ($P = 0.746$). Similar results were observed for the ION ($P = 0.465$).

Discussion

Controlling and reducing postoperative edema after orthognathic surgery is important for the surgical outcome and the patient's recovery. Even airway obstruction can occur in severe cases [22].

Three-dimensional face scans have opened the opportunity to measure the three-dimensional swelling in its complete extension without unnecessary radiation exposure [10, 23]. This procedure is described more and more frequently and has proven its precision and accuracy. The scan has to be taken with the same facial expression to ensure an adequate matching of the scans. In this study, all participants were asked to close their eyes and keep their mouths closed during image acquisition.

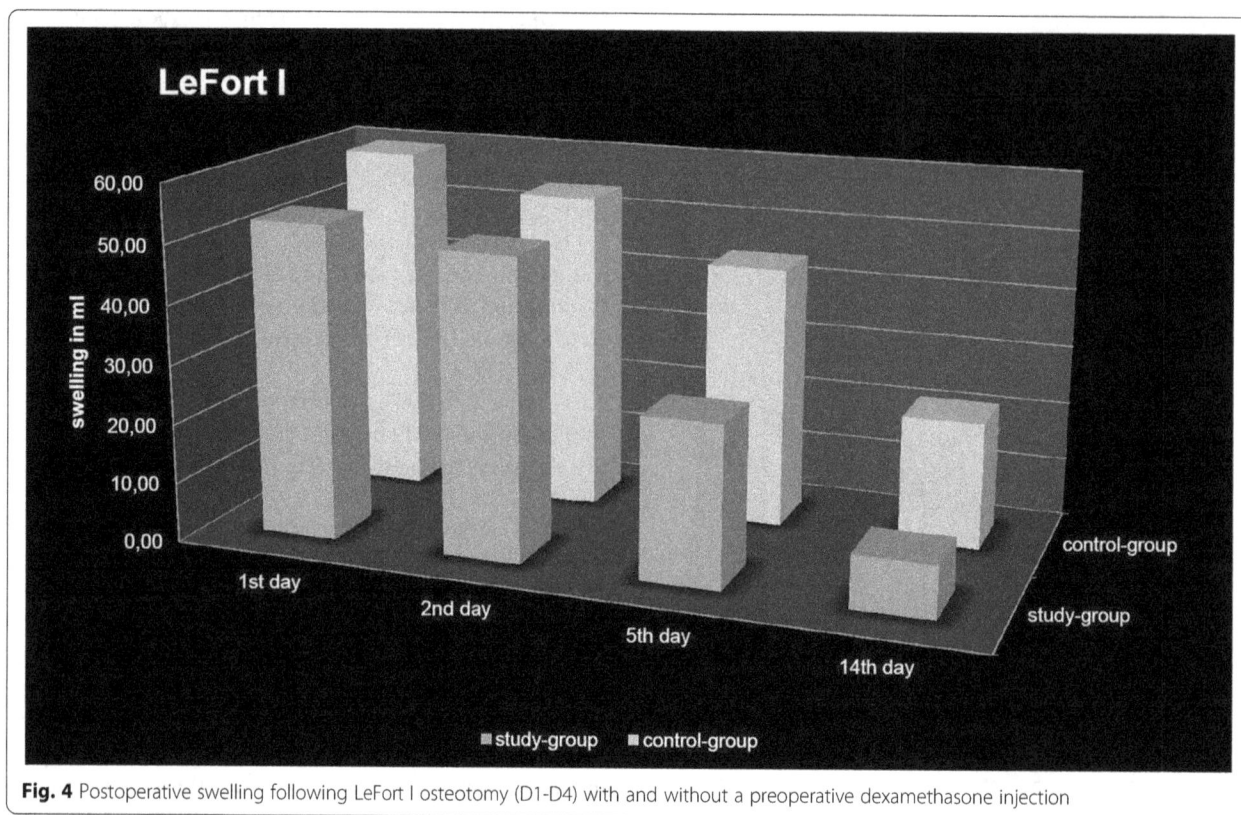

Fig. 4 Postoperative swelling following LeFort I osteotomy (D1-D4) with and without a preoperative dexamethasone injection

For the evaluation, the scan from postoperative day 90 (D = 90) was chosen as reference scan. Investigations confirm that only about 10% of the swelling can be observed at that time point and minimal facial changes occur in the following months [15, 24]. A preoperative scan would lead to wrong results as the surgery changes the patient's facial profile. Due to the general conditions of the patients and related immobility after bimaxillary osteotomies (subgroup C), the first postoperative face scan was taken on postoperative day 2. In two of three subgroups (BSSO and bimaxillary osteotomies), the maximum swelling was observed on postoperative day 2 confirming the results of Milles et al., Troullos et al. and Lin et al. [25–27].

In contrast to a study conducted by Lin et al., no glucocorticoids were administered to the control group to investigate the medication-related effect as described by several authors [5, 8, 20]. Glucocorticoids have not yet reached full acceptance in orthognathic surgery in all medical centers [5]. Long-term glucocorticoid therapy can cause several side effects if administered with high doses and for more than 5 days [20, 28] such as Cushing-Syndrome, adrenal insufficiency, temporarily increase of blood sugar level [22, 29] psychological impairment [30] or even decrease of wound healing [31]. However, there is no clear evidence, that a single preoperative administration of glucocorticoids shows the reported side effects.

Still, the dose having the highest capability in reducing swelling is unknown. The present study used 40 mg dexamethasone according to studies in traumatology. In these studies 40 mg dexamethasone is administered as antiemetic and opioid-sparing medication after surgery. Also in oncologic studies a high single dose of dexamethasone shows beneficial effects versus prednisolone. Regarding side effects, the results are somewhat contradictory. While one study showed a slight increase of complications after perioperative corticoid administration, most studies showed no side-effects of a single high-dose dexamethasone therapy [13, 32]. Due to these very positive effects, we decided in favor to the relatively high single dose amount, even if in former studies in orthognatic and oral surgery, a single shot administration of only 8-16 mg dexamethasone was used, which, however, shows only some beneficial effects concerning swelling and edema [11–14].

Regarding possible side effects of the glucocorticoids like decreased wound healing, increased infection rate hypotension, or even neurosensory disturbances, there was no difference between the control and the test group. However, the results confirm the assumption that glucocorticoids decrease postoperative edema after orthognathic surgery, which is a clear negative aspect of orthognathic surgery. The amount of swelling is inter-individually

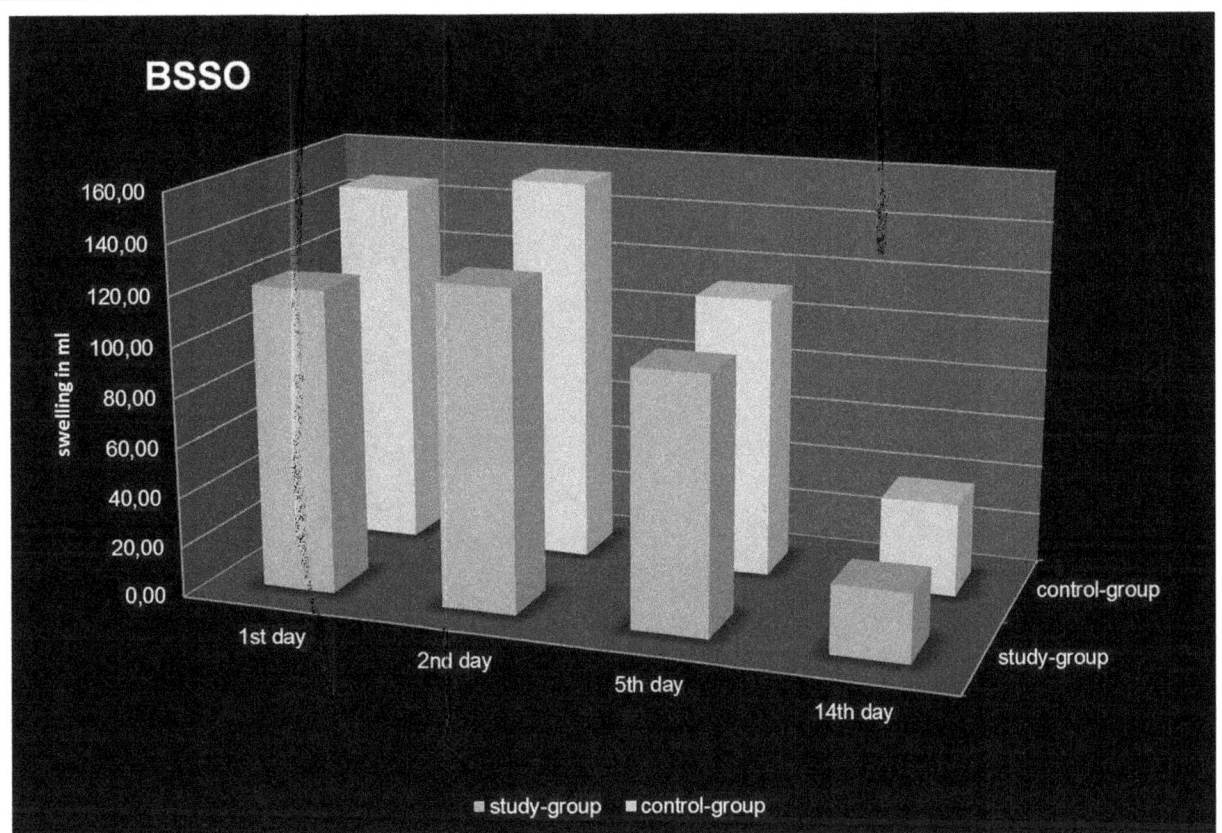

Fig. 5 Postoperative swelling following bilateral sagittal split osteotomy (BSSO) (D1-D4) with and without a preoperative dexamethasone injection

different and depends also on the surgical techniques. Differences in surgical techniques were excluded by including only cases treated by one surgeon. All in all, we were able to show that the single high dose of the glucocorticoid dexamethasone shows beneficial effects in reduction of postoperative edema, independent of the amount of swelling. Therefore, we can state that the single dose together with modern operation techniques can increase the patient's comfort after such elective surgery.

The administration of glucocorticoids is one possibility to reduce swelling. A continuously cooling of the surgery site, shows beneficial effects, too. For this reason a standardized cooling procedure was performed in all patients to ensure comparable conditions. As described by several authors, the patients of the study group showed less swelling in the initial postoperative phase than the patients of the control group [33–36]. Comparing three different cortisone drugs (methylprednisolone, betamethasone and dexamethasone), dexamethasone seems most suitable because of its high anti-inflammatory activity, no mineralocorticoid activity and its long biologic half-life of 36–48 h [5, 8, 9]. Intravenous injection is recommended preoperatively [20]. However, the ideal timing is uncertain [20]. The conversion of dexamethasone which is delivered as a prodrug takes 10 min [37]. To reach clinical effectiveness it takes about one to two additional hours [38, 39]. Therefore, an early injection 12 h preoperatively as described by Schaberg et al. does not seem to be necessary [9]. Additional postoperative injections showed no further decrease of edema [5, 8]. The different protocols as well as the different measuring methods do not allow a direct comparison of the results. Further trials with comparable and objective measurements of swelling are needed to achieve a consensus about the ideal dose and the injection time.

The present study did not approve a significant influence of dexamethasone on reduction of neurosensory disturbances. To detect possible effects, thermal stimulation was used. Many approaches of examining neurosensory disturbances have been made. They vary from analysis with visual analogue scales to the investigation of mechanical thresholds by Semmes aesthesiometer (measuring device for tactile sensitivity), thermal stimulation, light touch, static 2-point touch and pin-prick discrimination [6, 7, 18]. The variety of testing methods makes it difficult to compare the results. Al-Bishri et al. described less neurosensory disturbances after the administration of glucocorticoids. However, this trial was

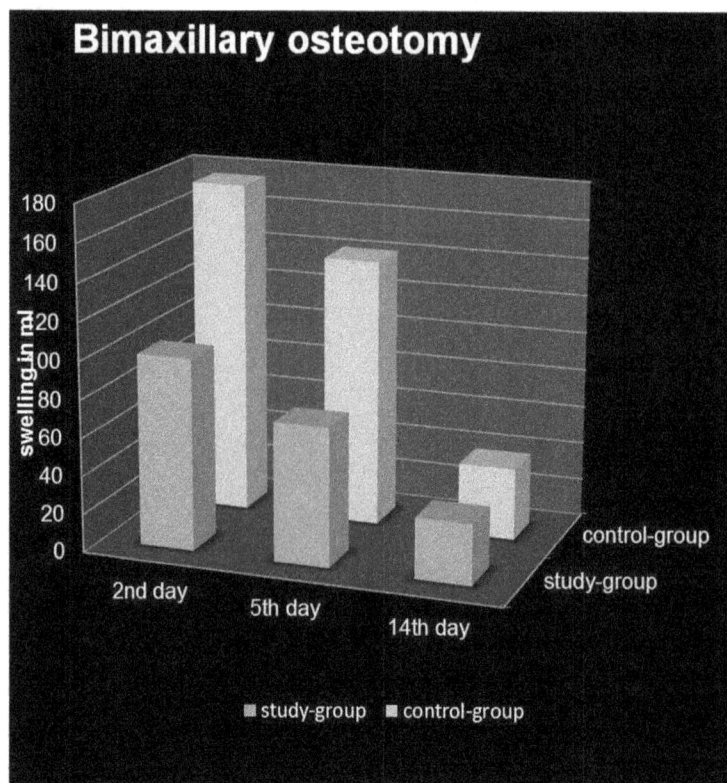

Fig. 6 Postoperative swelling following bimaxillary osteotomy (D2-D4) with and without a preoperative dexamethasone injection

only based on the patients' personal evaluation of neuro-sensory dysfunctions [18]. Seo et al. achieved significant less neurosensory disturbances with a glucocorticoid therapy over 2 weeks (30 mg prednisolone for 7 days, 15 mg for 4 days and 5 mg for 3 days), if started 3 weeks postoperative. A local intraoperative application of dexa-methasone on the nerve shows no clinical effect as well as a single preoperative application [5, 19]. The results were gained by using thermal stimulation as a simple and precise method to measure neurosensory disturbances. Limitations based on interindividual differences must be taken into account, if judging the results. Lacking of precise and easy to handle instruments, the thermal stimulation test seems to be appropriate to compare the study and the control group. Ongoing research must increase the evidence of glucocorticoids for reduction of neurosensory disturbances. Furthermore, postoperative nausea and vomiting (PONV) are common complications after orthognathic surgery and occur in 40% of cases during the first 24 h [40]. A large systematic literature re-search has revealed that a single dose of dexamethasone is additionally effective in decreasing the risk of PONV [41].

Conclusion

The present study demonstrates that dexamethasone sig-nificantly reduces postoperative swelling. In patients

with bimaxillary osteotomies, the greatest reduction in swelling was achieved. A promotion of nerve healing or less neurosensory disturbances after a single injection of glucocorticoids could not be observed. Further studies are needed to evaluate the ideal dose and timing of the administration of glucocorticoids to reach the maximum benefit from dexamethasone.

Abbreviations
BSSO: Bilateral sagittal split osteotomy; IAN: Inferior alveolar nerve; ION: Infraorbital nerve; PONV: Postoperative nausea and vomiting

Acknowledgements
The authors would like to thank A. Soranno for her great support and K. Vach for her help with the statistical analysis.

Funding
The article processing charge was funded by the German Research Foundation (DFG) and the Albert Ludwigs University Freiburg in the funding programme Open Access Publishing. There was no additional funding for this study.

Authors' contributions
WS-H interpreted the data and was a major contributor in preparing the manuscript. MAF was responsible for data evaluation, preparation of the figures and contributed in preparing and revising the manuscript. TWD was responsible for data acquisition and has been involved in drafting of the manuscript. CPC revised the manuscript critically. MCM was responsible for

conception and design of the study and gave the final approval of the manuscript. All authors read and approved the final manuscript.

Competing interests
The authors declare that they have no competing interests.

Author details
[1]Department of Oral and Craniomaxillofacial Surgery, Center for Dental Medicine, University Medical Center Freiburg, Hugstetter Straße 55 D, 79106 Freiburg, Germany. [2]Department of Oral and Maxillofacial Surgery, Ludwig-Maximilians-University Munich, Lindwurmstraße 2a D, 80337 München, Germany.

References
1. Schaubel HJ. The local use of ice after orthopedic procedures. Am J Surg. 1946;72:711–4.
2. Rana M, Gellrich N-C, von See C, Weiskopf C, Gerressen M, Ghassemi A, Modabber A. 3D evaluation of postoperative swelling in treatment of bilateral mandibular fractures using 2 different cooling therapy methods: a randomized observer blind prospective study. J Cranio-Maxillofac Surg. 2013;41:e17–23.
3. Dan AEB, Thygesen TH, Pinholt EM. Corticosteroid Administration in Oral and Orthognathic Surgery: a systematic review of the literature and meta-analysis. J Oral Maxillofac Surg. 2010;68:2207–20.
4. Nauck M, Karakiulakis G, Perruchoud AP, Papakonstantinou E, Roth M. Corticosteroids inhibit the expression of the vascular endothelial growth factor gene in human vascular smooth muscle cells. Eur J Pharmacol. 1998;341:309–15.
5. Widar F, Kashani H, Alsén B, Dahlin C, Rasmusson L. The effects of steroids in preventing facial oedema, pain, and neurosensory disturbances after bilateral sagittal split osteotomy: a randomized controlled trial. Int J Oral Maxillofac Surg. 2015;44:252–8.
6. Edelman JL, Lutz D, Castro MR. Corticosteroids inhibit VEGF-induced vascular leakage in a rabbit model of blood retinal and blood aqueous barrier breakdown. Exp Eye Res. 2005;80:249–58.
7. Koedam JA, Smink JJ. Van Buul-offers SC: Glucocorticoids inhibit vascular endothelial growth factor expression in growth plate chondrocytes. Mol Cell Endocrinol. 2002;197:35–44.
8. Weber CR, Griffin JM. Evaluation of dexamethasone for reducing postoperative edema and inflammatory response after orthognathic surgery. J Oral Maxillofac Surg. 1994;52:35–9.
9. Schaberg SJ, Stuller CB, Edwards SM. Effect of methylprednisolone on swelling after orthognathic surgery. J Oral Maxillofac Surg. 1984;42:356–61.
10. Munro I, Boyd J, Wainwright D. Effect of steroids in maxillofacial surgery. Ann Plast Surg. 1986;17:440–4.
11. Boonsiriseth K, Latt MM, Kiattavorncharoen S, Pairuchvej V, Wongsirichat N. Dexamethasone injection into the pterygomandibular space in lower third molar surgery. Int J Oral Maxillofac Surg. 2017;46:899–904.
12. Dereci O, Tuzuner-Oncul AM, Kocer G, Yuce E, Askar M, Ozturk A. Efficacy of immediate postoperative intramasseteric dexamethasone injection on postoperative swelling after mandibular impacted third molar surgery: a preliminary split-mouth study. JPMA. J. Pak. Med. Assoc. 2016;66:320–3.
13. Bergeron SG, Kardash KJ, Huk OL, Zukor DJ, Antoniou J. Perioperative dexamethasone does not affect functional outcome in total hip arthroplasty. Clin Orthop Relat Res. 2009;467:1463–7.
14. Esen E, Taşar F, Akhan O. Determination of the anti-inflammatory effects of methylprednisolone on the sequelae of third molar surgery. J. Oral Maxillofac. Surg.J. Am.A Oral Maxillofac. Surg. 1999;57:1201–6. discussion 1206-1208.
15. Kau CH, Cronin AJ, Richmond S. A three-dimensional evaluation of postoperative swelling following orthognathic surgery at 6 months. Plast Reconstr Surg. 2007;119:2192–9.
16. Panula K, Finne K, Oikarinen K. Incidence of complications and problems related to orthognathic surgery: a review of 655 patients. J Oral Maxillofac Surg. 2001;59:1128–36.
17. Seo K, Tanaka Y, Terumitsu M, Someya G. Efficacy of steroid treatment for sensory impairment after orthognathic surgery. J Oral Maxillofac Surg. 2004;62:1193 7.

18. Al-Bishri A, Rosenquist J, Sunzel B. On neurosensory disturbance after sagittal split osteotomy. J Oral Maxillofac Surg. 2004;62:1472–6.
19. Pourdanesh F, Khayampour A, Jamilian A. Therapeutic effects of local application of Dexamethasone during bilateral Sagittal split Ramus Osteotomy surgery. J Oral Maxillofac Surg. 2014;72:1391–4.
20. Chegini S, Dhariwal DK. Review of evidence for the use of steroids in orthognathic surgery. Br J Oral Maxillofac Surg. 2012;50:97–101.
21. Obwegeser HTR. Zur Operationstechnik bei der Progenie und anderen Unterkieferanomalien. Dtsch. Zahn Mund Kieferheilkd. 1955;23:232–41.
22. Alexander ETR. A review of perioperative corticosteroid use in dentoalveolar surgery. Orl Surg Oral Med Oral Pathol Oral Radiol Endod. 2000;90:406–15.
23. van der Meer WJ, Dijkstra PU, Visser A, Vissink A, Ren Y. Reliability and validity of measurements of facial swelling with a stereophotogrammetry optical three-dimensional scanner. Br J Oral Maxillofac Surg. 2014;52:922–7.
24. van Loon B, Maal TJ, Plooij JM, Ingels KJ, Borstlap WA, Kuijpers-Jagtman AM, Spauwen PH, Berge SJ. 3D Stereophotogrammetric assessment of pre- and postoperative volumetric changes in the cleft lip and palate nose. Int J Oral Maxillofac Surg. 2010;39:534–40.
25. Milles M, Desjardins PJ. Reduction of postoperative facial swelling by low-dose methylprednisolone: an experimental study. J Oral Maxillofac Surg. 1993;51:987–91.
26. Troullos ES, Hargreaves KM, Butler DP, Dionne RA. Comparison of nonsteroidal anti-inflammatory drugs, ibuprofen and flurbiprofen, with methylprednisolone and placebo for acute pain, swelling, and trismus. J Oral Maxillofac Surg. 1990;48:945–52.
27. Lin HH, Kim S-G, Kim H-Y, Niu L-S, Lo L-J. Higher dose of Dexamethasone does not further reduce facial swelling after Orthognathic surgery: a randomized controlled trial using 3-dimensional Photogrammetry. Ann Plast Surg. 2017;78:S61–9.
28. Gersema L, Baker K. Use of corticosteroids in oral surgery. J Oral Maxillofac Surg. 1992;50:270–7.
29. Butler R. Dosage effects of pulsed steroid therapy on serum cortisol levels in oral and maxillofacial surgery patients. J Oral Maxillfac Surg. 1993;51:750–3.
30. Fleming PS, Flood TR. Steroid-induced psychosis complicating orthognathic surgery: a case report. Br Dent J. 2005;199:647–8.
31. Joseph J, Tydd M. The effects of cortisone acetate on tissue regeneration in the rabbit's ear. J Anat. 1973;115:445–60.
32. Wei Y, Ji X-b, Wang Y-w, Wang J-x, Yang E-q, Wang Z-c, Sang Y-q, Bi Z-m, Ren C-a, Zhou F, et al. High-dose dexamethasone vs prednisone for treatment of adult immune thrombocytopenia: a prospective multicenter randomized trial. Blood. 2016;127:296–302. quiz 370
33. van der Vlis M, Dentino KM, Vervloet B, Padwa BL. Postoperative swelling after orthognathic surgery: a prospective volumetric analysis. J Oral Maxillofac Surg. 2014;72:2241–7.
34. Tozzi U, Santillo V, Tartaro GP, Sellitto A, Gravino GR, Santagata M. A prospective, randomized, double-blind, placebo-controlled clinical trial comparing the efficacy of anti-edema drugs for edema control in Orthognathic surgery using digitizer 3-D to measure facial swelling. J Maxillofac Oral Surg. 2015;14:386–92.
35. Dan AEB, Thygesen TH, Pinholt EM. Corticosteroid administration in oral and orthognathic surgery: a systematic review of the literature and meta-analysis. J. Oral Maxillofac. Surg. Off. J. Am.Assoc.Oral Maxillofac. Surg. 2010;68:2207–20.
36. de Lima VN, Lemos CAA, Faverani LP, Santiago Junior JF, Pellizzer EP. Effectiveness of corticoid Administration in Orthognathic Surgery for edema and Neurosensorial disturbance: a systematic literature review. J Oral Maxillofac Surg. 2017;75(1528):e1521–1528.e1528.
37. Rohdewald P, Möllmann H, Barth J, Rehder J, Derendorf H. Pharmacokinetics of Dexamethasone and its phosphatester. Biopharm Drug Dispos. 1987;8
38. Walther A, Böttinger B. Anaphylaktoide Reaktionen in der Prähospitalphase. Internist. 2004;45
39. Ring J, Grosber M, Möhrenschlager K, Brockow K. Anaphylaxis: acute treatment and management. Chem Immunol Allergy. 2010;95:201–10.
40. Silva AC, O'Ryan F, Poor DB. Postoperative nausea and vomiting (PONV) after Orthognathic surgery: a retrospective study and literature review. J Oral Maxillofac Surg. 2006;64:1385–97.
41. Henzi I, Walder B, Tramèr M. Dexamethasone for the prevention of postoperative nausea and vomiting: a quantitative systematic review. Annest Analg. 2000;90:186–94.

32

The efficacy of Er,Cr:YSGG laser supported periodontal therapy on the reduction of peridodontal disease related oral malodor: a randomized clinical study

Ömür Dereci[1*], Mükerrem Hatipoğlu[2], Alper Sindel[3], Sinan Tozoğlu[3] and Kemal Üstün[2]

Abstract

Background: This study aims to evaluate the efficacy of Er,Cr:YSGG laser assisted periodontal therapy on the reduction of oral malodor and periodontal disease.

Methods: Sixty patients with chronic periodontitis were included in the study and allocated into two groups each containing 30 patients. The study was planned in a double blind fashion. Conventional periodontal therapy was performed in group 1 and conventional periodontal therapy was performed in association with Er,Cr:YSGG application in group 2. Periodontal parameters of probing depth, clinical attachment level, plaque index and bleeding on probing were measured with a periodontal probe. Quantitative analysis of volatile sulphure compunds (VSCs) were measured with a calibrated halimeter at baseline level and at post-treatment 1st, 3rd and 6th months. P values <0.05 were accepted as statistically significant.

Results: There was a statistical significant reduction in VSC values in group 2 at post-treatment 3rd and 6th months ($p < 0.05$). Pocket depth values at post-treatment 1st month and bleeding on probing values at post-treatment 3rd and 6th months were significantly decreased in group 2 ($p < 0.05$). Intragroup statistical analysis revealed that there were statistically significant differences for all parameters ($p < 0.01$).

Conclusions: Er,Cr:YSGG laser assisted conventional periodontal therapy is more effective in reducing oral malodor and improving periodontal healing compared to conventional periodontal therapy alone.

Keywords: Halitosis, Periodontitis, Subgingival curettage, YSGG laser

Background

Periodontal treatment aims to reduce and remove periodontal diseases with a variety of techniques such as scaling and root plaining and flap procedures [1, 2]. Mechanical therapy of periodontal diseases have been applied securely with high success rates for years. The improvement in bacterial reduction in periodontal pocket and clinical healing appeared to be better in patients with conventional periodontal therapy assisted with adjunctive therapy than in patients with conventional periodontal therapy alone [2, 3].

Lately, there have been several improvements in the treatment of periodontal disease, such as the usage of hard and soft lasers as an adjunctive to conventional periodontal therapy for the effective reduction and elimination of pathogenic microorganisms in the periodontal pocket, thus, leading to a more effective and pain free treatment [3–7]. As a member of the erbium laser family, Er,Cr:YSGG lasers demonstrate a very shallow penetration in tissue with a wavelength of 2.78 μm posing minimal thermal risk to the deeper tissues when compared with other lasers and provide a better surface for the attachment of blood derived components on roots [8, 9]. It is also reported that ER,Cr:YSGG laser enhances cell attachment and migration on the root surfaces [10]. The morphological surface alterations

* Correspondence: omurdereci@hotmail.com; odereci@ogu.edu.tr
[1]Department of Oral and Maxillofacial Surgery, Faculty of Dentistry, Eskişehir Osmangazi University, Meşelik Campus, 26480 Eskişehir, Turkey
Full list of author information is available at the end of the article

promoted by Er,Cr:YSGG have been related to its high absorption in water [11, 12]. The utilization of Er,Cr:YSGG laser adjunctive to conventional periodontal therapy is reported to be more effective in bacterial reduction compared to conventional periodontal therapy [1, 8]. In addition to the bacterial reduction, Er,Cr:YSGG lasers are also successful in coagulating the opened blood vessels and de-epithelizing the gingival pocket [1, 13]. The laser assisted treatment is a better treatment modality compared to the coventional non-surgical periodontal treatment according to several studies [1, 4, 7, 14].

Oral malodor or halitosis is defined as an unpleasent odor originating from the oral cavity or extra-oral sources. The oral region is substantially responsible for oral malodor, which is a result of bacterial putrification of food debris in periodontal pockets or interdental regions [15, 16]. Volatile sulphur compounds (VSC) are sources of bad odor and production of specific oral bacteria such as Treponema denticola, Porphyromonas gingivalis, Prevotella intermedius and Porphyromonas endodontalis, which are promoted in the secluded regions of the oral cavity such as dental cavities and periodontal pockets in which bacterial growth is favoured due to accumalating debris [17, 18].

Oral malodor mostly originates from the oral region and there is a sound link between periodontal disease and oral malodor [19]. Several studies reported that effective periodontal therapy significantly reduced oral malodor [19, 20]. The efficacy of Er,Cr:YSGG laser assisted periodontal therapy on the reduction of oral malodor has not yet been reported. The hypothesis of this study is defined as Er,Cr:YSGG laser assisted periodontal therapy may be more effective in controling periodontal disease related oral malodor compared to conventional periodontal therapy. The aim of this study is to evaluate the efficacy of Er,Cr:YSGG laser assisted periodontal therapy on the reduction of oral malodor and periodontal disease.

Methods

This study was planned in a double blind fashion. Sixty-seven patients who were referred to the Department of Periodontology, Faculty of Dentistry of Akdeniz University for periodontal therapy due to the complaint of bad breath between October 2014 and December 2014 were enrolled into the study. Inclusion criteria for the study were as follows;

1- Chronic periodontitis with 5 mm or greater pocket depth in at least 2 teeth
2- Older than 18 years old
3- No administration of antibiotics in 6 months period before treatment
4- No history of previous periodontal therapy
5- At least 15 teeth present
6- No systemic diseases
7- No deep carious teeth

One patient refused to be included in the study. Six patients were excluded from the study because they did not meet the inclusion criteria. Sixty patients were included in the study. All patients signed written informed consent forms prior to the study. The study protocol was approved by the local Clinical Research Ethics Commitee with approval number 11/09/2014-46/3 and performed in accordance with the ethical standarts laid down in the 1964 Declaration of Helsinki and its later amendments.

Superficially carious teeth of all selected patients were examined and treated prior to the study. All treatments were performed under local anesthesia. All patients were allocated into group 1 and group 2 by random number generation in Microsoft Excel (Microsoft Corporation, Washington, USA) (Fig. 1). Group 2 comprised conventional scaling and root-plaining followed by immediate Er,Cr:YSGG application. Group 1 comprised conventional scaling root-plaining therapy. Patients did not know to which group they were assigned. Measurements for plaque index (PI), probing depth (PD), clinical attachment level (CAL) and bleeding on probing (BOP) were recorded before treatment (baseline) and after treatment at the 1st, 3rd and 6th months. All teeth with 5 mm or greater pocket depth were treated in the same patient and all measurements of periodontal parameters were performed at six sites per tooth (mesio-buccal, mid-buccal, disto-buccal, mesio-palatal, mid-palatal and disto-palatal) with a Williams 1 mm scaled periodontal probe by one researcher who is blinded to the allocation process. (MH) Plaque index was evaluated with criteria which is proposed by Löe [21]. PD was the distance between the free gingival margin and the deepest point of the pocket. CAL was the distance between the cemento-enamel junction and base of the pocket. BOP was scored as presence and abscence in a period of 30 seconds after probing. BOP presence was determined as a per cent value.

Halitosis scoring was done thru a portable sulfur monitor (Halimeter Interscan, Chatsworth, California, USA) Volatile sulphur compounds were detected with the aid of parts per billion unit (ppb) and ppb monitoring was performed as previously reported [18]. The halimeter was calibrated according to manufacturer's recommendations. Patients were instructed to hold their breaths and keep their mouths closed for 2 min and not to swallow prior to each measurement. A plastic straw connected to the monitor was inserted approximately 4 cm into the mouth of the patient as they inhaled and exhaled through the nose. Measurement was repeated

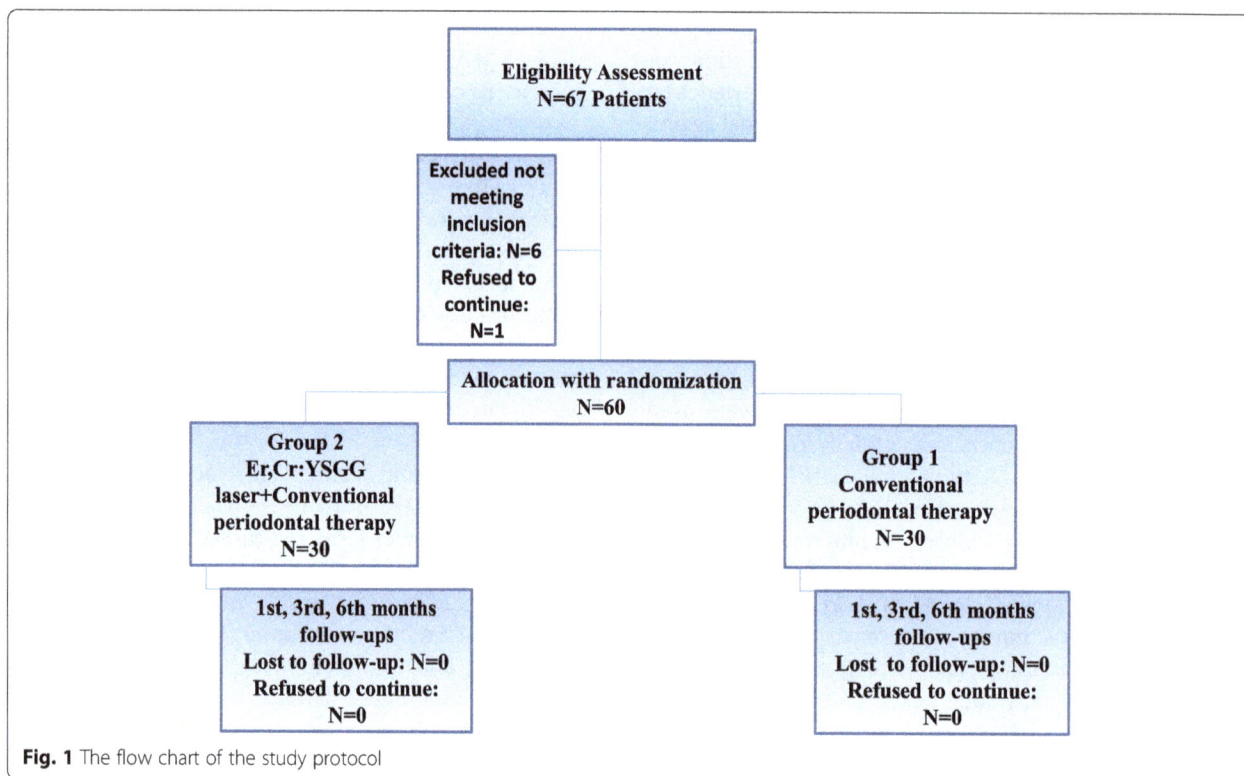

Fig. 1 The flow chart of the study protocol

three times for each patient and the highest value was recorded. All patients were instructed not to use alcohol, smoke, eat garlic or spicy food 1 day before the measurements. Halitosis scoring was done before and 1st, 3rd and 6th months after the ending of all treatment sessions in group 1 and group 2. All measurements were done on 10 a.m. and all patients were instructed to have their breakfast and perform oral hygiene procedures of teeth and tongue brushing 1 h before the measurements.

A Waterlase MD Er,Cr:YSGG laser (Biolase, Irvine, California, USA) with a RFPT 5-14 360° firing tip was used in the study. The firing tip of the laser was used with an angulation of 10° to the root surface and a bottom-up technique in which the laser was applied in a bottom to upward direction with circulation movements in contact with the pocket. Only inside of the pockets were irradiated and each pocket was irradiated once per session. The laser settings were 1.5 W, 30 Hz pulse rate, 11 % air, 20 % H_2O and H-Mode (Pulse Duration: 140 us). The laser irradiation was applied three times over a period of 7 days under local anesthesia (40 mg/ml articaine hydrochloride and 0.006 mg adrenaline hydrochloride). In both groups, second session was applied after 48 h after first session and third session was applied on the 7th day after first session. In group 2, laser irradiation was applied immediately after conventional periodontal treatment in session 1 and it was applied alone without conventional periodontal treatment in sessions 2 and 3. In group 1, conventional periodontal treatment was performed in all 3 sessions. For blindness purposes, in group 1, laser firing tip was positioned into the periodontal pockets as in group 2, but not activated.

An ultrasonic scaler and hand instruments (Gracey Curettes, Hu-Friedy, Chicago, IL, US) were used for full mouth subgingival and supragingival scaling and root-plaining. All patients received oral hygiene instructions at the time of the appointment and were given written and verbal recommendations to brush their teeth daily and maintain oral health measures after periodontal therapy.

Statistical analysis

SPSS version 20.0 (IBM, Chicago, IL, USA) was used for statistical analysis. A Shapiro-Wilk's test ($p < 0.05$) and a visual inspection of their histograms, normal Q-Q plots and box plots showed that the exam scores were not normally distributed for both groups. Friedman test was used to define the statistical difference level between follow-up time point measurements in the study and control groups seperately. Mann–Whitney-U test was used to define the statistical difference level between study and control groups. P values <0.05 were accepted as statistically significant.

Results

The mean age of all patients was 43.7 (±3.1). There were 31 males (51.7 %) and 29 females (48.3 %). All patients included in the study complied with the progress of the study and there were no drop-outs. Healing was uneventful in all patients and no adverse effects such as burning sensation, dentin hypersensitivity or pain were recorded.

The differences of baseline values of all periodontal parameters and ppb values between the study and control groups were not statistically significant. There was statistically significant improvement in all parameters of both group 1 and group 2 from baseline to post-treatment 1st, 3rd and 6th months ($p < 0.01$) (Table 1). Nevertheless, there was a statistically significant reduction in ppb levels at post-treatment 3rd and 6th month in group 2 comparing to group 1 ($p < 0.05$) (Table 1), while there was also a statistically significant reduction in PD at post-treatment 1st month and in BOP at post-treatment 3rd and 6th months in the group 2 comparing to group 1 ($p < 0.05$) (Table 1).

Discussion

Laser-assisted dentistry is a recent emerging trend. Dental lasers are frequently used in oral surgical procedures as well as restorative dentistry and prosthodontics. Er,Cr:YSGG lasers have been used since the last decade in dentistry and reported to have provided better periodontal tissue regeneration than that of conventional non-surgical periodontal therapy [5, 6]. Kelbauskiene et al. [5]. reported that a combination of Er,Cr:YSGG laser and conventional scaling and root plaining had better results compared to scaling root-plaining alone in terms of attachment level restoration. Other types of high intensity lasers such as Er:YAG and Nd:YAG lasers have been recently used in a way similar to Er,Cr:YSGG in the periodontal therapy [22, 23]. Er:YAG lasers are securely used as an alternative to non-surgical periodontal therapy or as an adjunct for pocket treatment [24, 25]. However, there is few evidence showing the superiority of ER:YAG lasers to others [23]. Quadri et al. [26] reported that SRP in combination with a single application of Nd:YAG laser significantly promotes periodontal healing compared to SRP alone. However, diode and Nd:YAG lasers are reported to have a profound complication of excessive heating of surrounding tissues [27]. It is reported that the damage of the termal side effects is prominently reduced in Er,Cr:YSGG laser and it can be safely and effectively used in non-surgical periodontal therapy [4]. Although there have been certain advantages of adjunctive use of lasers in periodontal therapy, recent studies suggest that the benefits of adjunctive lasers are questionable compared to other periodontal therapy methods. In a meta-analysis conducted by Smiley et al. [28], it is reported that photodynamic laser therapy with diode laser used as an adjunct to SRP is considered beneficial with a moderate level of certainty. In addition, Birang et al. [29] reported that adjunctive laser therapy

demonstrated minimal benefits compared to adjunctive photodynamic therapy in the treatment of chronic periodontitis.

In the current study, there was statistically significant improvement in all periodontal parameters in both group 1 and group 2 at all time points ($p < 0.01$). However, the difference between group 1 and group 2 was not significant in all time periods for periodontal parameters, especially in PI and CAL. This finding is not consistent with the literature [1, 5, 7]. Kelbauskiene et al. [5] reported that periodontal parameters of PD, BOP and PI in patients treated with Er,Cr:YSGG laser assisted periodontal therapy are significantly improved compared to patients treated with SRP alone. Gupta et al. [4] reported no significant difference between CAL and PI levels of two groups consisting of Er,Cr:YSGG assisted conventional periodontal therapy and open flap debridement. In the current study, there was a statistically significant decrease in PD at 1st month after treatment in the laser group. However, there was no statistically significant difference between PD values of group 1 and group 2 at the 3rd and 6th month after treatment. This finding is consistent with the study of Gutknecht et al. [1], who reported that laser irradiation did not have a significant effect on reducing pocket depth compared to non-laser conventional treatment. However, they concluded that the antibacterial effect of laser treatment was very effective. Similar to PD, a marked reduction of BOP scores was observed in the laser treatment group and this is in accordance with the literature findings [4, 5].

Halitosis is bad odor emanating from the oral region and majorly originates from the oral cavity [20]. Pham et al. [19] reported that oral malodor is directly correlated with periodontal disease. Oral malodor is evaluated by two main methods: one is a subjective and the other an objective evaluation method [30, 31]. Subjective evaluation is also called organoleptic evaluation which is performed by the researcher by means of inhaling the breath of the patient directly. Objective methods such as gas chromotography and quantitative analysis of VSCs are useful to obtain quantitative data regarding oral malodor. Although an organolaeptic method is cost-effective and easier to perform, it has a disadvantage of being subjective. In the current study, the objective method of quantitative measurement of VSC was preferred because it provided a numeric value. Yaegaki & Sanada [32] reported that VSC levels are directly related with periodontal bleeding. However, this finding does not support the idea that all patients with periodontitis will certainly have oral malodor or vice versa. In the current study, VSC levels showed a dramatic decrease in patients treated with Er,Cr:YSGG laser compared to conventional periodontal therapy, revealing that conventional periodontal therapy with the asisstance of Er,Cr:YSGG laser

Table 1 Mean values and standart derivations of study parameters halitosis (quantitative analysis of VSC volume), probing depth, clinical attachment level, plaque index and bleeding on probing on pre-treatment (baseline), 1st month, 3rd month and 6th month follow-up periods

Follow-up Time Points	Halitosis (ppb)			Probing depth (PD)(mm)			Clinical attachment Level (CAL)(mm)			Plaque index (PI)			Bleeding on probing (BOP)(per cent)		
	Group 1	Group 2	P*	Group 1	Group 2	P*	Group 1	Study	P*	Group 1	Group 2	P*	Group 1	Group 2	P*
Baseline values, mean (SD)	89.7 (13.9)	88.2 (15.2)	0.58	5.3 (1.8)	5.3 (1.8)	0.91	2.9 (0.4)	2.9 (0.6)	0.65	2.5 (0.5)	2.4 (0.5)	0.37	77.7 (7.4)	75.1 (7.2)	0.12
1 months, mean (SD)	63.8 (7.3)	60.6 (8.8)	0.10	2.7 (0.4)	2.3 (0.8)	**<0.05**	2.0 (0.2)	2.0 (0.5)	0.06	1.9 (0.4)	1.8 (0.4)	0.75	48.5 (7.7)	48.5 (9.4)	0.93
3 months, mean (SD)	69.2 (8.7)	54.4 (8.8)	**<0.001**	2.3 (0.6)	2.2 (0.6)	0.78	1.8 (0.4)	1.8 (0.7)	0.76	1.7 (0.4)	1.6 (0.4)	0.57	47.9 (6.6)	40.7 (11.0)	**<0.05**
6 months, mean (SD)	68.8 (10.2)	57.1 (12.2)	**<0.05**	2.1 (0.6)	1.9 (0.7)	0.13	1.9 (0.4)	1.8 (0.5)	0.20	1.5 (0.5)	1.5 (0.5)	0.71	41.6 (8.6)	37.8 (7.7)	**<0.05**
P**	**<0.01**	**<0.01**	-	**<0.01**	**<0.01**	-	**<0.01**	**<0.01**	-	**<0.01**	**<0.01**	-	**<0.01**	**<0.01**	-

Statistically significant data was shown in the bold emphasis

*p values in the columns represents significance between study and control groups ($p < 0.05$)

**p value in the rows represents significance between measurements on time periods in study and control groups separately ($p < 0.05$)

may be more effective than conventional periodontal therapy in reducing oral malodor. Similar to this study, in the study conducted by Silveira et al. [33] in which a sample size of 27 patients were included, it is reported that supragingival plaque control reduced halitosis in patients with periodontitis. In the study of Kara et al. [18], who compared the efficacy of a Nd: YAG laser on reducing oral malodor to conventional periodontal therapy in a population of 60 patients, it is suggested that Nd:YAG laser was superior in reducing oral malodor compared to conventional periodontal therapy.

Tongue coating is defined as one of the primary sites of oral malodor [34]. In the current study, patients were encouraged to cleanse their tongue by brushing the dorsal region of the tongue. However, a score for tongue coating was not recorded. This is one of the limitations of this study. Additionally, oral hygiene education regarding tongue cleansing might have contributed to the reduction of oral malodor.

The effectiveness of laser therapy on oral malodor has been reported in several studies in the literature [18, 35]. Kara et al. [18] reported that Nd:YAG lasers had an adjunctive role in reducing oral malodor compared to conventional periodontal therapy. They also concluded that oral malodor and periodontal disease levels are directly related. In the study of Lopez et al. [35], photodynamic therapy was applied to the dorsum of the tongue of teenager patients suffering from oral malodor and was observed to be effective in reducing oral malodor. However, the success of adjunctive use of diode laser with conventional periodontal therapy is emphasized to be questionable in recent studies [36, 37].

In the present study, a significant decrease in BOP and halitosis was observed in 3rd and 6th months in patients treated with Er,Cr:YSGG assisted conventional periodontal therapy. The significant change in these parameters brings up the assumption of the reduction in periodontal disease related halitosis may be associated with the reduction of BOP. VSCs are mainly produced from bacterial colonies residing in the periodontal pocket [38]. Thus, reduction in halitosis may be explained by the elimination of the VSC producing bacteria in the periodontal pocket. However, a more definite examination and a separate study protocol are needed to expose the true relationship between BOP and halitosis.

Conclusion

Although there is an ongoing debate about the benefits of the usage of adjunctive laser therapy with conventional periodontal treatment, the present study confirms that Er,Cr:YSGG assisted periodontal therapy improves periodontal parameters of PD and BOP in chronic periodontitis and reduces periodontal disease related oral malodor more effectively than conventional non-surgical

periodontal therapy. The current study to the best of our knowledge is the first to evaluate the efficacy of Er,Cr:YSGG laser on halitosis. The study population should be expanded in further studies in order to achieve more definite results.

Abbreviations
BOP: bleeding on probing; CAL: clinical attachment level; PD: probing depth; PI: plaque index; VSC: volatile sulphur compounds.

Competing interests
The authors declare that they have no competing interests.

Authors' contributions
ÖD conducted prospective data selection & statistical analysis, interpreted the analysis and wrote the manuscript, ST is supervisor of the study, helped to write the manuscript, MH performed periodontal measurements and helped to write the manuscript, AS performed VSC measuremens and helped in the interpretation of the data analysis, KÜ is the co-supervisor of the study and helped to draft the manuscript. All authors read and approved the final manuscript.

Acknowledgements
Authors declare that they had no funding.

Author details
[1]Department of Oral and Maxillofacial Surgery, Faculty of Dentistry, Eskişehir Osmangazi University, Meşelik Campus, 26480 Eskişehir, Turkey. [2]Department of Periodontology, Faculty of Dentistry, Akdeniz University, Antalya, Turkey. [3]Department of Oral and Maxillofacial Surgery, Faculty of Dentistry, Akdeniz University, Antalya, Turkey.

References
1. Gutknecht N, Van Betteray C, Ozturan S, Vanweersch L, Franzen R. Laser supported reduction of specific microorganisms in the periodontal pocket with the aid of an Er,Cr:YSGG laser: a pilot study. ScientificWorldJournal. 2015;2015:450258.
2. Quirynen M, Zhao H, Soers C, Dekeyser C, Pauwels M, Coucke W, et al. The impact of periodontal therapy and the adjunctive effect of antiseptics on breath odor-related outcome variables: a double-blind randomized study. J Periodontol. 2005;76:705–12.
3. Saglam M, Kantarci A, Dundar N, Hakki SS. Clinical and biochemical effects of diode laser as an adjunct to nonsurgical treatment of chronic periodontitis: a randomized, controlled clinical trial. Lasers Med Sci. 2014;29:37–46.
4. Gupta M, Lamba AK, Verma M, Faraz F, Tandon S, Chawla K, et al. Comparison of periodontal open flap debridement versus closed debridement with Er,Cr: YSGG laser. Aust Dent J. 2015;58:41–9.
5. Kelbauskiene S, Maciulskiene V. A pilot study of Er, Cr:YSGG laser therapy used as an adjunct to scaling and root planing in patients with early and moderate periodontitis. Stomatologija. 2007;9:21–6.
6. Pavone C, Perussi LR, de Oliveira GJ, Scardueli CR, Cirelli JA, Cerri PS, et al. Effect of Er, Cr:YSGG laser application in the treatment of experimental periodontitis. Lasers Med Sci. 2015;30:993–9.
7. Kelbauskiene S, Baseviciene N, Goharkhay K, Moritz A, Machiulskiene V. One-year clinical results of Er, Cr:YSGG laser application in addition to scaling and root planing in patients with early to moderate periodontitis. Lasers Med Sci. 2011;26:445–52.
8. de Oliveira GJ, Cominotte MA, Beraldo TP, Sampaio JE, Marcantonio RA. A microscopic analysis of the effects of root surface scaling with different power parameters of Er,Cr:YSGG laser. Microsc Res Tech. 2015;78:529–35.
9. Iwai K, Shi YW, Endo M, Ito K, Matsuura Y, Miyagi M, et al. Penetration of high-intensity Er:YAG laser light emitted by IR hollow optical fibers with sealing caps in water. Appl Opt. 2004;43:2568–71.
10. Hakki SS, Korkusuz P, Berk G, Dundar N, Saglam M, Bozkurt B, et al. Comparison of Er, Cr:YSGG laser and hand instrumentation on the attachment of periodontal ligament fibroblasts to periodontally diseased root surfaces: an in vitro study. J Periodontol. 2010;81:1216–25.

11. Matsumoto K, Hossain M, Hossain MM, Kawano H, Kimura Y. Clinical assessment of Er, Cr:YSGG laser application for cavity preparation. J Clin Laser Med Surg. 2002;20:17–21.

12. Franzen R, Esteves-Oliveira M, Meister J, Wallerang A, Vanweersch L, Lampert F, et al. Decontamination of deep dentin by means of erbium, chromium:yttrium-scandium-gallium-garnet laser irradiation. Lasers Med Sci. 2009;24:75–80.

13. Gilthorpe MS, Zamzuri AT, Griffiths GS, Maddick IH, Eaton KA, Johnson NW. Unification of the "burst" and "linear" theories of periodontal disease progression: a multilevel manifestation of the same phenomenon. J Dent Res. 2003;82:200–5.

14. Dyer B, Sung EC. Minimally invasive periodontal treatment using the Er, Cr: YSGG laser. A 2-year retrospective preliminary clinical study. Open Dent J. 2012;6:74–8.

15. Scully C, Greenman J. Halitosis (breath odor). Periodontol 2000. 2008;48:66–75.

16. Miyazaki H, Sakao S, Katoh Y, Takehara T. Correlation between volatile sulphur compounds and certain oral health measurements in the general population. J Periodontol. 1995;66:679–84.

17. Rosenberg M, McCulloch CA. Measurement of oral malodor: current methods and future prospects. J Periodontol. 1992;63:776–82.

18. Kara C, Demir T, Orbak R, Tezel A. Effect of Nd: YAG laser irradiation on the treatment of oral malodour associated with chronic periodontitis. Int Dent J. 2008;58:151–8.

19. Pham TA, Ueno M, Zaitsu T, Takehara S, Shinada K, Lam PH, et al. Clinical trial of oral malodor treatment in patients with periodontal diseases. J Periodontal Res. 2011;46:722–9.

20. Quirynen M, Mongardini C, van Steenberghe D. The effect of a 1-stage full-mouth disinfection on oral malodor and microbial colonization of the tongue in periodontitis. A pilot study. J Periodontol. 1998;69:374–82.

21. Löe H. The gingival index, the plaque index and the retention index systems. J Periodontol. 1967;38(Suppl):610–6.

22. Yoshino T, Yamamoto A, Ono Y. Innovative regeneration technology to solve peri-implantitis by Er:YAG laser based on the microbiologic diagnosis: a case series. Int J Periodontics Restorative Dent. 2015;35:67–73.

23. Aoki A, Mizutani K, Schwarz F, Sculean A, Yukna RA, Takasaki AA, et al. Periodontal and peri-implant wound healing following laser therapy. Periodontol 2000. 2015; 68:217–69.

24. Aoki A, Sasaki KM, Watanabe H, Ishikawa I. Lasers in nonsurgical periodontal therapy. Periodontol 2000. 2004;36:59–97.

25. Ishikawa I, Aoki A, Takasaki AA, Mizutani K, Sasaki KM, Izumi Y. Application of lasers in periodontics: true innovation or myth? Periodontol 2000. 2009;50:90–126.

26. Qadri T, Poddani P, Javed F, Tunér J, Gustafsson A. A short-term evaluation of Nd:YAG laser as an adjunct to scaling and root planing in the treatment of periodontal inflammation. J Periodontol. 2010;81:1161–6.

27. Sculean A, Schwarz F, Berakdar M, Windisch P, Arweiler NB, Romanos GE. Healing of intrabony defects following surgical treatment with or without an Er:YAG laser. J Clin Periodontol. 2004;31:604–8.

28. Smiley CJ, Tracy SL, Abt E, Michalowicz BS, John MT, Gunsolley J, et al. Systematic review and meta-analysis on the nonsurgical treatment of chronic periodontitis by means of scaling and root planing with or without adjuncts. J Am Dent Assoc. 2015;146:508–24.

29. Birang R, Shahaboui M, Kiani S, Shadmehr E, Naghsh N. Effect of nonsurgical periodontal treatment combined with diode laser or photodynamic therapy on chronic periodontitis: a randomized controlled split-mouth clinical trial. J Lasers Med Sci. 2015;6:112–9.

30. Kara C, Tezel A, Orbak R. Effect of oral hygiene instruction and scaling on oral malodour in a population of Turkish children with gingival inflammation. Int J Paediatr Dent. 2006;16:399–404.

31. Morita M, Wang HL. Association between oral malodor and adult periodontitis: a review. J Clin Periodontol. 2001;28:813–9.

32. Yaegaki K, Sanada K. Biochemical and clinical factors influencing oral malodor in periodontal patients. J Periodontol. 1992;63:783–9.

33. Silveira EM, Piccinin FB, Gomes SC, Oppermann RV, Rösing CK. Effect of gingivitis treatment on the breath of chronic periodontitis patients. Oral Health Prev Dent. 2012;10:93–100.

34. Moriyama T. Clinical study of the correlation between bad breath and subgingival microflora. Shikwa Gakuho. 1989;89:1425–39.

35. Lopes RG, de Santi ME, Franco BE, Deana AM, Prates RA, França CM, et al. Photodynamic therapy as novel treatment for halitosis in adolescents: a case series study. J Lasers Med Sci. 2014;5:146–52.

36. Nguyen NT, Byarlay MR, Reinhardt RA, Marx DB, Meinberg TA, Kaldahl WB. Adjunctive non-surgical therapy of inflamed periodontal pockets during maintenance therapy using diode laser: a randomized clinical trial. J Periodontol. 2015;86:1133–40.

37. Slot DE, Jorritsma KH, Cobb CM, Van der Weijden FA. The effect of the thermal diode laser (wavelength 808–980 nm) in non-surgical periodontal therapy: a systematic review and meta-analysis. J Clin Periodontol. 2014;41:681–92.

38. Lu RF, Feng L, Gao XJ, Meng HX, Feng XH. Relationship between volatile fatty acids and Porphyromonas gingivalis and Treponema denticola in gingival crevicular fluids of patients with aggressive periodontitis. Beijing Da Xue Xue Bao. 2013;45:12–6.

33

Stenting the Eustachian tube to treat chronic otitis media - a feasibility study in sheep

Friederike Pohl[1,2], Robert A. Schuon[1,2], Felicitas Miller[1,3], Andreas Kampmann[3], Eva Bültmann[4], Christian Hartmann[5], Thomas Lenarz[1,2] and Gerrit Paasche[1,2]*

Abstract

Background: Untreated chronic otitis media severely impairs quality of life in affected individuals. Local destruction of the middle ear and subsequent loss of hearing are common sequelae, and currently available treatments provide limited relief. Therefore, the objectives of this study were to evaluate the feasibility of the insertion of a coronary stent from the nasopharynx into the Eustachian tube in-vivo in sheep and to make an initial assessment of its positional stability, tolerance by the animal, and possible tissue reactions.

Methods: Bilateral implantation of bare metal cobalt-chrome coronary stents of two sizes was performed endoscopically in three healthy blackface sheep using a nasopharyngeal approach. The postoperative observation period was three months.

Results: Stent implantation into the Eustachian tube was feasible with no intra- or post-operative complications. Health status of the sheep was unaffected. All stents preserved their cylindrical shape. All shorter stents remained in position and ventilated the middle ear even when partially filled with secretion or tissue. One of the long stents became dislocated toward the nasopharynx. Both of the others remained fixed at the isthmus but appeared to be blocked by tissue or secretion. Tissue overgrowth on top of the struts of all stents resulted in closure of the tissue-lumen interface.

Conclusion: Stenting of the Eustachian tube was successfully transferred from cadaver studies to an in-vivo application without complications. The stent was well tolerated, the middle ears were ventilated, and clearance of the auditory tube appeared possible. For fixation, it seems to be sufficient to place it only in the cartilaginous part of the Eustachian tube.

Keywords: Auditory tube, Middle ear ventilation, Stent, Otitis media, Sheep as animal model, Tissue reaction

Background

Acute and chronic otitis media continue to be significant issues in human medicine [1]. Especially otitis media with effusion (OME), which is not only common in children under the age of 10, but also the most prevalent reason why advice and treatment from an otorhinolaryngology specialist are needed [2]. In approximately 20% of patients, symptoms become chronic [2], causing severe and often irreversible damage to middle ear structures, including the tympanic membrane and ossicular chain. In the development of these diseases, the Eustachian (or auditory) tube (ET) is one of the key factors [2, 3].

The ET forms the only connection between the middle ear and the nasopharynx. It consists of an inelastic bony part that begins at the protympanum of the middle ear and covers one third of the ET's full length in humans. This merges into an elastic cartilaginous part, which extends over the remaining two thirds and ends in the nasopharynx. The conjunction of both parts creates a narrow passage, the isthmus [4]. The most important functions of the ET are the transport of secretion, middle ear ventilation, and protection against pathogenic microorganisms [3], but also protection from nasopharyngeal

* Correspondence: paasche.gerrit@mh-hannover.de
[1]Department of Otolaryngology, Hannover Medical School, Carl-Neuberg-Str. 1, 30625 Hannover, Germany
[2]Hearing4all Cluster of Excellence, Hannover Medical School, Hannover, Germany
Full list of author information is available at the end of the article

sound and reflux [5]. If one or more of these functions cannot be maintained, this can lead to a dysfunctional Eustachian tube (ETD) and middle ear effusion, followed by middle ear inflammation.

To treat ETD and OME, several different approaches, such as a PVC tube with attached thread inserted via the perforated tympanic membrane [6], a Silastic® tube, inserted via the tympanic orifice of the ET [7], or a gold wire, remaining in-situ for years, with rare rejection and initially good functions [8] have been applied in patients but with limited long-term success [9, 10]. Current management includes conservative methods like the Valsalva maneuver for pressure equalization; nasal douching with saline solution, or nasal application of decongestants, antihistamines, or corticosteroids. The most common surgical approach is the insertion of a tympanostomy tube into the tympanic membrane [11].

Apart from this surgery, two more approaches are used: Eustachian laser tuboplasty, in which enlarged mucous membranes and cartilage are removed to avoid obstruction [12], and balloon dilatation, in which a balloon catheter is inserted into the cartilaginous part of the ET and inflated to loosen adhesions and dilate the lumen [13]. Additionally, the topical application of fluids directly into the ET [14] has recently emerged. Despite the fact that these numerous methods appear in practical use and literature, according to Llewellyn et al. [11], there is little consensus about indications of treatment and moreover, conclusions regarding efficacy have been questioned. In addition, the causes of dysfunction and the mechanisms of intervention and long-term clinical outcomes need to be fully assessed [5].

In preclinical research in chinchilla and rabbit, a poly-L-lactide ET stent, not adapted to the size of the animal, was implanted through the bulla and tympanic membrane and investigated, with moderate outcome [15, 16]. The sheep was also evaluated for preclinical assessment of middle and inner ear implants [17], and the feasibility of endoscopic implantation of a commercially available coronary stent through the nasopharyngeal orifice of the ET was proven in a cadaver study [18], in order to test stents sized for human application in a large animal model. To investigate the feasibility of this approach in-vivo, in the present study differently sized coronary stents were implanted into the ETs of blackface sheep.

In addition, it would be beneficial to have an adequate disease model available. There are models described in the literature using either cauterization of the ET, knock-out mice, or Streptococcus pneumonia in the rat [19, 20]. In chinchilla, aseptically triggered OME was induced [21] with inflammatory mediators, platelet activating factor (PAF) [22], and Prostaglandin E_2 [21], which provides an easily applied, reversible method, without the risk of uncontrolled infection of the animal.

Therefore, the objectives of the current study were to evaluate the feasibility of in-vivo insertion of a commercially available coronary stent from the nasopharynx into the ET, and to analyze how such stents are tolerated over the course of three months. Additionally, induced aseptic otitis media was evaluated as a potential disease model.

Methods

Ethics approval

The State Office for Consumer Protection and Food Safety, Dept. of Animal Welfare, in accordance with the German and European animal welfare legislation, approved this study under number 12/1089. With regard to the valid directives for accommodation, care, and usage of experimental animals, the sheep were cared for, and the experiments were performed in a central animal facility.

Stents

ProKinetik Energy® stents (Biotronik, Berlin, Germany) consisting of a non-degradable cobalt-chrome alloy, with a strut thickness of 60 μm and a recoil of less than 5 %, were implanted in two different sizes: 2.75 mm × 26 mm (left ear) and 2.0 mm × 20 mm (right ear). Stents were mounted on an expandable catheter for insertion (Rapid exchange catheter, length: 1.4 m).

Animals and study design

ETs of three healthy adult (2 to 4 years) female blackface sheep were stented bilaterally, with a delay of one week between sides. One week prior to the first implantation, an initial bilateral control of external and middle ears and endoscopic examination of the nasopharyngeal orifices of the ET was performed under general anesthesia. At the time of the first implantation, a sterile middle ear inflammation was triggered in the second ear followed by implantation of the second stent one week later. Regular endoscopic examinations of the nasopharyngeal orifices of the ET were performed according to the study design (Fig. 1). A second sterile inflammation was induced in the first implanted ear one week before euthanasia, after 12 weeks. The degree of inflammatory reaction was evaluated by a daily check on the general health of the sheep and an endoscopic score of the pharyngeal orifice of the ET as described below.

General anesthesia, implantation, and induction of inflammation

Implantation and induction of inflammation were performed under general anesthesia (GA) after sedation with Midazolam (0.2 mg/kg i.v.; Midazolam-ratiopharm® 5 mg/mL, Ratiopharm, Blaubeuren, Germany) and induction of GA with propofol (5–10 mg/kg i.v.; Propofol®-Lipuro 10 mg/mL, B. Braun Melsungen AG, Melsungen, Germany). For the maintenance of GA, Isoflurane (1.5–2.

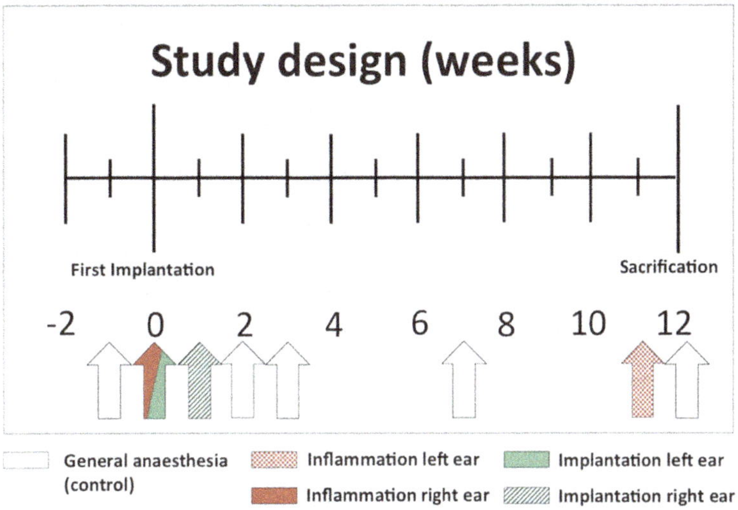

Fig. 1 Study design in weeks. The arrows indicate time points of general anesthesia with endoscopic control (white), instillation of inflammatory mediators, or stent implantation

0% end-tidal inhalation; Isofluran CP 1 mL/mL, CP-Pharma, Burgdorf, Germany) was used. To prevent bleeding and to provide local anesthesia, pointed swabs wetted with Naphazolin 10 mL (Privin® 1 mg, Novartis, München, Germany) and Lidocaine 5 mL (Xylocain 2%, AstraZeneca GmbH, Wedel, Germany) were applied into both nostrils prior to the endoscopic approach.

Stenting was performed via a nasopharyngeal endoscopic approach to the ET. The stent, mounted on the catheter, was completely inserted into the epipharyngeal orifice of the ET via the working canal of a flexible broncho-fiberscope (Broncho-Fiberskop: 3.7 mm diameter, 1.5 mm working canal, 0° angle of view, 110° opening angle, 54 cm length, Karl Storz, Tuttlingen, Germany). The balloon of the catheter was inflated with physiologic saline solution and thus the stent expanded, using a pressure of 10 bar for two minutes. Afterward, the balloon was deflated, held in position for one minute and slowly extracted from the orifice of the ET. While the short stent (2.0 mm × 20 mm) stayed only in the cartilaginous part of the ET, the longer stent (2.75 mm × 26 mm) reached through the isthmus between the bony and cartilaginous parts where it became clamped during the balloon inflation process.

Inflammation was initiated using platelet activating factor 10^{-5} mol/L (1-O-Hexadecyl-2-O-acetyl-sn-glycero-3-phosphocholine, Bachem GmbH, Weil am Rhein, Germany) and prostaglandin E_2 10^{-5} mol/L (Prostaglandin E_2, Sigma-Aldrich Chemie, Schnelldorf, Germany) delivered as a single treatment of 1 mL via a perforated balloon catheter at the time of first implantation in the unstented right ear and in a double concentration one week before euthanasia in the stented left ear. During the instillation of the fluid, no pressure occurred in the balloon or the ET, due to the

perforation of the balloon. Postoperative pain management was provided by Carprofen 1.4 mg/kg i.v. (Rimadyl® 50 mg/mL, Pfizer, Berlin, Germany) and protection from bacterial inflammation performed with Benzylpenicillin-Dihydrostreptomycin 0.04 mg/kg s.c. (Veracin Comp®, Albrecht GmbH, Aulendorf, Germany).

Health and endoscopic score

To ensure the health of the animals, a daily check on their general health status and periodic endoscopic examinations of the ear and ET according to Fig. 1 were conducted. The health score according to Otto and Short [23] was modified, and included parameters such as breathing frequency, rumination, intake of food and water, head tilt or nasal discharge ranged from a score of zero (unaffected constitution) to seven (severely affected constitution) (see table provided as Additional file 1). The quality of mucus, the degree of opening of the nasopharyngeal orifice of the ET, inflammatory erythema, and swelling were accessed in the endoscopic score (Table 1). This score ranged from a maximum of 12 (severe inflammation) to a minimum of zero (no inflammation), with a score of zero to three categorized as non-inflammatory, from four to six as mild

Table 1 Score for semi quantitative evaluation of the endoscopic images of the nasopharyngeal orifice of the ET

Criteria	Endoscopic score value			
	None	Mild	Moderate	Severe
Quality of mucus	0	1	2	3
Opening degree of n. orifice[a]	0	1	2	3
Inflammatory erythema	0	1	2	3
Inflammatory swelling	0	1	2	3

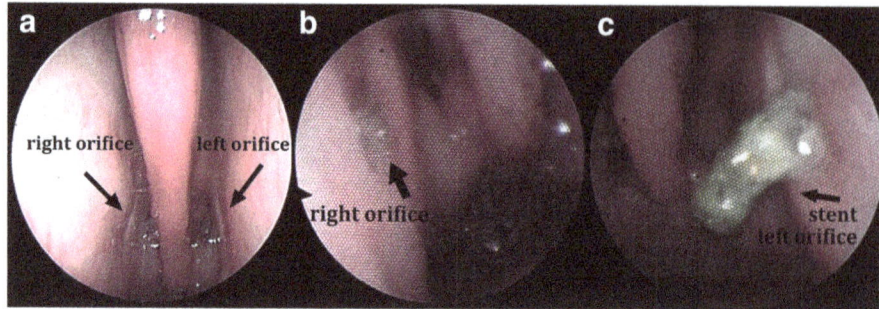

Fig. 2 Endoscopic view of the ET for the evaluation of stent position and inflammation. Examples of (**a**) no [endoscopic score 1–3], (**b**) mild [score 4–6] and (**c**) moderate [score 7–9] inflammation in the nasopharyngeal orifice region are shown

inflammation, from seven to nine as moderate inflammation, and from 10 to 12 as severe inflammation. Additionally, the visibility of the implanted stent in the proximity of the ET opening was documented. Examples of specific endoscopic images are presented in Fig. 2.

Fixation, embedding, and staining procedure

After 12 weeks of implantation, sheep were euthanized under GA by an overdose of pentobarbital i.v. (Release® 300 mg/mL, WDT, Garbsen, Germany) before decapitation behind the second cervical vertebrae.

Post-mortem, a spiral computed tomography (CT) scan was performed. On coronal reconstructions, the stent in its entire length as well as the middle ear and the external auditory canal were depicted (example shown in Fig. 3). The location of the stent and the degree of its obstruction (tissue or secretion) were determined. The middle ear, including the hypo-, meso- and epitympanum, was inspected regarding tissue formation and occurrence of effusion.

For histologic analysis, each ET with surrounding tissue was dissected, orienting on the nasopharyngeal opening and the opening to the middle ear, using a bone

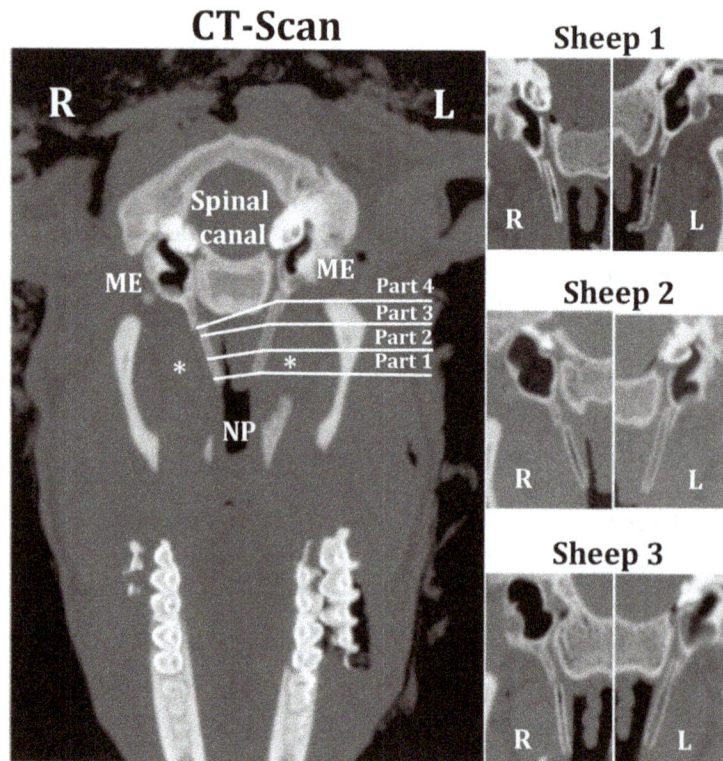

Fig. 3 Coronal CT sections of both stents (*) in-situ for each sheep. Tympanic cavity (ME), nasopharynx (NP) and spinal canal were used for orientation and evaluation. The lines indicate the regions of histologic evaluation

saw (FK23 bone saw, Bizerba, Balingen, Germany). Each specimen was washed in physiological saline solution (B. Braun Melsungen AG, Melsungen, Germany) and fixed in formalin (3.5%, pH 7.4; C. Roth, Karlsruhe, Germany) for two weeks. Prior to embedding in methylmethacrylate (MMA; Merck KGaA, Darmstadt, Germany) [24], dehydration of the specimen via an increasing ethanol series (70%, 80%, 90%, 100%; Merck) was performed. Each step was carried out overnight and finalized with MMA infiltration and polymerization in a water bath with increasing temperature (35 °C to 40 °C) for two to four days, depending on the status of polymerization. The excess MMA was removed with a plaster model trimmer (HSS 88, Wassermann Dental-Maschinen GmbH, Hamburg, Germany) until only the specimen remained. Specimen were cut into two halves and fixed on a specimen holder to cut slices of approx. 33 μm thickness with a saw microtome (Leica SP1600 ®, Leica Biosystems, Wetzlar, Germany), beginning in the middle of each ET and following the course of the ET in both directions. Additionally, slices of approx. 1 mm thickness were discarded at periodical intervals. Staining of the slices was performed with Alizarin red (Alizarin red S staining solution; Merck) and Methylene blue (Löffler's Methylene blue solution; Merck). The slices were incubated for 45 s with Methylene blue on a heating plate (80 °C). After rinsing with distilled water, the slices were incubated with Alizarin red for 1.5 min. Drying in an incubator at 37 °C overnight followed an additional rinsing step. After staining, each slice was mounted on microscopic slides with Entellan®-new (Merck) and covered with cover slips.

Histologic analysis and evaluation

Histologic analysis was performed with image editing software (NIS-Elements Imaging Software 4.20®, Nikon, Düsseldorf, Germany) after digitalization of the histologic slices under a microscope (SMZ1000 ®, Nikon, Düsseldorf, Germany, with a Nikon Digital Sight DS-Vi1 camera) at 2× magnification. In each set of slices, the end of the stent in the proximity of the nasopharynx was set as the starting point for the analysis while the end in the proximity of the middle ear opening was the endpoint of analysis. The position of the discarded slices was taken as reference to estimate the length of the tube and to divide the length of the stent in the tube into four parts. Part one represented the first third of the cartilaginous part of the ET and the beginning of the stent, following it from the nasopharyngeal opening. Part two adjoined it, representing the middle part, whereas part three covered the final third of the cartilaginous part of the tube in the direction of the middle ear. Due to the different lengths of the stents, the fourth part partially overlapped with the third part in the shorter stents but

was positioned in the isthmus region for the longer stents, and revealed the ending of each stent. In each part, three representative concurrent slices were analyzed. In each slice, the lumen (L) of the ET, the amount of secretion (S) and tissue (T), and the total area of the ET, excluding the chondral and bony parts, gland tissue, or fat (ROI), were assessed. The free lumen (L$_F$) was calculated by subtraction of the secretion from the lumen. Tissue, lumen, secretion and free lumen were given as percentages of the total ROI. The values of the three consecutive slices were averaged to obtain the results for a specific section of the ET. To calculate overall values averaged results were used.

An ellipse was positioned on the slices, such that the most visible struts of the stent were on or very close to the ellipse (Fig. 4). The stent diameter was determined via the stent area (the area of the ellipse) in the histological sections. The area was quantified in the slices for the four different parts of the ET and was compared to the references given by the manufacturer for each stent.

Results

Stent implantation and application of inflammatory mediators

In all three sheep, the endoscopic approach afforded a clear view on the pharyngeal orifice (Fig. 2), and implantation was easily completed on both sides. Furthermore, the insertion of the entire stent could be done without complication for both stent sizes. The application of inflammatory mediators using a perforated balloon was performed in the right ET prior to implantation and was not hampered by the previously implanted stent in the left ET at the end of the study.

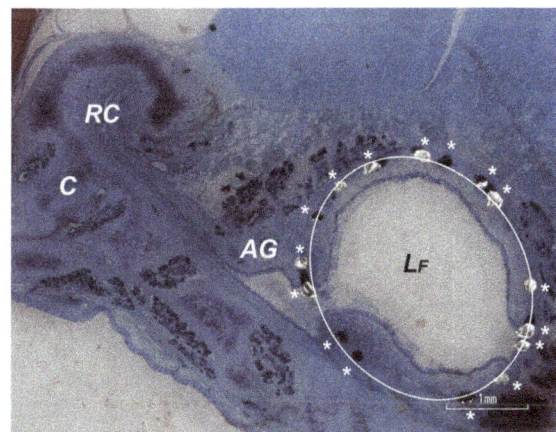

Fig. 4 Slice of the ET with plotted ellipse illustrating the region of analysis of stent expansion. Depicted are Rüdinger's safety canal (RC), auxiliary gap (AG), the tubal cartilage (C) and free lumen (L$_F$) of the ET. An ellipse is depicted on the struts (*) indicating the position of the stent

Health score and endoscopic score

During the entire period of the experiment, all three sheep displayed a health score of two or less from a maximum score of seven (see table in Additional file 2: summary of the specific findings for each sheep). Recurring periods of hot weather resulted in a 0.5 point increase due to the sheep's enhanced breathing frequency. In sheep 3, serous nasal discharge was observed three times: two weeks prior to the first manipulation, during the week after the first general anesthesia before stent implantation and triggering of inflammation, and three weeks after stent implantation and first application of inflammatory mediators.

The mean endoscopic score revealed no inflammatory signs for two of the short stents and one of the longer stents (Fig. 5). Mild inflammatory reactions occurred with one short and one long stent. A moderate reaction was detected for one long stent (Fig. 2c). Sporadic visibility in the pharyngeal orifice was apparent in all implanted stents. In sheep 1, the long stent was visible in all endoscopic examinations performed and in sheep 2, in four of the seven endoscopic examinations. In all three sheep an increase in secretion in the region of both ETs was detected relative to the first GA before implantation. Neither in the health score nor in the endoscopic score (Fig. 5), severe inflammation was detected in all three sheep showing a temporal connection to the instilled inflammatory mediators.

CT scans

Coronal reconstructions (Fig. 3) demonstrated ventilated middle ears with few or minimal accumulations of secretion and limited soft tissue formations. The CT scans displayed air filling with proximal obstruction in all short stents and one long stents (sheep 1). In contrast to this, the remaining longer stents appeared to be fully obstructed. All stents were located in the chondral part of the ET. In sheep 1, the long stent showed a proximal dislocation in the direction of the nasopharynx, and in sheep 2 the shorter stent was located directly in the nasopharyngeal orifice of the ET. Both accurately

positioned longer stents showed narrowing in the bony part and isthmus of the ET.

Histologic analysis

Tissue formation was assessed in the histologic analysis. The ET stented with the 2.75 mm × 26 mm sized implant covered on average an area (ROI) of 10.2 ± 2 mm^2 with 6.6 ± 2.2 mm^2 tissue (T) and 3.6 ± 0.3 mm^2 lumen (L). The lumen was filled with 1.2 ± 1 mm^2 secretion (S), leaving a free lumen (L_F) of 2.4 ± 1.1 mm^2. The ET implanted with the smaller stent showed a ROI of 7.2 ± 2.2 mm^2 with 4.9 ± 1.8 mm^2 tissue and 2.4 ± 0.8 mm^2 lumen, with the latter filled with 0.8 ± 0.4 mm^2 secretion, leaving a free lumen of 1.5 ± 0.7 mm^2. The values for each sheep are summarized in Additional file 2. When evaluating the tissue in the different parts (1 to 4) of the tube, in both ETs an increase in tissue as well as a decrease in lumen, secretion and free lumen was detected from the nasopharynx (part 1) to the middle ear (part 4) (Fig. 6), with only minor differences among parts 1 to 3 (not shown).

Stent dimensions and lumen-tissue interface

In general, both implanted stent sizes were expanded up to their nominal diameter (Additional file 2). In part one, close to the nasopharyngeal opening, five of the six stents were expanded almost to their full diameter. In contrast to this, all six stents displayed a smaller degree of expansion in part four, at or close to the bony isthmus (Fig. 7). The struts of both stents generally maintained their circular arrangement and could be detected in the sub-mucosal layer. However, in sheep 3, the struts in part 4 appeared to be deeper in the tissue, leaving the mucosal layer and becoming embedded in muscle and gland tissue. The general percentage of struts lying free in the lumen ranged from 6.5% to 43%, and was generally higher in the right ETs, i.e., the smaller stent (Fig. 8).

The first mucosal layer on the interface between mucosa and lumen of the ET consisted in each ET of

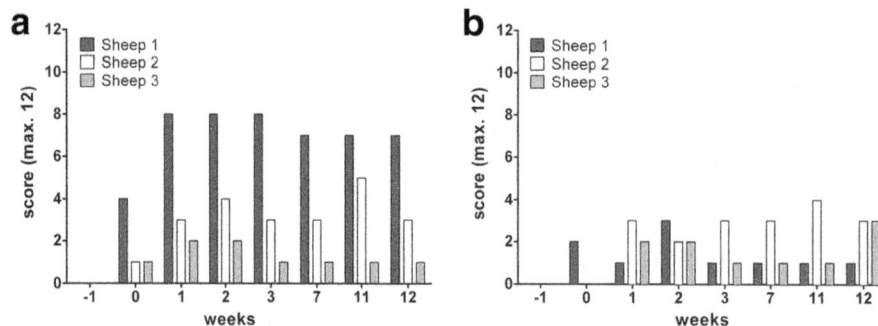

Fig. 5 Recorded endoscopic score values. **a** Left (long stent) and (**b**) right (short stent) ET of each sheep under general anesthesia in the course of the experiment. In the first GA (week − 1) a score of zero was observed

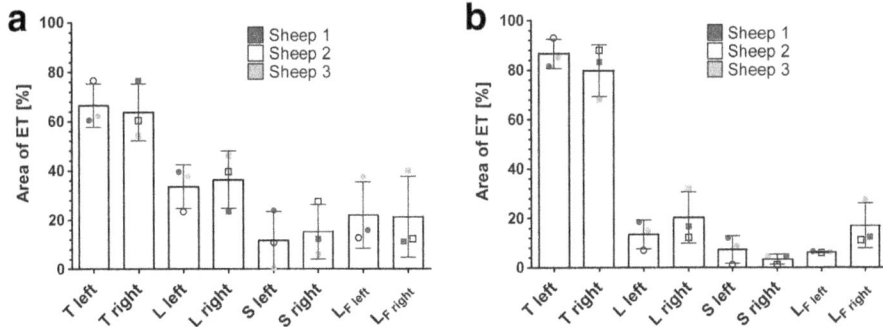

Fig. 6 Areas of tissue occurrence (T), lumen (L), secretion (S) and free lumen (L$_F$). Depicted are parts 1 (**a**) and 4 (**b**) of the ET for both stents (compare Fig. 3). The total area of the ET (ROI) was set as 100%

prismatic epithelium. The luminal side of this epithelium was covered with cilia, which could also be detected in the respiratory epithelium of the nasopharynx (Fig. 9). In sheep 3, both ETs showed moderate signs of mucosal detachment and autolysis, yet fragments of prismatic epithelium and cilia could be detected as well in both ETs in this sheep.

Discussion

Improvement of middle ear ventilation via ventilation tubes in the tympanic membrane causes tympanic membrane perforation and may create new pathways for entry of pathogenic microorganisms from the external auditory canal. If used repeatedly, atrophic scarring of the tympanic membrane, myringo- and tympanosclerosis, tympanic membrane retraction, persistent perforation, or granulation tissue formation become apparent with an incidence of 51% [25, 26]. Few therapeutic approaches utilize the ET itself with a nasopharyngeal approach for the treatment of chronic otitis media and ETD. Stenting the ET could improve ventilation of the middle ear and clearance of secretion through the ET itself, preventing tympanic membrane perforation and over the long term, middle ear destruction.

Thus, the primary aim of the present study was to investigate stent implantation from the nasopharynx into the ET in-vivo in blackface sheep, and to evaluate possible body reactions. The secondary aim was to develop a model of induced aseptic OME, as the need for an intervention only arises when the function of ET is impaired.

The application of inflammatory mediators into the middle ear of sheep via the ET was easily performed. As described in human practice [14], small amounts of fluid (one to two milliliters) could be instilled in the sheep through the working channel of the flexible endoscope using a catheter perforated at its tip. The amount of fluid deposited in the middle ear was difficult to determine precisely, because of an apparent efflux from the nasopharyngeal orifice. However, a considerable amount of fluid and therefore inflammatory mediators potentially reached the middle ear and ET, resulting in the physiological absorption from middle ear and tubal mucosa. In contrast to the findings in the chinchilla model of induced OME triggered by inflammatory mediators applied through the bulla [21], no signs of moderate or severe inflammation with a temporal connection to the instillation of PAF and prostaglandin E_2 were observed. The effective dosage of PAF necessary to induce middle ear effusion in mongrel dogs is reported to be between 10^{-7} mol/L and 10^{-6} mol/L [27],

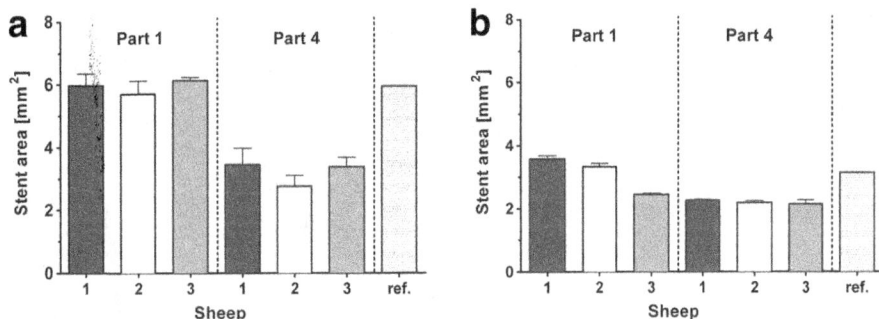

Fig. 7 Mean stent area. Parts 1 and 4 (compare Fig. 3) of the implanted 2.75 mm × 26 mm (**a**) and 2.0 mm × 20 mm (**b**) stents with the calculated reference for each stent size. The data are shown as mean + SD

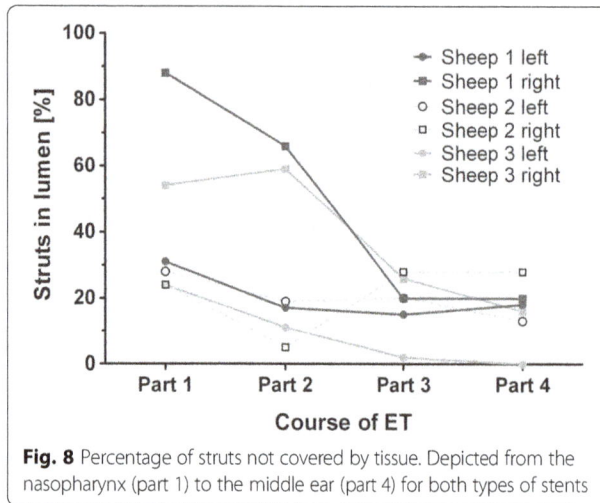

Fig. 8 Percentage of struts not covered by tissue. Depicted from the nasopharynx (part 1) to the middle ear (part 4) for both types of stents

indicating that the dosage of 10^{-5} mol/L first used in the current study and especially the doubled concentration in the second application, should have been sufficient to trigger the desired effect. According to a study investigating the inflammatory potency of PAF, induced OME lasts for up to 14 days in chinchillas due to the initiation of an inflammatory cascade, although the initial inflammatory mediator was already cleared from the body [22]. However, the peak of the inflammatory reaction was suggested to occur on day 4 post-inflammation [21]. For these reasons we expected the inflammation in the sheep to peak during the first week after application, and to still be visible on day seven. Due to species restraints regarding the frequency of anesthesia (limited to once a week), the follow up was performed on day seven after the instillation of PAF and

prostaglandin E_2. Unfortunately, use of the tympanometry method in sheep [28] was not available at the time the examination was performed, which would have facilitated monitoring of middle ear effusion or negative middle ear pressure [3] at shorter intervals. Therefore, we can only speculate about the reasons for missing inflammatory signs related to the application of the substances. Amongst the possible reasons are (i) clearance of all the inflammatory mediators through the ET, (ii) a lower susceptibility of the sheep to the substances, or (iii) a reaction that does not present symptoms detectable with the applied methods one week after instillation. Even though we failed in inducing detectable inflammation, this should have no impact on the other results of this study.

Stent implantation in-vivo was shown to be quite feasible, as in the cadaver (compare [18]). All sheep were healthy during the experiment and the sporadic incidences of serous secretion in sheep 3 may be explained by dust particles in hay and straw, irritating the mucous membrane. This phenomenon had already been observed before stent implantation, and in veterinary practice it is common in a variety of species living in dusty environments.

During stent implantation, no erosion of the carotid artery was observed. This was expected, as the same pressure recommended for balloon dilatation was used, the diameters of both stents were smaller than that of the balloon, and balloon dilatation does not have adverse effects on the bony part of the ET [29].

Five of the six inserted stents stayed in position where implanted. Fixation of the shorter stents only in the cartilaginous part of the ET was successful in all three instances, and fixation of the larger stent in the isthmus

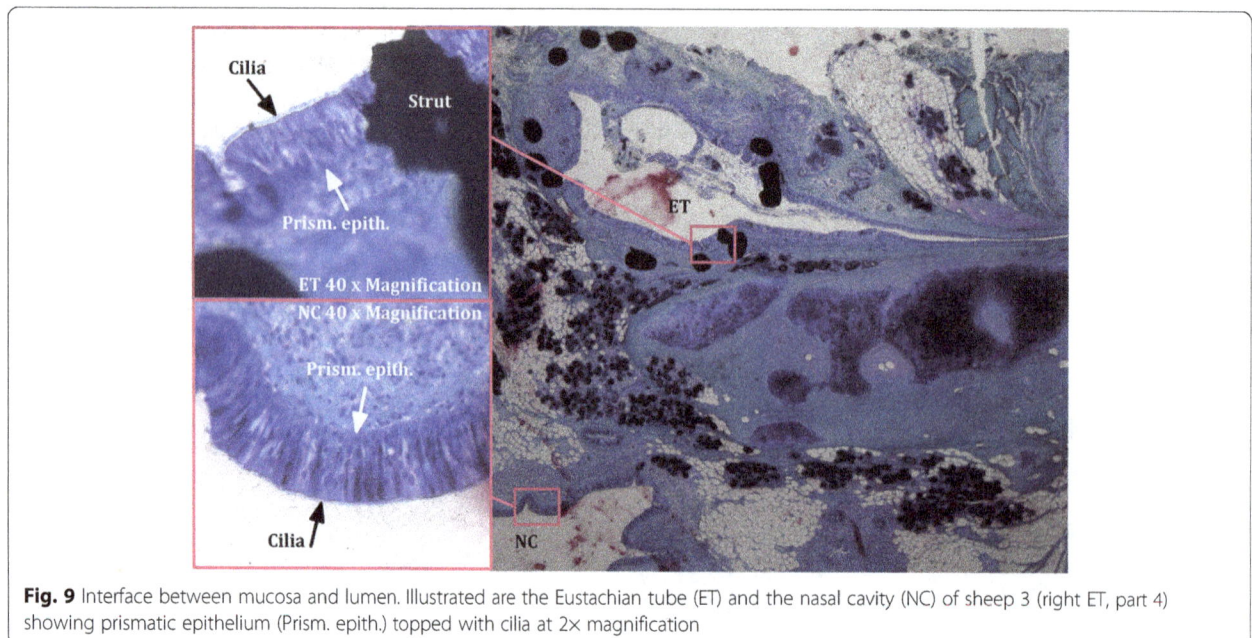

Fig. 9 Interface between mucosa and lumen. Illustrated are the Eustachian tube (ET) and the nasal cavity (NC) of sheep 3 (right ET, part 4) showing prismatic epithelium (Prism. epith.) topped with cilia at 2× magnification

was successful in two of three cases. In one sheep, shortly after implantation, the stent migrated in the direction of the nasopharynx, eventually reaching into the nasopharynx. However, the stent stayed in this position for the rest of the observation period. According to these findings, fixation at the isthmus may not be required. This fact is important particularly because consequences of stent placement in the isthmus seem to include a narrower stent diameter in the vicinity of the bony isthmus and local ET distortion with further impaired clearance function. This may have led to difficulty with mucus transport and resulted in the obstruction of the stents and finally the ET itself, although secretion was seen in all correctly positioned 26 mm stents on CT scans. Even though no signs of increased inflammation were found in the histology of these stents, it remains unclear whether the application of the inflammatory mediators might have contributed to the obstruction of the long stents at the isthmus. The single dislocated stent had a position closer to that of the 20 mm stents and showed similar ventilation with a smaller degree of narrowing compared to the other 26 mm stents.

In general, mild inflammation was detected in the endoscopic images of the ET orifice at the nasopharynx as well as moderate connective tissue encapsulation in the histologic slices. Additionally, rare signs of inflammation and minimal accumulation of secretion were seen in the middle ears. As the entrance of pathogenic microorganisms is limited to the pharynx and prevention of ascending infections to the middle ear is one of the main tasks of the ET [30], the protective function appears to be maintained, at least over the observation period of three months. However, dislocation of the stent should be avoided, as direct contact of the stent with bacterial flora in the nasopharynx might have led to an increase of purulent secretion and inflammation. Further, the extruded part of the stent is expected to cause continuous mechanical irritation during all epipharyngeal movements. Nonetheless, the middle ear itself appeared to be as unaffected as in the other sheep.

With the stents in this study we might have created a permanently open ET. A permanently open ET is a symptom of a patulous ET [31], allowing sounds of speech and nasopharyngeal sounds (autophony), reflux from the gastrointestinal tract [32], and pathogenic microorganisms [3] to ascend into the middle ear, leading to sickness of the patient as well as mucosal irritation and infections. Thus, migration into the nasopharynx and direct placement of the stent in the nasopharyngeal opening of the ET should be avoided. Ideally, a stent would be positioned in the ET such that it facilitates opening, but does not cause a permanently open ET.

The free lumen was calculated to be about 20% in both ET, which is 2.35 mm^2 in the cross section of the larger

and 1.5 mm^2 in the smaller stent. The isthmus, the narrowest portion of the ET, measures 1 mm in width × 3. 5 mm in height in the blackface sheep [18] and 1 mm × 2 mm [4] in humans, implying that the detected free lumen should be enough to promote permanent ventilation as it is described for Rüdinger's safety canal in the tubal cartilage, which measures only 0.4 to 0.5 mm [33]. In contrast, a stent diameter of 1.5 mm was not sufficient to maintain transport of secretion in an earlier study [8], thus, the obstruction with secretion in the longer stents might be caused by the narrowing of the stent diameter at the isthmus, explaining why the dislocated larger stent did not show total obstruction.

Additionally, the movement of the auxiliary gap, i.e. the movable space below the safety canal, which opens only in process of swallowing or yawning, is hampered by the ingrown stent (Fig. 4), limiting its opening diameter to the stent diameter. This part of the ET in humans physiologically provides an opening diameter of up to 6–10 mm [18], ensuring the clearance [33]. This diameter in sheep was reduced by the ingrown stent to 2.75 mm or less.

In coronary vessels, an overgrowth of the vascular graft with intima is desirable to prevent thrombus formation and re-establish a smooth surface, ideally mimicking the original surface of the endothelium [34]. This overgrowth was observed in all specimens in the current study, leaving only an average of 25.4% of the struts in the lumen. Furthermore, the appearance of ciliated epithelium and prismatic cells, in the epithelium of the nasopharynx and usually as well in the ET [35], indicates a reparation of the mucosal layer traumatized by the insertion of the stent and therefore closure of the tissue-lumen interface. Thus, the stent is incorporated and fixed in its position. This phenomenon may facilitate the clearance, but may also bear the risk of excessive growth of tissue. Finally, explantation of the stent is not advisable because surgical removal would be accompanied by the removal of mucosa, which may cause the ET to coalesce in the process of healing.

Conclusion

Application of fluids into the ET and middle ear of blackface sheep was feasible, but the reaction of the inflammatory mediators was not as extensive as expected. The nontraumatizing and minimally invasive procedure of stenting the ET was successfully transferred from cadaver studies to in-vivo application without complications. The stent was well tolerated by the sheep and did not hamper ventilation of the middle ear or clearance of the ET. Regarding the design of the stent, it seems to be sufficient to place it only in the cartilaginous part of the ET, but the length and/or positioning should be adjusted to prevent a permanently open, and therefore patulous, ET.

Abbreviations
CT: Computed tomography; ET: Eustachian tube; ETD: Eustachian tube dysfunction; GA: General anesthesia; MMA: Methylmethacrylate; OME: Otitis media with effusion; PAF: Platelet activating factor

Acknowledgements
The authors wish to thank Steffi Rausch (Cranio-Maxillo-Facial Surgery), Miriam Behrendt and Jasmin Bohlmann (Otolaryngology) for technical support. In addition, we thank the central animal facility for their support throughout the study.

Funding
This study was supported by the German Federal Ministry of Education and Research (BMBF) as part of REMEDIS: Higher quality of life through novel micro-implants (FKZ03IS2081E).

Authors' contributions
Conducted the experiments (stent implantation), FP, FM, RS, GP Data acquisition (health score, endoscopy, CT scan, histology), FM, FP, RS, EB, GP, AK Histologic examination and analysis, CH, FP, AK Analysis of in-vivo data (endoscopy, health score): FP, RS, GP Conducted and analyzed CT scan: EB, FP; RS Substantial contribution to preparation of manuscript: TL, FP, GP, RS Substantial contribution to study concept, and study design TL, GP, RS, FM, FP. All authors read and approved the final manuscript.

Competing interests
The authors declare that they have no competing interests.

Author details
[1]Department of Otolaryngology, Hannover Medical School, Carl-Neuberg-Str. 1, 30625 Hannover, Germany. [2]Hearing4all Cluster of Excellence, Hannover Medical School, Hannover, Germany. [3]Clinic for Cranio-Maxillo-Facial Surgery, Hannover Medical School, Hannover, Germany. [4]Institute of Diagnostic and Interventional Neuroradiology, Hannover Medical School, Hannover, Germany. [5]Department of Neuropathology, Hannover Medical School, Hannover, Germany.

References
1. Monasta L, Ronfani L, Marchetti F, Montico M, Brumatti LV, Bavcar A, et al. Burden of disease caused by otitis media: systematic review and global estimates. PLoS One. 2012;7:e36226.
2. Minovi A, Dazert S. Diseases of the middle ear in childhood. GMS Curr Top Otorhinolaryngol Head Neck Surg. 2014;13:1–29.
3. Di Martino EFN. Eustachian tube function tests: an update. HNO. 2013;61:467–76.
4. Proctor B. Embryology and anatomy of the eustachian tube. Arch Otolaryngol. 1967;86:503–14.
5. Adil E, Poe D. What is the full range of medical and surgical treatments available for patients with Eustachian tube dysfunction? Curr Opin Otolaryngol Head Neck Surg. 2014;22:8–15.
6. Zöllner F. The principles of plastic surgery of the sound-conducting apparatus. J Laryngol Otol. 1955;69:637–52.
7. Wright JWJ, Wright JW 3rd. Preliminary results with use of an eustachian tube prosthesis. Laryngoscope. 1977;87:207–14.
8. Steinbach E. Zur Einlage eines Tubenimplantates bei Belüftungsstörungen des Mittelohres. In: Fleischer K, Kleinsasser O. (eds) Teil II: Sitzungsbericht. Verhandlungsbericht der Deutschen Gesellschaft für Hals-Nasen-Ohren-Heilkunde, Kopf- und Hals-Chirurgie, vol 1991 / 2. Berlin: Springer; 1991.
9. Lesinski SGG, Fox JM, Seid AB, Bratcher GO, Cotton R. Does the Silastic Eustachian Tube prosthesis improve eustachian tube function? Laryngoscope. 1980;90:1413–28.
10. Schrom T, Kläring S, Sedlmaier B. Treatment of chronic tube dysfunction. Use of the tube conductor. HNO. 2007;55:871–5.
11. Llewellyn A, Norman G, Harden M, Coatesworth A, Kimberling D, Schilder A, et al. Interventions for adult Eustachian tube dysfunction: a systematic review. Health Technol Assess. 2014;18:1–180.
12. Poe DS, Grimmer JF, Metson R. Laser eustachian tuboplasty: two-year results. Laryngoscope. 2007;117:231–7.
13. Ockermann T. Die Ballondilatation der Eustachischen Röhre zur Behandlung der obstruktiven Tubendysfunktion. Dissertation. Ruhr-Universität Bochum. http://www-brs.ub.ruhr-uni-bochum.de/netahtml/HSS/Diss/Ockermann Thorsten/diss.pdf. 2009.
14. Todt I, Seidl R, Ernst A. A new minimally invasive method for the transtubal, microendoscopic application of fluids to the middle ear. Minim Invasive Ther Allied Technol. 2008;17:300–2.
15. Litner JA, Silverman CA, Linstrom CJ, Arigo JV, McCormick SA, Yu GP. Tolerability and safety of a poly-L-lactide eustachian tube stent using a chinchilla animal model. Int Adv Otol. 2009;5:290–3.
16. Presti P, Linstrom CJ, Silverman CA, Litner J. The Poly-L-Lactide Eustachian tube stent: tolerability, safety and resorption in a rabbit model. Int Adv Otol. 2011;7:1–3.
17. Schnabl J, Glueckert R, Feuchtner G, Recheis W, Potrusil T, Kuhn V, et al. Sheep as a large animal model for middle and inner ear implantable hearing devices: a feasibility study in cadavers. Otol Neurotol. 2012;33:481–9.
18. Miller F, Burghard A, Salcher R, Scheper V, Leibold W, Lenarz T, et al. Treatment of middle ear ventilation disorders: sheep as animal model for stenting the human Eustachian tube – a cadaver study. PLoS One. 2014;9:e113906.
19. Park MK, Lee BD. Development of animal models of otitis media. Korean J Audiol. 2013;17:9–12.
20. Piltcher OB, Swarts JD, Magnuson K, Alper CM, Doyle WJ, Hebda PA. A rat model of otitis media with effusion caused by eustachian tube obstruction with and without Streptococcus pneumoniae infection: methods and disease course. Otolaryngol Head Neck Surg. 2002;126:490–8.
21. Ganbo T, Hisamatsu K, Kikushima K, Inoue H, Kjxushima K, Murakami Y. Effects of platelet activating factor on mucociliary clearance of the eustachian tube. Ann Otol Rhinol Laryngol. 1996;105:140–5.
22. Rhee C-KM, Miller S, Jung TKTMP, Weeks D. Experimental otitis media with effusion induced by middle ear effusion. Laryngoscope. 1993;102:1037–42.
23. Otto KA, Short CE. Pharmaceutical control of pain in large animals. Appl Anim Behav Sci. 1998;59:157–69.
24. Kokemueller H, Spalthoff S, Nolff M, Tavassol F, Essig H, Stuehmer C, et al. Prefabrication of vascularized bioartificial bone grafts in vivo for segmental mandibular reconstruction: experimental pilot study in sheep and first clinical application. Int J Oral Maxillofac Surg. 2010;39:379–87.
25. Lous J, Burton MJ, Felding JU, Ovesen T, Rovers MM, Williamson I. Grommets (ventilation tubes) for hearing loss associated with otitis media with effusion in children. Cochrane Database Syst Rev. 2005;(1): CD001801.
26. Djordjević V, Bukurov B, Arsović N, et al. Long term complications of ventilation tube insertion in children with otitis media with effusion. Vojnosanit Pregl. 2015;72:40–3.
27. Minami T, Kubo N, Tomoda K, Kumazawa T. Effects of various inflammatory mediators on eustachian tube patency. Acta Otolaryngol. 1992;112:680–5.
28. Pohl F, Paasche G, Lenarz T, Schuon R. Tympanometric measurements in conscious sheep – diagnostic tool for pre-clinical middle ear implant studies. Int J Audiol. 2017;56:53–61.
29. Ockermann T, Reineke U, Ebmeyer J, Ebmeyer J, Sudhoff HH. Balloon dilation eustachian tuboplasty: a feasibility study. Otol Neurotol. 2010;31:1100–3.
30. Pau HW. Eustachian tube and middle ear mechanics. HNO. 2011;59:953–63.
31. Poe DS. Diagnosis and management of the patulous Eustachian tube. Otol Neurotol. 2007;28:668–77.
32. Sone M, Kato T, Nakashima T. Current concepts of otitis media in adults as a reflux-related disease. Otol Neurotol. 2013;34:1013–7.
33. Sudhoff H. Eustachian tube dysfunction. 1st ed. Bremen: UNI-MED Science; 2013.
34. Hoenig MR, Campbell GR, Campbell JH. Vascular grafts and the endothelium. Endothelium. 2006;13:385–401.
35. Pahnke J. Morphologie, Funktion und Klinik der Tuba Eustachii. Laryngo-Rhino-Otol. 2000;79:S1–S21.

Protective effect and related mechanisms of curcumin in rat experimental periodontitis

Chang-Jie Xiao[1,2], Xi-Jiao Yu[2], Jian-Li Xie[2], Shuang Liu[1] and Shu Li[1*]

Abstract

Background: Curcumin exhibits anti-inflammatory effects and has been suggested as a treatment for inflammatory diseases. The aim of this study was to investigate the effects of curcumin on the lipopolysaccharide induced inflammatory response in rat gingival fibroblasts in vitro and ligation-induced experimental periodontitis in vivo, and to speculate the possible anti-inflammatory mechanism of curcumin.

Methods: The gingival fibroblasts were incubated with different concentrations of curcumin in the absence or presence of lipopolysaccharide (LPS). Concentrations of interleukin-1β(IL-1β), tumor necrosis factor-α (TNF-α), osteoprotegerin (OPG) and soluble receptor activator of nuclear factor kappa-B ligand (RANKL) culture supernatants of rat gingival fibroblasts were determined by enzyme linked immunosorbent assay. The nuclear fraction of rat gingival fibroblasts was extracted and nuclear factor kappa-B (NF-κB) activation was assessed by western blotting to elucidate related mechanisms. Curcumin was given every two days by oral gavage. The gingival inflammation and alveolar bone loss between the first and second molars were observed by hematoxylin and eosin staining. Collagen fibers were observed by picro-sirius red staining. Alveolar bone loss was assessed by micro-CT analysis.

Results: Curcumin attenuated the production of IL-1β and TNF-α in rat gingival fibroblasts stimulated by LPS, and inhibited the LPS-induced decrease in OPG/sRANKL ratio and NF-κB activation. Curcumin significantly reduced gingival inflammation and modulated collagen fiber and alveolar bone loss in vivo.

Conclusions: curcumin modulates inflammatory activity in rat periodontitis by inhibiting NF-κB activation and decreasing the OPG/sRANKL ratio induced by LPS.

Keywords: Curcumin, NF-κB, OPG/RANKL, Periodontitis, Micro-CT

Background

Periodontitis is a prevalent oral inflammatory disease characterized by progressive gingival tissue inflammation, irreversible alveolar bone loss and deep periodontal pockets. It is caused by accumulation of profuse amounts of dental plaque. The conventional treatment for periodontitis is to reduce dental bacteria levels by scaling and root planing [1]. Antibiotics such as doxycycline have been used to alter the host response to the periodontal pathogens by disrupting the action of matrix metalloproteinase and to thus minimize host-mediated tissue

destruction [2], but systemic use of antibiotics can interfere with normal body systems and may cause several side effects,such as drug resistance [3].

Treatment of periodontitis in traditional Chinese medicine or natural substances is one of the research points in recent years. Several compounds extracted from spices and herbs exhibit anti-inflammatory effects, which suggest potential pharmacological uses. Curcumin, the principal curcuminoid in turmeric (*Curcuma longa*), has been used as a food additive and herbal supplement because of its potential medicinal properties [4]. Curcumin has been shown to exhibit anti-inflammatory biological activity [5–8]. Gingival tissues are the first tissues affected during the initial stage of periodontitis [9]. Gingival fibroblasts, as the major cell type in gingival

---

* Correspondence: lishu@sdu.edu.cn
[1]Shandong Provincial Key Laboratory of Oral tissue regeneration, Department of Periodontology, School and Hospital of Stomatology, Shandong University, 44-1# West Wenhua Road, Jinan, Shandong, China
Full list of author information is available at the end of the article

tissues, which stimulated by lipopolysaccharide (LPS) can activate the nuclear factor kappa-B (NF-κB) signaling pathway and products inflammatory cytokines such as IL-1β and TNF-α. Extensive research has demonstrated that the transcription factor NF-κB is a key component of the inflammatory process [10]. However, the anti-inflammatory effects of curcumin on LPS-stimulated rat gingival fibroblasts and the molecular mechanisms remain unclear. The expression and activation of OPG and RANKL are crucial for alveolar bone absorption and metabolism [11]. The present study was undertaken to investigated the hypothesis that curcumin would inhibit the LPS-induced inflammatory response in rats gingival fibroblasts in vitro and ligation-induced experimental periodontitis in vivo.

Methods
Reagents
LPS and curcumin were purchased from Sigma (USA). NF-κB p-p65 and p-IκBα were purchased from Cell Signaling Technology (USA). IL-1β, TNF-α, OPG and soluble RANKL (sRANKL) ELISA kits were obtained from R & D Systems (Minneapolis, MN, USA). Wistar rats for the ligation-induced experimental periodontitis model were obtained from the Laboratory Animal Center of Shandong University (Shandong, China). This study was approved by the Local Ethics Committee of the Animal Care and Use Committee of the School of Stomatology, Shandong University.

Cell culture
Normal gingival tissues were obtained from male Wistar rats (aged 5 weeks) that were clinically free of periodontal disease. Enzymatic digestion were adopted and maintained in Dulbecco's modified Eagle's medium (DMEM; Gibco, USA) containing 20% fetal bovine serum (FBS), 100 U/mL penicillin and 100 mg/mL streptomycin (Hyclone, Beijing, China). After reaching confluence, the cells were detached from the culture surface with 0.25% trypsin and subcultured in DMEM containing 10% FBS and antibiotic solution. The medium was changed every 48 h. Gingival fibroblasts between passages 4 and 7 were used in this study.

Cell viability
The cell viability of gingival fibroblasts was assessed using the MTT assay as previously described [12]. Briefly, gingival fibroblasts were seeded in 96-well plates (1×10^4 cells per well) and cultured for 12 h. The cells (LPS, LPS+ 10 μM curcumin, LPS+ 20 μM curcumin, 10 μM curcumin, 20 μM curcumin and normal fibroblasts as control)($n = 8$) were incubated with different concentrations of curcumin in the absence or presence of LPS (1 μg/ml) [13, 14] for 24 h. Then, 20 μl of MTT

(5 mg/ml) was added to each well and the cells were incubated for 4 h. The medium was then removed and 150 μl of DMSO was added to each well. Optical density was measured at 450 nm using a Bio-Rad microplate reader (model 680, Bio-Rad, USA).

ELISA assay
The concentrations of IL-1β, TNF-α, OPG and sRANKL in the culture supernatants of gingival fibroblasts incubated with different concentrations of curcumin in the absence or presence of LPS (1 μg/ml) for 24 h were measured using commercially available ELISA kits [15, 16]. ELISA assays were performed according to the manufacturer's instructions.

Protein extraction and western blotting
The nuclear fraction of gingival fibroblasts was extracted for NF-κB evaluation using an Ambion PARIS system (Thermo Fisher). Protein concentrations were measured using a bicinchoninic acid quantitative protein analysis assay kit (Boshe, China). Proteins were separated on 10% SDS gels and transferred onto polyvinylidene difluoride membranes (Millipore, USA). After being blocked in 0.1% Tween 20 in Tris-buffered saline containing 5% nonfat dried milk for 1 h at room temperature, the membranes were incubated with NF-κB, p-p65 and p-IκBα (all diluted 1:1000) overnight at 4 °C. The membranes were then rinsed with TBST for 10 min three times, and incubated with horseradish peroxidase-labeled second antibody (Beyotime). Immunoreactive bands were visualized on Canon film using enhanced chemiluminescence substrate solution (Millipore). Histone H3 (antibody diluted 1:10000) was used as an internal control.

Animals
Twenty-four male Wistar rats that had undergone this ligation procedure were randomly distributed into the following 3 groups: a ligation-only (L) group, a group treated with 30 μg/g body weight curcumin (L + C₃₀), and a group treated with 100 μg/g body weight curcumin (L + C₁₀₀). Curcumin diluted in corn oil vehicle was administered every 2 days by oral gavage, starting the day before ligation. Animals in the L group were administered the same volume of the corn oil vehicle. Food and water were provided ad libitum.

Ligation-induced experimental periodontitis
The procedure used for ligation-induced experimental periodontitis was as previously described [17]. Briefly, a 4–0 silk suture and an orthodontic ligature wire were passed through the interdentium between the first and second molars using Dumont forceps, and then the silk suture was wound tightly around the orthodontic

ligature wire to cover it. After the gingiva was lacerated by a dental probe, the orthodontic ligature wire was ligated firmly to the dental cervix of the right first lower molar.

Micro-computerized tomography (micro-CT) analysis

SkyScan 1176 (BRUKER, USA) at 65 kV and 380 μA was applied for micro-CT analysis. Mandibles were scanned at 9-μm resolution. Three-dimensional (3D) volume viewing and analysis software (DataViewer, CT-volume and CT-analyser, SkyScan, Bruker, USA) were used to visualize and quantify 2D and 3D data on a personal computer output, and a standardized gray-scale value was used to visualize mineralized tissues only.

Collagen fibers analysis

Sections were deparaffinized, hydrated and washed, then stained with 0.1% picro-sirius red for 60 min and rinsed with hydrochloric acid (0.01 M) for 2 min. The sections were dehydrated and sealed with mounting medium, and then the gingival fibers were analyzed under a polarizing microscope (Olympus BHSP, Japan).

Statistical analysis

All data are presented as means ± SD of three independent experiments. Data were statistically analyzed by one-way analysis followed by the Newman–Keuls post hoc test using SPSS 17.0 statistical software (SAS, Cary, NC, USA). $P < 0.05$ was considered statistically significant.

Results

Effects of curcumin on cell viability

The cytotoxic effect of curcumin on rat gingival fibroblasts was assessed by the MTT assay. There was no significant difference in cell viability in LPS + 10 μM curcumin-treated cells, LPS + 20 μM curcumin-treated

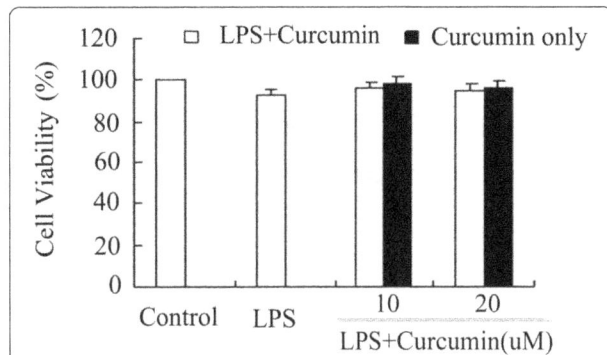

Fig. 1 Effects of curcumin on the cell viability of rat gingival fibroblasts. Cells were cultured with different concentrations of curcumin (0, 10 and 20 μM) in the presence or absence of 1 μg/ml lipopolysaccharide (LPS). Cell viability was determined by MTT assay. Curcumin was not cytotoxic to gingival fibroblasts at 10 or 20 μM ($P > 0.05$)

cells, 10 μM curcumin-treated cells or 20 μM curcumin-treated cells compared with control fibroblasts ($P > 0.05$). These results show that 10 and 20 μM curcumin were not cytotoxic to gingival fibroblasts (Fig. 1). Thus, curcumin was used at 10 and 20 μM in the subsequent in vitro studies.

Effects of curcumin on TNF-α and IL-1β expression in gingival fibroblasts

The culture supernatants of gingival fibroblasts treated with LPS, LPS + 10 μM curcumin, and LPS + 20 μM curcumin, and from the untreated control cells were tested. TNF-α and IL-1β in culture supernatants were markedly elevated in the LPS group comparing with the Control group ($P < 0.05$). 10 and 20 μM Curcumin decreased the levels of TNF-α and IL-1β stimulated by LPS in the culture supernatants of gingival fibroblasts ($P < 0.05$) (Fig. 2).

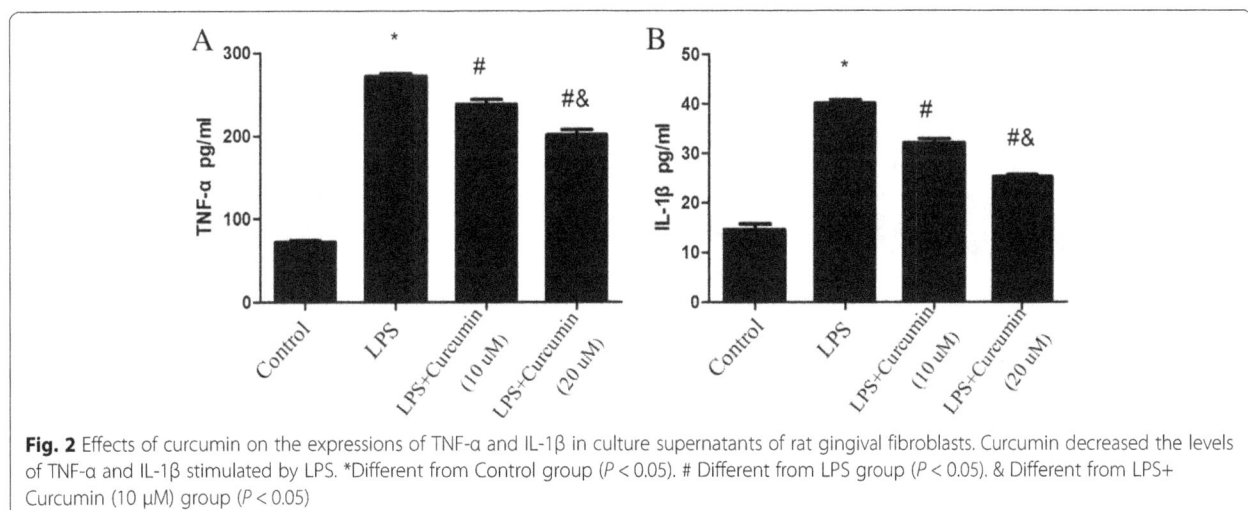

Fig. 2 Effects of curcumin on the expressions of TNF-α and IL-1β in culture supernatants of rat gingival fibroblasts. Curcumin decreased the levels of TNF-α and IL-1β stimulated by LPS. *Different from Control group ($P < 0.05$). # Different from LPS group ($P < 0.05$). & Different from LPS+ Curcumin (10 μM) group ($P < 0.05$)

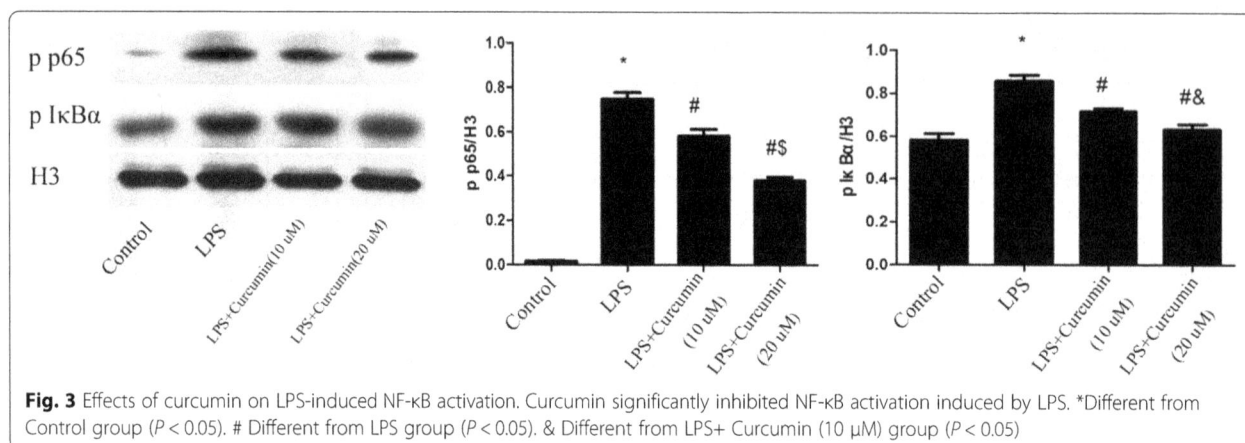

Fig. 3 Effects of curcumin on LPS-induced NF-κB activation. Curcumin significantly inhibited NF-κB activation induced by LPS. *Different from Control group ($P < 0.05$). # Different from LPS group ($P < 0.05$). & Different from LPS+ Curcumin (10 μM) group ($P < 0.05$)

Effects of curcumin on LPS-induced NF-κB activation in vitro

Cells were treated with curcumin (10, 20 μM) in the presence of LPS (1 μg/ml) for 24 h. Cell nuclear protein samples were analyzed by western blotting. The results showed that LPS significantly increased NF-κB, p-p65 and p-IκBα levels ($P < 0.05$). Moreover, curcumin significantly inhibited LPS-induced NF-κB activation ($P < 0.05$).*Different from Control group ($P < 0.05$). # Different from LPS group ($P < 0.05$). & Different from LPS+ Curcumin(10 μM) group ($P < 0.05$) (Fig. 3).

Effects of curcumin on OPG/sRANKL ratio in gingival fibroblasts

The level of sRANKL in LPS-treated cells was significantly higher than that in control cells ($P < 0.05$). OPG release was significantly decreased when gingival fibroblasts were treated with LPS. Therefore, the OPG/sRANKL ratio decreased significantly in the LPS-treated cells. Curcumin reduced sRANKL release from gingival fibroblasts, and also increased OPG release. Thus, curcumin

inhibited the LPS-induced decrease in the OPG/sRANKL ratio ($P < 0.05$) (Fig. 4).

Effects of curcumin on ligation-induced experimental periodontitis in vivo

Alveolar bone loss in the mandible between the first and second molars was observed by micro-CT (Fig. 5). Alveolar bone loss was observed in all three groups of rats. Alveolar bone crest height was obviously decreased, and notable alveolar bone loss between the first and second molars was observed in the L group (Fig. 6). Alveolar bone loss was reduced in the L + C_{30} and L + C_{100} groups.

The histological changes in rat experimental periodontitis with the treatment of curcumin. Histological analysis revealed gingival inflammation in all three groups. However, a significant reduction in gingival inflammation and bone loss was observed in the L + C_{30} and L + C_{100} groups (Fig. 7). According to Picrosirius red staining, seriously collagen fiber destructions were observed in the L group. The fiber bundles were scattered and

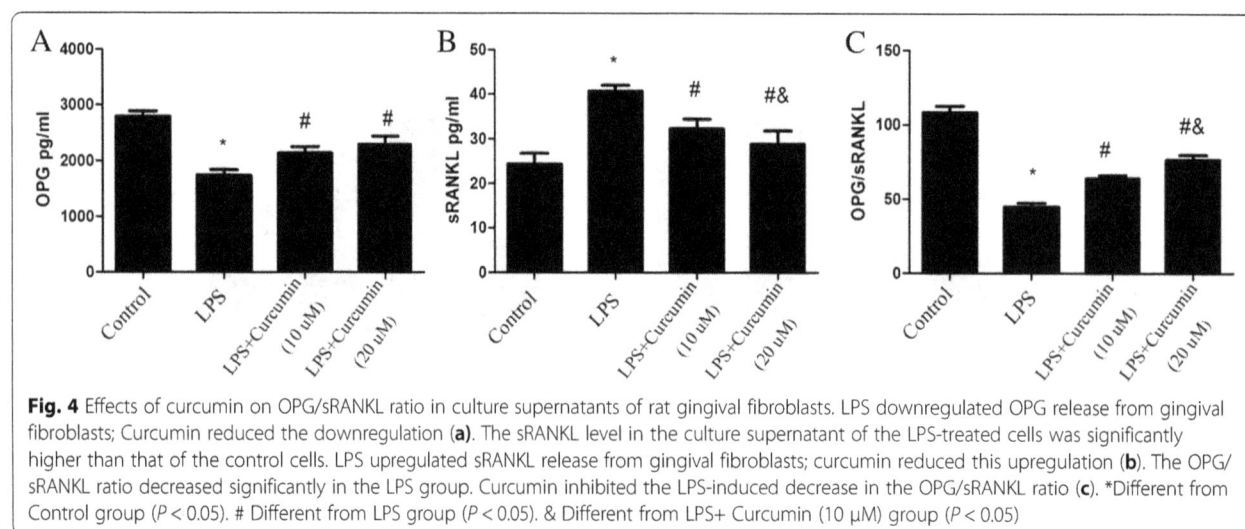

Fig. 4 Effects of curcumin on OPG/sRANKL ratio in culture supernatants of rat gingival fibroblasts. LPS downregulated OPG release from gingival fibroblasts; Curcumin reduced the downregulation (**a**). The sRANKL level in the culture supernatant of the LPS-treated cells was significantly higher than that of the control cells. LPS upregulated sRANKL release from gingival fibroblasts; curcumin reduced this upregulation (**b**). The OPG/sRANKL ratio decreased significantly in the LPS group. Curcumin inhibited the LPS-induced decrease in the OPG/sRANKL ratio (**c**). *Different from Control group ($P < 0.05$). # Different from LPS group ($P < 0.05$). & Different from LPS+ Curcumin (10 μM) group ($P < 0.05$)

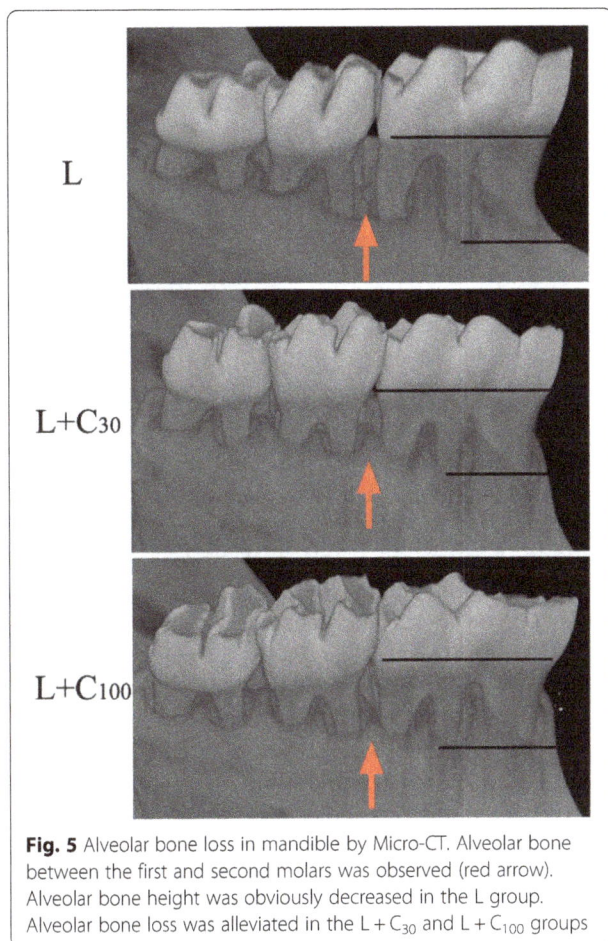

Fig. 5 Alveolar bone loss in mandible by Micro-CT. Alveolar bone between the first and second molars was observed (red arrow). Alveolar bone height was obviously decreased in the L group. Alveolar bone loss was alleviated in the L + C$_{30}$ and L + C$_{100}$ groups

disordered. This collagen fiber destructions were also alleviated in the L + C$_{30}$ and L + C$_{100}$ groups (Fig. 8).

Discussion

Curcumin has been demonstrated to have various biological properties, including anti-inflammatory, antioxidant, antimicrobial, and antiviral effects. Because of these properties, curcumin provides a very promising approach for the treatment of periodontitis [18, 19]. This study aimed to investigate the anti-inflammatory effects of curcumin on LPS-stimulated rat gingival fibroblasts and the underlying molecular mechanisms of these effects, which remain unclear. The cytotoxic effect of curcumin on rat gingival fibroblasts was assessed by the MTT assay in vitro. There was no significant difference between curcumin-treated fibroblasts and normal fibroblasts. So we did not use any negative or placebo controls in vivo for the consistency of experimental comparisons as we mainly aimed at the mechanism of curcumin in anti-inflammatory action.

TNF-α and IL-1β, as two of the important pro-inflammatory mediators, were significantly up-regulated in the process of periodontitis [20, 21], which are actively involved in jeopardizing periodontal tissues by affecting the activities of leukocytes, oteoclasts and collagenolytic enzyme MMPs to mediate alveolar bone resorption and collagen destruction [22, 23]. So, in this study we chose TNF-α and IL-1β to examine the effect of curcumin on the production of these cytokines, since these cytokines participate to various extent in the production and the

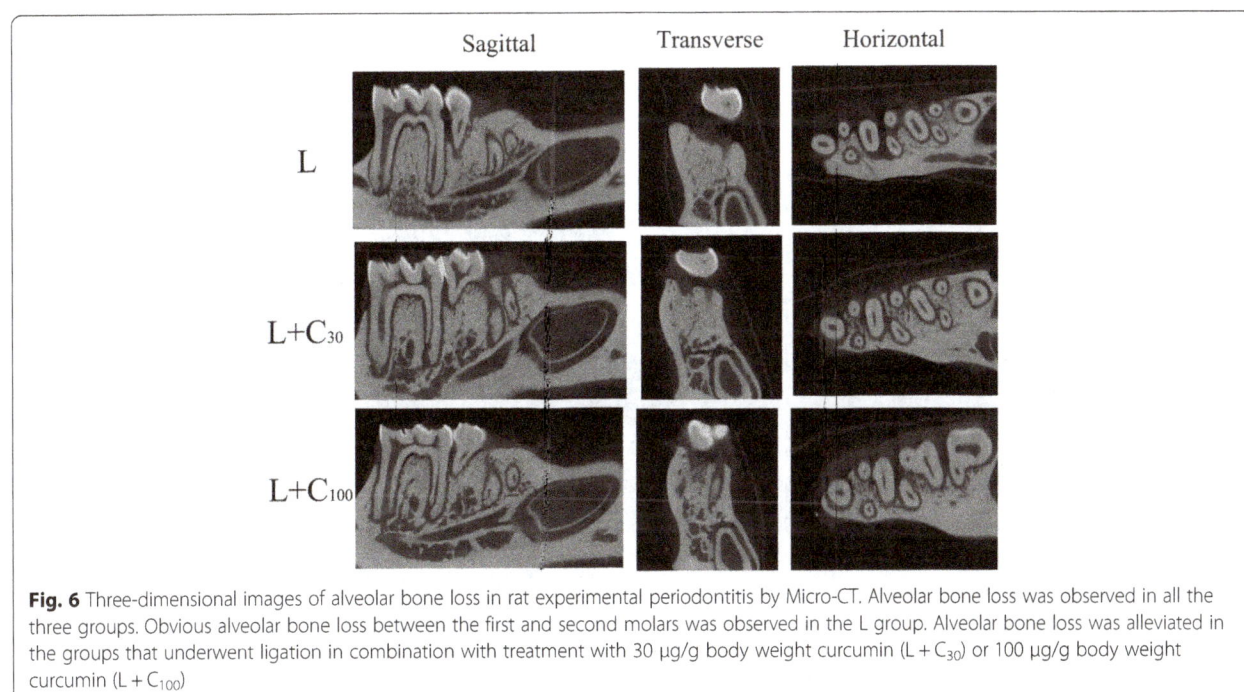

Fig. 6 Three-dimensional images of alveolar bone loss in rat experimental periodontitis by Micro-CT. Alveolar bone loss was observed in all the three groups. Obvious alveolar bone loss between the first and second molars was observed in the L group. Alveolar bone loss was alleviated in the groups that underwent ligation in combination with treatment with 30 μg/g body weight curcumin (L + C$_{30}$) or 100 μg/g body weight curcumin (L + C$_{100}$)

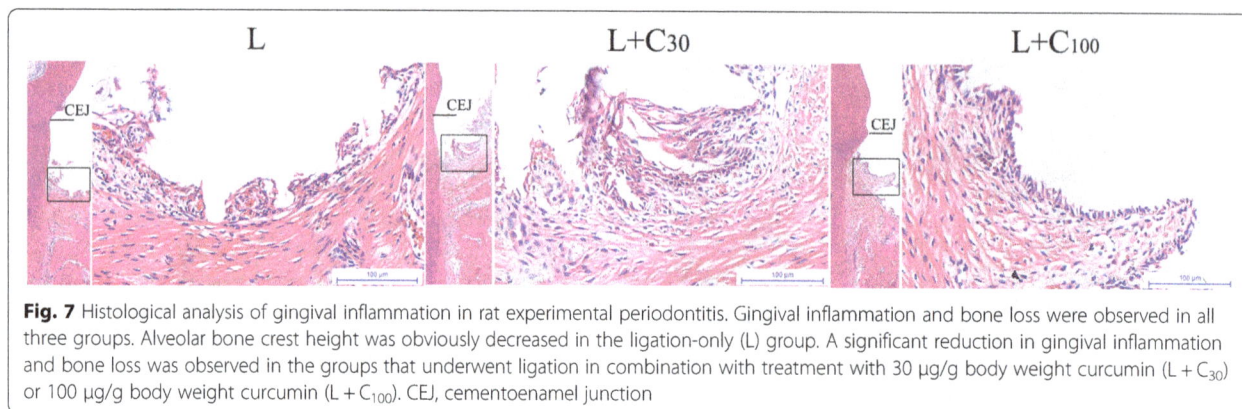

Fig. 7 Histological analysis of gingival inflammation in rat experimental periodontitis. Gingival inflammation and bone loss were observed in all three groups. Alveolar bone crest height was obviously decreased in the ligation-only (L) group. A significant reduction in gingival inflammation and bone loss was observed in the groups that underwent ligation in combination with treatment with 30 μg/g body weight curcumin (L + C$_{30}$) or 100 μg/g body weight curcumin (L + C$_{100}$). CEJ, cementoenamel junction

development of inflammation through recruitmnt and activation of inflammatory cells [24].

Gingival tissues were first invaded and stimulated by periodontal bacteria and their metabolic products in the initial process of periodontitis. The overproduction of IL-1β and TNF-α have been known to play important roles in periodontal inflammatory degradation [25]. According to our ELLSA results, curcumin inhibited the production of IL-1β and TNF-α in rat gingival fibroblasts induced by LPS, which showed that curcumin has potential role in modulating immune response associated with periodontal diseases.

To investigate the inflammatory mechanism, the effects of curcumin on LPS-induced NF-κB activation were detected by western blotting. Results showed that curcumin significantly inhibited upregulated NF-κB p65 and IκB phosphorylation induced by LPS.

NF-κB activation can stimulate a number of inflammatory events and amplify the inflammatory responses, including inducing adhesion molecules, and activating matrix metalloproteinase, which occur in periodontal disease process. NF-κB activation in gingival fibroblasts leads to the over-release of proinflammatory cytokines IL-1β and TNF-α, which further enhanced periodontal tissue destruction. IL-1 and TNF-α also promote the recruitment and activity of osteoclasts, by enhancing production of a crucial osteoclastogenic factor, the Receptor Activator of Nuclear Factor κ B Ligand (RANKL) and favor bone destruction [26].

The expression/activation of OPG and RANKL are crucial for alveolar bone absorption and metabolism [27, 28]. The osteoclast differentiates from monocyte/macrophage precursors under the regulation of RANKL/RANK signaling. OPG is a secreted protein that protects bone from excessive resorption by binding to RANKL and preventing it from binding to RANK [29–31]. Soluble RANKL (sRANKL) and OPG from gingival fibroblasts stimulated by LPS may interrupt alveolar bone metabolism by paracrine secretion. Thus, OPG/sRANKL ratio is a major determinant. According to our results, OPG/sRANKL ratio in culture supernatants of gingival fibroblasts was decreased when incubated with LPS, curcumin

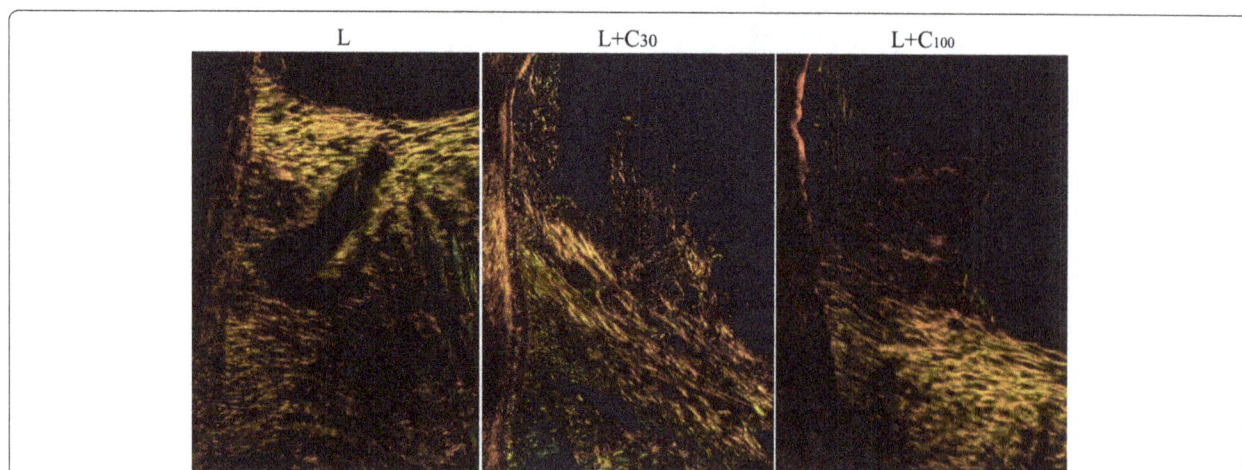

Fig. 8 Picro-sirius red staining. Marked collagen fiber destruction was observed in the ligation-only (L) group. The fiber bundles were scattered and disordered. Collagen fiber destruction was alleviated in the groups that underwent ligation in combination with treatment with 30 μg/g body weight curcumin (L + C$_{30}$) or 100 μg/g body weight curcumin (L + C$_{100}$)

alleviated LPS-induced down-regulated OPG/sRANKL ratio. Curcumin may alleviate LPS-induced osteoclast activation and alveolar bone absorption by down-regulating OPG/sRANKL ratio.

In vivo, histological observation and micro-CT results showed gingival inflammation and alveolar bone loss was observed in rat experimental periodontitis. Both 30 and 100 μg / g / body weight of curcumin could alleviate the gingival inflammation and alveolar bone loss [32–35]. According to Picrosirius red staining, the fiber bundles became scattered and disordered in rat experimental periodontitis. Collagen fiber destructions were also alleviated by curcumin.

Conclusion

In the present study, we provided new evidence on the inhibitory effect of curcumin on inflammatory activity. Curcumin significantly reduced gingival inflammation and modulated collagen fiber and alveolar bone loss in vivo. Curcumin can significantly inhibit NF-κB activation and decrease the OPG/sRANKL ratio induced by LPS. This study provides a new anti-inflammatory therapeutic for periodontal diseases.

Acknowledgements
The authors would like to thank all participants who willingly participated in this study. We thank Ruth Tunn, PhD, from Liwen Bianji, Edanz Editing China for editing the English text of a draft of this manuscript.

Funding
This work was partly supported by National Natural Science Foundation of China (81271138) awarded to Shu Li. Natural Science Foundation of Shandong Province (ZR2017QH007) awarded to Xijiao Yu.

Authors' contributions
SL and XJY carried out the conception and design of the study. CJX participated in the sequence alignment and drafted the manuscript. JLX and SL performed cell culture and statistical analysis. All authors read and approved the final manuscript.

Competing interests
The authors declare that they have no competing interests.

Author details
[1]Shandong Provincial Key Laboratory of Oral tissue regeneration, Department of Periodontology, School and Hospital of Stomatology, Shandong University, 44-1# West Wenhua Road, Jinan, Shandong, China. [2]Department of Endodontics, Jinan Stomatological Hospital, 101# Jingliu Road, Jinan, Shandong, China.

References
1. Ebersole JL, Kirakodu S, Novak MJ, Stromberg AJ, Shen S, Orraca L, Gonzalez-Martinez J, Burgos A, Gonzalez OA. Cytokine gene expression profiles during initiation, progression and resolution of periodontitis. J Clin Periodontol. 2014;41:853–61.
2. Goodson JM. Antimicrobial strategies for treatment of periodontal diseases. Periodontol 2000. 1994;5:142–68.
3. Garala K, Joshi P, Shah M, Ramkishan A, Patel J. Formulation and evaluation of periodontal in situ gel. Int J Pharm Investig. 2013;3:29–41.
4. Schaffer M, Schaffer PM, Bar-Sela G. An update on Curcuma as a functional food in the control of cancer and inflammation. Curr Opin Clin Nutr Metab Care. 2015;18:605–11.
5. Guimarães MR, de Aquino SG, Coimbra LS, Spolidorio LC, Kirkwood KL, Rossa C Jr. Curcumin modulates the immune response associated with LPS-induced periodontal disease in rats. Innate Immun. 2012;18:155–63.
6. Jurenka JS. Anti-inflammatory properties of curcumin, a major constituent of Curcuma longa: a review of preclinical and clinical research. Altern Med Rev. 2009;14:141–53.
7. Shehzad A, Ha T, Subhan F, Lee YS. New mechanisms and the anti-inflammatory role of curcumin in obesity and obesity-related metabolic diseases. Eur J Nutr. 2011;50:151–61.
8. Wang W, Sukamtoh E, Xiao H, Zhang G. Curcumin inhibits lymphangiogenesis in vitro and in vivo. Mol Nutr Food Res. 2015;59:2345–54.
9. Cobb CM. Non-surgical pocket therapy: mechanical. Ann Periodontol. 1996; 1:443–90.
10. Abe Y, Hashimoto S, Horie T. Curcumin inhibition of inflammatory cytokine production by human peripheral blood monocytes and alveolar macrophages. Pharmacol Res. 1999;39:41–7.
11. Yu XJ, Xiao CJ, Du YM, Liu S, Du Y, Li S. Effect of hypoxia on the expression of RANKL/OPG in human periodontal ligament cells in vitro. Int J Clin Exp Pathol. 2015;8:12929–35.
12. Wang QB, Sun LY, Gong ZD, Du Y. Veratric acid inhibits LPS-induced IL-6 and IL-8 production in human gingival fibroblasts. Inflammation. 2015;39: 237–42.
13. Oliveira JR, Jesus D, Figueira LW, Oliveira FE, Pacheco Soares C, Camargo SE, Jorge AO, Oliveira LD. Biological activities of *Rosmarinus officinalis* L. (rosemary) extract as analyzed in microorganisms and cells. Exp Biol Med (Maywood). 2017;242(6):625–34.
14. Aroonrerk N, Niyomtham N, Yingyoungnarongkul BE. Anti-inflammation of N-Benzyl-4-Bromobenzamide in lipopolysaccharide-induced human gingival fibroblasts. Med Princ Pract. 2016;25(2):130–6.
15. Wan J, Jiang F, Qingsong X, Chen D, He J. Alginic acidoligosaccharide accelerates weaned pig growth through regulating antioxidant capacity, immunity and intestinal development. RSC Adv. 2016;6(90):87026–35.
16. Wan J, Chen D, Yu B, Luo Y, Mao X. Leucine protects against skeletal muscle atrophy in lipopolysaccharide-challenged rats. J Med Food. 2017;20(1):93–101.
17. Yu X, Gong Z, Lin Q, Wang W, Liu S, Li S. Denervation effectively aggravates rat experimental periodontitis. J Periodontal Res. 2017; 52(6):1011–20.
18. Akram M, Uddin S, Ahmed A, Usmanghani K, Hannan A, Mohiuddin E, et al. Curcuma longa and curcumin: A review article. Rom J Biol Plant Biol. 2010; 55:65–70.
19. Motterlini R, Foresti R, Bassi R, Green CJ. Curcumin, an antioxidant and anti-inflammatory agent, induces heme oxygenase-1 and protects endothelial cells against oxidative stress. Free Radic Biol Med. 2000;28:1303–12.
20. Jiang ZL, Cui YQ, Gao R, Li Y, Fu ZC, Zhang B, Guan CC. Study of TNF-α, IL-1β and LPS levels in the gingival crevicular fluid of a rat model of diabetes mellitus and periodontitis. Dis Markers. 2013;34:295–304.
21. Noguchi T, Ebina K, Hirao M, Kawase R, Ohama T, Yamashita S, Morimoto T, Koizumi K, Kitaguchi K, Matsuoka H, Kaneshiro S, Yoshikawa H. Progranulin plays crucial roles in preserving bone mass by inhibiting TNF-α-induced osteoclastogenesis and promoting osteoblastic differentiation in mice. Biochem Biophys Res Commun. 2015;465:638–43.
22. Graves DT, Cochran D. The contribution of interleukin-1 and tumor necrosis factor to periodontal tissue destruction. J Periodontol. 2003;74:391–401.
23. Geivelis M, Turner DW, Pederson ED, Lamberts BL. Measurements of interleukin-6 in gingival crevicular fluid fromadults with destructive periodontal disease. J Periodontol. 1993;64:980–3.
24. Lapérine O, Cloitre A, Caillon J, Huck O, Bugueno IM, Pilet P, Sourice S, Le Tilly E, Palmer G, Davideau JL, Geoffroy V, Guicheux J, Beck-Cormier S, Lesclous P. Interleukin-33 and RANK-L interplay in the alveolar bone loss associated to periodontitis. PLoS One. 2016;11:e0168080.
25. Page RC. The role of inflammatory mediators in the pathogenesis of periodontal disease. J Periodontal Res. 1999;26:230–42.
26. Hienz SA, Paliwal S, Ivanovski S. Mechanisms of bone resorption in periodontitis. J Immunol Res. 2015;2015:615486.
27. Yuan H, Gupte R, Zelkha S, Amar S. Receptor activator of nuclear factor kappa B ligand antagonists inhibit tissue inflammation and bone loss in experimental periodontitis. J Clin Periodontol. 2011;38:1029–36.
28. Yu X, Lv L, Zhang J, Zhang T, Xiao C, Li S. Expression of neuropeptides and bone remodeling-related factors during periodontal tissue regeneration in denervated rats. J Mol Hist. 2015;46:195–203.

29. Boyce BF, Xing L. Functions of RANKL/RANK/OPG in bone modeling and remodeling. Arch Biochem Biophys. 2008;15:139–46.

30. Lv L, Wang Y, Zhang J, Zhang T, Li S. Healing of periodontal defects and calcitonin gene related peptide expression following inferior alveolar nerve transection in rats. J Mol Histol. 2014;45:311–20.

31. Tong W, Wang Q, Sun D, Suo J. Curcumin suppresses colon cancer cell invasion via AMPK-induced inhibition of NF-κB, uPA activator and MMP9. Oncol Lett. 2016;12:4139–46.

32. Zhang Y, Gu Y, Lee HM, Hambardjieva E, Vranková K, Golub LM, Johnson F. Design,synthesisand biological activity of new polyenolic inhibitors of matrixmetalloproteinases: a focus on chemically-modified curcumins. Curr Med Chem. 2012;19(25):4348–458.

33. Elburki MS, Moore DD, Terezakis NG, Zhang Y, Lee HM, Johnson F, Golub LM. A novel chemically modified curcumin reduces inflammation-mediated connective tissue breakdown in a rat model of diabetes: periodontal and systemic effects. J Periodontal Res. 2017;52(2):186–200.

34. Guimarães MR, Coimbra LS, de Aquino SG, Spolidorio LC, Kirkwood KL, Rossa C Jr. Potent anti-inflammatory effects of systemically administered curcumin modulate periodontal disease in vivo. J Periodontal Res. 2011; 46(2):269–79.

35. Elburki MS, Rossa C, Guimaraes MR, Goodenough M, Lee HM, Curylofo FA, Zhang Y, Johnson F, Golub LM. A novel chemically modified curcumin reduces severity of experimental periodontal disease in rats: initial observations. Mediators Inflamm. 2014:959471.

Permissions

List of Contributors

Michelle Pereira Costa Mundim Soares
Master degree of Dentistry School of Federal University of Uberlandia, Uberlandia, Minas Gerais, Brazil

Paulo Vinícius Soares
Associate Professor of Operative Dentistry and Dental Materials Department at the Dentistry School of Federal University of Uberlandia, Uberlandia, Minas Gerais, Brazil

Analice Giovani Pereira and Priscila Barbosa Ferreira Soares
Doctoral student of Dentistry School of Federal University of Uberlandia, Uberlandia, Minas Gerais, Brazil

Christian Gomes Moura
Adjunct Professor of Federal University of Triangulo Mineiro, Uberaba, Minas Gerais, Brazil

Lucas Zago Naves
Post Doctoral student of Dentistry School of Estadual University of Campinas, Piracicaba, São Paulo, Brazil

Denildo de Magalhães
Associate Professor of Histology of Periodontics and Implant Dentistry Department at the Dentistry School of Federal University of Uberlandia, Av. Para 1720, Campus Umuarama, Zip Code 38400-000 Uberlandia, Minas Gerais, Brazil

Charles Yat Cheong Yeung
Department of Paediatric Dentistry and Orthodontics, Faculty of Dentistry, The University of Hong Kong, Hong Kong SAR, China

Colman Patrick McGrath
Department of Periodontology and Public Health, Faculty of Dentistry, The University of Hong Kong, Hong Kong SAR, China

Ricky Wing Kit Wong
Department of Paediatric Dentistry and Orthodontics, Faculty of Dentistry, The University of Hong Kong, Hong Kong SAR, China

Erik Urban Oskar Hägg
Department of Paediatric Dentistry and Orthodontics, Faculty of Dentistry, The University of Hong Kong, Hong Kong SAR, China

John Lo
Department of Oral and Maxillofacial Surgery, Faculty of Dentistry, The University of Hong Kong, Hong Kong SAR, China

Yanqi Yang
Department of Paediatric Dentistry and Orthodontics, Faculty of Dentistry, The University of Hong Kong, Hong Kong SAR, China

Marthinus J Kotze and Kurt-W Bütow
Department Maxillo-Facial and Oral Surgery, Faculty of Health Sciences, University of Pretoria, Pretoria, South Africa

Kurt-W Bütow
College of Health Sciences, University of KwaZulu-Natal, Durban, South Africa

Steve A Olorunju
Medical Research Council of South Africa, Pretoria, South Africa

Harry F Kotze
Faculty of Health Sciences, University of The Free State, Bloemfontein, South Africa

Marc Philipp Dittmer
Center of Dentistry, Oral and Maxillofacial Medicine, Hannover Medical School, Carl-Neuberg-Strasse 1, Hannover 30625, Germany

Carolina Fuchslocher Hellemann, Rainer Schwestka-Polly and Anton Phillip Demling
Department of Orthodontics, Hannover Medical School, Carl-Neuberg-Strasse 1, Hannover 30625, Germany

Sebastian Grade, Wieland Heuer and Meike Stiesch
Department of Prosthetic Dentistry and Biomedical Materials Science, Hannover Medical School, Carl-Neuberg-Strasse 1, Hannover 30625, Germany

Michael Knösel
Department of Orthodontics, University Medical Center Göttingen (UMG), 37099 Göttingen, Germany

David Ellenberger
Department of Medical Statistics, University Medical Center Göttingen (UMG), 37099 Göttingen, Germany

Yvonne Göldner
Private Practice, Hannover, Germany

Paulo Sandoval
Department of Orthodontics, Universidad de la Frontera (UFRO), Temuco, Chile

Dirk Wiechmann
Orthodontic Practice, Lindenstrasse 44, 49152 Bad, Essen, Germany
Department of Orthodontics, Hannover Medical School (MHH), 30625 Hannover, Germany

Alice Chin
Hong Kong SAR, China

Suzanne Perry, Chongshan Liao and Yanqi Yang
Faculty of Dentistry, University of Hong Kong, Hong Kong SAR, China

Quan Shi, Shuo Yang, Fangfang Jia and Juan Xu
Department of Stomatology, Chinese People's Liberation Army General Hospital, 28 Fuxing Road, 100853 Beijing, China

Vanessa Paredes, Beatriz Tarazona and Natalia Zamora
Orthodontics Department, Faculty of Dentistry and Medicine, University of Valencia, Gasco Oliag n°1, 46010 Valencia, Spain

Rosa Cibrian
Physiology Department, Faculty of Medicine and Dentistry, University of Valencia, Spain, Valencia, Spain

Ning Zhao, Jing Feng, Zheng Hu, Rongjing Chen and Gang Shen
Department of Orthodontics, Shanghai Key Laboratory of Stomatology, Shanghai No. 9 Hospital, ShanghaiJiaotong University School of Medicine, Shanghai, China

Elena Krieger
Department of Orthodontics, Medical Centre of the Johannes-Gutenberg-University Mainz, Augustusplatz 2, 55131 Mainz, Germany

Heinrich Wehrbein
Department of Orthodontics, Medical Centre of the Johannes-Gutenberg-University Mainz, Augustusplatz 2, 55131 Mainz, Germany

Stefano Mummolo, Enrico Marchetti, Francesca Albani, Filippo Pugliese, Salvatore Di Martino and Giuseppe Marzo
Department MeSVA, University of L'Aquila, L'Aquila, Italy

Vincenzo Campanella
Unità Operativa Semplice Dipartimentale di Pronto Soccorso Odontoiatrico, con annessa Unità di Odontoiatria Conservativa, University of Tor Vergata, Roma, Italy

Simona Tecco
University Vita-Salute San Raffaele, Via Olgettina 60, 20132, Milano, Italy

Shengbin Huang
Department of Prosthodontics, Hospital of Stomatology, Wenzhou Medical University, Wenzhou, China

Weiting Chen, Zhenyu Ni and Yu Zhou
Department of Orthodontics, Hospital of Stomatology, Wenzhou Medical University, 113 West College Road, 325000 Wenzhou, China

Beatriz Vera-Sirera and Leopoldo Forner-Navarro
Departaments of Stomatology, University of Valencia, Valencia, Spain

Francisco Vera-Sempere
Departaments of Pathology, University of Valencia, Valencia, Spain
Service of Pathology, Hospital Universitario y Politécnico La Fe, Avda Campanar 21, Valencia 46009, Spain

Zhou Yu, Lin Jiaqiang, Chen Weiting, Yi Wang, MinLing Zhen and Zhenyu Ni
DDS, Hospital of Stomatology, Wenzhou Medical University, Wenzhou, China

Zhenyu Ni
Department of Orthodontics, Hospital of Stomatology, Wenzhou Medical University, Wenzhou, 113 west college road, 325000 Wenzhou, China

Andreas F. Hellak, Michael Schauseil and Heike M. Korbmacher-Steiner
Department of Orthodontics, University Hospital, Georg-Voigt-Strasse 3, Marburg 35039, Germany.

Bernhard Kirsten, Rolf Davids and Wolfgang M. Kater
Private Practice, Bad Homburg, Germany

Mehmet Muhtarogullari
Department of Prosthodontics, Faculty of Dentistry, Hacettepe University, Ankara, Turkey

Mehmet Avci
Private practice, Istanbul, Turkey

Bulem Yuzugullu
Department of Prosthodontics, Faculty of Dentistry, Baskent University, Ankara, Turkey

Pit Jacob Voss, Rainer Schmelzeisen, Andres Stricker, Gido Bittermann and Philipp Poxleitner
Department of Oral and Maxillofacial Surgery, Regional Plastic Surgery, Medical Center - University of Freiburg, Hugstetter Str. 55, 79106 Freiburg im Breisgau, Germany

Gustavo Vargas Soto
Department of Oral and Maxillofacial Surgery, Hospital San Juan de Dios, Universidad Latina, San José, Costa Rica

Kiwako Izumi
Department of Oral and Maxillofacial Surgery, Fukuoka Dental College, Fukuoka, Japan

Nadja Rohr and Jens Fischer
Division of Materials Science and Engineering, Clinic for Reconstructive Dentistry and Temporomandibular Disorders, University Center for Dental Medicine, Hebelstrasse 3, CH-4056 Basel, Switzerland

Rui Hou, Hongzhi Zhou, Kaijin Hu, Yuxiang Ding, Xia Yang, Guangjie Xu, Peng Xue, Chun Shan and Sen Jia
State Key Laboratory of Military Stomatology and National Clinical Research Center for Oral Diseases and Shaanxi Clinical Research Center for Oral Diseases, Department of Oral Surgery, School of Stomatology, the Fourth Military Medical University, Xi'an City, Shaanxi Province 710032, China

Yuanyuan Ma
Department of Stomatology, Research Institute of Surgery and Daping Hospital, The Third Military Medical University, Chongqing City 400042, China

Stefan Bürgin, Nadja Rohr and Jens Fischer
Division of Dental Materials and Engineering, Department of Reconstructive Dentistry and Temporomandibular Disorders, University Center for Dental Medicine Basel, University of Basel, Hebelstrasse 3, 4056 Basel, Switzerland

Jan Hourfar, Jörg Alexander Lisson and Björn Ludwig
Department of Orthodontics, Saarland University, Homburg, Germany

Dirk Bister
Department of Orthodontics, Guy's and St Thomas' NHS Foundation Trust and King's College Dental Institute, London, UK

Georgios Kanavakis
Department of Orthodontics, Tufts University School of Dental Medicine, Boston, USA

Björn Ludwig
Private Practice, Am Bahnhof 54, 56841 Traben-Trarbach, Germany

Nada Binmadi and Azza Elsissi
Department of Oral Diagnostic Sciences, King Abdulaziz University, Jeddah 21589, Saudi Arabia

Azza Elsissi and Nadia Elsissi
Oral Pathology Department, University of Mansoura, Mansoura, Egypt

Atsushi Musha, Masaru Ogawa and Satoshi Yokoo
Department of Oral and Maxillofacial Surgery, Plastic Surgery, Gunma University Graduate School of Medicine, Gunma, Japan

Darren Isfeld
Orthodontic Graduate Program, School of Dentistry University of Alberta, Edmonton, AB, Canada

Manuel Lagravere
School of Dentistry, University of Alberta, Edmonton, 11405 - 87th avenue, Edmonton, AB T6G 1C9, Canada

Vladimir Leon-Salazar
Division of Pediatric Dentistry, School of Dentistry, University of Minnesota Minneapolis, MN, USA
Orthodontic Graduate Program, School of Dentistry, University of Alberta, Edmonton, AB, Canada

Carlos Flores-Mir
School of Dentistry, University of Alberta, Edmonton, AB, Canada

Markus Martini, Anne Klausing and Nils Heim
Department of Maxillofacial and Plastic Surgery, University of Bonn, Sigmund-Freud Str. 25, 53127 Bonn, Germany

Guido Lüchters
Center for Development Research (ZEF), University of Bonn, Walter-Flex-Str. 3, 53113 Bonn, Germany

Martina Messing-Jünger
Department of Neurosurgery, Asklepios Children's Hospital, Arnold-Janssen-Str. 29, 53757 Sankt Augustin, Germany

Markus Martini
Department of Oral, Maxillofacial and Plastic Surgery, University of Bonn, Welschnonnenstraße 17, D – 53111 Bonn, Germany

Katharina Klaus and Sabine Ruf
Department of Orthodontics, Justus-Liebig University Giessen, Schlangenzahl 14, 35392 Giessen, Germany

Johanna Eichenauer
Private orthodontic practice, Rosengasse 2, 35305 Grünberg, Germany

Rhea Sprenger
Private orthodontic practice, Marktgasse 2, 72070 Tübingen, Germany

Wataru Katagiri, Masashi Osugi, Takamasa Kawai and Hideharu Hibi
Department of Oral and Maxillofacial Surgery, Nagoya University Graduate School of Medicine, 65 Tsuruma-cho, Showa-ku, Nagoya 466-8550, Japan

Jing Huang and Jiu-Hui Jiang
Department of Orthodontics, Peking University School and Hospital of Stomatology, 22 South Zhongguancun Avenue, Haidian District, Beijing 100081, China

Cui-Ying Li
Central Laboratory, Peking University School and Hospital of Stomatology, 22 South Zhongguancun Avenue, Haidian District, Beijing 100081, China

Jan Hourfar
Department of Orthodontics, University of Heidelberg, Heidelberg, Germany

Dirk Bister
Department of Orthodontics, Guy's and St Thomas' NHS Foundation Trust and King's College Dental Institute, London, UK

Jörg A. Lisson and Björn Ludwig
Department of Orthodontics, University of Saarland, Homburg/Saar, Germany

Björn Ludwig
Private Practice, Am Bahnhof 54, 56841 Traben-Trarbach, Germany

Ferdinand J. Kammerer, Benedikt Schlude, Michael A. Kuefner, Philipp Schlechtweg, Matthias Hammon, Michael Uder and Siegfried A. Schwab
Institute of Radiology, University Erlangen-Nuremberg, Maximiliansplatz 1, D-91054 Erlangen, Germany

W. Semper-Hogg, M. A. Fuessinger, T. W. Dirlewanger and M. C. Metzger
Department of Oral and Craniomaxillofacial Surgery, Center for Dental Medicine, University Medical Center Freiburg, Hugstetter Straße 55 D, 79106 Freiburg, Germany

C. P. Cornelius
Department of Oral and Maxillofacial Surgery, Ludwig-Maximilians-University Munich, Lindwurmstraße 2a D, 80337 München, Germany

Ömür Dereci
Department of Oral and Maxillofacial Surgery, Faculty of Dentistry, Eskişehir Osmangazi University, Meşelik Campus, 26480 Eskişehir, Turkey

Mükerrem Hatipoğlu and Kemal Üstün
Department of Periodontology, Faculty of Dentistry, Akdeniz University, Antalya, Turkey

Alper Sindel and Sinan Tozoğlu
Department of Oral and Maxillofacial Surgery, Faculty of Dentistry, Akdeniz University, Antalya, Turkey

Friederike Pohl, Robert A. Schuon, Felicitas Miller, Thomas Lenarz and Gerrit Paasche
Department of Otolaryngology, Hannover Medical School, Carl-Neuberg-Str.1, 30625 Hannover, Germany

Friederike Pohl, Robert A. Schuon, Thomas Lenarz and Gerrit Paasche
Hearing4all Cluster of Excellence, Hannover Medical School, Hannover, Germany

Felicitas Miller and Andreas Kampmann
Clinic for Cranio-Maxillo-Facial Surgery, Hannover Medical School, Hannover, Germany

Eva Bültmann
Institute of Diagnostic and Interventional Neuro-radiology, Hannover Medical School, Hannover, Germany

Christian Hartmann
Department of Neuropathology, Hannover Medical School, Hannover, Germany

Chang-Jie Xiao, Shuang Liu and Shu Li
Shandong Provincial Key Laboratory of Oral tissue regeneration, Department of Periodontology, School and Hospital of Stomatology, Shandong University, 44-1# West Wenhua Road, Jinan, Shandong, China

Chang-Jie Xiao, Xi-Jiao Yu and Jian-Li Xie
Department of Endodontics, Jinan Stomatological Hospital, 101# Jingliu Road, Jinan, Shandong, China

Index